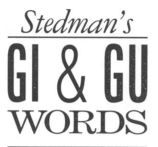

Stedman's

GI & GU
WORDS

SECOND EDITION

Edited by
Darla Haberer, CMT

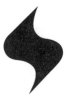

Stedman's
GI & GU
WORDS

SECOND EDITION

Including:

Nephrology

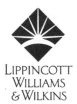

LIPPINCOTT
WILLIAMS
& WILKINS

Series Editor: Elizabeth B. Randolph
Associate Managing Editor: Maureen Barlow Pugh
Editor: Darla Haberer
Production Coordinator: Patricia Smith
Cover Design: Reuter & Associates

351 West Camden Street
Baltimore, Maryland 21201-2436 USA

Printed in the United States of America

First Editions, 1992 and 1993

Library of Congress Cataloging-in-Publication Data

Stedman's GI & GU words: including nephrology. / edited by Darla Haberer, CMT—2nd ed.
    p.   cm.
    Rev. ed. of: Stedman's GI words. © 1992, and Stedman's urology words. © 1993.
    Includes bibliographical references.
    1. Gastroenterology—Terminology.   2. Urology—Terminology.
  I. Stedman, Thomas Lathrop, 1853–1938.   II. Stedman's GI words.
III. Stedman's urology words.
    [DNLM: 1. Gastrointestinal Diseases—terminology.   2. Gastroenterology—
terminology.   3. Urogenital Diseases—terminology.   4. Urologic Diseases—
terminology.   5. Nephrology—terminology.   WI 13 S8115 1996]
RC802.S68 1996
616.3′3′0014—dc20
DNLM/DLC
for Library of Congress   96-15638
                                          CIP
Developed from the database of Stedman's medical dictionary and supplemented by terminology found in the current medical literature.
    Includes bibliographical references.
    ISBN 0-683-18145-9

99
5 6 7 8 9 10

Contents

Preface to the Second Edition

As medical language specialists, I often feel our jobs are similar to a detective's in a mystery novel. We are constantly learning new "clues," seeking answers, and using and extending our knowledge on a daily basis. We unravel the voices coming across the tapes and wires to determine who the main characters are, familiarize ourselves with the details of the situation, and choose which tools are needed to unravel the clues. Then, we put the pieces together to come up with the final results: the reports.

There continues to be a need to research information quickly, format it correctly, and go on to the next "case" as soon as possible, all the while being sure not to miss any pertinent information. Since there are many medical terms that are similar, but do not fit the particular situation at hand, we often need to search diligently for the correct answer. Sometimes this means relying on several references, our own past experiences (or those of our colleagues), or searching for that elusive information that may be hiding in the back of our minds, refusing for the moment to come to light.

Thankfully, the editors at Williams & Wilkins are a part of our team. They listen to our advice and requests and have published this word book to help solve the mysteries of gastrointestinal, genitourinary, and nephrology terminology. By nephrology, I also refer to the other systematic effects of uremia, which can affect every system in the body including the neurologic, ocular, cardiovascular, metabolic, musculoskeletal, dermatologic, endocrine, respiratory, hematology, gastrointestinal, and reproductive.

The need to make this book as comprehensive as possible and yet keep it to a user-friendly size made it necessary to have some guidelines about which terms to include and which to leave out. This was not an easy task. If we had been able to include all the terms that could be in a report related to these areas, we would have another dictionary-sized reference. We wanted to make this a reference book that you could comfortably reach for and use without the aid of a detective's magnifying glass, but which would be comprehensive enough for you to find the phrase or word you were "hunting" down.

I feel honored to have had a hand in bringing this book to you and to help in your quests for the proper terms needed to solve your "cases." Not a day goes by that we don't learn something new if we want to. My hope is that this book will help guide you down a path of learning and that you will find it to be a useful companion.

Darla Haberer, CMT

Acknowledgments

An important part of our editorial process is the involvement of medical transcriptionists—as advisors, reviewers, and/or editors.

Special thanks are due Darla Haberer, CMT, for editing and proofing the manuscript (and doing the necessary research involved with that large task), as well as helping to compile the appendices. We also would like to extend our thanks to our two other editors who worked on this book: Carolyn Wilkinson, CMT, who reviewed all the new terms that were added to this combined editon of *Stedman's GI & GU Words, Second Edition,* and Judy Johnson, CMT, who proofread the first editions of both *Stedman's GI Words* and *Stedman's Urology Words.*

Thanks also to our *Stedman's GI & GU Words* MT Editorial Advisory Board, consisting of Patty Barrett, CMT; Betsy Dearborn, CMT; Kathy Hefner, CMT; Brenda Hurley, CMT and Susan Kopec, RN of T-C Transcription, Inc.; Robin A. Koza; and Seamond Roberts. These medical transcriptionists served as editors and advisors, and spent hours perusing texts, journals, and manufacturer's information to compile the latest terms in gastroenterology, urology, and nephrology. Patty Barrett, CMT, and Carolyn Wilkinson, CMT, contributed to the appendices as well.

Other important contributors to this revised edition include: Debbie Frank; Carolyn Kromer; Helen Littrell, CMT; Norma Lopresti, CMT; Averill Ring, CMT; Ann Williams; and Debbie Zielinski, all of whom gathered new words and/or provided invaluable suggestions. Barb Ferretti played an integral role in the process by updating the database and providing a final quality check.

As with all our *Stedman's* word references, we have benefited from the suggestions and expertise of our many contacts in the medical transcriptionist community. Thanks to all our advisory board participants, reviewers, editors, AAMT meeting attendees, and others who have written in with requests and comments—keep talking, and we'll keep listening.

Explanatory Notes

Users of the first edition of *Stedman's GI Words* and *Stedman's Urology Words* will notice the merging of these two word books for this second edition. In this "combined" word book, we have edited, updated, and expanded the gastroenterology and urology content from the first editions and have added nephrology terms. *Stedman's GI & GU Words, Second Edition,* offers an authoritative assurance of quality and exactness to the wordsmiths of the health care professions—medical transcriptionists, medical editors and copy editors, health information management personnel, court reporters, and the many other users and producers of medical documentation.

Stedman's GI & GU Words, Second Edition, can be used to validate both the spelling and the accuracy of terminology specific to gastroenterology, urology, and nephrology. Gastroenterology-related terms include: GI endoscopy, hepatology (liver disease), clinical nutrition, and pediatric gastroenterology. Urology-related terms include: genitourinary surgery, laparoscopic urology, endourology, urolithology and lithotripsy, renography, ultrasonography, male infertility, urogynecology and fluorourodynamics, and pediatric urology. In addition, the user will find terminology related to these specialties, such as dialysis terms, endocrinology terms, and liver and renal transplant terms with related immunology.

The user will find listed thousands of drugs; diagnostic and therapeutic procedures; new techniques and maneuvers; lab tests; and equipment, instrument, and prosthesis names. Abbreviations and acronyms are also included. For quick reference, anatomy illustrations, a list of drug names by indication, a list of terms by commonly performed procedures, and sample reports of common procedures appear in the appendices at the back of the book.

Because our goal has been to provide a comprehensive, yet streamlined, reference tool, we have omitted terminology that is not specific to these specialties. Thus, some terms (such as anatomy and physiology terms) that are often dictated in these specialties are not included in this text, as they can be found in general medical dictionaries.

This compilation of over 82,500 entries, fully cross-indexed for quick access, was built from a base vocabulary of over 60,000 medical words, phrases, abbreviations, and acronyms. The extensive A-Z list was developed from the database of *Stedman's Medical Dictionary* and supplemented by terminology found in current medical literature (please see list of References on page xv).

Medical transcription is an art as well as a science. Both are needed to correctly interpret the dictation of a physician, whose language is a product of education, training, and experience. This variety in medical language means that there are several acceptable ways to express certain terms, including jargon. This second edition of *Stedman's GI & GU Words* provides variant spellings and phrasings for many terms. This, in addition to complete cross-indexing, makes *Stedman's GI & GU Words, Second Edition,* a valuable resource for determining the validity of terms as they are encountered.

Alphabetical Organization

Alphabetization of entries is letter by letter as spelled, ignoring punctuation, spaces, prefixed numbers, Greek letters, or other characters. For example:

acid-fast staining methods
acid formaldehyde hematin
α-acid glycoprotein
acid hematin

In subentries, the abbreviated singular form or the spelled-out plural form of the noun main entry word is ignored in alphabetization.

Format and Style

All main entries are in **boldface** to speed up location of a sought-after entry, to enhance distinction between main entries and subentries, and to relieve the textual density of the pages.

Irregular plurals and variant spellings are shown on the same line as the singular or preferred form of the word. For example:

scolex pl. **scoleces**

curette, curet

Hyphenation

For years we have followed a rule of style that hyphenated multiple eponyms (e.g., Green-Kenyon corneal marker). This style rule worked quite well and added consistency to the word list. We noticed, however, that many terms in the word list coupled manufacturer names with eponyms and that these terms were hyphenated inconsistently. We found that in some cases it was difficult to differentiate an eponym from a manufacturer name (after all, many companies are named after people). Therefore, we have decided that, as a rule of style, we will add a hyphen between a manufacturer and one or more eponyms (e.g., Vital-Metzenbaum dissecting scissors). Please note that hyphenation is a question of style, not of accuracy, and thus is a matter of choice.

Possessives

Possessive forms have been dropped in this reference for the sake of consistency and to conform to the guidelines outlined by the American Association for Medical Transcription (AAMT) and other groups. Please note, however, that retaining the possessive is a question of style, not of accuracy, and thus is a matter of choice. To form the possessive of a word, simply add the apostrophe or apostrophe "s" to the end of the word.

Cross-indexing

The word list is in an index-like main entry–subentry format that contains two combined alphabetical listings:

(1) A *noun* main entry-subentry organization that is typical of the A-Z section of medical dictionaries like *Stedman's:*

dyspepsia
　acid d.
　biliary d.
　gastric d.
　nervous d.

endoscope
　ACMI e.
　flexible fiberoptic e.
　Hirschowitz e.
　Welch Allyn video e.

(2) An *adjective* main entry–subentry organization that lists words and phrases as you hear them. The main entries are the adjectives or modifiers

in a multi-word term. The subentries are the nouns around which the terms are constructed and to which the adjectives or modifiers pertain:

metastatic
  m. dissemination
  m. lesion
  m. prostatic carcinoma
  m. renal cell carcinoma

endoscopic
  e. assessment
  e. Doppler probe
  e. gastrostomy tube
  e. monopolar electrocoagulation

This format provides the user with more than one way to locate and identify a multi-word term. For example:

nephritis
  hemorrhagic n.

hemorrhagic
  h. nephritis

balloon
  Fogarty b.
  Garren b.
  hydrostatic b.

Fogarty
  F. balloon
  F. biliary probe
  F. irrigation catheter

It also allows the user to see together all terms that contain a particular descriptor as well as all types, kinds, or variations of a noun entity. For example:

fluid
  f. absorptive capacity
  f. analysis
  ascitic f.
  bile-tinged f.
  cul-de-sac f.

colonoscopy
  cecal c.
  c. complication
  high-magnification c.
  c. screening
  splenic flexure c.

Wherever possible, abbreviations are separately defined and cross-referenced. For example:

AEG
  acute erosive gastritis

acute

a. erosive gastritis (AEG)

gastritis

acute erosive g. (AEG)

References

In addition to the manufacturers' literature we gather at various medical meetings, scientific reports from hospitals, and our MT Editorial Advisory Board members' lists (from their daily transcription work), we used the following sources for new words for *Stedman's GI & GU Words, Second Edition:*

Books

Lance LL. Quick look drug book. Baltimore: Williams & Wilkins, 1995.

Massry SG, Glassock RJ. Textbook of nephrology, volume 2, 3rd ed. Baltimore: Williams & Wilkins, 1995.

Stedman's medical dictionary, 26th ed. Baltimore: Williams & Wilkins, 1995.

Sloane SB. The medical word book, 3rd ed. Philadelphia: WB Saunders Company, 1991.

Stedman's GI words. Baltimore: Williams & Wilkins, 1992.

Stedman's medical equipment words. Baltimore: Williams & Wilkins, 1993.

Stedman's urology words. Baltimore: Williams & Wilkins, 1993.

Journals

American Journal of Gastroenterology. Baltimore: Williams & Wilkins, 1993–1995.

Contemporary Gastroenterology. Montvale, NJ: Medical Economics, 1992.

Contemporary Urology. Montvale, NJ: Medical Economics, 1992–1993.

Gastroenterology. Philadelphia: WB Saunders Company, 1992–1993.

Gastrointestinal Endoscopy. St. Louis: Mosby-Yearbook, Inc. 1992–1995.

Gastroenterology Nursing. Baltimore: Williams & Wilkins, 1994–1995.

Internal Medicine. Montvale, NJ: Medical Economics, 1995.

Journal of the American Society of Nephrology. Baltimore: Williams & Wilkins, 1994–1995.

Journal of Urology. Baltimore: Williams & Wilkins, 1992–1995.

The Latest Word. Philadelphia: WB Saunders Company, 1994.

Perspectives on the Medical Transcription Profession. Modesto: Health Professions Institute, 1993–1995.

Your Medical Word Publisher

We strive to provide you with the most up-to-date and accurate word references available. Your use of this word book will prompt new editions, which will be published as often as justified by updates and revisions. We welcome your suggestions for improvements, changes, corrections, and additions—whatever will make this *Stedman's* product more useful to you. Please use the postpaid card at the back of this book to send your recommendations care of "Stedmans" at Williams & Wilkins.

α_1
 α_1 adrenoreceptor
 α_1 agonist
$\alpha_2\beta_1$
 alpha-2-beta-1 integrin cell-surface
 collagen
A
 A bile
 A ring
 A ring of esophagus
A-4 protein
AAA
 abdominal aortic aneurysm
 aromatic amino acid
AAC
 antibiotic-associated colitis
AAG
 antral atrophic gastritis
AAH
 atypical adenomatous hyperplasia
AAL
 anterior axillary line
AAPBDS
 anomalous arrangement of
 pancreaticobiliary ductal system
Aaron sign
AAT
 androgen ablation therapy
AATD
 α_1-antitrypsin disease
 AATD-related emphysema
AAV
 adeno-associated virus
abate
Abbe operation
Abbott
 A. esophagogastroscopy
 A. esophagogastrostomy
 A. HCV EIA 2nd generation
 kit
 A. HCV 2.0 test kit
 A. IMx PSA assay
 A. LifeCare pump
 A. Lifeshield needleless system
 A. TDx monoclonal
 fluorescence polarization
 immunoassay
 A. tube
Abbott-Miller tube

Abbott-Rawson double-lumen
 gastrointestinal tube
ABC
 alkaline phosphatase Vectastain
 ABC
 ABC reagent -
abdomen
 acute a.
 acute surgical a.
 board-like rigidity of a.
 boat-shaped a.
 carinate a.
 diffusely tender a.
 distended a.
 doughy a.
 dull to percussion a.
 exquisitely tender a.
 flabby a.
 flat a.
 flat plate of a.
 hyperresonant a.
 navicular a.
 nondistended a.
 a. obstipum
 pendulous a.
 plain film of a.
 protuberant a.
 resonant a.
 rigid a.
 rotund a.
 scaphoid a.
 silent a.
 soft a.
 splinting of a.
 surgical a.
 tight a.
 tympanitic a.
abdominal
 a. abscess
 a. angina
 a. aortic aneurysm (AAA)
 a. aortography
 a. apoplexy
 a. apron
 a. bruits
 a. canal
 a. cavity
 a. colectomy
 a. compression belt
 a. contents

1

abdominal *(continued)*
  a. desmoid tumor
  a. distention
  a. dropsy
  a. ectopic pregnancy
  a. esophagus
  a. fasciocutaneous flap
  a. fat
  a. fat pad
  a. fistula
  a. fluid wave
  a. fullness
  a. girth
  a. guarding
  a. incision dehiscence
  a. laparotomy pad
  a. lavage
  a. mass
  a. migraine
  a. muscle deficiency syndrome
  a. nephrectomy
  a. pad
  a. pain
  a. paracentesis
  a. partitioning
  a. patch electrode
  a. peritoneum
  a. pool
  a. pressure
  a. pressure technique
  a. procedure
  a. pulse
  a. rectopexy
  a. rigidity
  a. ring
  a. section
  a. situs inversus
  a. stoma
  a. tap
  a. testis
  a. tympany
  a. typhoid
  a. ultrasonography
  a. ultrasound
  a. vascular accident
  a. viscus
  a. wall
  a. wall hernia
  a. wall mass
  a. wall venous pattern
  a. zone
abdominalis
  pulsus a.

abdominal-perineal resection
abdominis
  angina a.
  diastasis recti a.
  rectus a.
abdominocentesis
abdominopelvic orocecal transit
  time
abdominoperineal
  a. excision
  a. resection (APR)
abdominoscopy
abdominoscrotal
  a. hydrocele
abenteric
aberrant
  a. obturator vein
  a. pancreas
  a. umbilical stomach
aberration
aberrations by scintigraphy
ABG
  arterial blood gas
ability
  renal autoregulatory a.
Ablaser laser delivery catheter
ablation
  androgen a.
  carbon dioxide laser plaque a.
  cold forceps a.
  cold snare a.
  cryogenic a.
  cryosurgical a.
  homogeneous a.
  laser a.
  neoadjuvant total androgen a.
  transurethral needle a. (TUNA)
  tumor a.
  valve a.
  visual laser a.
ablative laser therapy
abnormality
  amino acid a.
  chromosomal a.
  clotting a.
  coloboma-heart disease-atresia
    choanae-retarded growth-
    genital ear a.'s (CHARGE)
  diminished branching a.
  electrolyte a.
  hematologic a.
  hepatic a.
  a. of hepatic artery

immunologic a.
mucosal a.
ocular a.
omphalocele, exstrophy of the
bladder, imperforate anus and
spinal a.'s (OEIS)
platelet a.
pruning a.
vascular a.
ABO barrier
Abocide disinfectant
ABO-incompatible
AB/PAS
Alcian blue and periodic acid-Schiff
Abrikosov tumor
abrogate
abrupt pulse
abscess
abdominal a.
amebic a.
anorectal a.
appendiceal a.
cavernosal a.
cortical a.
crypt a.'s
cuff a.
deep interloop a.
diaphragmatic a.
Douglas a.
echinococcal a.
echinococcal liver a.
Entamoeba histolytica a.
enteroperitoneal a.
fecal a.
a. formation
fungal a.
fungal liver a.
gallbladder wall a.
gas a.
hepatic a.
high intermuscular a.
horseshoe a.
interloop a.
intermesenteric a.
intersphincteric perirectal a.
intra-abdominal a.
intrahepatic a.

intramesenteric a.
intraperitoneal a.
ischiorectal perirectal a.
liver a.
midabdominal a.
non-gas-forming liver a.
pancreatic a.
pancreatic pseudocyst a.
paracolic a.
paranephric a.
pararectal a.
pelvic a.
perianal a.
perianal fistula a.
pericecal a.
pericholecystic a.
pericolic a.
pericolonic a.
perineal a.
perinephric a.
perirectal a.
perirenal a.
peritoneal cavity a.
periureteral a.
periurethral a.
phlegmonous a.
pilonidal perirectal a.
postoperative a.
psoas a.
pyogenic a.
rectal a.
renal a.
renal cortical a.
retrocecal a.
retroperitoneal-iliopsoas a.
splenic a.
stercoral a.
subacute a.
subcapsular hepatic a.
subdiaphragmatic a.
subhepatic a.
subphrenic a.
supralevator perirectal a.
urachal a.
absent
a. ankle jerk
a. bowel sounds

NOTES

absent *(continued)*
    a. gag reflex
    a. peristalsis
Absidia
    A. corymbifera
    A. ramosum
absolute
    a. alcohol
    a. alcohol sclerosant
    a. diet
    a. erythrocytosis
absorbable
    a. clip
    a. gelatin sponge
    a. sponge
    a. suture
absorptiometry
    dual-energy x-ray a.
    dual-photon a.
absorption
    alcohol a.
    dual-energy x-ray a. (DEXA)
    gastrointestinal a.
    impaired gastric a.
    paracetamol a.
    reservoir mucosal a.
absorptive
    a. cell
    a. hyperoxaluria
abstinence
A/B switch box
abuse
    alcohol a.
    ethanol a.
    intravenous drug a.
    ipecac a.
    laxative a.
    phencyclidine a.
    salicylate a.
    substance a.
AC
    adenylate cyclase
    Pepcid AC
ACA
    adenocarcinoma
    anticardiolipin antibody
acalculous
    a. cholecystitis
    a. gallbladder disease
acanthosis
    glycogenic a.
    a. nigricans
Acarbose

Ac-5-ASA
    N-acetyl-5-ASA
Acationox
ACBE
    air contrast barium enema
accelerated
    a. hypertension
    a. transplant rejection
access
    peritoneal a.
    vascular a.
accessory
    a. adrenal
    a. duct of Luschka
    a. pancreas
    a. pancreatic duct
    a. phallic urethra
    a. trocar
    a. vessel
accident
    abdominal vascular a.
accumulation
    gamma-aminobutyric acid a.
    glycoprotein a.
    tubular iron a.
Accurate catheter
Accuratome pre-curved papillotome
AccuSharp endoscope
Accuson-128 color flow Doppler machine
Accutorr oscillometric device
ACE
    angiotensin converting enzyme
    antegrade continence enema procedure
    BICAP silver ACE
    ACE inhibitor
ACEI
    angiotensin-converting enzyme inhibitor
acetabulum
acetaldehyde
acetaminophen
    a. hepatotoxicity
    a. overdose
acetate
    anaritide a.
    buserelin a.
    calcium a.
    cortisone a.
    cyproterone a. (CPA)
    desmopressin a.
    free a.

goserelin a.
hydrocortisone a.
leuprolide a.
medroxyprogesterone a.
megestrol a.
methylprednisolone a.
octreotide a.
phorbol myristate a. (PMA)
roxatidine a.
uranyl a.
acetazolamide
acetic acid
acetohydroxamic
  a. acid
  a. acid irrigation
acetonitrile eluate
acetowhite
  a. lesion
acetylcholine
acetylcholinesterase
acetyl-Co-hypoglycin A
acetylcysteine
acetylsalicylic
  a. acid
  5-a. acid
ACG
  American College of
  Gastroenterology
achalasia
  a. balloon dilation
  a. cardia
  classic a.
  cricopharyngeal a.
  a. dilator
  esophageal a.
  idiopathic a.
  pelvirectal a.
  secondary a.
  sphincteral a.
  vigorous a.
achalasia-like esophagus
ache
  stomach a.
Achiever
  A. balloon dilation catheter
  A. balloon dilator

achlorhydria
  gastric a.
  histamine-resistant a.
  medically-induced a.
acholangic biliary cirrhosis
acholia
acholic
  a. stool
acholuric jaundice
achoresis
Achromycin
Achromycin V
achylia
  a. gastrica
  a. pancreatica
achylous
acid
  acetic a.
  acetohydroxamic a.
  acetylsalicylic a.
  5-acetylsalicylic a.
  amino a.
  aminocaproic a.
  5-aminosalicylic a. (5-ASA)
  arachidonic a.
  aromatic amino a. (AAA)
  ascorbic a.
  a. base imbalance
  bile a. (BA)
  branched-chain amino a.
    (BCAA)
  caustic a.
  a. cell
  chenodeoxycholic a. (CDCA)
  cholic a. (CA)
  a. clearance test (ACT)
  cocarcinogenic fecal bile a.
  complementary
    deoxyribonucleic a. (cDNA)
  conjugated bile a.
  deoxycholic a.
  deoxyribonucleic a. (DNA)
  diethylenetriamine pentaacetic a.
    (DTPA)
  diisopropyl iminodiacetic a.
    (DISIDA)
  dimercaptosuccinic a. (DMSA)

NOTES

acid *(continued)*
 disopropyliminodiacetic a.
 a. dyspepsia
 eicosapentaenoic a. (EPA)
 7β-epimer of
  chenodeoxycholic a.
 epsilon-aminocaproic a.
 essential amino a.
 essential fatty a.
 esterified fecal a.
 ethacrynic a.
 ethylenediaminetetraacetic a.
  (EDTA)
 ethylene glycol tetraacetic a.
  (EGTA)
 fatty a.
 fecal bile a. (FBA)
 folic a.
 folinic a.
 free fatty a.
 free fecal bile a.
 gamma-aminobutyric a.
 gastric a.
 genomic deoxyribonucleic a.
 glutamic a.
 a. guanidine thiocyanate-phenol-
  chloroform method
 a. hemolysis test
 hepato-iminodiacetic a. (HIDA)
 homovanillic a. (HVA)
 hyaluronic a.
 hydrochloric a. (HCl)
 hydroxyeicosatetraenoic a.
  (HETE)
 5-hydroxyindoleacetic a.
 a. hypersecretion
 iminodiacetic a. (IDA)
 a. indigestion
 a. ingestion
 a. injury
 iocetamic a.
 iopanoic a.
 ^{131}I para-aminohippuric a.
 isovaleric a.
 keto a.
 lactic a.
 Lewis a.'s
 lithocholic a. (LCA)
 luminal a.
 medium-chain fatty a.'s
  (MCFA)
 messenger ribonucleoprotein a.
  (mRNA)

 methylaminoisobutyric a.
  (MeAIB)
 a. microclimate
 mucosal fatty a.
 nalidixic a.
 N-benzoyl-L-tyrosyl-P-
  aminobenzoic a.
 nonsulfated bile a.
 Novamine amino a.
 oral bile a. (OBA)
 p-amino-hippuric a.
 pantothenic a.
 para-aminobenzoic a. (PABA)
 para-isopropyliminodiacetic a.
  (PIPIDA)
 a. peptic ulcer
 a. perfusion test
 polyglycolic a.
 pteroylglutamic a.
 a. reflux
 a. reflux test
 a. regurgitation
 renal messenger
  ribonucleoprotein a.
 reptilase a.
 ribonucleic a. (RNA)
 saponifiable fecal bile a.
 a. secretion
 serum uric a.
 short-chain fatty a. (SCFA)
 sulfuric a.
 a. suppression
 tannic a.
 taurocholic a.
 ^{99m}Tc pentetic a.
 technetium-99m
  diethylenetriamine penta-
  ascetic a. (^{99m}Tc-DPTA)
 technetium-99m Tc-99m
  iminodiacetic a.
 tranexamic a.
 Travasol amino a.
 tricarboxylic a. (TCA)
 trichloroacetic a. (TCA)
 trihydrocoprostanic a. (TCA)
 uric a.
 ursodeoxycholic a. (UDCA)
 valproic a.
 vanillacetic a. (VLA)
 vanillylmandelic a. (VMA)
acid-ash diet
acid-base
 a.-b. balance

a.-b. disturbance
a.-b. equilibrium
acidemia
 isovaleric a.
acidic fibroblast growth factor
acidification
 a. defect
 a. of stool test
acidity
 circadian gastric a.
 gastric a.
 intracellular a.
 intragastric a.
 urinary a.
acid-labile
acidophilic
 a. body
 a. PAS-positive granule
acidophilus
 a. capsule
 Lactobacillus a.
 a. milk
acidosis
 acute a.
 chronic metabolic a.
 congenital lactic a.
 distal renal tubular a. (dRTA)
 high anion-gap metabolic a.
 hyperchloremic metabolic a.
 hypokalemic renal tubular a.
 lactic a.
 non-anion-gap metabolic a.
 renal tubular a.
 renal tubular a. I (RTA-I)
 respiratory a.
 uremic a.
 winter a.
acidotic
acid-pepsin reflux esophagitis
acid-peptic
 a.-p. disease
 a.-p. esophagitis
 a.-p. juice
acid-provoked spasm
acid-Schiff
 Alcian blue and periodic a.-S.
 (AB/PAS)

periodic a.-S. (PAS)
 a.-S. stain
acid-suppressed stomach
acid-suppression therapy
Acidulin
aciduria
 3-hydroxy 3-methylglutaric a.
acification
 intracellular a.
acinar
 a. cell
 a. cell carcinoma
 a. gradient
 a. tissue
acinarization
Acinetobacter calcoaceticus
acini
 pancreatic a.
acinous adenoma
acinus, pl. **acini**
acipimox
ACKD
 acquired cystic kidney disease
ackee fruit poisoning
ACLA
 anticardiolipin antibody
ACMI
 ACMI cystourethroscope
 ACMI endoscope
 ACMI fiberoptic colonoscope
 ACMI fiberoptic esophagoscope
 ACMI gastroscope
 ACMI Martin endoscopy
  forceps
 ACMI monopolar electrode
 ACMI ulcer measuring device
acnes
 Propionibacterium a.
acne vulgaris
acontractile detrusor
acorn-tipped
 a.-t. bougie
 a.-t. catheter
acorn treatment
acoustically transparent cradle
acoustic blink

NOTES

acquired
  a. cystic kidney disease (ACKD)
  a.. diverticulosis
  a. gastric ectopy
  a. hyperlipoproteinemia
  a. hyperoxaluria
  a. immunodeficiency
  a. immunodeficiency syndrome (AIDS)
  a. lactose deficiency
  a. megacolon
  a. neutrophil chemotaxis defect
  a. pancreatitis
acquisita
  epidermolysis bullosa a.
acrobystitis
acrocyanosis
acromegalic
acrophase
acroposthitis
acrosin
acrosome-reacted spermatozoa
acrosome reaction
ACT
  acid clearance test
ACTH
  adrenocorticotropic hormone
Actidose-Aqua
Actigall
actin
  a. filament
  smooth muscle isoform a.
β-actin
  β-a. cDNA probe
  β-a. mRNA
  β-a. mRNA signal
Actinomyces
  A. naeslundii
actinomycin C
actinomycin D
actinomycosis
  biliary a.
  gastric a.
actinomycotic esophageal disease
action
  cytolytic a.
  immunomodulatory a.
  virus-like a. (VLA)
activated
  a. alkaline glutaraldehyde
  a. charcoal

  a. partial thromboplastin time
  a. thromboplastin time
activation
  complement a.
  nuclear transcriptional a.
  very late a. (VLA)
activator
  plasminogen a. (PA)
  tissue plasminogen a. (TPA)
  tissue-type plasminogen a. (t-PA)
  urokinase plasminogen a.
  vascular plasminogen a. (v-PA)
Active
active
  a. bowel sounds
  a. chronic hepatitis
  a. congestion
  a. duodenal ulcer
  A. Living incontinence pad
  A. Living incontinence shield
  a. renin
  a. source of bleeding
  a. systemic bacterial infection
actively bleeding varix
Activin A
activity
  adenosine deaminase a.
  ATPase a.
  brush-border disaccharidase specific a.
  brush-border enzyme a.
  brush-border hydrolase a.
  complement hemolytic a.
  disaccharidase enzyme a.
  efferent renal sympathetic nerve a. (ERSNA)
  endogenous peroxidase a.
  fibrinolytic a.
  β-galactosidase a.
  gastric myoelectrical a.
  gastric urease a.
  intrinsic enzymatic a.
  mitotic a.
  motor a.
  muscarinic a.
  myoelectric a.
  NA+/H+ antiporter a.
  Na/K-ATPase a.
  opsonic a.
  oxidoreductase a.
  phospholipase A2 catalytic a.
  plasma renin a. (PRA)

protein serine/threonine
kinase a.
PyNPase a.
renal sympathetic a.
renal xanthine oxidase-xanthine
dehydrogenase a.
serum cholinesterase a.
single potential analysis
cavernous electrical a.
(SPACE)
specific a.
spike-burst electrical a.
succinate dehydrogenase a.
(SDH)
sympathetic nervous system a.
tumorigenesis a.
tyrosine kinase a.
Actril disinfectant
Acucise
   A. balloon
   A. endopyelotomy catheter
**AcuClip endoscopic multiple clip
   applier**
acuity
acuminatum, pl. **acuminata**
   condyloma a.
   esophageal condyloma a.
acupuncture
AcuSnare
acute
   a. abdomen
   a. abdominal vascular disease
   a. acalculous cholecystitis
   a. acidosis
   a. alcoholic hepatitis
   a. appendicitis
   a. cellular rejection
   a. cholecystitis
   a. diverticulitis
   a. drug-induced cholestasis
   a. erosive gastritis (AEG)
   a. fatty liver
   a. fatty liver of pregnancy
   (AFLP)
   a. flank pain syndrome
   a. focal bacterial nephritis
   (AFBN)

a. gallstone pancreatitis
a. gastric anisakiasis
a. gastric mucosal lesion
a. gastroenteritis (AGE)
a. glomerulonephritis
a. graft-vs-host disease
a. hemorrhagic gastritis
a. hemorrhagic pancreatitis
a. hepatic coma
a. hepatic failure
a. hepatic rupture
a. hepatic toxicity
a. hepatitis (AH)
a. hepatocellular degeneration
a. hydramnios
a. idiopathic inflammatory
   bowel disease
a. infectious colitis
a. infectious diarrhea
a. infectious gastroenteritis
a. infectious nonbacterial
   gastroenteritis
a. intermittent porphyria (AIP)
a. interstitial nephritis (AIN)
a. intrinsic renal failure
a. lead poisoning
a. leukopenia
a. mercury poisoning
a. mononucleosis-like hepatitis
a. myelomonocytic leukemia
a. nephritis
a. nephrosis
a. nonocclusive bowel
   infarction
a. nonvariceal upper
   gastrointestinal hemorrhage
a. obstructive cholangitis
a. obstructive suppurative
   cholangitis (AOSC)
a. pancreatitis
a. pancreatitis prevention
a. parenchymatous hepatitis
a. polycystic disease
a. porphyria
a. proctitis
a. pyelonephritis
a. recurrent pancreatitis (ARP)

NOTES

acute *(continued)*
  a. rejection of liver transplant
  a. relapsing pancreatitis
  a. renal failure (ARF)
  a. renal transplant vasculopathy
  a. sclerosing hyaline necrosis (ASHN)
  a. scrotum
  a. self-limited colitis (ASLC)
  a. self-limited hepatitis
  a. suppurative cholangitis (ASC)
  a. surgical abdomen
  a. tubular necrosis
  a. urethritis
  a. vascular rejection
  a. viral hepatitis (AVH)
Acutrim
acyclovir
  a. sodium
acyltransferase
  lecithin-cholesterol a.
ADA
  American Diabetes Association
  ADA diet
Adair-Allis forceps
Adalat CC
adapter, adaptor
  camera a.
  c-mount a.
  friction-fit a.
  Olympus a.
  Polaroid SX-70 with ACMI a.
Adaptic
  A. dressing
  A. packing
adaptive relaxation
adaptor *(var. of* adapter)
  Cook plastic Luer lock a.
  friction-fit a.
  Tuohy-Borst a.
ADCC
  antibody-dependent cell-mediated cytotoxicity
ADD
  angled delivery device
Addison
  A. clinical planes
  A. disease
  A. point
  A. syndrome
addressins
ADD'Stat laser

adductor
  a. brevis muscle
  a. longus muscle
adelomorphous cell
adenemphraxis
Aden fever
adenitis
  mesenteric a.
adenoacanthoma
adeno-associated virus (AAV)
adenocarcinoma (ACA)
  annular a.
  appendiceal a.
  clear cell a.
  colloid-producing a.
  colonic a.
  colorectal a.
  duodenal a.
  esophageal a.
  exophytic a.
  gastric a.
  giant cell a.
  hepatoid a.
  infiltrating a.
  invasive a.
  metastatic a.
  mucinous a.
  mucin-producing a.
  mucosal a.
  papillary a.
  Paris renal a.
  peritoneal a.
  prostatic a.
  renal a.
  scirrhous a.
  a. in situ
  ulcerating a.
adenofibromyoma
adenoid cystic carcinoma
adenoleiomyofibroma
adenolysis
adenoma
  acinous a.
  aggressive a.
  bile duct a. (BDA)
  Brunner gland a.
  colonic a.
  colorectal villous a.
  cortical a.
  depressed a.
  a. destruens
  duodenal a.
  embryonal a.

flat a.
hepatic a.
hepatocellular a. (HCA)
incidental a.
islet cell a.
Leydig cell a.
liver cell a. (LCA)
metachronous a.
moderately differentiated a.
mucinous a.
nephrogenic a.
nonpolypoid a.
papillary a.
Pick tubular a.
poorly differentiated a.
prostatic a.
rectal villous a.
renal cortical a.
a. sebaceum
sessile a.
testicular tubular a.
tubulovillous a.
undifferentiated a.
villoglandular a.
villous colorectal a.
well-differentiated a.
adenoma-carcinoma sequence
adenoma-hyperplastic polyp ratio
adenoma-nonadenoma ratio
adenomas
synchronous a.
adenomatoid tumor
adenomatosis
multiple endocrine a. type I (MEA-I)
multiple endocrine a. type II (MEA-II)
adenomatous
a. colorectal polyp
a. epithelium
a. gastric polyp
a. hyperplasia (AH)
a. polyp (AP)
a. polyp-cancer sequence
a. polyposis
a. polyposis coli (APC)
a. polyposis coli gene

adenomyoma of gallbladder
adenomyomatosis
adenomyosarcoma
adenomyosis
adenopapillomatosis
gastric a.
adenopathy
axillary a.
inguinal a.
lymph node a.
palpable a.
paraductal a.
adenosine
a. deaminase
a. deaminase activity
a. diphosphatase (ADPase)
a. diphosphate (ADP)
a. monophosphate (AMP)
a. triphosphatase (ATPase)
a. triphosphate (ATP)
adenosinergic
adenosis
sclerosing a.
adenosquamous carcinoma
adenovirus
a.-12 viral protein
a. colitis
enteric a.
human a. 12
a. infection
adenylate
a. cyclase (AC)
a. cyclase complex
adenyl cyclase stimulation
ADF
aortoduodenal fistula
ADH
alcohol dehydrogenase
antidiuretic hormone
adherence
bacterial a.
adherent clot
adhesion
antigen-independent a.
attic a.
bacterial a.
banjo-string a.

NOTES

adhesion (*continued*)
    cell-cell a.
    coronal a.
    dense a.
    a. dyspepsia
    filmy a.
    a. formation
    freeing up of a.'s
    hard a.
    hepatic a.
    intra-abdominal a.
    intraperitoneal a.
    lysis of a.'s
    a. molecule
    omental a.
    pelvic a.
    perihepatic a.
    peritoneal a.
    postcholecystitis a.
    postoperative a.
    taking down of a.'s
    T-cell a.
    thick a.
    thin a.
    tight a.
    violin-string a.
adhesive
    a. band
    Comfeel skin a.
    a. dressing
    fibrin tissue a.
    a. ileus
    a. protein receptor
    a. tape
    Uro-Bond skin a.
Adipex-P
adiphenine
adipose tissue
adiposus
    ascites a.
adjuvant
    anesthesia a.
    a. chemotherapy
    a. drug therapy
    Freund a.
    a. nephrectomy
    a. treatment
administration
    percutaneous bacille Calmette-
    Guérin a.
adnexal
    a. fullness
    a. mass

    a. tenderness
    a. torsion
    a. tumor
ADP
    adenosine diphosphate
ADPase
    adenosine diphosphatase
ADPKD
    autosomal dominant polycystic
    kidney disease
    oligosymptomatic ADPKD
ADPKD1
    A. gene
    A. genotype
ADPKD2
    ADPKD2 gene
    ADPKD2 genotype
ADR
    Adriamycin
adrenal
    accessory a.
    a. cortex
    a. corticoadenoma
    a. disease
    a. hirsutism
    a. hyperplasia
    a. myelolipoma
    a. rest
    a. scintigraphy
adrenalectomy
    ipsilateral a.
    transperitoneal laparoscopic a.
    (TLA)
adrenalin
    a. chloride
    a. injection therapy
adrenergic
    a. neuron
    a. receptor
adrenergic-cholinergic agonist
adrenocortical macrocyst
adrenocorticotropic
    a. hormone (ACTH)
adrenogenital syndrome
adrenoreceptor
    α_1 a.
Adriamycin (ADR)
    A. glomerulopathy
    A.-induced nephrosis
Adrucil
Adson
    A. clamp

A. forceps
  A. tissue forceps
Adson-Brown tissue forceps
adsorption
adult
  a. familial hyaline membrane
    disease
  a. hypolactasia
  a. phimosis
  a. polycystic disease (APCD)
  a. polycystic kidney disease
    (APKD)
  a. polycystic liver disease
    (APLD)
  a. respiratory distress syndrome
  a. sigmoidoscope
adult-onset obesity
advance
  A. formula
  a. to regular diet
advanced
  a. glycation end (AGE)
  A. surgical suture applier
  a. therapeutic endoscopy
advancement
  Duckett meatal a.
  Glenn-Anderson a.
  meatal a.
  a. of rectal flap
  sleeve a.
Advantx digital system
adventitia
  fibrofatty a.
adverse prognostic factor
adynamic
  a. ileus
  a. intestinal obstruction
Adzorbstar
AEG
  acute erosive gastritis
AER
  albumin excretion rate
AERD
  atheroembolic renal disease
aerobic
  a. culture
  a. glycolysis

aerobilia
**Aerochamber pediatric spacer
  device**
aerocystoscope
aerocystoscopy
aerogastria
  blocked a.
aerogenes
  Enterobacter a.
aerogenosum
  sputum a.
Aeromonas
  A.-associated enterocolitis
  A. caviae
  A. diarrhea
  A. hydrophila
  A. liquefaciens
  A. punctata
  A. salmonicida
  A. sobria
aerophagia, aerophagy
aerosol
  inhalation a.
  ^{99m}Tc DTPA a.
aeruginosa
  Pseudomonas a.
AESOP
  automated endoscopic system for
  optimal positioning
  AESOP ReView feature
AFBN
  acute focal bacterial nephritis
afferent
  a. arteriolar vasoconstriction
  a. arteriole
  a. fiber
  a. limb
  a. loop
  a. loop syndrome
  a. neuron
  a. projection
  a. renal nerve
  splanchnic primary a.
affinity
  boronate a.
affinity-avidity hypothesis

NOTES

AFIP
    Armed Forces Institute of Pathology
aflatoxin
AFLP
    acute fatty liver of pregnancy
AFP
    alpha fetoprotein
    α-fetoprotein
African hemochromatosis
AFTP
    ascitic fluid total protein
agalactiae
    Streptococcus a.
agammaglobulinemia
    Bruton-type a.
    X-linked infantile a.
aganglionic
    a. bowel
    a. segment of colon
aganglionosis
    congenital a.
agar
    brain-heart infusion a.
    a. bridge
    a. dilution
    a. gel
    MacConkey a.
    phenyl ethyl alcohol a.
    Sabouraud glucose a.
    vancomycin/nalidixic acid a.
    Wilkins-Chilgren a.
agarose
    a. gel
    a. gel electrophoresis
AGE
    acute gastroenteritis
    advanced glycation end
agenesis
    corpus callosum a.
    renal a.
    scrotal a.
agent
    anticholinergic a.
    antidiarrheal a.
    antifungal a.
    antihypertensive a.
    antimicrobial a.
    antimotility a.
    antimuscarinic a.
    antisecretory a.
    antispasmodic a.
    5-ASA a.
    azole antifungal a.

beta-sympathomimetic
    tocolytic a.
bulking a.
carbon dioxide trapping a.
central adrenergic a.
contrast a.
cyanocobalamin radioactive a.
cytotoxic a.
distal tubular acting a.
embolic a.
hemostatic a.
imidoacetic acid radioactive a.
interleukin-2 receptor-
    blocking a.
iodinated contrast a.
mucolytic a.
Norwalk a.
parasympathomimetic a.
peripheral adrenergic a.
progesteronal a.
prokinetic a.
Racobalamin-57 radioactive a.
Robengatope radioactive a.
rose bengal sodium ^{131}I
    radioactive a.
Rubratope-57 radioactive a.
sclerosing a.
selenomethionine radioactive a.
Sethotope radioactive a.
test-yolk buffer
    cryopreservation a.
thrombolytic a.
virucidal a.
ageusia
ageusic
agglutinin
    peanut a. (PNA)
aggregate
    lymphoid a.
aggregation
    erythrocyte a.
    familial a.
aggressive adenoma
agonist
    α_1 a.
    adrenergic-cholinergic a.
    alpha-2-adrenergic a.
    beta-adrenergic a.
    dopamine a.
    5-HT4 a.
    muscarinic cholinergic a.
    nicotinic a.
Agoral

agranulocytic ulcer
AH
    acute hepatitis
    adenomatous hyperplasia
AID
    artificial insemination donor
AIDS
    acquired immunodeficiency
      syndrome
AIDS-related complex (ARC)
AIH
    artificial insemination husband
AIN
    acute interstitial nephritis
AIO
    all-in-one
      AIO parenteral solution
AIP
    acute intermittent porphyria
air
    biliary a.
    blood gas on room a.
    a. contrast barium enema
      (ACBE)
    a. cyst
    free a.
    a. insufflation
    intramural colonic a.
    intraperitoneal a.
    a. pressure enema reduction
    a. swallowing
    a. thermometer
air-filled loop
airflow obstruction
air/fluid level
airfuge
    Beckman a.
airway
    a. epithelium
    a. obstruction
    patent a.
AJCC TNM tumor classification
AJCC/UICC
    American Joint Committee on
    Cancer/International Union against
    Cancer
    AJCC/UICC staging system

Ajmalin liver injury
Akerlund
    diverticulum of A.
Alagille syndrome
alanine
    a. aminotransferase (ALT)
alarm
    bed-wetting a.
    a. clock voiding
    enuresis a.
    glutaraldehyde a.
Alazide
alba
    linea a.
Albarran
    A. laser cystoscope
    A. mechanism
    A. reflecting bridge
    A. test
albendazole
Albert suture
albicans
    Candida a.
albuginea
    tunica a.
albumin
    ^{125}I-a.
    bovine serum a. (BSA)
    a. excretion rate (AER)
    fatty acid-free bovine serum a.
    glycated a.
    a. gradient
    human a.
    human serum a.
    intravenous a.
    macroaggregated a. (MAA)
    a. messenger RNA
    a. metabolism
    nonglycated a.
    plasma a.
    a. plasma concentration
    serum a.
    a. synthesis
    technetium-99m
      macroaggregated a. (^{99m}Tc-
      MAA)
albumin-coated resin hemoperfusion

NOTES

albuminuria
albuminuric
albuterol
alcalifaciens
　　Providencia a.
Alcian
　　A. blue
　　A. blue dye
　　A. blue and periodic acid-
　　　　Schiff (AB/PAS)
　　A. blue stain
Alcock
　　A. canal
　　A. syndrome
alcohol
　　absolute a.
　　a. absorption
　　a. abuse
　　a. consumption
　　a. cooling bath
　　a. dehydrogenase (ADH)
　　ethyl a.
　　graded a.
　　isoamyl a.
　　polyvinyl a.
　　a. potentiation
　　a. sclerosis
　　a. thermometer
alcohol-fixed gastric biopsy
alcoholic
　　a. cirrhosis
　　a. fatty liver
　　a. fibrosis
　　a. hemorrhagic gastritis
　　a. hepatitis
　　a. hyalin
　　a. liver disease (ALD)
　　a. pancreatitis
　　a. prognostic factor
　　a. varix
alcohol-induced
　　a.-i. extracellular volume
　　　　contraction
　　a.-i. gastrointestinal symptom
alcoholism
Alconefrin
ALD
　　alcoholic liver disease
Aldactazide
aldehyde dehydrogenase
Alden loop gastric bypass
aldesleukin
　　Proleukin a.

Aldoclor
aldolase
Aldomet
Aldoril
aldose reductase (AR)
aldosterone
aldosteronism
Aleo meter
Alert
　　Sears Wee A.
Alexander elevator
alexandrite
　　a. laser
　　a. and rhodamine
alexithymia
alfa
　　epoetin a.
alfa-2a
　　interferon a.
　　recombinant interferon a.
alfa-2b
　　interferon a.
　　interferon a.
alfa-n1
　　interferon a.-n.
alfa-n3
　　interferon a.-n.
Alferon N
alfuzosin
Al-Ghorab
　　A.-G. modification
　　A.-G. modification shunt
　　A.-G. procedure
Algicon
algid malaria
algorithm
　　management a.
alimentary
　　a. apparatus
　　a. bolus
　　a. canal
　　a. diabetes
　　a. glycosuria
　　a. hyperinsulinism
　　a. obesity
　　a. system
　　a. tract
　　a. tract duplication
alimentation
　　central venous a.
　　enteral a.
　　forced a.
　　parenteral a.

A

peripheral intravenous a.
rectal a.
total parenteral a.
Alimentum
aliquot
alkali
  caustic a.
  a. ingestion
alkaline
  a. injury
  a. milk drip
  a. phosphatase (ALP, AP)
  a. phosphatase test
  a. phosphatase Vectastain ABC
  a. reflux esophagitis
  a. reflux gastritis
alkaline-ash diet
alkalinization
  a. test
alkaloid
  ergot a.'s
  indolalkylamine a.
  Veratrum a.'s
alkalosis
  hypochloremic hypokalemic
    metabolic a.
  hypokalemic metabolic a.
  metabolic a.
  respiratory a.
Alka-Mints
alkane
  breath a.
Alka-Seltzer
Alken approach
Alkets
allantoic cyst
allele
  HLA-DP a.
allelic
  DC locus a.
allelotyping
  p53 a.
Allen
  A. anastomosis clamp
  A. intestinal clamp
  A. intestinal forceps
  A. test

Allen-Kocher clamp
Allen-Masters syndrome
allergen
  food a.
allergic
  a. colitis
  a. enteropathy
  a. interstitial nephritis
  a. proctitis
  a. vasculitis
allergy
  cow's milk protein a.
  food a.
  latex a.
  medication a.
all four quadrants
Alliance integrated inflation system
alligator jaws forceps
alligator-type grasping forceps
all-in-one (AIO)
Allis
  A. catheter
  A. clamp
  A. forceps
  A. inhaler
  A. tooth grasper
Allison gastroesophageal reflux
  repair
alloantigen
  a. response
allochezia, allochetia
allogenic, allogeneic
  a. kidney transplant
  a. liver perfusion
allograft
  hepatic a.
  kidney a.
  a. parenchyma
  a. rejection
  renal a.
  a. survival rate
allograft-mediated hypertension
alloplastic
  a. biomaterial
  a. prostatic bladder
allopurinol
allotransplantation

NOTES

17

allowance
    recommended daily a. (RDA)
alloy
    shape memory a. (SMA)
Aloka MP-PN ultrasound probe
alopecia
ALP
    alkaline phosphatase
alpha
    a. blockade
    a. heavy-chain disease
    A. I inflatable penile prosthesis
    a. interferon
    interferon a.
    a. interferon therapy
    a. interferon treatment
    a. loop
    a. motor neuron
    prostaglandin F2 a.
    a. sigmoid loop
    a. sympathetic blockade
alpha-1 blocker
alpha-2 globulin
alpha-adrenergic
    a.-a. antagonist
    a.-a. receptor
alpha-2-adrenergic agonist
alpha$_1$-adrenergic receptor
alpha-amylase
    pancreatic a.-a.
alpha-1-antitrypsin
alpha-2-beta-1 integrin cell-surface collagen ($\alpha_2\beta_1$)
alpha-chain disease
alpha fetoprotein (*var. of* α-fetoprotein) **(AFP)**
alpha-gliadin fraction
alpha-glucosidase inhibitor
alpha-1-glycero-monooctanoin
alpha-hemolytic streptococcus
alpha-interferon
alpha-loop maneuver
alphaprodine
alpha-receptor antagonist
alpha *Streptococcus viridans*
Alport syndrome
alprazolam
alprostadil
ALR cystoresectoscope
Alseroxylon-Alkavervir
Alstrom disease

ALT
    alanine aminotransferase
    ALT test
alteration
    genetic a.
    molecular genetic a.
    nuclear matrix a.
altered sperm motility
ALternaGEL
alternate-day treatment
alternate mRNA splicing
alternative cell attachment domain
Altertome
    Microvasive A.
Altmann pulse
ALTRA-FLUX hemodialyzer
Aludrox
alum curd
aluminum
    a. hydroxide
    a. hydroxide, magnesium hydroxide, and simethicone
    a. hydroxide and magnesium trisilicate
    a. toxicity
Alupent
Alutabs
alvei
    Hafnia a.
alveolar
    a. hydatid cyst
    a. rhabdomyosarcoma
AlveoSampler
    Quintron A.
alverine citrate
alvine calculus
alvinolith
Alzer Model 2001 osmotic minipump
AMA
    antimitochondrial antibody
    AMA inflatable cylinder
Amadori products
amalonaticus
    Citrobacter a.
Amanita
    Amanita mushroom
    Amanita mushroom hepatotoxicity
Amaryl
amastigote
amaurosis
    Leber a.

ambenonium chloride
amber
Ambicor penile prosthesis
ambiguous external genitalia
Ambilhar
AmB-induced reduction GFR
ambiothermic
ambulation
ambulatory
   a. hemorrhoidectomy
   a. monitoring
   a. pH monitoring
   a. probe
   a. urodynamic monitoring
   a. urodynamics
amebiasis
   hepatic a.
   indigenous a.
amebic
   a. abscess
   a. appendicitis
   a. colitis
   a. dysentery
   a. granuloma
   a. hepatitis
   a. ulcer
amebism
ameboma
ameliorate
ameliorated vasodilating response
America
   Crohns and Colitis Foundation
   of A. (CCFA)
American
   A. ACMI (S3565, TX-915)
   flexible fiberoptic
   sigmoidoscope
   A. Anorexia/Bulimia
   Association
   A. College of Gastroenterology
   (ACG)
   A. Diabetes Association (ADA)
   A. Dilation System dilator
   A. Endoscopy automatic
   reprocessor
   A. Endoscopy dilator

   A. endoscopy mechanical
   lithotriptor
   A. Joint Committee on
   Cancer/International Union
   against Cancer (AJCC/UICC)
   A. Society for Gastrointestinal
   Endoscopy (ASGE)
   A. trypanosomiasis
   A. type culture collection
   A. Urological Association
   (AUA)
   A. Urological Association
   symptom index
   A. Urological Association
   symptom index for BPH
americanus
   Necator a.
Amerlex-M second antibody
Ames
   semiquantitative agglutination
   SERA-TEK A.
   A. test
Ames Hemastix reagent strips
AMF
   autocrine motility factor
Amicar
Amicon D-20 filter
amidation
amifloxacin
amikacin
Amikin
amiloride
   a. hydrochloride
amiloride-sensitive, electroneutral
   Na+/H+antiporter
Amin-Aid
   A.-A. powdered feeding
amine
   aromatic a.
   biogenic a.
   a. precursor uptake and
   decarboxylation (APUD)
   a. precursor uptake and
   decarboxylation cell (APUD
   cell)
Amino
   A. Mel Hepa

NOTES

amino
  a. acid
  a. acid abnormality
  a. acid-based dialysate solution
  a. acid-glucose mixture
  a. terminus
aminoacidopathy
  dibasic a.
aminoaciduria
aminobenzoate
  butyl a.
  a. potassium
4-Aminobiphenyl
aminocaproic acid
Aminofusin L Forte amino acid
  solution
aminoglutethimide
aminoglycoside
aminoguanidine
aminonucleoside
  glomerular epithelial cell toxin
    puromycin a.
  puromycin a.
aminopeptidase
  leucine a. (LAP)
aminophylline
aminopyrine
  a. breath test
  a. clearance
aminorex
5-aminosalicylic
  -a. acid (5-ASA)
  -a. acid enema
amino-terminal undecapeptide
aminotransferase
  alanine a. (ALT)
  aspartate a. (AST)
amiodarone
Amipaque
amitriptyline
  a. hydrochloride
amlodipine
  a. besylate
ammonia
  arterial a.
  blood a.
  a. level
  plasma a.
  a. production
  serum a.
  a. toxicity
ammoniagenesis

ammonium
  a. hydroxide
amnesia
  antegrade a.
  procedural a.
  retrograde a.
amnion
amniopeptidase
  leucine a.
amodiaquine
amoeba
amorphous filling defect
amoxicillin
  luminal a.
  a. trihydrate
amoxicillin/omeprazole treatment
amoxicillin-tinidazole-ranitidine
  therapy
Amoxil
AMP
  adenosine monophosphate
  AMP level
  urinary cyclic AMP
amperage
amphetamine
amphibolic fistula
amphibolous fistula
amphiregulin
Amphojel
amphotericin
  a. B-induced reduction
    glomerular filtration rate
    (AmB-induced reduction GFR)
  a. B therapy
ampicillin
Amplatz
  A. catheter
  A. fascial dilator
  A. sheath
  A. Super Stiff guidewire
  A. TractMaster system
amplitude
  mean distal contraction a.
  (MDCA)
amplitude-acrophase vector
ampulla
  invagination of the a.
  rectal a.
  a. of Vater
ampullary
  a. carcinoma
  a. granulation tissue
  a. hamartoma

a. stenosis
a. stone
a. tumor
ampulloma
ampullopancreatic carcinoma
amputation
    penile a.
AMS
    AMS controlled expansion
    penile prosthesis cylinder
    (AMS 700CX penile prosthesis
    cylinder)
    AMS 700CX penile prosthesis
    cylinder
    AMS Hydroflex penile
    prosthesis
    AMS 700 inflatable penile
    prosthesis
    AMS 600 malleable penile
    prosthesis
    AMS 700-series double-cuff
    Silastic artificial urinary
    sphincter
    AMS 800-series double-cuff
    Silastic artificial urinary
    sphincter
    AMS Ultrex penile prosthesis
amsacrine (mAMSA)
Amsterdam biliary stent
Amsterdam-type biliary stent
Amussat
    A. incision
    A. operation
amyl
    a. nitrate
    a. nitrite
amylase
    ascitic a.
    a. concentration
    pancreatic a.
    P-type a.
    salivary a.
    serum a.
    Somogyi units to measure a.
    S-type a.
    a. unit
    urinary a.

amylase/creatinine clearance ratio
amylo-1,6-glucosidase deficiency
amyloglucosidase
amyloid
    a. nephropathy
    a. nephrosis
    serum a. P (SAP)
amyloid-like glomerulopathy
amyloidoma
amyloidosis
    hepatic a.
    localized a.
    rectal a.
    renal a.
    secondary a.
    systemic a.
    a. type AA
    type IV a.
amyloidotic glomerulus
amylopectinosis
amylorrhea
AN69 membrane dialyzer
ANA
    antinuclear antibody
anabolic
    a. steroid
    a. steroid treatment
anacidic stomach
anacidity
anaerobe
    obligate a.
anaerobic
    a. culture
    a. glycolysis
anal
    a. anastomosis
    a. atresia
    a. bulging
    a. canal
    a. column
    a. condyloma
    a. crypt
    a. dilation
    a. dilator
    a. discharge
    a. disk
    a. effluent

NOTES

anal *(continued)*
- a. electrical stimulation
- a. encirclement
- a. endoscopy
- a. fissure
- a. fistula
- a. foreign body
- a. gland
- a. ileostomy with preservation of sphincter
- a. intramuscular gland
- a. lesion
- a. manometry
- a. mapping
- a. pit
- a. pitting
- a. plate
- a. pouch
- a. pressure
- a. procidentia
- a. prolapse
- a. protrusion
- a. sinus
- a. sphincter
- a. sphincter contraction
- a. sphincter dysfunction
- a. sphincter function
- a. sphincter reconstruction
- a. sphincter repair
- a. sphincter squeeze pressure
- a. sphincter tone
- a. stenosis
- a. stricture
- a. transition zone
- a. ulceration
- a. valve
- a. verge
- a. wart
- a. wound

analeptic enema
analgesic
- a. nephropathy
- a. requirement

analgesic-antipyretic
analog, analogue
- arginine a.
- prostaglandin a.

analysis
- anthropometric a.
- bioelectrical impedance a. (BIA)
- Bland-Altman a.
- body composition a.
- cineradiographic a.
- contexture a.
- cosinor a.
- cost a.
- cytogenetic a.
- cytometric a.
- Diacyte DNA ploidy a.
- electrophoresis immunoblot a.
- energy dispersive x-ray a.
- enzymatic spectrophotometric a.
- fecal a.
- flow cytometric a.
- fluid a.
- gastric a.
- gene-linkage a. (GLA)
- heteroduplex a.
- histochemical-ultrastructural a.
- image a.
- Kaplan-Meier a.
- logistic regression a.
- monoclonality by genetic a.
- multivariate a.
- Northern blot a.
- pentagastrin stimulated a.
- ploidy a.
- prefreeze semen a.
- p53 tumor suppressor gene a.
- pulse-width a.
- real-time spectral a.
- regression a.
- renal morphometric a.
- sequencing a.
- single-parameter DNA a.
- single strand conformation polymorphism a.
- Southern blot a.
- spectral a.
- spectrophotometric a.
- step-wise regression a.
- trace-gas a.
- two-dimensional flow cytometric a.
- univariate a.
- a. of variance (ANOVA)
- Vindelov method flow cytometry a.
- Western blot a.
- x-ray a.

analyzer
- automatic chemical a.
- Beckman ion-selective a.
- Cell Soft 2000 semen a.
- C-Trak a.

Hamilton-Thorn motility a.
Hitachi 717 a.
Menuet Compact primary
  urodynamic a.
Olympus SP-series image a.
Orion model AE 940 ion a.
Packard Auto-Gamma 5650 a.
reflectance TS-200 spectrum a.
RJL Model 10 bioelectrical
  impedance a.
sequential multiple a. (SMA)
Siemens Somatom DRH CT a.
SYNCHRON CX-5, CX-7
  automated a.
Anandron
anaphylactic reaction
anaphylactoid
  a. food sensitivity
  a. purpura
anaphylaxis
anaplasia
anaplastic
  a. seminoma
  a. tumor
  a. Wilms tumor
Anaprox
anaritide   acetate
anasarca
Anaspaz
anastalsis
  ureteroileourethral a.
anastomose
anastomosis, pl. **anastomoses**
  anal a.
  antecolic a.
  biliodigestive a.
  Billroth I a., Billroth II a.
  bladder neck-to-urethra a.
  Brackin ureterointestinal a.
  Braun a.
  Carrel aortic patch a.
  choledococaval a. (CDCA)
  Coffey ureterointestinal a.
  coloanal a. (CAA)
  colocolonic a.
  Couvelaire ileourethral a.
  crunch stick a.

curved end-to-end a. (CEEA)
Daines-Hodgson a.
dismembered a.
dog-ear of a.
end-to-end a. (EEA)
end-to-side a.
esophagocolic a.
extravesical a.
Hofmeister a.
Hofmeister-Pólya a.
homocladic anastomoses
Horsley a.
H-shaped ileal pouch-anal a.
ileal pouch-anal a. (IPAA)
ileal pouch distal rectal a.
ileoanal a.
ileorectal a. (IRA)
ileotransverse colon a.
ileovesical a.
intestinal a.
intravesical a.
J-shaped ileal pouch-anal a.
Kocher a.
Lich-Gregoire a.
mesocaval a.
mucosa-to-mucosa a.
nondismembered a.
Parks ileoanal a.
Politano-Leadbetter a.
Pólya a.
primary a.
rectosigmoid a.
right-angled end-to-side a.
Roux-en-Y a.
Schoemaker a.
side-to-side a.
splenorenal venous a.
S-shaped ileal pouch-anal a.
State end-to-end a.
sutureless bowel a.
tension-free a.
transureteroureteral a.
two-layer a.
ureterocolonic a.
ureteroileal a.
ureterosigmoid a.
ureterotubal a.

NOTES

anastomosis *(continued)*
ureteroureteral a.
urethrocecal a.
vascular a.
vesicourethral a.
Von Haberer-Finney a.
wide elliptical a.
W-shaped ileal pouch-anal a.
anastomotic
a. leakage
a. material
a. recurrence
a. stoma
a. stricture
a. suture
a. ulcer
a. ulceration
anastomotic/stomal ulcer
anatomical radical retropubic
prostatectomy
anatomic stress incontinence
anatomy
anomalous a.
Billroth II a.
congenitally altered a.
peritoneal a.
Anatrast barium sulfate paste
anatrophic
a. nephrolithotomy
a. nephroscopy
a. nephrotomy
ANCA
antineutrophil cytoplasmic antibody
Ancef
anchor
Mitek bone a.
anchoring suture
Ancylostoma duodenale
ancylostomiasis
Andersen disease
Anderson
A. classification
A. gastric tube
Anderson-Hynes
A.-H. dismembered pyeloplasty
A.-H. pyeloplasty
androblastoma
androgen
a. ablation
a. ablation therapy (AAT)
a. ablative monotherapy
a. blockade
a. deprivation

a. deprivation therapy
a. priming
a. receptor
androgen-independent prostate
cancer
andrology
androstenedione
basal a.
androstenedione-to-testosterone ratio
anechoic
anejaculation
anemia
autoimmune hemolytic a.
B_{12} a.
a. of chronic renal failure
deficiency a.
febrile pleomorphic a.
folate a.
hemolytic a.
homozygous sickle cell a.
hypovolemic a.
iron deficiency a.
macroangiopathic hemolytic a.
megaloblastic a.
pernicious a.
posthepatitis aplastic a.
sickle cell a.
anephric
aneroid manometry
Anestacon
anesthesia
a. adjuvant
general a.
general endotracheal a.
(GETA)
local a.
pharyngeal a.
Ponka technique for local a.
preperitoneal a.
topical a.
topical oropharyngeal a.
(TOPA)
anesthetic
Cetacaine topical a.
EMLA a.
a. hepatitis
a. hepatotoxicity
lidocaine topical a.
topical a.
Xylocaine topical a.
aneuploidy
DNA a.
mucosal a.

aneurysm
  abdominal aortic a. (AAA)
  aortic a.
  arterial a.
  arteriosclerotic a.
  bilobate false a.
  Dieulafoy cirsoid a.
  dissecting abdominal a.
  hepatic artery a.
  mycotic a.
  perforating a.
  renal artery a.
  ruptured a.
  saccular a.
aneurysmal dilation
aneurysmectomy
ANF
  atrial natriuretic factor
Angelchik
  A. antireflux prosthesis
  A. ring prosthesis
Anger scintillation camera
angina
  abdominal a.
  a. abdominis
  intestinal a.
anginal attack
anginiform
anginose, anginous
angiocatheter
angiocholecystitis
angiocholitis
angiodysplasia
  bleeding colonic a.
  diffuse a.
angiodysplastic lesion
angioedema
  hereditary a. (HAE)
angiofibroma
  nasopharyngeal a.
angiogenesis
  tumor a.
Angiografin
angiogram
  celiac a.
  cystic duct a.
  splenic a.

angiographic
  a. embolization
  a. end hole catheter
  a. intervention
  a. portacaval shunt
  a. variceal embolization
angiographically
angiography
  a. catheter
  celiac a.
  diagnostic a.
  digital subtraction a.
  dynamic fluorescein a.
  fluorescence a.
  intra-arterial digital
    subtraction a.
  intraoperative ultrasonography
    and a.
  magnetic resonance a.
  mucosal a.
  renal a.
  selective mesenteric a.
  subtraction a.
  superior mesenteric a.
  therapeutic a.
angioinfarction
angioma, pl. **angiomata**
  bleeding a.
  cherry a.
  gastric a.
  petechial a.
  spider a.
  telangiectatic a.
  umbilicated a.
angiomata
  UGI a.
  upper gastrointestinal a.
angiomatoid tumor
angiomatous lymphoid hamartoma
Angiomed
  A. blue stent
  A. Puroflex stent
angiomyolipoma
  gastric a.
angioneurectomy

NOTES

25

angioneurotic
   a. edema
   a. hematuria
angioplasia
angioplasty
   a. balloon
   a. balloon catheter
   percutaneous transluminal
   renal a. (PTRA)
angiosarcoma
   hepatic a.
   radiation-induced a.
angiostrongyliasis
angiotensin
   a. converting enzyme (ACE)
   a. I, II, III
   a. II infusion test
angiotensin-converting enzyme
   inhibitor (ACEI)
Angiovist
angle
   anopouch a.
   anorectal a.
   cardiohepatic a.
   epigastric a.
   hepatorenal a.
   a. of His
   a. of incidence
   mesangial a.
   splenorenal a.
angled delivery device (ADD)
angled dissecting forceps
angularis
   a. body
   incisura a.
angular velocity
angulation
angulus
   a. on the lesser curve
   a. of stomach
anhaustral colonic gas pattern
anhemolytic strep
anhepatic stage of liver
   transplantation
anheptic
anhydrase
   carbonic a. (CA)
ani (*gen. of* anus)
   levator a.
   pruritus a.
anicteric
   a. hepatitis
   a. sclera

   a. skin
   a. viral hepatitis
anileridine
anion
   a. exchange resin
   a. gap
anionic
   a. ferritin
   a. IgG 4 fraction
aniridia
anisakiasis
   acute gastric a.
   gastric a.
anismus
anisocoria
anisokaryosis
anisotropine
   a. methylbromide
anisoylated plasminogen
   streptokinase activator complex
anitidine
ankle jerk
ankyloproctia
ankylosing spondylitis
ankylostomiasis
ankylurethria
anlage
   a. of pancreas
   splenic a.
anlagen
   prepancreatic a.
Ann
   A. Arbor cancer staging
   A. Arbor classification
annexin
annular
   a. adenocarcinoma
   a. esophageal stricture
   a. pancreas
ano
   fissure-in-a.
   fistula-in-a.
anococcygeal raphe
anocutaneous
   a. reflex
   a. stimulation
anoderm
anomalous
   a. anatomy
   a. arrangement of
   pancreaticobiliary ductal
   system (AAPBDS)
   a. genitalia

a. pancreaticobiliary
communication
a. pancreaticobiliary duct
(APBD)
a. pancreaticobiliary ductal
union (APBDU)
anomaly
Cruveilhier-Baumgarten a.
duplication a.
fixation a.
vitelline duct a.
a. of Zahn
anoplasty
cutback a.
house advancement a.
houseflap a.
Martin a.
a. treatment
Y-V a.
anopouch angle
anorchia
anorchism
anorectal
a. abscess
a. angle
a. atresia
a. band
a. carcinoma
a. disease
a. dysgenesis
a. fistula
a. foreign body
a. inhibitory reflex
a. junction
a. malformation
a. manometry
a. measurement
a. myectomy
a. physiology
a. physiology testing
a. ring
a. sensorimotor dysfunction
a. sepsis
a. space
a. sphincter
a. stenosis
a. surgery

a. test
a. varix
anorectic, anoretic
a. drug
anorectoplasty
Laird-McMahon a.
anorectum
anoretic (*var. of* anorectic)
anorexia
a. nervosa
anorexia-cachexia syndrome
anorexiant
anorexic
anorexigenic
anoscope
Bacon a.
Hirschmann a.
slotted a.
anoscopic
anoscopy
anosigmoidoscopy
anospinal center
ANOVA
analysis of variance
anoxia
chemical a.
gastric a.
ANP
atrial natriuretic peptide
ANP receptor
ANS
autonomic nervous system
Ansaid
ansa pancreatica
antacid
liquid a.
antagonist
alpha-adrenergic a.
alpha-receptor a.
beta-adrenergic a.
BQ123 receptor a.
calcium a.
calcium channel a. (CCA)
cytokine a.
EtA a.
EtB a.
histamine$_2$ receptor a. (H2RA)

NOTES

antagonist *(continued)*
  hormone a.
  H2 receptor a. (H2RA)
  5HTM3 receptor a.
  interleukin-1 receptor a.
  opiate a.
  PIVKA-II a.
  potassium-canrenoate a.
  serotonin a.
  TxA2 receptor a.
antagonistic drug
antagonist-II
antalgic gait
antecedent pancreatic injury
antecolic
  a. anastomosis
  a. long-loop isoperistaltic
    gastrojejunostomy
antecubital arteriovenous fistula
anteflexed uterus
antegrade
  a. amnesia
  a. approach
  a. continence enema procedure
    (ACE)
  a. contrast study
  a. cystography
  a. ejaculation
  a. enema
  a. pyelogram
  a. urography
antepartum constipation
anterior
  a. abdominal wall
  a. abdominal wall syndrome
  a. approach
  a. axillary line (AAL)
  a. band of colon
  a. cord syndrome
  a. duodenal ulcer
  a. exenteration
  a. fecal incontinence
  a. hemiblock
  a. innominate osteotomy
  a. nephrectomy
  a. pelvic exenteration
  a. rectopexy
  a. rectus fascia
  a. rectus sheath
  a. renal fascia
  a. resection
  a. rib impingement syndrome
  a. transabdominal approach

  a. urethra
  a. wall antral ulcer
anterior-posterior cystoresectoscope
anterolateral thoracotomy incision
antero-oblique position
anteverted uterus
antevesical hernia
anthracene-type laxative
anthraquinone
anthrax
  intestinal a.
anthrone
  a. colorimetric technique
  a. method
anthropometric
  a. analysis
  a. marker
  a. measurement
anthropometry
anthropomorphic parameter
anti-ABO antibody
anti-actin antibody
antialgesic
antiandrogen
anti-basement membrane antibody
antibiotic
  beta-lactam a., β-lactam a.
  broad-spectrum a.
  perioperative a.
  preoperative a.
  prophylactic a.
  a. prophylaxis
  a. therapy
  topical a.
antibiotic-associated
  a.-a. colitis (AAC)
  a.-a. diarrhea
antibiotic-coated stent
antibiotic-induced
  a.-i. diarrhea
  a.-i. enterocolitis
antibody
  Amerlex-M second a.
  anti-ABO a.
  anti-actin a.
  anti-basement membrane a.
  antibrush border a.
  anticardiolipin a. (ACA, ACLA)
  anticolonic a.
  anticytokeratin a.
  anti-DCP monoclonal a.
  antidelta IgM a.

antidesmin monoclonal a.
anti-double-stranded
deoxyribonucleic acid a.
(anti-dsDNA)
antiendomysial a. (EMA)
antiendothelial a.
antiepithelial membrane
antigen a.
anti-GBM a.
antigliadin a.
antiglomerular basement
membrane a.
anti-HA a.
anti-HAV IgM a.
anti-HB a.
anti-HBc IgM a.
anti-HBe a.
anti-HBs a.
anti-HCV core a.
anti-HD a.
anti-HGF a.
anti-idiotype a.
antimicrosomal a.
antimitochondrial a. (AMA)
antineutrophil cytoplasmic a.
(ANCA)
antinuclear a. (ANA)
anti-PCNA/cyclin monoclonal a.
antiphospholipid a. (APA)
antiphospholipid/anticardi-
olipin a.
anti-RAP a.
anti-RAP-GST a.
antireticulin a.
antirotavirus a.
anti-smooth muscle a.
anti-somatostatin a.
antisperm a.
anti-TBM a.
anti-Thy-1 a.
antithyroglobulin a. (ATA)
anti-TNF α a.
antivimentin a.
basal cell-specific anti-
cytokeratin a.
4B4 monoclonal a.
B72.3 murine monoclonal a.

cagA a.
CD14 monoclonal a.
CM1 polyclonal a.
a. to core peptide 9 (anti-
CP9)
a. to core peptide 10 (anti-
CP10)
a. to c100 protein
a. directed cytotoxic response
eluted a.
a. to EMA
enzyme-conjugated anti-IgA a.
fibronectin monoclonal a.
fluorescein isothiocyanate-
conjugated a.
fluorescein isothiocyanate-
labeled monoclonal a.
fluorescent antinuclear a.
(FANA)
Fx1A a.
a. to GOR (anti-GOR)
a. to GOR epitope
HBe a.
HCV a.
a. to hepatitis C virus (anti-
HCV)
a. to hepatitis D virus (anti-
HDV)
heterologous anti-GBM a.
Heyman a.
a. to HTLV-I (anti-HTLV-I)
hybridoma-derived
monoclonal a.
IgG2a a.
immunoglobulin G2a antibody
IgG α-gliadin a.
IgG reticulin a.
IgM a.
IgM anti-HAV a.
IgM anti-HBc a.
IgM-HA a.
immunoglobulin G2a a. (IgG2a
antibody)
infectious mononucleosis
heterophil a.
IOT29, clone K20
monoclonal a.

NOTES

29

antibody *(continued)*
  islet cell a.
  4KB5 monoclonal a.
  a. to keratin
  a. to Leu M1
  liver-kidney microsomal a.
  lymphocytotoxic a.
  M a.
  microsome a. (MCHA)
  milk protein a.
  mitochondrial a.
  monoclonal a. (MAB, mAb,
    MoAb)
  mycelial a.
  mycobacterial a.
  OKT3 anti-T-cell a.
  OKT3 monoclonal a.
  p53 a.
  PAb 1801 monoclonal a.
  p-ANC a.
  panel-reactive a. (PRA)
  PBC-associated a.
  PC10 monoclonal a.
  phosphotyrosine a.
  polyclonal epidermal growth
    factor a.
  protein a. (PAb)
  serum virus a.
  smooth muscle a. (SMA)
  thyroglobulin a. (TGHA)
  thyroid microsomal a.
  a. to B72.3
  a. to c100 (anti-c100)
  a. to C22-3
  UCHL-1 monoclonal a.
  xenoreactive a.
**antibody-dependent cell-mediated
  cytotoxicity (ADCC)**
anti-BrDu
anti-BrdU
antibrush border antibody
anti-c100
  antibody to c100
anticardiolipin
  a. antibody (ACA, ACLA)
  a. antibody syndrome
antiCD3
anti-CD45
anticholinergic
  a. agent
  a. drug
  a. medication
  a. medicine therapy

anticholinesterase
  parasympathomimetic a.
anti-class II mAb
anti-CMV antiserum
anticoagulant
  lupus a. (LA)
anticoagulation
  a. therapy
anticolonic antibody
anticonvulsant agent hepatotoxicity
anti-CP9
  antibody to core peptide 9
anti-CP10
  antibody to core peptide 10
anticytokeratin antibody
anti-DCP monoclonal antibody
antidelta IgM antibody
antidepressant
  a. drug hepatotoxicity
  tricyclic a.
antidesmin monoclonal antibody
antidiabetic agent hepatotoxicity
antidiarrheal
  a. agent
  opioid a.
antidiuretic
  a. arginine vasopressin V2
    receptor (AVPR2)
  a. hormone (ADH)
anti-DNA immunological study
antidopaminergic
**anti-double-stranded deoxyribonucleic
  acid antibody (anti-dsDNA)**
anti-dsDNA
  anti-double-stranded
    deoxyribonucleic acid antibody
antidysenteric
antielastase
antiemetic
  a. drug
anti-ENA immunological study
antiendomysial antibody (EMA)
antiendothelial antibody
antiendotoxin measure
**antiepithelial membrane antigen
  antibody**
antifol
  Baker a.
antifungal
  a. agent
  a. esophageal infection
**antifungal-resistant opportunistic
  infection**

anti-GBM
  a.-G. antibody
  a.-G. disease
antigen
  anti-viral capsid a. (VCA)
  Australian a.
  basement membrane a.
  C100-3 a.
  Ca50 a.
  cancer-associated sialyl-Lea a.
  carbohydrate a. 19-9 (CA 19-9)
  carcinoembryonic a. (CEA)
  cell membrane epithelial a.
  circulating tumor-associated a.
  class I a.
  class II a.
  delta a.
  endogenous renal a.
  enterobacterial common a.
    (ECA)
  ethylchlorformate
    polymerized a.
  extracted nuclear a. (ENA)
  extrarenal a.
  fetal sulfoglycoprotein a. (FSA)
  gastrointestinal cancer-
    associated a. (GICA)
  hepatitis B a. (HBAg)
  hepatitis B core a. (HBcAg)
  hepatitis Be a. (HBeAg)
  hepatitis B surface a. (HBsAg)
  hepatitis B virus-encoded a.
  hepatitis D a. (HDAg)
  hidden a.
  histocompatibility a.
  HIV P24 a.
  HLA class II a.
  HLA-DR a.
  human leukocyte a. (HLA)
  human lymphocyte a. (HLA)
  immunobead-reacting a.
  leukocyte common a.
  Lewis A blood group a.
  Lewis B a.
  Lewis X a.
  Lewis Y a.
  liver membrane a.

  liver-specific a.
  a. marker
  MHC class I a.
  MHC class II a.
  MHC class II a.
  monoclonal a.
  nuclear protein cyclin
    proliferating cell nuclear a.
  P24 a.
  486p 3/12 a.
  pancreatic oncofetal a. (POA)
  pHCV31 a.
  pHCV34 a.
  polysaccharide a.
  proliferating cell nuclear a.
    (PCNA)
  prostate-specific a. (PSA)
  sialyl Lewis A a.
  soluble liver a. (SLA)
  a. specific
  stage-specific embryonic a.
  a. stimulation
  tissue polypeptide a.
  tumor-associated a. (TAA)
  Ulex europeus I a.
antigen-antibody system
antigen-dependent pathway
antigenic
  a. determinant
  a. phenotype
antigen-independent
  a.-i. adhesion
  a.-i. pathway
antigen-positive
antigen-presenting cell
antigen-specific
  nucleocapsid a.-s.
antigliadin
  a. antibody
antiglomerular
  a. basement membrane
  a. basement membrane
    antibody
  a. basement membrane disease
  a. basement membrane
    glomerulonephritis
  a. basement membrane-negative

NOTES

antiglomerular *(continued)*
    crescentric glomerular
    nephritis
    a. basement membrane
    nephritis
anti-GOR
    antibody to GOR
anti-gp330 immunoglobulin G
anti-HA antibody
anti-HAV
    IgM a.-H.
    a.-H. IgM antibody
anti-HAV-positive
    IgG a.-H.-p.
anti-HB antibody
anti-Hbc
    anti-HBc IgM antibody
    monoclonal a.-H.
anti-HBe antibody
anti-HBs antibody
anti-HCV
    antibody to hepatitis C virus
    anti-HCV core antibody
anti-HD antibody
anti-HDV
    antibody to hepatitis D virus
anti-*Helicobacter pylori* IgM
anti-*Helicobacter pylori* treatment
anti-hepatitis A-IgM immunological
    study
anti-HGF antibody
antihistamine
anti-HSV IgM Ab titer
anti-HTLV-I
    antibody to HTLV-I
antihydropic
antihypertensive agent
anti-icteric
anti-idiotype antibody
anti-incontinence procedure
anti-inhibin
antilipemic drug
anti-liver microsomal antibody
    detection
antilymphocyte
    a. globulin
    a. heteroconjugate
    a. therapy
anti-M2 antimitochondrial antibody
    level
antimajor histocompatibility complex
antimegalin antiserum

antimesenteric
    a. border
    a. border of distal ileum
    a. enterotomy
    a. fat pad
antimesocolic side of the cecum
antimicrobial
    a. agent
    macrolide a.
    a. prophylaxis
    a. therapy
antimicrosomal antibody
Antiminth
antimitochondrial antibody (AMA)
antimony pH electrode
antimotility
    a. agent
    a. drug
anti-müllerian derivative syndrome
antimuscarinic agent
antimycobacterial drug
antinatriuresis
antinauseant
antineoplastic drug hepatotoxicity
antinephrocalcin antiserum
antineutrophil
    a. cytoplasmic antibody
    (ANCA)
    a. cytoplasmic antibody titer
antinociceptive effect
antinuclear
    a. antibody (ANA)
    a. antibody immunological
    study
antioxidant
    endogenous lipophilic a.
anti-PCNA/cyclin monoclonal
    antibody
antiperistalsis
antiperistaltic
antiphospholipid
    a. antibody (APA)
    a. syndrome
antiphospholipid/anticardiolipin
    antibody
antiplasmin
    α-21 a.
antiporter
    Na+/H+ a.
antipsychotic drug hepatotoxicity
antipyrine clearance
anti-RAP antibody
anti-RAP-GST antibody

antireflux
- a. double-J stent
- a. flap-valve mechanism
- a. operation
- a. procedure
- a. prosthesis
- a. regimen
- a. surgery
- a. therapy
- a. ureteral implantation technique

antirefluxing colonic conduit
antireticulin antibody
antirotavirus antibody
antiruminant
anti-Schiff stain
antisecretory
- a. agent
- a. drug
- a. opioid
- a. therapy

antisense
- a. DNA inhibition
- a. RNA probe
- ^{35}S a. fibronectin riboprobe

antiseptic dressing
antiserum, pl. **antisera**
- anti-CMV a.
- antimegalin a.
- antinephrocalcin a.
- galanin a.
- nephrotoxic a.
- VIP a.

anti-SLA test
anti-smooth muscle antibody
anti-somatostatin antibody
antispasmodic
- a. agent
- a. drug

antisperm antibody
anti-SSA immunological study
anti-SSB immunological study
antistreptolysin O
antistreptolysin-O titer
anti-Tamm-Horsfall protein
anti-TBM antibody

antithrombin
- a. III
- a. III deficiency

anti-Thy-1
- a.-T.-1 antibody
- a.-T.-1 nephritis

antithymocyte
- a. gamma-globulin (ATGAM)
- a. globulin (ATG)

antithyroglobulin antibody (ATA)
antithyroid
- a. autoantibody
- a. drug hepatotoxicity

anti-TNF α **antibody**
α_1**-antitrypsin**
- α_1-a. deficiency
- α_1-a. deficiency disease
- α_1-a. disease (AATD)
- α_1-a. disease-related emphysema
- α_1-a. globulin
- α_1-a. level

antitubular basement membrane
antiulcer
Antivert
antivimentin antibody
anti-viral capsid antigen (VCA)
antral
- a. atrophic gastritis (AAG)
- a. biopsy
- a. D-cell
- a. EC-cell
- a. edema
- a. gastric cell
- a. gastrin
- a. gastrin cell hyperfunction
- a. gastritis
- a. G-cell hyperplasia
- a. membrane
- a. mucosa
- a. peptide
- a. polyp
- a. pressure transducer
- a. somatostatin
- a. stasis
- a. stenosis
- a. stricture

NOTES

antral *(continued)*
  a. ulcer
  a. vascular ectasia
antral-predominant gastritis
AntraR
antrectomy
  Roux-en-Y biliary bypass
    with a.
Antrenyl
Antrocol
antroduodenal ulcer
antroduodenectomy
antrofundal mucosa
antromotility
antro-pyloro-duodenal region
antrostomy
antrotomy
antrum
  cardiac a.
  gastric a.
  a. gastritis
  prepyloric a.
  retained a.
  a. of stomach
  a. of Willis
anucleate fragment
anuresis
anuretic
anuria
anuric
anus
  imperforate a.
Anusol-HC
Anusol-HC-1
anvil portion of EEA stapler
anxiety-related diarrhea
anxiolytic
  a. sedative
Anzemet
aorta
  supraceliac a.
aortic
  a. aneurysm
  a. dissection
  a. graft
  a. patch
  a. punch
  a. stenosis
  a. valvular stenosis
aortica
  dysphagia a.

aortic/superior mesenteric artery bypass
aortoduodenal fistula (ADF)
aortoenteric
  a. fistula
  a. graft
aortoesophageal fistula
aortogastric fistula
aortograft duodenal fistula
aortography
  abdominal a.
  biplanar a.
aortohepatic arterial graft
aortoiliac
aortorenal
  a. bypass
  a. reimplantation
aortosigmoid fistula
aortotomy
AOSC
  acute obstructive suppurative cholangitis
AP
  adenomatous polyp
  alkaline phosphatase
  AP marker enzyme
AP1
  transcription factor AP1
APA
  antiphospholipid antibody
APACHE-II
  A.-II point
  A.-II score
apancreatic
apatite
  a. calculus
  carbonate a.
APBD
  anomalous pancreaticobiliary duct
APBDU
  anomalous pancreaticobiliary ductal union
APC
  adenomatous polyposis coli
APCD
  adult polycystic disease
apellous
apenteric
apepsinia
aperistalsis
aperistaltic esophagus
Apert syndrome
aperture

apex
   a. of duodenal bulb
   a. of external ring
aphasia
apheresis
Aphrodyne
aphtha, pl. **aphthae**
aphthoid
   a. proctocolitis
   a. ulcer
aphthous
   a. gastropathy
   a. stomatitis
   a. ulcer
aphthous-type lesion
apical
   a. duodenal ulcer
   a. polar nephrectomy
   a. sound
   a. thickening
APKD
   adult polycystic kidney disease
aplasia
   bone marrow a.
   pure red cell a. (PRCA)
aplastic bone disease
APLD
   adult polycystic liver disease
apnea
apo
   apolipoprotein
   a. A-I
   a. A-IV
   a. B
apolipoprotein (apo)
   a. B-containing lipoprotein
   a. CII-CIII ratio
apomorphine
aponeurosis
   external oblique a.
   a. of external oblique
   a. of internal oblique
apoplexy
   abdominal a.
   mesenteric a.
apoptosis
apparatus, pl. **apparatus**

   alimentary a.
   digestive a.
   GIA autosuture a.
   Golgi a.
   juxtaglomerular a.
   Manifold II slot-blot a.
   Von Petz suturing a.
   Wangensteen suction a.
appearance
   cobblestone-like a.
   ground-glass a.
   picket fence a.
   stack of coins a.
   tadpole-like a.
Appedrine
appendage
   epiploic a.
   torsion of a.
appendalgia
appendectomy (appy)
   colonoscopic a.
   emergency a.
   emergent a.
   incidental a.
   interval a.
   inversion a.
   a. tape
appendiceal
   a. abscess
   a. adenocarcinoma
   a. intussusception
   a. Kaposi sarcoma
   a. mass
   a. opening
   a. orifice
   a. perforation
   a. stump
appendicitis
   acute a.
   amebic a.
   chronic a.
   fulminating a.
   gangrenous a.
   helminthic a.
   lumbar a.
   nonperforated a.
   a. obliterans

NOTES

appendicitis *(continued)*
  obstructive a.
  pelvic a.
  perforated a.
  recurrent a.
  retrocecal a.
  retroileal a.
  segmental a.
  stercoral a.
  subperitoneal a.
  suppurative a.
  traumatic a.
appendicocele
appendicocystostomy
  continent cutaneous a.
  dismembered reimplanted a.
  nonplicated a.
  orthotopic a.
  plicated a.
  reversed reimplanted a.
appendicoenterostomy
appendicolithiasis
appendicolysis
appendicopathy
appendicostomy
appendicovesicostomy
  Mitrofanoff a.
appendicular colic
appendix
  base of a.
  cecal a.
  a. epididymis
  epiploic a.
  a. fibrosa
  gangrenous a.
  hot a.
  indurated a.
  inflamed a.
  Morgagni a.
  nonperforated a.
  normal a.
  paracecal a.
  perforated a.
  preileal a.
  retrocecal a.
  retroileal a.
  ruptured a.
  subcecal a.
  suppurative a.
  a. testis
  vermiform a.
  xiphoid a.
appendolithiasis

appetostat
apple-core lesion
apple-peel bowel syndrome
appliance
  external a.
  external cooling a.
  Karaya ring ileostomy a.
  ostomy a.
application
  laparoscopic clip a.
applicator
  Mick TP-200 a.
  multifire clip a.
  multiload occlusive clip a.
  resorbable thread clip a.
Applied Biosystems 340A nucleic acid extractor
applier
  AcuClip endoscopic multiple clip a.
  Advanced surgical suture a.
  multiloaded clip a.
  Stone clamp a.
Appolito suture
approach
  Alken a.
  antegrade a.
  anterior a.
  anterior transabdominal a.
  case-by-case a.
  choledochofiberscopic a.
  consortial a.
  fascial sling a.
  flank a.
  gasless laparoscopic a.
  Kraske parasacral a.
  percutaneous transhepatic a.
  peroral a.
  posterior a.
  posterior lumbar a.
  preperitoneal a.
  Redman a.
  retroperitoneal a.
  supraduodenal a.
  thoracoabdominal extrapleural a.
  thoracoabdominal intrapleural a.
  transduodenal a.
  transmural a.
  transpapillary a.
  vaginal wall a.
approximation
  a. suture

tissue a.
wound a.
approximator clamp
appy
appendectomy
APR
abdominoperineal resection
apraxia
constructional a.
Apresoline
aproctia
apron
abdominal a.
fatty omental a.
a. skin incision
aprotinin
APS
arterioportal vein shunting
Apt-Downey alkali denaturation test
APUD
amine precursor uptake and
decarboxylation
APUD cell
APUDoma
Aquachloral
AquaMEPHYTON
Aquatag
aquatosis coli
Aquazide-H
aqueous phenol
AR
aldose reductase
AR mRNA
arachidonic
a. acid
a. acid metabolite
a. acid oxidation
arachis oil
arachnoid fibrosis
Aralen
Aramine
Arandel cell harvester
arbacet
arbaprostil
arbitrary unit (AU)
arborization of ducts

ARC
AIDS-related complex
arcade
gastroepiploic a.
arch
pubic a.
archaea
methanogenic a.
architecture
hepatic a.
intestinal villous a.
lobular a.
arcuate
a. artery
a. vein
arcus tendineus fasciae pelvis
area, pl. **areae**
cell surface a.
choledochoduodenal a.
a. gastrica
gastrohepatic bare a.
high-echoic a.
midepigastric a.
midrectal a.
Paget disease of perianal a.
perianal a.
pericolostomy a.
peripancreatic a.
periportal a.
peristomal a.
postcricoid a.
punctate a.
skip a.
subhepatic a.
watershed a.
areflexia
detrusor a.
areflexic bladder
ARF
acute renal failure
mercuric chloride-induced ARF
argentaffin
a. cell
a. reaction test
a. stain
argentaffinity
cytoplasmic a.

NOTES

37

arginase deficiency
arginine
   a. analog
   a. vasopressin (AVP)
arginosuccinate
argon
   a. beam coagulation
   a. beam coagulator
   a. ion laser
   a. laser therapy
argon-pumped dye laser
Argyle
   A. chest tube
   A. Medicut R catheter
Argyle-Salem sump tube
argyrophilia
   cytoplasmic a.
argyrophilic
   a. and argyophobic neuron
   a. cell
Arias syndrome
Aristocort
ARKD
   autosomal recessive kidney disease
arm
   cell-mediated a.
   humoral a.
Armanni-Ehrlich degeneration
Armed Forces Institute of
   Pathology (AFIP)
Army-Navy retractor
Arndorfer
   A. capillary perfusion system
   A. pneumohydraulic capillary
     infusion system
aromatic
   a. amine
   a. amino acid (AAA)
Aronson esophageal retractor
ARP
   acute recurrent pancreatitis
arrest
   spermatogenic a.
arrhythmogenicity
Arrow
   A. Raulerson syringe
   A. UserGard injection cap
     system
ARROWgard Blue hemodialysis
   catheter
Artane
arterial
   a. ammonia

   a. aneurysm
   a. blood gas (ABG)
   a. blood sample
   a. circulation
   a. embolization
   a. line
   a. oxygen desaturation
   a. portography
   a. priapism
   a. saturation
   a. spider
   a. steal
   a. thrombosis
   a. underfilling
arterial-enteric fistula
arterialization
arteria lusoria
arteriogenic impotence
arteriogram
   hepatic a.
   superior mesenteric a.
arteriography
   hepatic a.
   mesenteric a.
   renal a.
   selective left gastric a.
   superselective a.
   visceral a.
arteriohepatic dysplasia
arteriolar
   a. hyalinosis
   a. nephrosclerosis
arteriole
   afferent a.
   efferent a.
   juxtamedullary a.
   preglomerular a.
arteriolopathy
   cyclosporine a.
arterioportal
   a. fistula
   a. vein shunting (APS)
arterioportographical examination
arteriosclerosis
arteriosclerotic aneurysm
arteriotomy
   end-to-side a.
arteriovenous (AV)
   a. catheter
   a. fistula
   a. hemofiltration
   a. malformation (AVM)
   a. shunt

arteritis
Takayasu a.
artery
abnormality of hepatic a.
arcuate a.
bulbar a.
colic a.
cystic a.
deep a.
gastroduodenal a. (GDA)
gastroepiploic a. (GEA)
hepatic a.
hypogastric a.
iliac a.
inferior mesenteric a. (IMA)
interlobar a.
internal iliac a.
internal pudendal a.
mesenteric a.
middle colic a. (MCA)
proximal superior mesenteric a.
retrograde vascularization of
  superior mesenteric a.
splenic a.
superior mesenteric a.
umbilical a.
a. weld strength
arthralgia
arthritis
reactive a.
rheumatoid a.
temporomandibular a.
arthropathy
psoriatic a.
arthroplasty
arthrosia
exanthesis a.
artifact
mirror-image a.
artificial
a. anus
a. bezoar
a. erection
a. erection test
a. gut
a. hepatic support
a. insemination donor (AID)

a. insemination husband (AIH)
a. kidney
a. organ
a. sphincter
a. urinary sphincter
aryepiglottic
a. fold
arylamine
arytenoid cartilage
AS
AS 800 balloon
AS 800 cuff
AS 800 male bulbous urethra
AS 800 pump
4-ASA
5-ASA
5-aminosalicylic acid
5-ASA agent
5-ASA enema
Asacol
A. delayed-release tablet
ASA-induced gastric ulceration
ASAP
ASAP channel cut automated
  biopsy needle
ASAP prostate biopsy needle
ASAP Stacker automated
  multi-sample biopsy system
asbestos
ASC
acute suppurative cholangitis
ascariasis
biliary a.
endobiliary a.
intrahepatic a.
pancreatic a.
Ascaris **infestation**
Ascaris lumbricoides
ascending
a. cholangitis
a. colon
a. limb
a. pyelonephritis
ascites
a. adiposus
bile a.
biliary a.

NOTES

ascites *(continued)*
blood-tinged a.
bloody a.
chyliform a.
chylous a., a. chylosus
cirrhotic a.
cloudy a.
culture-negative neutrocytic a.
(CNNA)
demeclocycline-induced a.
dialysis-related a.
a. drainage tube
eosinophilic a.
exudative a.
fatty a.
gelatinous a.
hemodialysis-associated a.
hemorrhagic a.
hydremic a.
idiopathic a.
malignant a.
McNemar test for a.
milky a.
myxedema a.
narrow albumin gradient a.
nephrogenic a.
neutrocytic a.
nonchylous a.
pancreatic a.
pseudochylous a.
refractory a.
resistant a.
straw-colored a.
tense a.
transudative a.
urinary a.
wide albumin gradient a.
ascitic
a. amylase
a. fluid
a. fluid total protein (AFTP)
ascitogenous
ascorbic acid
Ascriptin A/D
asecretory
Aselli pancreas
aseptic wound
Asepti-steryl disinfectant
Asepto irrigation syringe
ASGE
American Society for
Gastrointestinal Endoscopy
Asherson syndrome

ASHN
acute sclerosing hyaline necrosis
Ashton
A. briefs
A. pants
asialoglycoprotein
a. receptor
Asiatic
A. cholera
A. schistosomiasis
ASID Bonz PP infusion pump
ASI prostatic stent
asitia
Ask-Upmark
A.-U. kidney
A.-U. renal segment
ASLC
acute self-limited colitis
asparaginase
aspartate
a. aminotransferase (AST)
a. transferase
aspect
paraspinous a.
spinous a.
aspergillosis esophagitis
Aspergillus
A. flavus
A. fumigatus
A. infection
aspermatism
aspermatogenic
a. sterility
aspermia
aspirate
gastric a.
heme-positive NG a.
nasogastric a.
NG a.
aspirated sample
aspirating needle
aspiration
a. biopsy
a. biopsy cytology
a. catheter
corporeal a.
CT-guided fine-needle a.
a. and dissection tube
endoscopic transesophageal
fine-needle a.
epididymal sperm a. (ESA)
fine-needle a. (FNA)
gastric a.

A

microscopic epididymal
sperm a.
microsurgical epididymal
sperm a. (MESA)
percutaneous balloon a.
percutaneous CT-guided a.
percutaneous epididymal
sperm a.
percutaneous needle a.
peritoneal a.
a. pneumonia
pulmonary a.
real-time endoscopic ultrasound-
guided fine-needle a.
real-time fine-needle a.
(RTFNA)
seminal vesicle a.
silent a.
sonography-guided a.
sperm a.
a. syringe
Aspirator
Cavitron Ultrasonic Surgical A.
(CUSA)
aspirin
enteric-coated a.
aspirin-induced gastritis
Aspisafe nasogastric tube
asplenia syndrome
Assam fever
assay
Abbott IMx PSA a.
AUSAB EIA a.
Bio-Rad protein a.
BioWhittaker a.
Ciba-Corning ACS PSA a.
Clostridium difficile toxin a.
competitive protein binding a.
electroimmunodiffusion a.
enhanced reverse transcriptase
polymerase chain reaction a.
enzyme-linked
immunosorbent a. (EIA)
Galacto-light a.
HemoQuant a.
Hybritech Tandem prostate
specific antigen a.

Hybritech Tandem-R PSA a.
immunoradiometric a.
IMX Hg a.
indirect immunofluorescence a.
inhibition a.
intact hormone a.
liquid chromatographic a.
Pros-Check PSA a.
PTH-rP by
immunoradiometric a.
qualitative microculture a.
radioenzymatic a
radioimmunoinhibition a.
radioimmunoprecipitation a.
recombinant immunoblot a.
(RIBA)
second-generation recombinant
immunoblot a.
solution hybridization RNAse
protection a.
Tandem-E-PSA
immunoenzymetric a.
Tandem-ERA PSA
immuenzymetric a.
tandem PSA a.
Tandem-R PSA a.
tissue culture a.
TNF-α a.
tumor necrosis factor-α assay
toxin a.
transcriptase polymerase chain
reaction a.
tumor necrosis factor-α a.
(TNF-α assay)
Yang polyclonal a.
Yang Pros-Check PSA a.
assembly
dilating catheter-gastrostomy
tube a.
Konigsberg 5-channel solid-state
catheter a.
8-lumen catheter a.
assessment
blood flow a.
endoscopic a.
endoscopic color Doppler a.
extrapyramidal function a.

NOTES

assessment *(continued)*
> outcome and process a.
> penile vascular function a.

ASSI laparoscopic electrode assistant
> gastrointestinal a. (GIA)

assisted reproduction
association
> American Anorexia/Bulimia A.
> American Diabetes A. (ADA)
> American Urological A. (AUA)
> megacystis-megaureter a.
> United Ostomy A. (UOA)

AST
> aspartate aminotransferase
> AST test

AST-ALT ratio
astemizole
asterixis
asteroid body
asthenospermia
asthenoteratospermia
asthma
Astler-Coller classification (A, B1, B2, C1, C2)
ASTRA
> A. profile
> A. profile test

Astra/Merck Group
astrovirus gastroenteritis
Astwood-Coller staging system for carcinoma
asymmetrical
asymmetric pupils
asymmetry
asymptomatic
> a. bacteriuria
> a. gallstone
> a. mass
> a. urolithiasis

asystole
> lavage-induced cardiac a.

ATA
> antithyroglobulin antibody

Atabrine
ataxia
> late-onset a.

ataxic gait
atelectasis
atelectatic
atenolol
ATG
> antithymocyte globulin

ATGAM
> antithymocyte gamma-globulin

atheroemboli
atheroembolic renal disease (AERD)
atherogenesis
atheromatous
atherosclerosis
atherosclerotic
> a. plaque
> a. renal artery stenosis
> a. renovascular disease
> a. stenosis

Ativan
Atkinson
> A. introducer
> A. prosthesis
> A. scoring system for dysphagia
> A. silicone rubber tube

Atlantic ileostomy catheter
atomic absorbance spectrophotometer
atonic
> a. bladder
> a. constipation
> a. dyspepsia
> a. esophagus

atony
> gastric a.
> intestinal a.
> sphincter a.
> ureteral a.

atorvastatin
ATP
> adenosine triphosphate

ATPase
> adenosine triphosphatase
> ATPase activity

atraumatic
> a. clamp
> a. grasper
> a. locking/grasping forceps
> a. suture

atresia
> anal a.
> anorectal a.
> biliary a.
> congenital biliary a.
> congenital duodenal a.
> duodenal a.
> esophageal a.
> extrahepatic biliary a. (EBA)
> follicular a.

gastric a.
intestinal a.
intrahepatic a. (IHA)
jejunoileal a.
prepyloric a.
suprapubic cystotomy tract
  urethral a.
urethral a.
vaginal a.
atrial
  a. liver pulse
  a. natriuretic factor (ANF)
  a. natriuretic peptide (ANP)
atrium
Atrocholin
atrophia
atrophic
  a. gastritis
  a. vagina
atrophicus
  lichen sclerosus et a.
atrophied
atrophy
  fundic gland a.
  gastric a.
  lobar a.
  mucosal a.
  multiple system a.
  muscle a.
  sclerotic a.
  skin a.
  splenic a.
  tubular a.
  villous a.
  white a.
  yellow a. of the liver
atropine
  a. methylnitrate
  a. sulfate
Atrovent
ATS
  autotransfusion
  ATS canister
attachment
  mesenteric a.
  peritoneal a.

attack
  anginal a.
attenuated
attenuation
attic adhesion
atubular glomeruli
atypia
  cellular a.
  hepatocellular a.
atypical
  a. adenomatous hyperplasia
    (AAH)
  a. ductular cell
  a. gallbladder disease
AU
  arbitrary unit
AUA
  American Urological Association
  AUA symptom index
Auerbach
  A. and Meissner plexus
  A. mesenteric plexus
augmentation
  a. cystoplasty
  gastroileac a.
  ileocecocystoplasty bladder a.
  Mainz pouch a.
  a. plaque
  ureteral a.
  ureteral bladder a.
augmented bladder
Augmentin
aureus
  methicillin-resistant
    Staphylococcus a. (MRSA)
    Staphylococcus a.
Auriculin
AUSAB EIA assay
auscultation of bowel sounds
auscultatory sound
Ausonics OPUS-1
Australian antigen
autacoid
autemesia
autoanalyzer
  Beckman 2 a.
  Hitachi 737 a.

NOTES

autoantibody
  antithyroid a.
  circulating a.
  a. production
autoaugmentation
  bladder a.
autoclave
  heat-sterilized by a.
  steam a.
  a. sterilized
autoclaved India ink
autoclaving
autocoid
autocrine
  a. motility factor (AMF)
  a. regulation
autocystoplasty
autoerotic rectal trauma
autogenous
  a. tunica vaginalis graft
autografting
autoimmune
  a. cirrhosis
  a. connective tissue disorder
  a. deficiency syndrome
  a. disease
  a. hemolytic anemia
  a. hepatitis
  a. interstitial nephritis
  a. thyroid disease
  a. thyroiditis
autoimmunity
  thyroid a.
autointoxicant
autointoxication
autologous
  a. HBcAg-specific CD4+
  a. liver cell
  a. transfusion
autolymphocyte therapy
automated endoscopic system for optimal positioning (AESOP)
automatic
  a. chemical analyzer
  a. needle driver
auto-nephrectomy
  silent a.-n.
autonomic
  a. dysfunction
  a. dysreflexia
  a. nervous system (ANS)
  a. neurogenic bladder
  a. neuropathy

autopepsia
autophosphorylation
autopoisonous
autoradiogram
autoradiography
autoreactivity
  liver-directed a.
autoregressive
autoregulation
  renal a.
autosomal
  a. dominant disorder
  a. dominant polycystic kidney disease (ADPKD)
  a. recessive kidney disease (ARKD)
autosomally
  a. inherited forms of nephrolithiasis
  a. recessively inherited disease
autostapling device
autosuture
  A. stapler
  a. technique
autotoxic
autotoxicosis
autotoxin
autotransfusion (ATS)
autotransplantation
  colostomy pyloric a.
  posttraumatic a.
  pyloric a.
  renal a.
  a. of splenic fragment
autourethrography
AV
  arteriovenous
  AV fistula
  AV shunt
avascular
  a. necrosis
Aventyl
average flow rate
AVF
AVF-induced renal ischemia
AVH
  acute viral hepatitis
avian myeloblastosis virus reverse transcriptase
avidin-biotin complex
avidin-biotin-peroxidase
  a.-b.-p. complex
  a.-b.-p. complex method

Avihepadnavirus
avium
   Mycobacterium *a.* (MAI)
avium-intracellulare
   Mycobacterium *a.-i.*
AVM
   arteriovenous malformation
avoidance maneuver
AVP
   arginine vasopressin
AVPR2
   antidiuretic arginine vasopressin V2
   receptor
avulsion
   splenic a.
axial
   a. hiatal hernia
   a. image
Axid
axillary adenopathy
Axiom double sump tube
axis
   bowel a.
   brain-gut a.
   cardiopyloric a.
   celiac a.
   a. deviation
   enteroinsular a.
   hypothalamic-pituitary a. (HPA)
   hypothalamic-pituitary-testicular-
     penile a.
   macrophage-TGF-β a.
   neurohumoral-immune a.
   pituitary-gonadal a.
   renin-angiotensin-aldosterone a.
axon
   a. reflex
axonopathy
Axxcess ureteral catheter
Aylett operation
Ayre brush

aywl (or 2-4)
Aza
   azathioprine
Aza-antilymphocyte globulin
azamethonium
azan stain
azapetine
Aza-Pred therapy
azasteroid inhibitor
azathioprine (Aza)
AzBF
   azygos blood flow
azide
   sodium a.
azidothymidine (AZT)
azithromycin
azlocillin
Azo
   A. Gantanol
   A. Gantrisin
azole
   a. antifungal agent
azoospermia
   excretory a.
   occlusive a.
   steroid-induced a.
   unreconstructable obstructive a.
Azo-Standard
azotemia
   prerenal a.
AZQ
   diaziquone
AZT
   azidothymidine
Aztec two-step
Azulfidine
Azulfidine-EN
azygos
   a. blood flow (AzBF)
   coronary a.
   a. vein

NOTES

45

β

β adrenergic blocker
Bates-corrected β
transforming growth factor β (TGF-β)

B

B bile
B cell
B cell line
B lymphocyte
B protein
B ring
B ring of esophagus

B1 integrins

B-1

Dukes B-1

B2

bromobenzene
B2 integrins

B5 tumor marker

B$_{12}$

B$_{12}$ anemia
^{57}Co B$_{12}$ excretion
B$_{12}$ immunological study
vitamin B$_{12}$

B72.3

antibody to B.
B. murine monoclonal antibody

b558 membrane-bound cytochrome

BA

bile acid

Babcock

B. clamp
B. forceps
B. intestinal forceps

Babinski

B. reflex
B. sign

baby

b. Balfour retractor
b. scope

BAC

benzalkonium chloride

bacillary

b. dysentery
b. peliosis

bacille Calmette-Guérin (BCG, bCG)

bacilli

curved b.

bacillus

Calmette-Gúerin b.
coliform b.
Friedländer b.

Bacillus cereus

bacitracin

backflow

pyelolymphatic b.
pyelovenous b.

background

mucosal b.

Backhaus towel forceps

backwash ileitis

baclofen

Bacon anoscope

bacterascites

monomicrobial b.
polymicrobial b.

bacteremia

bacteria (*pl. of* bacterium)

bacterial

b. adherence
b. adhesion
b. biofilm
b. cast
b. cholangitis
b. cleavage
b. colitis
b. complication
b. cystitis
b. endotoxin
b. enterocolitis
b. esophagitis
b. factor
b. flora
b. food poisoning
b. infection
b. metabolism in intestines
b. mucosal infiltration
b. overgrowth
b. overgrowth syndrome
b. peritonitis
b. vaginosis
b. vector

bactericidal

b. function of phagocytes
b. stomach environment

bactericide

bacteriocholia

bacteriology

B

bacteriospermia
bacteriostatically
bacteriostatic barrier
bacterium, pl. **bacteria**
  Chauveau b.
  coliform b.
  colonic b.
  Gram-negative b.
  Gram-positive b.
  human gut b.
  intestinal b.
  mesophilic b.
  pathogenic b.
  pyogenic b.
  spiral b.
  toxigenic b.
bacteriuria
  asymptomatic b.
  catheter-associated b.
Bacteroides
  B. distasonis
  B. eggerthii
  B. fragilis
  B. ovatus
  B. praeacutus
  B. putredinis
  B. splanchnicus
  B. thetaiotaomicron
  B. uniformis
  B. ureolyticus
  B. vulgatus
bactibilia
Bactrim
  B. DS
baculovirus
BAD
  benign anorectal disease
BA-EDTA solution
Baermann
  B. stool filter
  B. stool test
bag
  bile b.
  Biohazard b.
  bowel b.
  colostomy b.
  DeRoyal Surgical grab b.
  EndoMate grab b.
  Hollister urostomy b.
  ileostomy b.
  intestinal b.
  Lahey liver transplant b.
  Le B.

  ostomy b.
  perfusate b.
  Perry b.
  Petersen b.
  Plummer b.
  pneumatic b.
  stomal b.
  Vacutainer b.
  Whitmore b.
BAGF
  brachioaxillary bridge graft fistula
Bagley helical basket
Bainbridge intestinal clamp
Bakamjian flap
Baker
  B. antifol
  B. intestinal decompression
  tube
  B. jejunostomy tube
Bakes common duct dilator
BAL
  blood alcohol level
balance
  acid-base b.
  chloride b.
  electrolyte b.
  equal fluid b.
  B. lavage solution
  metabolic b.
  negative nitrogen b.
  nitrogen b.
  positive nitrogen b.
  potassium b.
  sodium b.
  vagosympathetic b.
balanced
  b. diet
  b. electrolyte solution
balanic
  b. hypospadias
balanitic epispadias
balanitis
  b. circinata
  circinate b.
  b. circumscripta plasmacellularis
  b. diabetica
  plasma cell b.
  trichomonal b.
  b. xerotica obliterans (BXO)
  yeast b.
  b. of Zoon
balanoblennorrhea
balanocele

B

balanoplasty
balanoposthitis
balanopreputial
balanorrhagia
balanorrhea
balantidial dysentery
balantidiasis
Balantidium coli colitis
balantidosis
Balch 1 broth medium
bald gastric fundus
Balfour
    B. abdominal retractor
    B. gastroenterostomy
    B. retractor
    B. self-retaining retractor
Balkan
    B. nephrectomy
    B. nephropathy
ball
    b. electrode
    fungal b.
    hair b.
    b. myoma
    ureteropelvic fungus b.
    wool b.
Ballance sign
Ballenger forceps
Ballobes gastric balloon
balloon
    Acucise b.
    angioplasty b.
    AS 800 b.
    Ballobes gastric b.
    banana-shaped b.
    barostat b.
    BILISYSTEM stone removal b.
    centering b.
    b. cholangiogram
    cylindrical b.
    b. cystoscope
    b. cytology
    b. decompression
    b. defecation
    b. dilating catheter
    b. dilation
    b. dilation of the papilla

b. dilator
dissecting b.
doughnut-shaped b.
esophageal b.
esophageal single b.
b. expulsion test
extraction b.
Extractor XL triple lumen
    retrieval b.
Fogarty b.
French Swan-Ganz b.
Garren b.
Garren-Edwards b.
gastric b.
Gau gastric b.
Grüntzig b.
Helmstein b.
high-compliance latex b.
hydrostatic b.
intragastric b.
b. kymography
low-compliance b.
MaxForce TTS b.
mercury-containing b.
Microvasive retrieval b.
Microvasive Rigiflex through-
    the-scope b.
occlusion b.
b. occlusion cholangiography
Percival gastric b.
b. photodynamic therapy
b. proctogram
Provocative sensitivity b.
rectal b.
b. reflex manometry
retrieval b.
Riepe-Bard gastric b.
Rigiflex achalasia b.
Rigiflex TTS b.
scintigraphic b.
Sengstaken-Blakemore
    esophageal b.
stone retrieval b.
b. tamponade
b. tamponade prosthesis
Taylor gastric b.
b. therapy

NOTES

balloon *(continued)*
> through-the-scope b.
> b. topogram
> b. tube tamponade
> b. ureteral occlusion
> water displacing b.
> Wilson-Cook dilating b.
> Wilson-Cook esophageal b.
> Wilson-Cook gastric b.
> windowed esophageal b.
> wire-guided hydrostatic b.

balloon-catheter and basket-retrieval technique

ballooning
> b. degeneration of hepatocyte
> eosinophilic b.
> b. esophagoscope
> hepatocellular b.

balloon-occluded retrograde transvenous obliteration (B-RTO)
ballotable liver
ballottement
> b. tenderness

Balneol
Balser fatty necrosis
Balthazar grading system
BAM
> bile acid malabsorption

Bamethan
banana
> b. peel effect
> b. plug dipolar generator

banana-shaped balloon
bananas, rice, cereal, applesauce, tea, & toast (BRATT)
bananas, rice, cereal, applesauce, & toast (BRAT)
band
> adhesive b.
> anorectal b.
> anterior b. of colon
> dysgenetic fibrous b.
> b. form
> free b. of colon
> Harris b.
> Henle b.
> Ladd b.
> Lane b.
> b. ligation
> Lyon ring-constrictive b.
> Marlex b.
> mesocolic b.

> omental b.
> omphalodiverticular b.
> pecten b.
> peritoneal b.
> b. placement
> b. 3 protein
> silicone elastomer b.
> snap gauge b.
> WBC b.'s

bandage
> Sureseal pressure b.
> suspensory b.
> T-b.

banding
> b. cylinder
> esophageal b.
> hemorrhoid b.
> hemorrhoidal b.

Banff classification
banjo-string adhesion
Banthine
Banti
> B. disease
> B. syndrome

BAO
> basal acid output

BAR
> biofragmentable anastomotic ring
> Valtrac BAR

bar
> cricopharyngeal b.
> inter-symphyseal b.
> Mercier b.
> symphyseal b.

barber pole sign
Barbidonna
barbital-acetate buffer
barbotage
Barcat technique
Barcoo vomitus
Bard
> B. automatic reprocessor
> B. Biopty gun
> B. Biopty instrument
> B. BladderScan
> B. BladderScan bladder volume instrument
> B. button
> B. Extra Ileo B pouch
> B. gastrostomy catheter
> B. gastrostomy feeding tube
> B. Integrale pouch

B PEG
B PEG tube
B protective barrier
B Urolase fiber laser system
Bardex-Foley catheter
Bard-Parker
  B.-P. blade
  B.-P. knife
Bard-Stiegmann-Goff variceal ligation kit
bariatric
  b. operation
  b. surgery
Baricon
  B. contrast medium
barium
  b. bezoar
  b. burger
  b. contrast radiography
  double tracking of b.
  b. enema (BE)
  b. enema reduction
  b. enema with air contrast
  b. esophagram
  b. granuloma
  b. meal
  b. peritonitis
  residual b.
  retained b.
  b. retention
  b. sediment in urine
  b. study
  b. sulfate
  b. suspension
  b. swallow
barium-impregnated marshmallow
Baro-CAT
Baroflave
  B. contrast medium
barogenic perforation
Barophen
baroreceptor
  high-pressure arterial b.
  low-pressure
    cardiopulmonary b.
  renal b.
  sinoaortic b.

baroreceptor-mediated mesenteric arterial vasoconstriction
baroreflex
  cardiopulmonary b.
Barosperse
  B. contrast medium
barostat
  b. balloon
  b. method
barotrauma
Barr
  B. fistula hook
  B. fistula probe
  B. rectal retractor
  B. rectal speculum
Barracuda flexible cystoscopic hot biopsy forceps
barrel chest
Barrett
  B. carcinoma
  B. disease
  B. dysplasia
  B. epithelium
  B. esophagitis
  B. esophagus (BE)
  B. intestinal forceps
  B. metaplasia
  B. syndrome
  B. ulcer
Barrett-Donovan-Mayo artificial bladder
barrier
  ABO b.
  bacteriostatic b.
  Bard protective b.
  blood-liquor b.
  blood-urine b.
  Coloplast skin b.
  Comfeel skin b.
  Dansac skin b.
  gastric mucosal b.
  Hollister Guardian F skin b.
  Nu-Hope Adhesive waterproof skin b.
  Sween-A-Peel skin b.
  United XL 14 skin b.
Barrington third reflex

B

NOTES

Barron
    B. ligation
    B. rubber band ligator
Barr-Shuford rectal speculum
Bartel cytotoxicity
Barth hernia
Bartholin cyst
Bartter syndrome
bar-type esophageal varix
BAS-300 transurethral
  thermotherapy device
basal
    b. acid output (BAO)
    b. acid secretion
    b. anal canal pressure
    b. anal sphincter pressure
    b. androstenedione
    b. cell carcinoma
    b. cell nevus syndrome
    b. cell-specific anti-cytokeratin
      antibody
    b. diet
    b. granular cell
    b. interferon-gamma
    b. metabolic rate (BMR)
    b. pressure
    b. renal excretion
    b. renal vascular resistance
    b. secretion
    b. secretory flow rate (BSFR)
    b. secretory flow rate test
    b. testosterone
Basaljel
base
    b. of appendix
    erythromycin b.
    b. excess
    ulcer b.
baseball stitch
baseline
    delta over b. (DOB)
    b. tenting
basement
    b. membrane
    b. membrane antigen
    b. membrane protein
bas-fond
basic
    b. diet
    b. dye
basket
    Bagley helical b.
    Dormia stone b.

    ELIMINATOR stone
      extraction b.
    b. forceps
    Gemini paired wire helical b.
    laser lithotriptor b.
    Olympus stone retrieval b.
    Positrap mini-retrieval b.
    Pursuer helical b.
    Segura-Dretler laser b.
    six-wire spiral tip Segura b.
    sphincterotomy b.
    stone b.
    stone retrieval b.
basketing
basket-type crushing forceps
baso
    basophil
    WBC basos
basolateral membrane (BLM)
basophil (baso)
Bassen-Kornzweig syndrome
Bassini
    B. inguinal hernia repair
    B. inguinal herniorrhaphy
    B. operation
Bates-corrected β
bath
    alcohol cooling b.
    HydraClense sitz b.
    sitz b.
bathroom privileges
battery
    button b.
    b. ingestion
battery-powered endoscope
Battle
    B. incision
    B. operation
    B. sign
bat-wing catheter
Bauhin
    valve of B.
Baumrucker urinary incontinence
  clamp
Baxter
    B. CA-210 filter
    1550 B. hemodialyzer
    B. Interline IV system
Baylor bleeding score
bayonet/stylet
bayonet-type forceps
BBM
    brush-border membrane

B

BBMV
  brush-border membrane vesicle
BBS
  brown bowel syndrome
BCAA
  branched-chain amino acid
BCAA/AAA plasma ratio
B-cell
  B-c. antigen CD20
  B-c. differentiation factor
  B-c. epitope
  B-c. PHSL
B-cellular phenotype
BCG, bCG
  bacille Calmette-Guérin
  Mycobacterium bovis BCG
  BCG vaccine
BCM
  body cell mass
BCR
  bulbocavernosus reflex
BDA
  bile duct adenoma
BDL
  bile duct ligation
bDNA
  branched chain DNA
B-D Safety-Gard needle
BE
  barium enema
  Barrett esophagus
bead
  b. chain study
  Percoll b.
  PMMA b.'s
  Septopal b.'s
beaded hepatic duct
beading sign
beaker cell
Beamer
  B. ejection stent
  B. injection stent
  B. injection stent system
bear claw ulcer
Beardsley esophageal retractor
Bearn-Kunkel-Slater syndrome
Beasley-Babcock forceps

BEB
  blind esophogeal brushing
becanechol
Beck
  B. gastrostomy
  B. method
Beckman
  B. airfuge
  B. 2 autoanalyzer
  B. ion-selective analyzer
  B. 39042 pH probe
Beckwith-Wiedemann syndrome
Béclard hernia
beclomethasone
bed
  gallbladder b.
  graft b.
  hepatic b.
  liver b.
  nail b.
  portal vascular b.
  raw surface of liver b.
  suburothelial vascular b.
  ulcer b.
Bedge pillow
bed-wetting alarm
beef tapeworm
Beelith
B.E. Glass abdominal retractor
behavior
  binge-purge b.
behavioral treatment
Behçet
  B. colitis
  B. disease
  B. syndrome
Behrend cystic duct forceps
beigelli
  Trichosporon b.
belch
bell
  b. clapper deformity
Belladenal
belladonna
  tincture of b.
Bellafoline
Bellergal-S

NOTES

belli

Isospora b.
bell-shaped orifice
Bell suture
bellyache
Belsey
B. Mark IV antireflux operation
B. Mark IV 240-degree fundoplication
B. Mark IV repair
B. partial fundoplication
B. two-thirds wrap fundoplication
belt
abdominal compression b.
B. technique
b. test
Belt-Fuqua hypospadias repair
Belzer
B. machine
B. solution
B. UW liver preservation solution
Benadryl
benazepril HCl
Bence Jones protein
bench
b. surgery
b. surgical technique
Benchekroun
B. hydraulic valve
B. ileal valve
B. pouch
B. stoma
bend
cautery b.
bendroflumethiazide
Benedict gastroscope
Benedict-Talbot body surface area method
Benelux Multicentre Trial Study Group
Benemid
benign
b. adenomatous polyp
b. anorectal disease (BAD)
b. bile duct stricture
b. biliary stricture
b. cystic mesothelioma
b. cystic teratoma
b. duodenocolic fistula
b. familial hematuria
b. familial icterus
b. gastric ulcer
b. hyperplastic gastropathy
b. mesothelioma of genital tract
b. mucous membrane pemphigoid
b. neoplastic precursor
b. papillary stenosis
b. paroxysmal peritonitis
b. pneumatic colonoscopy complication
b. pneumatic problem
b. pneumoperitoneum
b. postoperative jaundice
b. prostatic hyperplasia (BPH)
b. prostatic hypertrophy (BPH)
b. recurrent intrahepatic cholestasis
b. stenosis
b. stricture
b. tumor
b. ulcer
Béniqué sound
benoxaprofen
Benson pylorus separator
bentiromide
b. test
Bentle button
bent nail syndrome
bentonite flocculation test
Bentson
B. floppy-tipped guidewire
B. guidewire
B.-type Glidewire guidewire
Bentyl
benzalkonium chloride (BAC)
benzathine
b. penicillin
benzidine
benzimidazole
benzoate
benzocaine
benzodiazepine
b. conscious sedation
benzodiazepine-induced hypoventilation
benzoin
tincture of b.
benzphetamine
benzquinamide
benzthiazide
benztropine

B

benzydamine
benzylpenicillin
Beppu score
Berci-Shore
    B.-S. choledochoscope
    B.-S. choledochoscopy
Berens esophageal retractor
Berger
    B. disease
    B. nephropathy
Bergkvist grading system
Berlin
    B. blue
    B. blue staining
Bernard-Sergent syndrome
Bernard-Soulier syndrome
Bernstein
    B. acid perfusion test
    B. gastroscope
Bertin
    hypertrophy of column of B.
berylliosis
Besnier-Boeck-Schaumann disease
BESP
    Bipolar EndoStasis probe
Bessauds-Hilmand-Augier syndrome
Bessey-Lowry unit for alkaline
    phosphatase
Best
    B. bite block
    B. gallstone forceps
    B. right-angle colon clamp
bestatin
besylate
    amlodipine b.
beta
    b. chain
    growth factor b.
    interferon b.
    b. interferon
beta-1
    b.-1 chain
    b.-1 chain integrins
beta-2
    interferon b.-2
beta-1a
    interferon b.-1a

beta-adrenergic
    b.-a. agonist
    b.-a. antagonist
    b.-a. receptor
beta-3-agonist
beta-aminopropionitrile
beta-1b
Beta-Cap
    B.-C. catheter closure
    B.-C. II closure
Betadine
    B. gel
    B. scrub
beta-endorphin peptide YY (PYY)
beta-galactosidase
Betagan
beta-HCG, beta-hCG
beta-hemolytic strep
beta-lactam antibiotic
beta-lactamase-resistant penicillin
beta-lactam-associated diarrhea
betamethasone
    topical b.
beta-sympathomimetic tocolytic
    agent
beta-thromboglobulin
betazole stimulation test
bethanechol
    b. chloride
    b. hydrochloride
bethanidine
Bethesda System for cervicovaginal
    sample
Bevan
    B. abdominal incision
    B. gallbladder forceps
    B. orchiopexy
beveled speculum
bezoar
    artificial b.
    barium b.
    fungal b.
    gastric b.
    medication b.
    persimmon b.
BFR
    blood flow rate

NOTES

B2 glycoprotein I
b-hydroxylase
dopamine b.-h.
BIA
bioelectrical impedance analysis
Biaxin
BIB
biliointestinal bypass
bibasilar
bicalutamide
BICAP
Bipolar Circumactive probe
BICAP bipolar diathermy
BICAP bipolar hemostasis
probe
BICAP cautery
BICAP coagulation
BICAP electrocoagulation probe
BICAP electrode probe
BICAP endoscopic probe
BICAP hemostatic system
BICAP monopolar
BICAP probe
BICAP silver ACE
bicarb
bicarbonate
Bicarbolyte
bicarbonate (bicarb)
b. dialysate
b. electrolyte
saliva b.
sodium b.
bicarotid truncus
BiCart dialysis fluid
bicho
Bicitra
bicornuate uterus
bicoudé catheter
bi-curved needle
bidirectional ligation
Biebl loop
bieneusi
Enterocytozoon b.
Biermer disease
Biethium ostomy rod
bifid
b. clitoris
b. penis
b. scrotum
b. tongue
bifida
spina b.
Bifidobacterium

bifidus
Lactobacillus b.
bifurcation
b. of common bile duct
b. tumor
bigeminy
biglycan
proteoglycan b.
bihisdin
Bihrle
B. dorsal clamp
B. dorsal clamp-T-C needle
holder
bilabe
bilaminar embryonic disk
Bilarcil
bilateral
b. hydronephrosis
b. incision
b. lithotomy
b. nephroureterectomy
b. pudendal artery embolization
b. renal tumor
b. renal vein thrombosis
b. subcostal incision
b. transabdominal incision
b. ureterostomy takedown
b. vagotomy
bilayer
phospholipid b.
bile
A b.
b. acid (BA)
b. acid binder
b. acid breath test
b. acid-EDTA solution
b. acid malabsorption (BAM)
b. acid pool
b. acid therapy
b. acid tolerance test
b. ascites
B b.
b. bag
C b.
clear b.
cloudy b.
b. concretion
b. duct
b. duct adenoma (BDA)
b. duct brushing
b. duct canaliculus
b. duct cancer
b. duct cannulation

b. duct carcinoma
b. duct dyskinesia
b. duct epithelial cell
b. duct hypoplasia
b. duct ligation (BDL)
b. duct lumen
b. duct paucity
b. duct pressure
b. duct proliferation
b. duct stone
b. duct stricture
b. duct trauma
b. duct type cytokeratin
inspissated b.
b. lake
limy b.
lithogenic b.
b. peritonitis
b. pleuritis
b. plug
b. pulmonary embolism
b. reflux
b. reflux gastritis
b. salt diarrhea
b. salt-losing enteropathy
b. salt-phospholipid ratio
b. salts
SI of b.
b. solubility test
stagnant b.
b. stasis
supersaturated b.
thick b.
b. thrombus
turbid b.
viscid b.
viscous b.
white b.
bile-laden macrophage
bile-salt binding resin
bile-stained
b.-s. fluid
b.-s. vomitus
bile-tinged fluid
Bilezyme

bilharzial
b. dysentery
b. worm
bilharziasis
bili
bilirubin
biliary
b. actinomycosis
b. air
b. ascariasis
b. ascites
b. atresia
b. balloon catheter
b. balloon dilator
b. balloon probe
b. calculus
b. cannulation
b. carcinoma
b. cholesterol secretion
b. cirrhosis
b. clonorchiasis
b. colic
b. cyst
b. decompression
b. dilation
b. dilator catheter
b. diverticulum
b. drainage
b. dyskinesia
b. dyspepsia
b. echinococcosis
b. endoprosthesis
b. endoprosthesis insertion
b. excretion
b. fibroadenomatosis
b. fistula
b. hypercholesterolemia
  xanthomatosis
b. infestation
b. instrumentation
b. leakage
b. lipid
b. lithotripsy
b. manometry
b. microhamartoma
b. mud
b. pain

B

NOTES

biliary *(continued)*
- b. pancreatitis
- b. papillomatosis
- b. passages
- b. piecemeal necrosis
- b. plexus
- b. prosthesis
- b. radicle
- b. saturation index
- b. scintiscan
- b. sclerosis
- b. sepsis
- b. sludge
- b. sphincter
- b. sphincterotomy
- b. stasis
- b. steatorrhea
- b. stent
- b. stenting
- b. stent patency
- b. stricture
- b. structure
- b. tract
- b. tract disease
- b. tract obstruction
- b. tract pressure
- b. tract stone
- b. tract stricture
- b. tract torsion
- b. tract tumor
- b. tree
- b. xanthomatosis

biliary-bronchial fistula
biliary-cutaneous fistula
biliary-duodenal
- b.-d. fistula
- b.-d. pressure gradient

biliary-enteric fistula
biliary-like
bilifaction, bilification
biliferous
biligenesis
biligenic
Biligrafin
- B. contrast medium

biliodigestive anastomosis
bilioduodenal prosthesis
bilioenteric
- b. bypass
- b. fistula

biliointestinal bypass (BIB)
biliopancreatic
- b. bypass (BPB)

- b. diversion
- b. shunt

bilious
- b. diarrhea
- b. emesis
- b. remittent fever
- b. remittent malaria
- b. stool
- b. vomiting

biliousness
biliptysis
bilirachia
bilirubin (bili)
- conjugated b.
- direct b.
- b. encephalopathy
- fat-soluble b.
- fractionation of b.
- indirect b.
- b. pigment gallstone
- serum b.
- b. test
- total b.
- unconjugated b. (UCB)
- urine b.
- water-soluble b.

bilirubinate stone
bilirubinemia
bilirubinuria
Biliscopin
- B. contrast medium

BILISYSTEM
- B. ERCP cannula
- B. stone removal balloon
- B. wire-guided papillotome

bilitherapy
biliverdin
Bilivist
- B. contrast medium

Billingham-Bookwalter rectal fenestrated blade
Billroth
- B. forceps
- B. I anastomosis
- B. I gastrectomy
- B. I gastroduodenostomy
- B. I gastroenterostomy
- B. I reconstruction
- B. II anastomosis
- B. II anastomotic scar
- B. II anatomy
- B. II gastrectomy
- B. II gastroenterostomy

B. II gastrojejunostomy
B. II reconstruction
bilobar
    b. hyperplasia
    b. hypertrophy
bilobate false aneurysm
bilobed
    b. gallbladder
    b. polypoid lesion
bilocular stomach
biloma
Bilopaque
    B. contrast medium
Biloptin
    B. contrast medium
Biltricide
binary factor
binder
    bile acid b.
    Dale abdominal b.
    T-b.
    b. test
binding
    phosphotyrosine-SH2 b.
    sperm-immunobead b.
    vasoactive intestinal
        polypeptide b.
binge
bingeing
binge-purge behavior
BIO101MERmaid kit
bioartificial liver support device
bioassay
    mink cell b.
biochemical marker
biocompatibility
Biodan Prostathermer
biodegradable microsphere
biodistribution of N-isopropyl-p-
    iodoamphetamine
bioeffect
bioelectrical impedance analysis
    (BIA)
Bio-Enzabead test

biofilm
    bacterial b.
biofragmentable anastomotic ring
    (BAR)
BioGel P4
Bio-Gen
    B.-G. urine test strip
Biogenex antigen retrieval method
biogenic amine
Bioglass
Biohazard bag
Biolab
    Malakit *Helicobacter pylori* B.
biologic
    b. response modifier therapy
    b. therapy
biological marker
biomarker
    intermediate b.
biomaterial
    alloplastic b.
Biomox
Biomydrin
bio-occlusive dressing
Bioplastique
bioplug
bio potential skin electrode
biopsy
    alcohol-fixed gastric b.
    antral b.
    aspiration b.
    bite b.
    blind percutaneous liver b.
    bone marrow b.
    brush b.
    brush and b.
    b. channel
    CLO b.
    cold b.
    cold cup b.
    colonoscopic b.
    colorectal b.
    core needle b.
    corporal b.
    Crosby-Kugler capsule for b.
    CT-guided liver b.
    CT-guided needle-aspiration b.

B

NOTES

biopsy *(continued)*
    cub bladder b.
    cytologic b.
    diathermic loop b.
    digitally-guided b.
    direct vision liver b.
    endoscopic b.
    endoscopic small bowel b.
    ERCP-guided b.
    esophageal b.
    fine-needle b.
    b. forceps
    b. of gastric mucosa
    guided transcutaneous b.
    guillotine needle b.
    b. gun
    hot b.
    ileal b.
    incisional b.
    b. instrument
    jumbo b.
    laparoscopic b.
    large-particle b.
    lift-and-cut b.
    liver b.
    Menghini technique for
      percutaneous liver b.
    mucosal b.
    multiple b.
    native renal b.
    needle b.
    open b.
    paracollicular b.
    percutaneous b.
    percutaneous fine-needle
      pancreatic b.
    percutaneous liver b.
    percutaneous native renal b.
    percutaneous pancreas b.
    peritoneal b.
    pinch b.
    pouch b.
    b. punch
    punch b.
    random bladder b.
    rectal b.
    renal b.
    saucerized b.
    scan-directed b.
    shave b.
    skinny-needle b.
    small-bowel b.
    snap-frozen b.

    snare excision b.
    snare loop b.
    sonoguided b.
    strip b.
    suction b.
    systematic sextant b.
    tangential b.
    transcutaneous b.
    transgastric fine-needle-
      aspiration b.
    transitional zone b.
    transjugular liver b.
    transpapillary b.
    transrectal ultrasound-guided-
      sextant b.
    transvenous liver b.
    Tru-Cut b.
    Tru-Cut needle b.
    ultrasound-guided b.
    Vim-Silverman technique for
      liver b.
    Watson capsule b.
    wedge hepatic b.
biopsy-verified chronic
    glomerulonephritis
Biopty
    B. cut needle
    B. gun
Bio-Rad protein assay
Biotel home screening test
biothesiometry
    penile b.
biotin
    endogenous b.
biotinylated
    b. DNA probe
biotransformation
BioWhittaker
    B. assay
    B. assay test
BIP biopsy instrument
biperiden
biphasic diurnal rhythm
4,5-biphosphate
    phosphatidyl inositol 4,5-b.
biplanar aortography
biplane sector probe
bipolar
    b. bleeding
    B. Circumactive probe
    (BICAP)
    B. Circumactive Probe
    coagulation

b. coagulation
b. electrocautery
b. electrocoagulation (BPEC)
B. EndoStasis probe (BESP)
b. glass electrode
b. hemostasis probe
b. neuron
b. probe
b. sphincterotome
bipolar coagulating forceps
bird-beak
 b.-b. configuration
 b.-b. narrowing
birefringence
Birtcher Hyfricator cautery wire
bisacodyl
 b. tannex
bismuth
 b. benign bile duct stricture
 classification
 b. compound
 b. salt
 b. subsalicylate
bismuthate
 tripotassium dicitrato b.
bismuth-free triple therapy
bismuth, metronidazole, tetracycline
 (BMT)
bistable
bistriazole fluconazole
bitartrate
 cysteamine b.
bite
 b. biopsy
 b. biopsy forceps
Bitome
 B. bipolar sphincterotome
 B. bipolar system
 B. catheter
bivalve
black
 B. Beauty ureteral stent
 b. clot
 b. faceted stone
 b. hairy tongue
 b. jaundice
 b. liver disease

b. pigment gallstone
b. pigment stone
b. sickness
b. tarry stool
b. vomitus
bladder
 alloplastic prostatic b.
 areflexic b.
 atonic b.
 augmented b.
 b. autoaugmentation
 autonomic neurogenic b.
 Barrett-Donovan-Mayo
 artificial b.
 b. calculus
 b. cancer
 b. capacity
 b. carcinoma
 b. chimney procedure
 b. compliance
 compliance of b.
 congenital bifid b.
 b. cooling reflex
 cord b.
 b. descensus
 distended b.
 b. diverticulectomy
 double b.
 dropped b.
 b. exstrophy
 fasciculate b.
 b. fistula
 Gilchrist ileocecal b.
 b. hernia
 hyperreflexic b.
 hypertonic b.
 hypotonic b.
 ileal b.
 ileocecal b.
 ileocolonic b.
 b. incontinence
 b. inhibition
 irritable b.
 low-compliance b.
 b. mapping
 b. neck contracture
 b. neck preserving technique

NOTES

bladder *(continued)*
    b. neck suspension
    b. neck-to-urethra anastomosis
    b. neoplasm
    nervous b.
    neurogenic b.
    neuropathic b.
    b. neurosis
    nonneurogenic b.
    orthotopic b.
    b. outflow obstruction
    b. outlet
    b. outlet obstruction (BOO)
    b. outlet reconstruction
    pancreatic b.
    b. perforation
    b. pillar block
    poorly compliant b.
    b. pressure (BP)
    b. pressure sensor
    b. prolapse
    prosthetic b.
    pseudoneurogenic b.
    reflex neurogenic b.
    reflex neuropathic b.
    b. replacement
    b. replacement urinary pouch
    stammering of the b.
    b. stone
    b. substitution
    b. support
    trabeculated b.
    transitional cell cancer of
      the b. (TCCA)
    b. tumor
    uninhibited neurogenic b.
    uninhibited overactive b.
    unstable b.
    urinary b.
    valve b.
    b. volume
    b. washing
    b. worm
    b. xanthoma
BladderScan
    Bard B.
blade
    Bard-Parker b.
    Billingham-Bookwalter rectal
      fenestrated b.
    Bookwalter-Cook anal rectal b.
    Bookwalter malleable
      retractor b.

    Bookwalter-Mayo b.
    Bookwalter-Parks anal
      sphincter b.
    Bovie b.
    knife b.
    malleable b.
    razor b.
    scalpel b.
Blair silicone drain
Blake gallstone forceps
Blakemore-Sengstaken tube
Blakemore tube
blanching of mucosa
bland
    b. diet
    b. food
    b. thrombosis
Bland-Altman analysis
blanket
    Gaymar water-circulating b.
blast
    b. cell
    b. injury
    WBC b.'s
blastocyst hatching
Blastocystis hominis
blastoid transformation
blastomere
blastomycosis
    peritoneal b.
bleb
bleed
    gastrointestinal b.
    GI b.
    herald b.
    postgastrectomy b.
    postpolypectomy b.
bleeder
bleeding
    b. acid-peptic disease
    active source of b.
    b. angioma
    bipolar b.
    b. colonic angiodysplasia
    colorectal b.
    b. control
    diverticular b.
    duodenal b.
    dysfunctional b.
    esophageal variceal b.
    esophagogastric variceal b.
    excessive b.
    functional b.

B

gastric b.
gastric variceal b.
b. gastritis
gastrointestinal b. (GIB)
GI b.
b. hemorrhoid
jet-like b.
b. lesion
lower GI b.
occult b.
occult GI b.
painless rectal b.
pancreatitis-related b.
peptic ulcer b.
b. per rectum
b. point
b. polyp
rectal b.
b. site
b. site localization
b. time
b. tumor
b. ulcer
upper gastrointestinal b.
   (UGIB)
vaginal b.
variceal b.
blend
b. waveform
b. waveform desiccation
blended current
blended cut
blenderized diet
blennemesis
bleomycin
bleomycin, etoposide and cisplatin
blepharitis
blepharospasm
blind
b. cautery
b. enema
b. esophogeal brushing (BEB)
b. limb
b. lithotripsy
b. loop
b. loop syndrome
b. percutaneous liver biopsy

b. stump
b. technique
b. upper esophageal pouch
blink
acoustic b.
blinking reflex
BLM
basolateral membrane
bloc
harvesting en b.
Blocadren
Bloch-Paul-Mikulicz operation
block
Best bite b.
bladder pillar b.
caudal b.
celiac plexus b.
nerve b.
neurolytic celiac plexus b.
OB-10 Comfort bite b.
transitory b.
Block-Ace solution
blockade
alpha b.
alpha sympathetic b.
androgen b.
cavernosal alpha b.
maximal androgen b. (MAB)
muscarinic b.
blockage
complete hormonal b.
blocked aerogastria
blocker
β adrenergic b.
alpha-1 b.
calcium channel b.
calcium entry b.
H2 b.
nicotinic receptor b.
proton pump b.
starch b.
β-blocker
Blom-Singer
B.-S. esophagoscope
B.-S. tracheoesophageal fistula
blood
b. admixed with stool

NOTES

63

blood *(continued)*
 b. agar plate
 b. alcohol level (BAL)
 b. ammonia
 bright red b.
 b. calculus
 b. clot
 clotted b.
 b. coagulation
 b. coagulation disorder
 crossmatched b.
 b. culture
 b. flow
 b. flow assessment
 b. flow rate (BFR)
 frank b.
 b. gas on oxygen
 b. gas on room air
 non-hemolyzed b.
 nostril b.
 occult b.
 b. on surface of stool
 oozing b.
 b. passed with stool
 b. pressure (BP)
 b. sample
 spurting b.
 stool for occult b.
 b. stream infection (BSI)
 b. transfusion
 b. type
 typed b.
 b. urea level
 b. urea nitrogen (BUN)
 b. vessel
 whole b.
blood-borne
 b.-b. non-A, non-B hepatitis
 b.-b. pathogen
 b.-b. transmission
blood-contactin catheter
blood-liquor barrier
blood in stool
blood-streaked stool
blood-testis-epididymis
blood-tinged
 b.-t. ascites
blood urea nitrogen (BUN)
blood-urine barrier
bloody
 b. ascites
 b. diarrhea
 b. discharge

 b. peritoneal fluid
 b. stool
 b. vomitus
blooming
 b. effect
blot
 Southern b.
blotting
 ECL Western b.
  enhanced chemiluminescence
  Western blotting
 enhanced chemiluminescence
  Western b. (ECL Western
  blotting)
 Western b.
Blount disease
blow-hole ileostomy
blown pupil
blue
 Alcian b.
 Berlin b.
 b. diaper syndrome
 b. dot sign
 B. Max balloon catheter
 methylene b.
 PAS-Alcian b.
 b. rubber-bleb nevus syndrome
 b. rubber nevus syndrome
 toluidine b.
 Urolene B.
 b. varices
Bluemle pump
Blumberg sign
Blumer rectal shelf
blunt
 b. abdominal trauma
 b. dissection
 b. liver trauma
 b. needle
 b. pancreatic trauma
 b. probe
 b. and sharp dissection
 b. trauma
blunting
 costophrenic b.
 haustral b.
 b. of valve
blunt-tipped obturator
B-lymphocyte system
BM
 bowel movement
BMD
 bone mineral densitometry

BMI
> body mass index

B-mode
>> B-m. imaging
>> B-m. ultrasonography
>> B-m. ultrasound image

BMR
> basal metabolic rate

BMT
> bismuth, metronidazole, tetracycline
> bone marrow transplantation

board-like
>> b.-l. rigidity
>> b.-l. rigidity of abdomen

Boari
>> B. bladder flap
>> B. bladder flap procedure
>> B. ureteral flap repair

Boari-Ockerblad
>> B.-O. flap
>> B.-O. principle

Boas point
boat-shaped abdomen
Bochdalek
>> foramen of B.
>> B. hernia

Boden-Gibb tumor staging
Bodenhammer rectal speculum
body
>> acidophilic b.
>> anal foreign b.
>> angularis b.
>> anorectal foreign b.
>> asteroid b.
>> Call-Exner b.
>> b. cell mass (BCM)
>> CMV inclusion b.
>> coccidian b.
>> colonic foreign b.
>> b. composition analysis
>> corneal foreign b.
>> Councilman b.
>> cyanobacterium-like b.
>> Donovan b.
>> duodenal foreign b.
>> epithelial inclusion b.
>> esophageal foreign b.

>> esophageal Lewy b.
>> foreign b.
>> gastric foreign b.
>> b. habitus
>> Howell-Jolly b.
>> inclusion b.
>> ingested foreign b.
>> intracytoplasmic CMV
>>> inclusion b.
>> intraepithelial b.
>> intranuclear CMV inclusion b.
>> Jaworski b.
>> ketone b.
>> Lafora b.
>> lower GI tract foreign b.
>> Mallory hyaline b.
>> malpighian b.
>> b. mass index (BMI)
>> Michaelis-Gutmann b.
>> polar b.
>> b. position
>> rectal foreign b.
>> Schaumann b.
>> S-shaped b.
>> upper GI tract foreign b.
>> vaginal foreign b.
>> vermiform b.
>> viral inclusion b.

Boehringer kit
Boerema anterior gastropexy
Boerhaave syndrome
boggy
>> b. prostate

Bogros space
bolster
>> b. suture

bolus
>> alimentary b.
>> b. challenge test
>> b. dressing
>> b. feeding
>> food b.
>> marshmallow b.

bombesin
bombesin-receptor
bone
>> b. marrow aplasia

B

NOTES

bone *(continued)*
- b. marrow biopsy
- b. marrow-derived B cell
- b. marrow stem cell
- b. marrow transplantation (BMT)
- b. marrow transplantation-related problem
- b. mineral densitometry (BMD)
- b. mineral density
- b. scan

Bonine
Bonney test
bony
- b. defect
- b. dysraphism
- b. landmarks
- b. spicule
- b. tenderness

BOO
  bladder outlet obstruction
Bookler swivel-ball laparoscope holder
Bookwalter
- B. malleable retractor blade
- B. retractor
- B. retractor system
- B. ring retractor

Bookwalter-Cook anal rectal blade
Bookwalter-Goulet retractor
Bookwalter-Hill-Ferguson rectal retractor
Bookwalter-Mayo blade
Bookwalter-Parks anal sphincter blade
Bookwalter-St. Mark deep pelvic retractor
borborygmus, pl. **borborygmi**
border
- antimesenteric b.
- brush b.
- b. cell
- fundopyloric mucosal b.
- mucosal b.
- b. zone

bore
- magnetic b.

Borge clamp
boring pain
boronate
- b. affinity
- b. affinity chromatography
- b. gel

Boros esophagoscope
Borrmann
- B. gastric cancer
- B. gastric cancer classification
- B. Type IV scirrhous carcinoma

Bors
- B. ice water test

Bosniak classification
B&O suppository
Botkin disease
Botox
botryoid sarcoma
bottle
- McGaw plastic b.
- b. operation
- Vacutainer b.

botulinum
- *Clostridium b.*
- b. toxin

botulism
Bouchard
- B. disease
- B. index

bougie
- acorn-tipped b.
- b. à boule
- bulbous b.
- Celestin dilator b.
- b. dilator
- elastic b.
- elbowed b.
- filiform b.
- following b.
- French b.
- Hegar b.
- Hurst mercury b.
- Hurst-type b.
- Jackson esophageal b.
- large-diameter b.
- Maloney b.
- Maloney-type b.
- mercury-weighted rubber b.
- polyvinyl b.
- Savary b.
- Savary-Gilliard Silastic flexible b.
- Savary-Gilliard wire-guided b.
- tapered rubber b.
- through-the-scope b.
- Trousseau esophageal b.
- wax-tipped b.
- wire-guided polyvinyl b.

bougienage
    esophageal b.
    Hurst b.
    peroral b.
    transgastric esophageal b.
Bouin
    B. fixative solution
    B. solution
boulardii
    Saccharomyces b.
boule
    bougie à b.
bouquet fever
Bourne test
Bourneville disease
bouton
    b. en chemise
Bouveret
    B. syndrome
    B. ulcer
Bovie
    B. blade
    B. coagulation
    B. electrocautery
    B. electrocoagulation unit
    B. holder
bovied
bovine
    b. graft
    b. serum albumin (BSA)
    b. thrombin
    b. trypsin
bovis
    Mycobacterium b.
    Streptococcus b.
bowed sternum
bowel
    b. adherent to omentum
    aganglionic b.
    b. axis
    b. bag
    b. bypass
    b. bypass syndrome
    b. contents
    b. continuity
    dead b.
    dilated loops of b.

    b. dilation
    b. disease
    b. displacement
    entrapment of b.
    fixed segment of b.
    fluid-filled small b.
    b. forceps
    b. function
    gangrenous b.
    b. gas
    b. grasper
    b. habit
    incarcerated b.
    b. incontinence
    infarcted b.
    b. intussusception
    ischemic b.
    kink in b.
    large b.
    b. loop
    b. lumen
    b. movement (BM)
    b. necrosis
    necrotizing vasculitis of b.
    Noble surgical plication of b.
    b. obstruction
    b. perforation
    b. plate
    pleating of small b.
    b. preparation (bowel prep)
    b. preparation complication
    prolapsed b.
    b. pseudo-obstruction
    b. refashioning procedure
    b. resection
    b. rest
    small b.
    b. sounds
    b. stoma
    strangulated b.
    b. tone
    b. wall
bowel prep
    bowel preparation
    Colonlite bowel prep
    COLyte bowel prep
    Dulcolax bowel prep

B

NOTES

bowel prep *(continued)*
Emulsoil bowel prep
Evac-Q-Kit bowel prep
Evac-Q-Kwik bowel prep
Fleet bowel prep
GoLYTELY bowel prep
inadequate bowel prep
OCL bowel prep
Tridrate bowel prep
X-Prep bowel prep
Bowen
B. disease
B. papule
B. patch
bowenoid papulosis
Bower PEG tube
bowler hat sign
Bowman
B. capsule
B. space
box
A/B switch b.
Boyarsky
B. BPH symptom score
B. symptom scoring system
Boyce
longitudinal nephrotomy of B.
B. modification of Sengstaken-
Blakemore tube
B. sign
Boyce-Vest procedure
Boyden
B. meal
B. sphincter
boydii
Pseudallescheria b.
Boyle and Goldstein saline test
Bozeman-Fritsch catheter
Bozeman operation
Bozicevich test
BP
bladder pressure
blood pressure
BPB
biliopancreatic bypass
BPEC
bipolar electrocoagulation
BPH
benign prostatic hyperplasia
benign prostatic hypertrophy
American Urological
Association symptom index
for BPH

BQ123 receptor antagonist
BR96
monoclonal antibody B.
Braasch
B. catheter
B. direct catheterization
cystoscope
**Braasch-Kaplan direct vision
cystoscope**
**brachioaxillary bridge graft fistula
(BAGF)**
brachioradialis
**brachiosubclavian bridge graft
fistula (BSGF)**
brachytherapy
interstitial b.
Brackin
B. technique
B. ureterointestinal anastomosis
Bradley
B. disease
B. loop
bradyarrhythmia
bradycardia
reflex b.
sinus b.
bradygastria
bradykinin
bradypepsia
bradyphagia
bradyspermatism
bradystalsis
bradyuria
brain
b. metastasis
b. stem-sacral loop
b. tumor
brain-gut
b.-g. axis
b.-g. peptide
brain-heart infusion agar
bran
branched
b. calculus
b.-chain amino acid (BCAA)
b. chain DNA (bDNA)
b. vascular graft
brancher
b. deficiency
b. deficiency glycogenosis
b. enzyme
b. glycogen storage disease
branching tubule formation

branchiogenous cyst
branch renal artery disease
Brandel cell harvester
brash
    sour b.
    water b.
    weaning b.
BRAT
    bananas, rice, cereal, applesauce, &
      toast
    BRAT diet
BRATT
    bananas, rice, cereal, applesauce, tea,
      & toast
    BRATT diet
Braun
    B. anastomosis
    B. stent
Braun-Jaboulay gastroenterostomy
BRBPR
    bright red blood per rectum
BrDu, BrdU, BrdUrd
    bromodeoxyuridine
breakage
    intracorporeal needle b.
breakbone fever
Break-cluster homology gene
breakfast
    Ewald b.
    test b.
Breakstone lithotriptor
breakthrough dose
breast
    b. cancer
    b. cancer-associated protein
      pS2 expression
breath
    b. alkane
    b. ethane level
    b. hydrogen test
    b. isotope bacterial urease
      detection
    b. odor
    b. pentane test
    b. sound

    b. test
    uremic b.
breathing
    deep b.
    diaphragmatic b.
    intermittent positive pressure b.
      (IPPB)
    mouth b.
    sleep-disordered b. (SDB)
Breisky-Navratil straight retractor
Brennemann syndrome
brequinar sodium
Brescia-Cimino shunt
Breslow-Day test
Brethine
Bretschneider histidine tryptophan
    solution
bretylium
Brevibloc
Brewer infarcts
Bricanyl
Bricker
    B. operation
    B. pouch
    B. ureteroileostomy
    B. urinary diversion
bridge
    agar b.
    Albarran reflecting b.
    colostomy b.
    loop ostomy b.
    mucosal b.
    suture b.
bridging
    mucosal b.
    b. necrosis
    portal-to-portal b.
bridle
    control b.
briefs
    Ashton b.
    Holyoke b.
    Suretys incontinence b.
bright
    B. disease
    b. red blood

B

NOTES

bright *(continued)*
    b. red blood per rectum
    (BRBPR)
    b. red vomitus
brim
    pelvic b.
Brinkerhoff rectal speculum
broad-based
    b.-b. gait
    b.-b. polyp
broadening
    spectral b.
broad-spectrum antibiotic
Brodel line
Broder index
broken stent retrieval device
bromide
    cetyldimethylethyl
      ammonium b.
    emepronium b.
    ethidium b.
    hexamethonium b.
    mepenzolate b.
    methantheline b.
    methscopolamine b.
    prifinium b.
    propantheline b.
bromobenzene (B2)
bromocriptine
    b. dopaminergic medication
bromodeoxyuridine (BrDu, BrdU, BrdUrd)
    b. cell kinetics
5-bromo-deoxyuridine
bromodiphenhydramine
Bromo Seltzer
brompheniramine
Bromsulphalein (BSP)
bronchial
    b. carcinoid
    b. sound
Broncho-Cath double-lumen endotracheal tube
bronchoesophageal fistula
bronchoesophagology
bronchoesophagoscopy
bronchophony
bronchopleurofistula
bronchopulmonary foregut malformation
bronchoscope
    Savary b.
bronchospasm

bronchus
Bronkosol
Brooke ileostomy
bropirimine
broth
    cysteine Brucella b.
    tryptic soy b.
Broviac catheter
brown
    b. bowel syndrome (BBS)
    B. dietary method for colon
      preparation
    b. pigment gallstone
    b. pigment stone
    b. stool
    B. and Wickham pressure
      profile method
Brown-Buerger cystoscope
Brown-McHardy
    B.-M. pneumatic dilator
    B.-M. pneumatic mercury
      bougie dilation
Brown-Mueller
    B.-M. T-bar fastener
    B.-M. T-fastener
Broyle
    B. esophagoscope
    B. retrograde cystoscope
B-RTO
    balloon-occluded retrograde
    transvenous obliteration
Brucella
    B. melitensis
brucellosis
Brudzinski sign
Bruel-Kjaer
    B.-K. axial transducer
    B.-K. scanner
    B.-K. 1846 ultrasound system
Bruening esophagoscope
bruisability
    easy b.
bruit
    abdominal b.'s
    carotid b.'s
    femoral b.'s
    vascular b.'s
Brunings esophagoscope
Brunner
    B. gland
    B. gland adenoma
    B. gland of duodenum
    B. gland hamartoma

B. gland hyperplasia
B. intestinal forceps
brunneroma
    b. of duodenum
Brunn nest
Brunschwig operation
brush
    Ayre b.
    b. biopsy
    b. and biopsy
    b. border
    b. catheter
    Combo Cath wire-guided
      cytology b.
    cytology b.
    b. cytology
    Endovations disposable
      cytology b.
    Geenen cytology b.
    Olympus cytology b.
    sheathed cytology b.
brush-border
    b.-b. digestion
    b.-b. disaccharidase specific
      activity
    b.-b. enzyme activity
    b.-b. hydrolase activity
    b.-b. marker enzyme
    b.-b. membrane (BBM)
    b.-b. membrane vesicle
      (BBMV)
brushing
    bile duct b.
    blind esophogeal b. (BEB)
    b. urea breath test
Bruton disease
Bruton-type agammaglobulinemia
Bryan-Leishman stain
BSA
    bovine serum albumin
BSA-induced overload proteinuria
B-scanner
BSFR
    basal secretory flow rate
    BSFR test

BSGF
    brachiosubclavian bridge graft
      fistula
BSI
    blood stream infection
BSP
    Bromsulphalein
    BSP retention
    BSP test
BT-PABA test
bubble
    Garren-Edwards gastric b.
    Garren gastric b.
    gastric air b.
    GEG b.
    intragastric b.
    b. therapy
bubble-free
buccal
    b. mucosa
    b. mucosal patch graft
    b. mucosal urethral
      replacement
bucket-handle incision
Buck fascia
Bucladin-S
buclizine
bucrylate
    b. sclerosant
bud
    dorsal b.
    ureteric b.
    ventral b.
Budd
    B. cirrhosis
    B. disease
    B. jaundice
Budd-Chiari syndrome
BUD drainage catheter
buffer
    barbital-acetate b.
    cacodylate b.
    guanidinium thiocyanate b.
    HEPES b.
    Krebs-Henseleit bicarbonate b.
      (KHB)
    Krebs-Ringer bicarbonate b.

NOTES

buffer *(continued)*
    Rapid-hyb b.
    b. solution
Bugbee
    B. electrocautery
    B. electrode
Buie
    B. clamp
    B. fistula probe
    B. forceps
    B. pile clamp
    B. pile forceps
    B. position
    B. rectal scissors
    B. rectal suction tip
    B. rectal suction tube
    B. suction tip
Buie-Smith retractor
Build Up enteral feeding
bulb
    apex of duodenal b.
    b. deformity
    duodenal b.
    genital end b.
    b. suction
    b. tip retrograde study
bulbar
    b. artery
    b. peptic ulcer
    b. urethral carcinoma
bulbi (*pl. of* bulbus)
bulbocavernosus
    b. fat pad
    b. reflex (BCR)
**bulbocavernous reflex latency
  measurement**
bulbomembranous
    b. stricture
    b. urethra
    b. urethral squamous cell
      carcinoma
bulbourethral stricture
bulbous
    b. bougie
bulb-tipped retrograde ureterogram
bulbus, pl. **bulbi**
    b. penis
    b. urethrae
bulgaricus
    Lactobacillus b.
bulge
    inguinal b.

bulging
    anal b.
    b. flank
bulimia nervosa
bulimorexia
bulking agent
bulk laxative
bulky
    b. dressing
    b. stool
bulla
bulldog
    b. clamp
    b. forceps
bullet
    b. probe
    b.-tip catheter
bullosa
    epidermolysis b.
bullous
    b. edema
    b. edema vesicae
    b. pemphigoid
bull's eye lesion
bumetanide
Bumex
bumper
    Cloverleaf internal b.
    dome-shaped internal b.
    gastrostomy b.
    PEG b.
BUN
    blood urea nitrogen
bunching maneuver
bundle
    coherent b.
    fiber b.
    fiberoptic b.
    b. of His
    image guide b.
    b. of Itis
    light guide b.
    master IG b.
    microfilament b.
    neovascular b.
BUN-to-creatinine ratio
bupivacaine
    b. hydrochloride
buprenorphine
    b. narcotic analgesic therapy
bur, burr
    Ultrasonic oscillating b.
Burch colposuspension

burden
    stone b.
Burdwan fever
burger
    barium b.
Bürger-Grütz syndrome
Burhenne steerable catheter
buried
    b. bumper syndrome
    b. penis
    b. suture
Burkitt lymphoma
burn
    thermal b.
    transmural b.
burned-out
    b.-o. mucosa
    b.-o. testis cancer
    b.-o. tumor
burnetii
    Coxiella b.
Burnett syndrome
burning pain
Burnishine disinfectant
burp
burr (*var. of* bur)
bursa
    b. of Fabricius
    infrapatellar b.
bursoscopy
    supragastric b.
burst
    phagocyte respiratory b.
    respiratory b.
bursula
Buschke-Löwenstein tumor
Busch umbilical scissors
Buscopan
Buselmeier shunt
buserelin
    b. acetate
buski
    Fasciolopsis b.
BuSpar
buspirone
    b. hydrochloride
butalbital

1-butanol
Butibel
butorphanol
butter
    b. meal
    b. stool
Butterfield cystoscope
butterflies in the stomach
butterfly needle
buttock
button
    Bard b.
    b. battery
    b. battery ingestion
    Bentle b.
    compression b.
    b. drainage
    b. of duodenum
    b. electrode
    b. gastrostomy
    gastrostomy b.
    Murphy b.
    One-Step gastric b.
    peritoneal b.
    Surgitek b.
    b. suture
buttonhole
    b. incision
    b. preputial transposition
button-type G-tube
buttress
    fascia lata b.
butyl aminobenzoate
butylscopolamine
butyl-silane extraction column
butyricum
    Clostridium b.
BXO
    balanitis xerotica obliterans
Byars flap
Byler disease
bypass
    Alden loop gastric b.
    aortic/superior mesenteric
      artery b.
    aortorenal b.
    bilioenteric b.

NOTES

bypass *(continued)*
    biliointestinal b. (BIB)
    biliopancreatic b. (BPB)
    bowel b.
    duodenoileal b. (DIB)
    gastric b. (GBP)
    b. graft
    Greenville gastric b.
    Griffen Roux-en-Y b.
    Hallberg biliointestinal b.
    hepatorenal b.
    iliorenal b.

    jejunal b.
    jejunoileal b. (JIB)
    mesenterorenal b.
    partial ileal b.
    Payne-DeWind jejunoileal b.
    Roux-en-Y gastric b.
    Scopinaro pancreaticobiliary b.
    Scott jejunoileal b.
    splenorenal b.
    superior mesenterorenal b.
    thoracic aortorenal b.
    b. wire

C

C bile
C graft
C of Hosmer-Lemeshow ratio
   test
C-1 esterase inhibitor
C1q nephropathy
C2

stage C2
C3

C. C4
C. convertase
C. deposit
C. immunological study
C. receptor
C3a

plasma-activated complement 3
C3a complement
C3b receptor
C4

C3 C.
leukotriene C.
C4a

plasma-activated complement 4
C4b receptor
C5a

plasma-activated complement 5
C5 receptor
C18 Sep-Pack column
C22-3

antibody to C.
c100

antibody to c. (anti-c100)
C100-3 antigen
CA

carbonic anhydrase
cholic acid
   CA cellulose acetate membrane
   hollow-fiber dialyzer
   CA 19-9 test
Ca2+
Ca2+-activated K+
CA 19-9

carbohydrate antigen 19-9
CA110 dialyzer
CA-125

cancer antigen 125
Ca50 antigen
CAA

coloanal anastomosis

cable

fiberoptic light c.
internal fiberoptic c.
leakage bypass c.
light c.
Cabot-Nesbit orchiopexy
CaC3 crystal
cachectic

c. fever
cachexia

c. aphthosa
malignant c.
tumor c.
vascular c.
cacodylate buffer
cadaver

c. kidney
c. renal preservation
cadaveric

c. renal transplant
c. transplant
cadaveris

Clostridium c.
cadmium-induced nephrotoxicity
**cadmiumselenide-vidicon video
   camera**
cafe

c. coronary
c. coronary syndrome
Cafergot
caffeine

c. clearance
c. gut
**caffeine, alcohol, pepper, spicy
   foods (CAPS)**
caffeinism
CAG

chronic atrophic gastritis
cagA

c. antibody
c. gene
CAGEIN

catheter-guided endoscopic
   intubation
CAH

chronic active hepatitis
chronic aggressive hepatitis
congenital adrenal hyperplasia
CAI

carbonic anhydrase inhibitor

Cajal
  interstitial cells of C.
Calan
calbindin-D
calbindin-D9k
  vitamin D-dependent c.-D.
calcereous pancreatitis
Calcibind
Calcidrine syrup
calcification
  carbonate apatite c.
  dystrophic c.
  pancreatic c.
  tram-line c.
calcific pancreatitis
calcified
  c. enterolith
  c. gallstone
calciform cell
calcifying pancreatitis
Calcijex
calcinosis
  c. cutis, Raynaud phenomenon,
    esophageal motility disorder,
    sclerodactyly, and
    telangiectasia (CREST)
  c. cutis, Raynaud phenomenon,
    sclerodactyly, and
    telangiectasia (CRST)
calcite
calcitonin
  c. gene-related peptide (CGRP)
  serum c.
calcitriol
Calcitrol
calcium
  c. acetate
  c. antagonist
  c. ATPase pump
  c. bilirubinate stone
  c. carbonate
  c. carbonate and simethicone
  c. channel antagonist (CCA)
  c. channel blocker
  c. chloride
  c. concentration
  cytosolic c.
  c. electrolyte
  c. entry blocker
  exogenous c.
  extracellular c.
  c.-free dialysate
  c. gluconate

  c. hydrogen phosphate
  c. infusion test
  intracytoplasmic c.
  c. oxalate
  c. oxalate calculus
  c. oxalate dihydrate stone
  c. oxalate monohydrate stone
  c. oxalate nephrolithiasis
  c. oxalate stone
  c. oxaluria
  c. phosphate calculus
  plasma ionized c.
  c. stone
  c. supplementation
calcium-calmodulin complex
Calcivirus
calcoaceticus
  Acinetobacter c.
calculous
  c. cholecystitis
  c. cirrhosis
  c. formation
  c. gallbladder disease
calculus, gen. and pl. **calculi**
  alvine c.
  apatite c.
  biliary c.
  bladder c.
  blood c.
  branched c.
  calcium oxalate c.
  calcium phosphate c.
  caliceal diverticular c.
  carbonate apatite c.
  cat's eye c.
  cholesterol c.
  combination c.
  coral c.
  cystine c.
  decubitus c.
  dendritic c.
  c. disease
  encysted c.
  fusible c.
  gallbladder c.
  gastric c.
  hepatic c.
  impacted c.
  indigo c.
  infection c.
  intestinal c.
  matrix c.
  metabolic c.

midureteral c.
c. migration
mulberry c.
nephritic c.
nonstruvite c.
oxalate c.
pancreatic c.
pocketed c.
preputial c.
primary renal c.
prostatic c.
renal c.
secondary renal c.
staghorn c.
stomach c.
struvite c.
submucosal c.
uric acid c.
urinary c.
vesical c.
Volkmann spoon for
pancreatic c.
weddellite c.
whewellite c.
**Calcutript electrohydraulic
lithotriptor**
caldesmon
Calgocide disinfectant
calibrate
calibration of the cardia
calibrator serum
caliceal
c. diverticular calculus
c. diverticulum
c. extension
c. fornix
c. infundibulum
calicectasis
calicectomy
calices (*pl. of* calix)
Caliciviridae virus family
calicivirus gastroenteritis
calicoplasty
calicotomy
caliectasis, calycectasis, calyectasis
caliectomy, calycectomy
calioplasty, calycoplasty, calyoplasty

caliorrhaphy, calyorrhaphy
caliotomy, calycotomy, calyotomy
caliper
Lange skin-fold c.'s
calix, calyx, pl. **calices**
c. puncture
Call-Exner body
Calmette-Guérin
bacille C.-G. (BCG, bCG)
C.-G. bacillus
calmodulin
Calogen LCT emulsion
caloric
c. intake
c. supplement
calorie
high c. (HC)
calorimeter
Calot triangle
calponin
calretinin
Caluso PEG gastrostomy tube
calyceal
c. filling time
c. fistula
calycectasis (*var. of* caliectasis)
calycectomy (*var. of* caliectomy)
calycoplasty (*var. of* calioplasty)
calycotomy (*var. of* caliotomy)
calyectasis (*var. of* caliectasis)
calyoplasty (*var. of* calioplasty)
calyorrhaphy (*var. of* caliorrhaphy)
calyotomy (*var. of* caliotomy)
calyx (*var. of* calix)
Camalox
camera
c. adapter
Anger scintillation c.
cadmiumselenide-vidicon
video c.
charge-coupled device
monochrome c.
Circon-ACMI MicroDigital-I c.
endoscopic c.
FG-110 Fuginon c.
field-of-view c.

NOTES

camera *(continued)*
Fujinon FG-series
endoscopic c.
gamma c.
instant c.
motion picture c.
Olympus OM-series
endoscopic c.
Olympus OM-2 c. with SM-45
enlarging adapter
Olympus OTV-S-series
miniature c.
Olympus SCA-series
endoscopic c.
Pen-F half-frame c.
Pentax endoscopic c.
Polaroid c.
positron c.
γ-scintillation c.
single-lens reflex c.
still c.
television c.
Urocam video c.

Cameron
C. gastroscope
C. omni-angle gastroscope

Cameron-Miller
C.-M. electrocoagulation unit
C.-M. electrode
C.-M. monopolar probe
C.-M. suction-coagulator

Camey
C. enterocystoplasty
C. enterocystoplasty urinary
diversion
C. I, II operation
C. ileocystoplasty
C. neobladder
C. procedure
C. urinary pouch

cAMP
cyclic adenosine monophosphate
5′-cyclic adenosine monophosphate
vasopressin-induced cAMP

Campbell
C. sound
C. technique
C. trocar

Campy-BAP culture medium
Campylobacter
C. cinaedi
C. coli
C. colitis

C. enteritis
C. fetus
C. fetus colitis
C. fetus enteritis
C. hyointestinalis
C. jejuni
C. lari
C. pylori
C. pyloridis gastritis
C. test (CLOtest)
Campylobacter-**like**
C.-l. organism
C.-l. organism test (CLOtest)
Camwrap plastic covering
Canada-Cronkhite syndrome
canal
abdominal c.
Alcock c.
alimentary c.
anal c.
epidermoanal c.
femoral c.
c. of Hering
inguinal c.
c. of Nuck
pancreatobiliary c.
pleuroperitoneal c.
canalicular cholestasis
canaliculi
pili torti et c.
canaliculus, pl. **canaliculi**
bile duct c.
cancelling A's test
cancer
American Joint Committee on
Cancer/International Union
against C. (AJCC/UICC)
androgen-independent
prostate c.
bile duct c.
bladder c.
Borrmann gastric c.
breast c.
burned-out testis c.
colon c.
colorectal c. (CRC)
de novo liver c.
duodenal c.
esophageal c.
European Organization for
Research and Treatment
of C. (EORTC)
extrahepatic c.

extrahepatic bile duct c.
c. family syndrome
gastric c.
gastrointestinal c.
GI c.
hereditary nonpolyposis
  colorectal c. (HNPCC)
hypoechoic c.
hypopharyngeal c.
intraepithelial c.
intramucosal c.
Japanese classification of c.
liver c.
lung c.
metastatic c.
Mostofi grade prostate c.
mucin-producing c.
nonpolyposis colorectal c.
ovarian c.
pancreatic c. (PC)
pancreatoduodenal c.
polypoid c.
postgastrectomy c.
primary colorectal c. (PCRC)
prostate c. (PCa)
rectal c.
recurrent colorectal c. (RCRC)
restaging of c.
c. screening
squamous cell c.
staging of c.
suburothelial infiltrative c.
superficial bladder c.
teratoma testicular c.
testis c.
transplanted c.
urologic system c.
Whitmore classification
  prostate c.
cancer antigen 125 (CA-125)
cancer-associated sialyl-Lea antigen
cancerous erosion
Candela
  C. MDA-200 Lasertripter
  C. Miniscope
  C. MiniScope Plus

  C. Model MDL 2000 laser
  C. 405-nm pulsed dye laser
Candida
  C. albicans
  C. esophagitis
  C. glabrata
  C. immitis
  C. immunological study
  C. krusei
  C. neoformans
  C. peritonitis
  C. tropicalis
candidal
  c. cellulitis
  c. esophagitis
  c. infection
candidemia
candidiasis
  esophageal c. (EC)
  vulvovaginal c.
candidosis
canine
canister
  ATS c.
canker sore
cannula
  BILISYSTEM ERCP c.
  contour ERCP c.
  double-lumen irrigation c.
  ERCP c.
  Flexicath silicone subclavian c.
  Fluoro Tip ERCP c.
  Franklin-Silverman biopsy c.
  Hasson c.
  Hasson open laparoscopy c.
  Intraducer peritoneal c.
  laparoscopic c.
  large-bore c.
  Makler c.
  Mayo-Ochsner suction trocar c.
  Olympus monopolar c.
  perfusion c.
  polyethylene c.
  portal c.
  Ramirez Silastic c.
  Tandem XL triple-lumen
    ERCP c.

NOTES

C

cannula *(continued)*
    Teflon ERCP c.
    Veress c.
    washout c.
    c. with pre-loaded 0.35-inch
      guidewire
cannulation, cannulization
    bile duct c.
    biliary c.
    c. of the biliary tree
    c. catheter
    endoscopic retrograde c.
    endoscopic transpapillary c.
    ERCP c.
    ex vivo c.
    post-sphincterotomy ERCP c.
    retrograde c.
    selective c.
    selective ductal c.
    transpapillary c.
cannulatome
    Cotton c.
Can-Opt
    C.-O. dual lumen ERCP
      system
    C.-O. stand-alone dual lumen
      ERCP catheter
C-ANP
    C-type atrial natriuretic peptide
Cantil
Cantor tube
Cantwell-Ransley
    C.-R. epispadias repair
    C.-R. urethroplasty
CAP
    carcinoma of prostate
cap
    Coloplast Flange Mini c.'s
    ConvaTec Active Life
      stoma c.
    duodenal c.
    phrygian c.
    c. polyposis
    pyloric c.
    Sur-Fit Stoma c.
capacitive coupling
capacity
    bladder c.
    cystometric bladder c.
    fluid absorptive c.
    functional bladder c.
    galactose elimination c. (GEC)
    gastric c.

    maximum bladder c.
    maximum cystometric c.
    peritoneal membrane solute
      transport c.
    PMN oxidative burst c.
    pressure-specific bladder c.
    total iron binding c. (TIBC)
capacity-limited kinetics
CAPD
    chronic ambulatory peritoneal
      dialysis
    continuous ambulatory peritoneal
      dialysis
Cape Town technique
cap-fitted panendoscope
capillariasis
    intestinal c.
capillary
    c. dilation
    c. endothelial cell
    glomerular c.
    c. hyperfiltration
    c. network
    peritubular c.
    c. permeability
    c. refill
    C. System slide holder
    c. wall
capillary-leak phenomenon
capillary-lymphatic invasion
capistration
capita (*pl. of* caput)
capitis (*gen. of* caput)
capitonnage
Capmul 8210
capnography
capnometry
Capoten
Capozide
CAPS
    caffeine, alcohol, pepper, spicy
      foods
Caps
    ZE C.
capsaicin
CAPS-free diet
capsid-encoding region
capsular
    c. blood vessel
    c. cirrhosis of liver
    c. flap pyeloplasty
    c. penetration
    c. tear

capsulatum
    Histoplasma c.
capsule
    acidophilus c.
    Bowman c.
    Crosby c.
    enteric-coated c.
    c. flap technique
    Gerota c.
    Glisson c.
    hepatic c.
    liver c.
    Max-EPA c.'s
    pH-sensitive radiotelemetry c.
    polysaccharide c.
    prostatic c.
    pyxigraphic sampling c.
    radioisotope c.
    splenic c.
    Watson c.
capsulotomy
    renal c.
Captiflex polypectomy snare
Captivator polypectomy snare
captopril
    c. renography
    c. test
captopril-DTPA
    c.-D. scanning
caput, gen. **capitis**, pl. **capita**
    c. epididymis
    c. medusae
    c. pancreatis
Carafate
Cara-Klenz skin cleanser
carbachol
carbamazepine
    c. hepatotoxicity
carbamoyl phosphate synthetase deficiency
carbenicillin
carbenoxolone
carbidopa dopaminergic medication
carbohydrate
    c. antigen 19-9 (CA 19-9)
    c. antigen 19-9

    immunohistochemical expression
carbohydrate-induced hyperlipidemia
carbon
    c. dioxide insufflator
    c. dioxide laser
    c. dioxide laser plaque ablation
    c. dioxide trapping agent
    c. tetrachloride
    c. tetrachloride-induced liver regeneration
    c. 14 urea breath test
carbon-14 urinary excretion test
carbonate
    c. apatite
    c. apatite calcification
    c. apatite calculus
    c. apatite stone
    calcium c.
carbonic
    c. anhydrase (CA)
    c. anhydrase inhibitor (CAI)
carboplatin
carboprost tromethamine
Carbowax
carboxykinase
    phosphoenolpyruvate c. (PEPCK)
carboxypeptidase B-like enzyme
carboxy-terminal noncollagenous domain
carboxyterminal PTH
carbuncle
    kidney c.
    renal c.
carbuterol
carcinoembryonic antigen (CEA)
carcinogenesis
    colorectal c.
    oncogene-induced c.
carcinogenicity
carcinogenic nitrosamine
carcinoid
    bronchial c.
    duodenal c.
    c. flush

C

NOTES

carcinoid *(continued)*
 gastric c.
 gastroduodenal c.
 hindgut c.
 c. secretory granule
 c. syndrome
 c. tumor
**carcinoma, pl. carcinomas,
carcinomata**
 acinar cell c.
 adenoid cystic c.
 adenosquamous c.
 ampullary c.
 ampullopancreatic c.
 anorectal c.
 Astwood-Coller staging system
  for c.
 Barrett c.
 basal cell c.
 bile duct c.
 biliary c.
 bladder c.
 Borrmann Type IV
  scirrhous c.
 bulbar urethral c.
 bulbomembranous urethral
  squamous cell c.
 cervical c.
 cholangiocellular c. (CCC)
 cholangitis c.
 clear cell hepatocellular c.
 clear cell c. of kidney
 clear cell nonpapillary c.
 collecting duct c.
 colon c.
 colorectal c.
 Dukes classification of c.
 Edmondson grading system for
  hepatocellular c.
 embryonal testicular c.
 encapsulated renal cell c.
 encephaloid gastric c.
 endometrial c.
 epidermoid c.
 esophageal c.
 esophageal squamous cell c.
 excavated gastric c.
 fibrolamellar c.
 fibrolamellar hepatocellular c.
  (FL-HCC)
 flat c.
 gallbladder c.
 gastric c.

 genitourinary c.
 germ cell c.
 hepatocellular c. (HCC)
 hereditary nonpolyposis
  colorectal c.
 hilar c.
 intramucosal c.
 invasive c.
 islet cell c.
 large bowel c.
 laryngeal c.
 linitis plastica c.
 medullary thyroid c.
 metastatic c.
 metastatic prostatic c.
 metastatic renal cell c.
  (MRCC)
 microtrabecular hepatocellular c.
 mucinous c.
 mucoepidermoid c.
 mutated colorectal c. (MCC)
 non-germ cell c.
 nonseminomatous testicular c.
 oat cell c.
 obstructing c.
 oropharyngeal c.
 ovarian c.
 pancreatic c. (PCA)
 pancreatic acinar cell c.
 pancreatic islet cell c.
 papillary gastric c.
 papillary renal cell c.
 papillary transitional cell c.
 pediatric c.
 penile c.
 perforated c.
 periampullary c.
 polypoid c.
 primary transitional cell c.
 c. of prostate (CAP)
 prostatic c.
 prostatic urethral transitional
  cell c.
 rectal c.
 renal cell c. (RCC)
 renal medullary c.
 renal pelvic transitional cell c.
 sarcomatoid squamous cell c.
 scirrhous c.
 sclerosing hepatic c. (SHC)
 secondary metastatic c.
 sessile nodular c.
 sigmoid colon c.

signet-ring cell c.
c. in situ (CIS)
splenic flexure c.
squamous cell c. (SCC)
stage B c.
stage C c.
superficial esophageal c. (SEC)
superficial gastric c.
supraglottic squamous cell c.
testicular c.
TNM classification of c.
transitional cell c.
transthoracic resection of
  esophageal c.
tubular c.
ulcerating c.
unresectable hepatocellular c.
ureteral c.
urethral c.
urothelial c.
verrucous c.
vulvar c.
yolk sac c.
carcinomatosis
peritoneal c.
c. peritonei
carcinosarcoma
gastric c.
polypoid exophytic non-
  ulcerating c.
renal c.
cardia
achalasia c.
calibration of the c.
crescent gastric c.
patulous c.
c. of stomach
cardiac
c. antrum
c. beta-adrenoreceptor
  hyporesponsiveness
c. beta receptor
c. cirrhosis
c. decompression
c. impression on the liver
c. output/cardiac index (CO/CI)
c. sphincter

c. stomach
c. stomach mucosa
c. sympathovagal tone
cardiac-type
c.-t. gland
c.-t. mucosa
cardiectomy
cardinal suture
cardiochalasia
cardiodiosis
cardioesophageal
c. junction (CE)
c. mucosal junction
c. reflux
c. relaxation
c. sphincter
cardiofundic gastropathy
cardiohepatic
c. angle
c. triangle
cardiomegaly
cardiomyopathy
uremic c.
cardiomyotomy
Heller c.
cardioplasty
cardiopulmonary
c. baroreflex
c. baroreflex dysfunction
c. baroreflex function
c. complication
cardiopyloric axis
cardiorespiratory complication
cardiospasm
cardiotomy
cardiotoxicity
ipecac-induced c.
cardiovascular
c. complication
c. disorder
c. drug hepatotoxicity
Cardizem
Cardura
**Carey-Coons biliary endoprosthesis
  kit**
caribi
carina

C

NOTES

carinate abdomen
carinii
    Pneumocystis c.
carious teeth
Carle analytic gas chromatograph
Carmalt
    C. clamp
    C. forceps
    C. hemostat
C-arm fluoroscope
carminative
carmine
    contrast chromoscopy using
      indigo c. (CCIC)
    indigo c.
carmustine
Carnett sign
Carney complex
Caroid
Caroli
    C. disease
    C. syndrome
Caroli-Sarles classification
carotene
    serum c.
carotenemia
carotid bruits
Carpenter syndrome
carphenazine
Carrel
    C. aortic patch
    C. aortic patch anastomosis
carrier
    Deschamps ligature c.
    Endo-Assist disposable
      ligature c.
    gene c.
    Goldwasser suture c.
    hepatitis c.
    nongene c.
    Pereyra ligature c.
    Semb ligature c.
Carson
    C. internal/external
      endopyelotomy stent
    C. Zero Tip balloon dilation
      catheter
cart
    Fujinon video endoscopy c.
carteolol
Carter-Horsley-Hughes syndrome
cartilage
    arytenoid c.

cartridge
    Clark hemoperfusion c.
Cartrol
caruncle
    urethral c.
carvedilol
CAS
    Cell Analysis system
    CAS 200 image cytometer
cascade
    clotting c.
    fibrogenic c.
    intrarenal matrix-degrading
      enzyme c.
    MAP kinase signaling c.
    metastatic c.
    c. stomach
cascara
caseation
case-by-case approach
Casec
    C. calcium supplement
casei
    Lactobacillus c.
casein refeeding
CaSki cell line
Casodex
Casoni skin test
cast
    bacterial c.
    coarse granular c.
    esophageal c.
    fine granular c.
    granular c.
    hematin c.
    hyaline c.
    c. nephropathy
    proteinaceous c.
    red blood cell c.
    c. syndrome
    urinary c.
    white blood cell c.
Castleman
    C. disease
    C. tumor
cast-like tube
castor oil
castrate
castration
    functional c.
catabolism
catalase
Catapres

catarrhal
   c. gastritis
   c. jaundice
catecholamine
catecholamines
   urinary c.
catgut
   chromic c.
catharsis
cathartic
   c. colon
catheter
   Ablaser laser delivery c.
   Accurate c.
   Achiever balloon dilation c.
   acorn-tipped c.
   Acucise endopyelotomy c.
   Allis c.
   Amplatz c.
   angiographic end hole c.
   angiography c.
   angioplasty balloon c.
   Argyle Medicut R c.
   ARROWgard Blue
    hemodialysis c.
   arteriovenous c.
   aspiration c.
   Atlantic ileostomy c.
   Axxcess ureteral c.
   balloon dilating c.
   Bardex-Foley c.
   Bard gastrostomy c.
   bat-wing c.
   biliary balloon c.
   biliary dilator c.
   Bitome c.
   blood-contactin c.
   Blue Max balloon c.
   Bozeman-Fritsch c.
   Braasch c.
   Broviac c.
   brush c.
   BUD drainage c.
   bullet-tip c.
   Burhenne steerable c.
   cannulation c.

Can-Opt stand-alone dual
  lumen ERCP c.
Carson Zero Tip balloon
  dilation c.
central venous c.
Chemo-Port c.
cholangiocath c.
cholangiographic c.
Clay-Adams (PE-10, PE-50) c.
coaxial c.
cobra c.
coil c.
Coil-Cath c.
colon motility c.
combination biliary brush c.
cone-tip c.
conical c.
Cook TPN c.
Cope loop nephrostomy c.
coudé c.
Councill c.
Curl Cath c.
decompression c.
à demeure c.
Dent sleeve c.
de Pezzer c.
dilating c.
Dormia stone basket c.
double-J c.
double-lumen balloon c.
Dow-Corning ileal pouch c.
Dowd, Dowd II prostatic
  balloon dilatation c.
dual-lumen c.
Duo-Flow c.
eight-lumen esophageal
  manometry c.
elbowed c.
end-hole ureteral c.
endoscopic retrograde
  cholangiopancreatography c.
EndoSound endoscopic
  ultrasound c.
Entract c.
epidural c.
ERCP c.
esophageal motility perfused c.

C

NOTES

catheter *(continued)*
esophageal perfusion c.
exdwelling ureteral occlusion
    balloon c.
exit site of c.
external ureteral c.
Extractor three-lumen retrieval
    balloon c.
female c.
femoral hemodialysis c.
fiberoptic c.
Flexxicon II PC internal
    jugular c.
Fogarty c.
Fogarty balloon biliary c.
Fogarty irrigation c.
Foley c.
four-lumen polyvinyl
    manometric c.
French Cope loop
    nephrostomy c.
French mushroom tip c.
French pigtail nephrostomy c.
French Teflon pyeloureteral c.
Gauder Silicon PEG c.
Glidex coated Percuflex c.
Gold Probe Direct bipolar
    hemostasis c.
Gold Probe
    electrohemostasis c.
Gore-Tex c.
Gouley c.
Graham c.
Greenfield caval c.
Grüntzig balloon c., Grüntzig
    balloon c.
c. guide
guiding c.
Handi-Cath c. kit
Hemoject injection c.
Hickman c.
Hydromer grafted c.
hydrostatic balloon c.
indwelling c.
Inmed whistle tip urethral c.
intra-arterial chemotherapy c.
intracholedochal manometric c.
Intraducer peritoneal c.
intraductal imaging c.
Jackson-Pratt c.
Jelco c.
Konigsberg c.
Kumpe c.

large-bore c.
LeVeen c.
Lifemed c.
lumen-seeking c.
Mahurkar c.
male c.
Malecot reentry c.
Mallinckrodt c.
manometric c.
MaxForce TTS biliary balloon
    dilatation c.
MaxForce TTS high
    performance balloon
    dilatation c.
Medicut c.
Medina ileostomy c.
Medi-Tech bipolar c.
Memokath c.
Mentor straight c.
metal ball-tip c.
metallic-tip c.
Mewissen infusion c.
micro-tip sensor c.
Microvasive balloon c.
Millar c.
MiniBard c.
Missouri c.
MS Classique balloon
    dilatation c.
multifiber c.
multilumen manometric c.
mushroom c.
nasobiliary drainage c.
nasocystic c.
nasopancreatic c.
nasovesicular c.
needle tip c.
Nélaton c.
nephrostomy c.
10 o'clock selector c.
olive-tipped c.
Olympus PW-1L wash c.
open-ended ureteral c.
oral suction c.
Oreopoulos Zellerman c.
over-the-wire balloon c.
passage biliary dilatation c.
Passport Balloon-on-a-Wire
    dilatation c.
PE-MV balloon dilatation c.
Percuflex c.
percutaneous drainage c.
percutaneous femoral vein c.

percutaneous nephrostomy
  Malecot c.
percutaneous transhepatic biliary
  drainage c.
percutaneous transhepatic
  pigtail c.
peritoneal c.
peritoneal dialysis c.
PermCath dual lumen c.
Pezzer c.
Phantom 5 Plus ST balloon
  dilatation c.
Phillips c.
pigtail c.
polyethylene c.
polyurethane nasoenteric c.
Porges c.
portal c.
prostatic c.
pulse spray c.
pusher c.
pyeloureteral c.
Quinton c.
Quinton Mahurkar dual-lumen
  peritoneal c.
radiopaque ERCP c.
Ranfac c.
red rubber c.
red rubber Robinson c.
retrograde occlusion balloon c.
Rigiflex ABD balloon
  dilatation c.
Rigiflex biliary balloon
  dilatation c.
Rigiflex OTW balloon
  dilatation c.
Rigiflex TTS balloon
  dilatation c.
Ring c.
Robinson c.
Sacks QuickStick c.
Sacks Single-Step c.
self-retaining c.
shepherd's hook c.
Siegel-Cohen dilating c.
Silastic c.

silicone rubber Dacron-
  cuffed c.
silver c.
Simplastic c.
c. sinography
Soehendra dilating c.
solid-state esophageal
  manometry c.
Sonicath endoluminal
  ultrasound c.
spiral tip c.
Stamey Malecot c.
Stamey open tip ureteral c.
standard ERCP c.
stenting c.
subclavian c.
Supra-Foley c.
Surgitek c.
Swan-Ganz pulmonary artery c.
swan-neck c.
swan-neck Coil-Cath c.
swan-neck Missouri c.
swan-neck pediatric Coil-
  Cath c.
synthetic 5-channel, water-
  perfused motility c.
Tandem thin-shaft
  transureteroscopic balloon
  dilatation c.
tapered-tip hydrophilic-coated
  push c.
taper-tip c.
Teflon c.
Tenckhoff c.
Tenckhoff 2-cuff c.
Tenckhoff peritoneal c.
Texas style two-piece c.
three-way irrigating c.
Toronto-Western c.
Trabucco double balloon c.
Tracker c.
translumbar inferior vena
  cava c.
Tratner c.
Trilogy low profile balloon
  dilatation c.
triple-lumen manometry c.

NOTES

87

catheter *(continued)*
    c. tunnel infection
    Tyshak c.
    ureteral occlusion balloon c.
    Urocath external c.
    urodynamic c.
    UroMax II high-pressure
      balloon c.
    Uro-San Plus external c.
    van Sonnenberg gallbladder c.
    Von Andel dilating c.
    VTC biliary c.
    Vygon Nutricath S c.
    washing c.
    water-infusion esophageal
      manometry c.
    whistle-tip c.
    Willscher c.
    Wilson-Cook fine-needle-
      aspiration c.
    winged c.
    Witzel enterostomy c.
    Z-Med c.
catheter-associated bacteriuria
catheter-guided endoscopic
   intubation (CAGEIN)
catheterization
    clean intermittent c. (CIC)
    cystic duct c.
    in-and-out c.
    intermittent c.
    Seldinger cystic duct c.
    selective c.
    subclavian vein c.
    transnasal bile duct c.
    transpapillary c.
    umbilical vein c.
    ureteral c.
    urinary c.
catheterize
Cath-Secure
    C.-S. catheter holder
    C.-S. tape
cation
    c. exchange
    c. exchanger
    c. transport
cationic
    c. colloidal gold (CCG)
    c. dye
cationized ferritin
cat's eye calculus

cauda
    c. epididymis
    c. equina
    c. equina lesion
    c. equina syndrome
caudal
    c. block
    c. pancreaticojejunostomy
    c. regression syndrome
caudate
    c. lobe
    c. lobe of liver
caustic
    c. acid
    c. alkali
    c. colitis
    c. esophagitis
    c. ingestion
    c. substance
cauterization
cauterize
cautery
    c. bend
    BICAP c.
    blind c.
    endoscopic laser c.
    c. knife
    looped c.
    c. pencil
    snare c.
cava
    inferior vena c. (IVC)
    infrahepatic vena c.
    retrohepatic vena c.
    suprahepatic vena c.
    vena c.
caveola
cavernitis
    fibrous c.
cavernosal
    c. abscess
    c. alpha blockade
    c. alpha blockade technique
cavernositis
cavernosogram
cavernosometry
    dynamic infusion c.
    Menuel c.
cavernosonography
    dynamic infusion
      cavernosometry and c.
cavernosorum
    tunica albuginea corporum c.

cavernospongiosum shunt
cavernous
    c. autonomic nerve dysfunction
    c. fibrosis
    c. hemangioma
    c. nerve-sparing prostatectomy
    c. transformation of the portal
      vein (CTPV)
    c. vein
cavernovenous leakage
CAVH
    chronic active viral hepatitis
    continuous arteriovenous
      hemofiltration
CAVH-B
    chronic active viral hepatitis, type B
CAVH-NAB
    chronic active viral hepatitis, non-A,
      non-B
caviae
    Aeromonas c.
cavitation
    pulmonary c.
Cavitron Ultrasonic Surgical
  Aspirator (CUSA)
cavity
    abdominal c.
    intraperitoneal c.
    nephrotomic c.
    peritoneal c.
    retroperitoneal c.
cavography
    synchronous inferior c.
    synchronous superior c.
    vena c.
cavotomy
CAVU
    continuous arteriovenous
      ultrafiltration
CBC
    complete blood count
CBD
    common bile duct
      CBD 2 Choledochoscope
      CBD stone
CBDE
    common bile duct exploration

CBI
    continuous bladder irrigation
^{13}C-bicarbonate breath test
CBP
    copper-binding protein
      CBP test
CBS
    colloidal bismuth subcitrate
CC
    Adalat C.
CCA
    calcium channel antagonist
CCC
    cholangiocellular carcinoma
    cylindrical confronting cisterna
CCD
    charge-coupled device
    cortical collecting duct
      CCD perfusion
CCE
    cholesterol crystal embolization
CCFA
    Crohns and Colitis Foundation of
      America
CCG
    cationic colloidal gold
C-cholyl-glycine breath test
CCIC
    contrast chromoscopy using indigo
      carmine
CCK
    cholecystokinin
CCK-8
    cholecystokinin octapeptide
CCK-LI
    cholecystokinin-like
      immunoreactivity
CCK-OP
    cholecystokinin octapeptide
CCK-PZ
    cholecystokinin-pancreozymin
CCl4-induced cirrhosis
CCL-64 cell
CCNU
    chloroethyl-cyclohexyl-nitrosourea
      (Lomustine)

NOTES

CCNU *(continued)*
  Lomustine
    methyl CCNU
CCP
  chronic calcifying pancreatitis
  colitis cystica profunda
CCPD
  continuous cycling peritoneal
    dialysis
CD
  Clostridium difficile
  collecting duct
  Crohn disease
    CD activity index
CD2
CD3+
CD4+
    autologous HBcAg-specific
      CD4+
    CD4+ cell
    CD4+ T-cell count
CD4
    CD4 count
    CD4 lymphocyte count
    CD4 molecule
    CD4 phenotype
    CD4 T cell
CD8+
    CD8+ cell
    CD8+ T lymphocyte
CD8
    CD8 lymphocyte
    CD8 lymphocyte count
    CD8 molecule
    CD8 phenotype
CD20
    B-cell antigen CD20
CD29
CD45
CD14 monoclonal antibody
CD23 enterocyte
CD3+T cell
CDAD
  Clostridium difficile-associated
    diarrhea
CDAI
  Crohn disease activity index
CDC
  Centers for Disease Control
  complement-dependent cytotoxicity
  Crohn disease of colon
CDC42 protein

CDCA
  chenodeoxycholic acid
  choledococaval anastomosis
CD4+-CD8+ T-cell ratio
CDE
  common duct exploration
  cystine dimethylester
CDEIS
  Crohn Disease Endoscopic Index of
    Severity
cDNA
  complementary deoxyribonucleic
    acid
    HSP-70 cDNA
    cDNA probe
CD45RA
CD45RO
    CD45RO lymphocyte
CDS
  commercial dialysis solution
CD3– T cell receptor complex
CDY
  cystoduodenostomy
CE
  cardioesophageal junction
CE-24 needle
CEA
  carcinoembryonic antigen
    CEA test
cecal
    c. appendix
    c. colonoscopy
    c. fissure
    c. fold
    c. hernia
    c. homogenate
    c. imbrication procedure
    c. mucosal nodule
    c. serosa
    c. ulcer
    c. vascular ectasia
    c. volvulus
cecectomy
Cecil
    C. procedure
    C. urethroplasty
cecitis
Ceclor
cecocolic intussusception
cecocolostomy
cecocystoplasty
cecofixation
cecoileostomy

cecopexy
cecoplication
cecoproctostomy
cecorrhaphy
cecosigmoidostomy
cecostomy
    percutaneous catheter c.
    tube c.
cecotomy
cecoureterocele
cecum
    antimesocolic side of the c.
    coned c.
    cone-shaped c.
    watermelon c.
CEEA
    curved end-to-end anastomosis
    CEEA stapler
cefaclor
cefadroxil monohydrate
CE-FAST
    contrast-enhanced fast sequence
cefazolin
    c. sodium
cefoperazone
cefotaxime
Cefotetan disodium
cefoxitin
cefpirome
cefpodoxime
    c. proxetil
cefsulodin
Ceftin
ceftriaxone
    c. pseudolithiasis
    c. sodium
cefuroxime
cEGF
    concentration epidermal growth
    factor
celectome
Celestin
    C. dilator bougie
    C. endoprosthesis
    C. esophageal tube
    C. graduated dilator
    C. latex rubber tube

    C. prosthesis
    C. tube
celiac
    c. angiogram
    c. angiography
    c. axis
    c. lymph node
    c. plexus block
    c. plexus reflex
    c. rickets
    c. sprue
    c. sprue disease
    c. trunk
    c. tumor
celiagra
celiocentesis
celioenterotomy
celiogastrostomy
celiogastrotomy
celiomyalgia
celiomyomotomy
celioparacentesis
celiopathy
celiorrhaphy
celioscopy
celiotomy
    exploratory c.
    c. incision
cell
    absorptive c.
    acid c.
    acinar c.
    adelomorphous c.
    amine precursor uptake and
      decarboxylation c. (APUD
      cell)
    C. Analysis system (CAS)
    C. Analysis system 200 image
      cytometer
    antigen-presenting c.
    antral gastric c.
    APUD c.
      amine precursor uptake and
        decarboxylation cell
    argentaffin c.
    argyrophilic c.
    atypical ductular c.

NOTES

cell *(continued)*
    autologous liver c.
    B c.
    basal granular c.
    beaker c.
    bile duct epithelial c.
    blast c.
    bone marrow-derived B c.
    bone marrow stem c.
    border c.
    calciform c.
    capillary endothelial c.
    CCL-64 c.
    CD4+ c.
    CD8+ c.
    CD3+T c.
    CD4 T c.
    central c.
    centroacinar c.
    chalice c.
    chief c.
    chromogranin A-
      immunoreactive c.
    columnar-cuboidal
      adenocarcinoma c.
    crypt c.
    c. culture transwell
    cytotoxic T c.
    D c.
    Davidoff c.
    delomorphous c.
    dendritic reticular c.
    DNA haploid c.
    Dukes A, B, C, signet c.
    ECL c.
    endocrine c.
    endodermic c.
    endothelial c.
    enteric ganglion c.
    enterochromaffin c.
    enterochromaffin-like c.
    epithelial c. (EC)
    epithelial endocrine c.
    F9 c.
    fat c.
    fat-storing liver c.
    fetal liver-derived B c.
    flare c.
    foam c.
    G c.
    gastric pacemaker c.
    gastrin c.
    gastrin-secreting c.

    Gaucher c.
    giant c.
    glomerular contractile c.
    glomerular epithelial c.
    gluconeogenic-competent human
      proximal tubule c.
    goblet c.
    Grimelius-positive c.
    ground-glass c.
    GTL-16 gastric carcinoma c.
    HBV-specific T c.
    Heidenhain c.
    HeLa c.'s
    helper T c.
    hematopoietic c.
    HGF-stimulated renal
      epithelial c.
    histamine-producing mast c.
    hobnailed c.
    human cytotoxic T c.
    human intestinal epithelial c.
    IEL T c.
    IgA-producing c.
    IgG-producing c.
    intercalated c.
    interstitial c.
    interstitial mononuclear c.
    intestinal epithelial c. (IEL)
    islet c.
    Ito c.
    killer T c.
    Kulchitsky c.
    Kupffer c.
    L c.
    LAK c.
    lamina propria lymphoid c.
    Langerhans c.
    Langhans c.
    LE c.
    Leydig c.
    c. line
    lipid-laden clear c.
    littoral c.
    liver-deprived epithelial
      clonic c.
    LLC-PK1-FBPase+ c.
    LLCPK renal tubular c.
    lymphocyte-target c.
    lymphokine-activated killer c.
      (LAK cell)
    lymphomononuclear c.
    M c.
    mast c.

MDCK epithelial c.
c. membrane
c. membrane epithelial antigen
memory T c.
mesangial c. (MC)
MN c.
mucous neck c.
mucus-secreting c.
murine B16 c.
murine lymphoid c.
murine mesangial c. (MMC)
murine proximal tubule c.
myenteric ganglion c.
natural killer c.
c. necrosis
neuroendocrine c.
NK c.
non-alpha, non-beta pancreatic
  islet c.
non-antigen expressing target c.
noncleaved B c.
nonrosetted c.
nuclear-tagged c.
oat c.
OK c.
osteoclast-like giant c. (OCLG)
oxyntic c.
P c.
pacemaker c.
packed red blood c.'s
pale c.
pancreatic acinar c.
pancreatic islet c.
Paneth c.
PAP-HT25 c.
paracrine c.
parietal c.
peptic c.
peripheral blood
  mononuclear c. (PBMC)
peripheral T c.
phagocytic stellate c.
Pick c.
plasma c.
PMN c.
Pockel c.
polymorphonuclear c.

postreceptor signaling of
  parietal c.
PP-immunoreactive c.
primed c.
principal c. (PC)
proliferating c.
proliferating tubular c.
c. proliferation
ptyocrinous c.
pulpar c.
purified T c.
Q c.
rectal epithelial c.
red blood c. (RBC)
renal collecting duct c.
renal cortical tubule c.
renal epithelial c.
renal proximal tubular c.
renomedullary interstitial c.
S c.
C. Saver
Schwann c.
schwannian spindle c.
senescent c.
c. separation technique
serotonin c.
Sertoli-Leydig c.
signet-ring c.
silver c.
sinusoid-lining c.
small granule c.
C. Soft 2000 semen analyzer
C. Soft system
somatostatin c.
spillage of tumor c.'s
spindle c.
squamous c.
stellate c.
suppressor T c.
c. surface area
c. surface receptor
c. swelling
T c.
target c.
T effector c.
thymus-derived c.
trans-blotting c.

C

NOTES

cell *(continued)*
    transitional c.
    Trypan blue-stained c.
    tubular epithelial c.
    tumor c.
    undifferentiated c.
    units of packed red blood c.'s
     (UPRBC)
    vascular permeation of
     tumor c.
    vascular smooth muscle c.
     (VSMC)
    von Hanseman c.
    von Kupffer c.
    white blood c. (WBC)
    xanthoma c.
    XL1-Blue c.
    zymogenic c.
cell-cell
    c.-c. adhesion
    c.-c. contact
    c.-c. interaction
Cellcept
cell-mediated
    c.-m. arm
    c.-m. hepatic injury
    c.-m. immunity
    c.-m. immunohistological
     response
    c.-m. mechanism
    c.-m. suppression
cell-positive margin
cell-substratum
Cell-Track
cellular
    c. atypia
    c. differentiation
    c. enzyme
    c. immune response
    c. immunity
    c. infiltration
    c. peptide
    c. proliferation
cellules
cellulitis
    candidal c.
    vaginal cuff c.
cellulosae
    Cysticercus c.
cellulose-based membrane
celomic epithelium
celotomy
Celsius thermometer

cement
    Wacker Sil-Gel 604 silicone c.
center
    anospinal c.
    free-standing ambulatory
     surgical c.
    organized germinal c.
    pontine micturition c.
    rectovesical c.
    swallowing c.
    vomiting c.
centering balloon
Centers for Disease Control (CDC)
centigrade thermometer
centimeter
    joules per c. (J/cm)
centipoise
central
    c. adrenergic agent
    c. cell
    c. echogenicity
    c. hyaline sclerosis
    c. hyperalimentation
    c. necrosis
    c. nervous system (CNS)
    c. spot
    c. vagal nerve stimulation
    c. venous alimentation
    c. venous catheter
    c. venous pressure (CVP)
    c. venous pressure line
centrifugal pump
centrifugation
    Ficoll-Hypaque gradient c.
    Polyprep c.
centrifuged
centrilobular
    c. acidophilic necrosis
    c. cholestasis
    c. pancreatitis
    c. region of liver
centroacinar cell
Century bicarbonate dialysis control unit
cephalad traction
cephalexin
cephalin-cholesterol flocculation test
cephalosporin
    prophylactic c.
cephalothin
cephalo-trigonal technique
cephradine
Cephulac

cerclage
    McDonald c.
    Shirodkar cervical c.
cerebelloretinal
  hemangioblastomatosis
cerebral
    c. fluid shunt
    c. hemangioblastoma
    c. perfusion pressure (CPP)
cerebral-brain stem circuit
cerebral-sacral loop
cerebrohepatorenal syndrome
cerebrotendinous xanthomatosis
cerebrovascular complication
Cerespan
cereus
    Bacillus c.
Cerezyme
ceroid-laden macrophage
cerulein
    exogenous cholecystokinin
      or c.
ceruloplasmin
    serum c.
cerumen obstruction
cervical
    c. carcinoma
    c. discharge
    c. erosion
    c. esophagus
    c. friability
    c. inflammation
    c. intraepithelial neoplasia
      (CIN)
    c. irregularity
    c. lymphadenopathy
    c. motion tenderness
    c. polyp
    c. position
    c. spasm
    c. ulcer
    c. wart
cervicitis
    mucopurulent c.
CESD
    cholesterol ester storage disease
cesium

cesium-137 wire
Cestoda **tapeworm**
cestode
cestodiasis
Cetacaine
    C. topical anesthetic
CETP
    cholesterol ester transfer protein
cetrimidesuboptimal
cetyldimethylethyl ammonium
  bromide
CF
    cystic fibrosis
    CF epithelia
CF-HM
    C.-H. endoscope
    C.-H. fiberscope
    C.-H. magnifying colonoscope
CF-LB3R colonoscope
C-Flex
    C.-F. Amsterdam stent
    C.-F. ureteral stent
c-fos proto-oncogene
CFTR
    cystic fibrosis transmembrane
      conductance regulator
CFU
    colony forming unit
CF-UHM colonoscope
CF-UM3 echocolonoscope
Cβ gene
C-glycocholic acid breath test
CGM
    coffee-grounds material
cGMP
    cyclic guanosine monophosphate
    5'-cyclic guanosine monophosphate
cGMP-mediated relaxant
CGN
    chronic glomerulonephritis
CGRP
    calcitonin gene-related peptide
c-GVHD
    chronic graft-versus-host disease
CGY
    cystogastrostomy
cGy radiation measure

C

NOTES

CH
chronic hepatitis
CH-40 activated charcoal
Chaffin-Pratt drain
Chagas-Cruz disease
Chagas disease
Chagasic megaesophagus
chain
α_5-c.
α_4-c.
α_3-c.
beta c.
beta-1 c.
c. cystogram
food c.
J c.
kappa light c.
γ light c.
monoclonal light c.
obturator lymphatic c.
c. suture
sympathetic c.
chain-of-lakes
c.-o.-l. deformity
c.-o.-l. filling defect
c.-o.-l. sign
chain-terminating inhibitor
chair
Hausted all purpose c.
Vess c.
chalazion
chalice cell
challenge
c. diet
food c.
gluten c.
rectal gluten c.
solid bolus c.
chamber
deglutitive pharyngeal c.
Makler counting c.
Microcell c.
Ussing c.'s
chancre
chancroid
change
degenerative c.
enzyme c.
erosive prepyloric c.
fibrocystic c.
fractional weight c.
mesenchymal c.
orthostatic c.

pancreatic ductal
morphological c.
phlegmonous c.
postsurgical c.
segmental c.
sensorium c.
spatial c.
trophic c.
ultrastructural basket-weave c.
channel
biopsy c.
common c.
8-c. cross-sectional anal
sphincter probe
gastric c.
ligand-gated c.
lymph c.
Mitrofanoff catheterizable c.
pancreaticobiliary common c.
pyloric c.
Sonotrode c.
stoma-like c.
treatment c.
voltage-gated c.
characteristic
receiver-operating c. (ROC)
c-Ha-ras gene
Charcoaid
charcoal
activated c.
CH-40 activated c.
c. filter
c. hemoperfusion
hemoperfusion with c.
mitomycin adsorbed onto
activated c. (M-CH)
C. Plus
c. suspension
CharcoCaps
Charcodote
Charcot
C. cirrhosis
C. intermittent fever
C. triad
C. triangle
Chardonna-2
CHARGE
coloboma-heart disease-atresia
choanae-retarded growth-genital
ear abnormalities
CHARGE syndrome
charge
c. selectivity

charge-coupled
  c.-c. device (CCD)
  c.-c. device monochrome
    camera
Charrière scale
ChAT
  choline acetyl transferase
Chauffard point
Chauveau bacterium
Cheatle-Henry hernia
Cheatle slit
checklist
  Hopkins symptom c.
cheilosis
Chelsea-Eaton anal speculum
chemical
  c. anoxia
  c. cholecystitis
  cystogenic c.
  c. gastritis
  c. litholysis
  c. peritonitis
  c. prostatitis
  c. splanchnicectomy
chemical-induced esophagitis
chemically defined diet
chemiluminescence
  luminol-enhanced c.
chemise
  bouton en c.
chemistry
  phosphoramidite c.
chemoattractant
chemoembolization
chemolysis
  intrarenal c.
Chemo-Port catheter
chemoprophylaxis
  travelers' c.
chemoradiation therapy
chemoradiotherapy
chemoreceptor
chemosensitivity
chemosis
chemotactic
  c. factor
  c. peptide

chemotaxis
  c. of polymorphonuclear
    leukocytes
chemotherapeutic agent
  hepatotoxicity
chemotherapy
  adjuvant c.
  continuous infusion c.
  cytotoxic c.
  intraperitoneal c.
  intrathecal c.
  intravesical c.
  platinum-based consolidation c.
  polyantibiotic c.
chemotherapy-induced vomiting
Chenix
chenodeoxycholate
chenodeoxycholic acid (CDCA)
chenodiol
Chenofalk
Cherchevski disease
Cherney incision
Chernez incision
cherry
  c. angioma
  c. sponge
Cherry-Crandall method for testing
  serum lipase
cherry-red spot (CRS)
chest
  barrel c.
  flail c.
  c. pain
  c. tube
  c. tube scar
Chester-Winter procedure
Chevalier
  C. Jackson esophagoscope
  C. Jackson gastroscope
chevron incision
chew-and-spit test
CHF
  congenital hepatic fibrosis
CHI
  creatinine height index

C

NOTES

Chiari
   C. disease
   C. malformation
Chiba
   C. needle
   C. percutaneous cholangiogram
chief cell
Chilaiditi
   C. sign
   C. syndrome
child
   C. class A
   C. class A patient
   C. class B
   C. class B patient
   C. class C
   C. class C patient
   C. classification
   C. classification of liver
     disease
   C. C-minus patient
   C. criteria
   C. esophageal varices
     classification
   c. esophagoscope
   C. hepatic dysfunction
     classification
   C. intestinal forceps
   C. liver criterion
   C. liver disease classification
   C. pancreaticoduodenostomy
Child-Phillips
   C.-P. bowel plication
Child-Pugh
   C.-P. classification
   C.-P. criteria
   C.-P. score
children's
   c. coma scale
   C. Hospital intestinal forceps
Child-Turcotte classification (CTC)
chili bean pseudopolyp
chips
   prostatic c.
Chiron
   C. RIBA HCV test
   C. RIBA HCV test system
     second generation
Chi-square test
chiufa
Chlamydia
   C. *trachomatis*
   C. *trachomatis* infection

chlamydia urethritis
chlorambucil
chloramphenicol
chlorhydria
chloride
   adrenalin c.
   c. balance
   benzalkonium c. (BAC)
   bethanechol c.
   calcium c.
   choline c.
   c. electrolyte
   mercury c. (HgCl2)
   mivacurium c.
   oxybutynin c.
   potassium c. (KCl)
   sodium c.
   strontium-89 c.
   tetramethyl ammonium c.
   titanous c.
   tridihexethyl c.
chlorisondamine
chlormethazine
chlorodontia
chloroethyl-cyclohexyl-nitrosourea
   (Lomustine) (CCNU)
chloroform
   c. toxicity
chlorohydrate
   linsidomine c.
chloroma
   gastric c.
chloromyceth sodium succinate
chloroprocaine
chloroquine
   c. phosphate
chloroquine-induced damage
chlorothiazide
chlorpheniramine
chlorphenoxamine
chlorpromazine
chlorpromazine-induced cholestasis
chlorprothixene
chlorthalidone
chlorzoxazone toxicity
choana, pl. **choanae**
chocolate agar medium
CHOD-PAP cholesterol reagent
Cho/Dyonics two-portal endoscope
choking
   Heimlich maneuver for c.
cholagogic
cholagogue

cholaneresis
cholangeitis
cholangiectasis
cholangiocarcinoma
    metastatic c.
    peripheral c. (PCC)
    peripheral intrahepatic c.
    type III c.
cholangiocath catheter
cholangiocatheter
    cystic duct c.
    saline-filled c.
cholangiocellular carcinoma (CCC)
cholangiodysplastic pseudocirrhosis
cholangioenterostomy
cholangiofibroma
cholangiofibromatosis
cholangiogastrostomy
cholangiogram, cholangiography
    balloon c.
    Chiba percutaneous c.
    common duct c.
    contrast selective c.
    cystic duct c.
    endoscopic retrograde c.
    fine-needle percutaneous c.
    fine-needle transhepatic c.
    intraoperative c.
    intravenous c. (IVC)
    operative c.
    percutaneous transhepatic c.
      (PTHC)
    pernasal c.
    serial c.
    thin-needle percutaneous c.
    transgastric c.
    transhepatic c.
    T-tube c. (TTC)
cholangiographic
    c. catheter
    c. finding
cholangiography
    balloon occlusion c.
    direct c.
    drip infusion c. (DIC)
    endoscopic c.
    endoscopic retrograde c. (ERC)

    fine-needle transhepatic c.
    intravenous c. (IVC)
    percutaneous c.
    percutaneous transhepatic c.
      (PTC)
    retrograde c.
    transhepatic c. (TC, THC)
cholangiohepatitis
    Oriental c.
    recurrent pyogenic c. (RPC)
cholangiole
cholangiolitic
    c. cirrhosis
    c. hepatitis
cholangiolitis
cholangiopancreatography
    endoscopic retrograde c.
      (ERCP)
cholangiopancreatoscopy
    peroral c. (PCPS)
cholangiopathy
    eosinophilic c.
cholangiophytiasis
cholangioscope
    prototype c.
cholangioscopy
    intraductal c.
    percutaneous transhepatic c.
    peroral c. (PCS)
cholangiostomy
cholangiotomy
cholangiovenous
    c. communication
    c. reflux
cholangitic biliary cirrhosis
cholangitis
    acute obstructive c.
    acute obstructive suppurative c.
      (AOSC)
    acute suppurative c. (ASC)
    ascending c.
    bacterial c.
    c. carcinoma
    chronic nonsuppurative
      destructive c.
    fibrous obliterative c.
    granulomatous c.

C

NOTES

cholangitis *(continued)*
    idiopathic autoimmune c.
    intrahepatic sclerosing c.
    lymphoid c.
    nonsuppurative destructive c.
    pleomorphic destructive c.
    postendoscopic c.
    primary sclerosing c. (PSC)
    progressive suppurative c.
    pyogenic c.
    sclerosing c.
    secondary c.
    septic c.
    suppurative c.
    transient c.
    viral c.
cholascos
cholate
Cholebrine
    C. contrast medium
cholecystagogic
cholecystagogue
cholecystatony
cholecystectasia
cholecystectomy
    laparoscopic c. (LC)
    minilaparoscope c.
    prophylactic c.
    c. treatment
cholecystendysis
cholecystenteric fistula
cholecystenterostomy
cholecystenterotomy
cholecystitis
    acalculous c.
    acute c.
    acute acalculous c.
    calculous c.
    chemical c.
    chronic c.
    emphysematous c.
    erythromycin-induced c.
    follicular c.
    gangrenous c.
    gaseous c.
    perforated c.
    c. with cholelithiasis
    xanthogranulomatous c.
cholecystocholangiography
cholecystocholedochal fistula
cholecystocolonic fistula
cholecystocolostomy

cholecystoduodenal
    c. fistula
    c. ligament
cholecystoduodenocolic
    c. fistula
    c. fold
cholecystoduodenostomy
    Jenckel c.
cholecystoendoprosthesis
    endoscopic retrograde c. (ERCCE)
cholecystoenterostomy
cholecystogastrostomy
cholecystogram
    oral c. (OCG)
cholecystography
cholecystoileostomy
cholecystojejunostomy
cholecystokinetic
    c. food
cholecystokinin (CCK)
    c. octapeptide (CCK-8, CCK-OP)
    c. test
cholecystokinin-like immunoreactivity (CCK-LI)
cholecystokinin-pancreozymin (CCK-PZ)
cholecystolithiasis
cholecystolithotomy
    percutaneous c.
cholecystolithotripsy
cholecystomy
cholecystoparesis
cholecystopathy
cholecystopexy
cholecystorrhaphy
cholecystoscopy
    percutaneous transhepatic c.
cholecystostomy
    laparoscopy-guided subhepatic c.
    percutaneous c.
cholecystotomy
    transpapillary endoscopic c. (TEC)
cholecystoxeransis
choledochal
    c. basal pressure
    c. cyst
    c. cystorigin
    c. region
    c. sphincter

choledochectomy
choledochendysis
choledochiarctia
choledochocele
choledochocholedochostomy
choledochocolonic fistula
choledochocyst
choledochoduodenal
    c. area
    c. fistula
    c. fistulotomy
    c. junctional stenosis
choledochoduodenostomy
choledochoenteric fistula
choledochoenterostomy
choledochofiberoscopy
    T-tube tract c.
choledochofiberscope
    Olympus URF-P2 c.
choledochofiberscopic approach
choledochojejunostomy
    end-to-side c.
    loop c.
    retrocolic end-to-side c.
    Roux-en-Y c.
choledocholith
choledocholithiasis
choledocholithotomy
choledocholithotripsy,
    choledocholithotrity
choledochopancreatic ductal junction
choledochoplasty
choledochorrhaphy
choledochoscope
    Berci-Shore c.
    CBD 2 C.
    flexible fiberoptic c.
    Hopkins rod-lens system for
      rigid c.
    Machida c.
    Olympus CHF-P-series c.
    URF-P2 c.
choledochoscopic guidance
choledochoscopy
    Berci-Shore c.
    cystic duct c.
    jejunostomy tract c.

    operative c.
    postoperative c.
    T-tube tract c.
choledochostomy
choledochotomy
    c. incision
    longitudinal c.
choledococaval anastomosis (CDCA)
cholelith
cholelithiasis
    cholecystitis with c.
    cholesterol c.
    intrahepatic c.
    c. prevalence
cholelithic dyspepsia
cholelitholysis
cholelithoptysis
cholelithorrhea
cholelithotomy
cholelithotripsy, cholelithotrity
cholemesis
cholemia
    familial c.
    Gilbert c.
cholepathia
    c. spastica
choleperitoneum
cholera
    Asiatic c.
    c. morbus
    pancreatic c.
    c. sicca
    c. toxin
    c. toxin-induced diarrhea
cholerae
    Vibrio c.
choleraic
    c. diarrhea
choleresis
choleretic
    c. effect
cholerheic
choleriform
cholerigenic, cholerigenous
cholerine
choleroid
cholerrhagia

C

NOTES

cholerrhagic
cholescintigram
cholescintigraphy
cholestasia, cholestasis
cholestasis
    acute drug-induced c.
    benign recurrent intrahepatic c.
    canalicular c.
    centrilobular c.
    chlorpromazine-induced c.
    drug-induced c.
    estrogen-induced c.
    extrahepatic c.
    familial c.
    hepatocanalicular c.
    hepatocellular c.
    high-grade c.
    intrahepatic c.
    methyltestosterone-induced c.
    neonatal c.
    tolbutamide-induced c.
cholestatic
    c. hepatitis
    c. hypersensitivity
    c. jaundice
    c. liver disease
    c. reaction
    c. syndrome
    c. viral hepatitis
cholesteatoma
cholesterol
    c. calculus
    c. cholelithiasis
    c. crystal embolization (CCE)
    dietary c.
    c. embolism
    c. ester
    c. ester storage disease
    (CESD)
    c. ester transfer protein
    (CETP)
    high-density lipoprotein c.
    (HDL-C)
    low-density lipoprotein c.
    (LDL-C)
    c. monohydrate crystal
    c. polyp
    radioactive c.
    c. saturation index (CSI)
    serum c.
    c. stone
    very-low-density lipoprotein c.
    VLDL c.

cholesterol-cholesteroloxidase-phenol
    4-aminophenazone method
cholesterol-containing gallstone
cholesterolosis
    c. of gallbladder
    c. of mucosal surface
cholestyramine
    c. therapy
cholic
    c. acid (CA)
    c. acid clearance
cholicele
choline
    c. acetyl transferase (ChAT)
    c. chloride
    c. deficiency liver disease
    phosphatidyl c.
cholinergic
    c. innervation
    c. neuron
Cholografin contrast medium
chololith
chololithiasis
chololithic
cholorrhea
choloscopy
cholotriansene
chondrogenic differentiation
Chooz
chordee
choreoathetosis
choriocarcinoma
chorionic
chorista
choristoma
Christie gallbladder retractor
Christmas
    C. tree appearance of pancreas
    C. tree sign
Christopher-Williams overtube
chromaffin tissue
chromagranin A
chromatograph
    Carle analytic gas c.
    Quintron Microlyzer 12 c.
chromatography
    boronate affinity c.
    column c.
    gas c.
    gel filtration c.
    high-performance liquid c.
    (HPLC)
    high-pressure liquid c. (HPLC)

ion c.
solid-phase extraction c.
thin-layer c. (TLC)
Varian model 3600 gas c.
chromic
    c. catgut
    c. catgut suture
    c. gut suture
    c. suture
chromium
    51-c.-labeled
    ethylenediaminetetraacetate
    (^{51}Cr-EDTA)
chromocystoscopy
chromoendoscope
chromogen
chromogranin A-immunoreactive cell
chromophobe cell tumor
chromophore
    c. enhanced laser welding
chromoscopy
chromosomal abnormality
chromosome
    human c. 6
    Y c.
chronic
    c. active gastritis
    c. active hepatitis (CAH)
    c. active liver disease
    c. active viral hepatitis
    (CAVH)
    c. active viral hepatitis, non-A,
    non-B (CAVH-NAB)
    c. active viral hepatitis, type
    B (CAVH-B)
    c. aggressive hepatitis (CAH)
    c. alcoholic cirrhosis
    c. alcoholic pancreatitis
    c. ambulatory peritoneal
    dialysis (CAPD)
    c. anoplasty treatment
    c. appendicitis
    c. atrophic duodenitis
    c. atrophic gastritis (CAG)
    c. autoimmune hepatitis
    c. bacterial enteropathy
    c. calcifying pancreatitis (CCP)

c. cholecystitis
c. cholestatic liver disease
c. cicatrizing enteritis
c. cystic gastritis
c. diarrhea
c. diverticulitis
c. erosion
c. erosive gastritis
c. fibrosing hepatitis
c. follicular gastritis
c. functional constipation
c. functional gastrointestinal
symptom
c. functional symptomatology
c. gastritis
c. glomerular disease
c. glomerulonephritis (CGN)
c. graft-versus-host disease (c-GVHD)
c. hepatitis (CH)
c. hepatitis B
c. idiopathic constipation
c. idiopathic intestinal pseudo-obstruction (CIIP)
c. idiopathic jaundice
c. inflammatory disease
c. interstitial hepatitis
c. intestinal dysmotility (CID)
c. intestinal ischemic syndrome
c. intestinal pseudo-obstruction
syndrome
c. lead poisoning
c. liver disease
c. lobular hepatitis (CLH)
c. mercury poisoning
c. metabolic acidosis
c. nonsuppurative destructive
cholangitis
c. obstructive uropathy
c. pancreatitis (CP)
c. pancreatitis Kasugai
c. parenchymal liver disease
c. peptic esophagitis
c. persistent hepatitis (CPH)
c. progressive hepatitis
c. progressive tubulointerstitial
disease

C

NOTES

chronic *(continued)*
    c. prostatitis
    c. pyelonephritis
    c. regurgitation
    c. relapsing pancreatitis
    c. renal failure (CRF)
    c. sclerosing hyaline fibrosis
    c. superficial gastritis (CSG)
    c. transplant rejection
    c. tubular damage
    c. type B hepatitis
    c. ulcer
    c. ulcerative colitis (CUC)
    c. ulcerative proctitis
    c. viral hepatitis
chronically inflamed gallbladder
chronic-continuous type
chronobiological parameter
chronotropism
Chronulac
CHRP
    coagulation and hemostatic resection of the prostate
chyle
    c. cyst
chyli
    cisterna c.
chylifaction
chylifactive
chyliferous
    c. vessel
chylification
chyliform
    c. ascites
chylocele
    parasitic c.
chyloderma
chylomicron
    c. production
    c. retention disease
chyloperitoneum
chylophoric
chylopoiesis
chylopoietic disease
chylorrhea
chylosis
chylothorax
chylous
    c. ascites
    c. ascitic fluid
    c. leukemia
chyme
Chymex

chymification
chymobilia
    iatrogenic c.
chymopoiesis
chymorrhea
Ciba-Corning ACS PSA assay
CIC
    clean intermittent catheterization
cicatricial
    c. stricture
    c. tissue
cicatrix
cicatrization
CID
    chronic intestinal dysmotility
Cidex
    C. activated dialdehyde solution
    C. Plus solution
cigarette drain
cigar-shaped hyperchromatic nucleus
ciguatera
CIIP
    chronic idiopathic intestinal pseudo-obstruction
cimetidine
CIN
    cervical intraepithelial neoplasia
cinaedi
    Campylobacter c.
cinedefecogram
cinedefecography
cine-esophagogram
cine-esophagoscope
cine-esophagoscopy
cinefluorographic study
cinefluoroscopic method
cinegastroscopy
cineradiographic analysis
cineurography
Cinobac Pulvules
Cipro
ciprofloxacin
    c. hydrochloride
circadian
    c. gastric acidity
    c. periodicity
    c. rhythm
    c. rhythmicity
    c. testosterone pattern
circadian-shaped infusion
circinata
    balanitis c.

circinate balanitis
circle
  c. needle
  Pagenstecher c.
Circon-ACMI
  C.-ACMI lithotriptor
  C.-ACMI MicroDigital-I camera
  C.-ACMI (MR-6, MR-9)
    ureteroscope
  C.-ACMI uteroscope
circuit
  cerebral-brain stem c.
  enteric neuronal c.
  extracorporeal
    cardiopulmonary c.
circular
  c. dichroism
  c. muscle fibers
  c. myotomy
  c. stapler
  c. stapling device
  c. suture
  c. tape
circulares
  plicae c.
circulating
  c. autoantibody
  c. enzyme
  c. immunocomplexes
    immunological study
  c. tumor-associated antigen
circulation
  arterial c.
  collateral abdominal c.
  cutaneous collateral c.
  hepatic c.
  herpkinetic c.
  hyperdynamic c.
  mesenteric c.
  portal-collateral c.
  venous c.
circulatory embarrassment
circumcise
circumcised
circumcision
  Plastibell c.

  routine neonatal c.
  sleeve-type c.
circumductive
circumference
circumferential
  c. mucosal dissection
circumlocution
circum-umbilical incision
cirrhogenous, cirrhogenic
cirrhosis
  acholangic biliary c.
  alcoholic c.
  autoimmune c.
  biliary c.
  Budd c.
  calculous c.
  capsular c. of liver
  cardiac c.
  CCl4-induced c.
  Charcot c.
  cholangiolitic c.
  cholangitic biliary c.
  chronic alcoholic c.
  compensated c.
  CPH-CAH c.
  Cruveilhier-Baumgarten c.
  cryptogenic c.
  decompensated alcoholic c.
  drug-induced c.
  end-stage c.
  fatty c.
  fatty micromedionodular c.
  focal biliary c.
  frank c.
  glabrous c.
  Glisson c.
  Hanot c.
  hemochromatotic c.
  hepatic c.
  histologic c.
  hypertrophic c.
  incomplete c.
  juvenile c.
  Laënnec c.
  liver c. (LC)
  macronodular c.

NOTES

cirrhosis *(continued)*
    medionodular c.
    micromedionodular c.
    micronodular c.
    mixed c.
    necrotic c.
    nutritional c.
    obstructive biliary c.
    pigmentary c.
    pipe stem c.
    portal c.
    posthepatic c., posthepatitic c.
    postnecrotic c.
    primary biliary c. (PBC)
    progressive familial c.
    secondary biliary c.
    stasis c.
    c. of stomach
    syndrome of primary biliary c.
    Todd c.
    toxic c.
    type C c.
    unilobular c.
    vascular c.
cirrhotic
    c. ascites
    c. gastritis
    c. hydrothorax
    hypochlorhydric c.
    c. liver
    nonazotemic c.
    c. patient
cirsocele
cirsoid
cirsomphalos
CIS
    carcinoma in situ
cisapride
CISCA
    cisplatin, cyclophosphamide and
    Adriamycin
    CISCA protocol
cisplatin
    c. nephropathy (CPN)
cisplatin, cyclophosphamide and
    Adriamycin (CISCA)
cisplatin, methotrexate and Velban
    (CMV)
cisplatinum
cisplatinum-Lipiodol-Spongel (CLS)
cisterna
    c. chyli

cylindrical confronting c.
    (CCC)
CIT
    cold ischemia time
Citra Forte
citrate
    lead c.
    c. of magnesia
    magnesium c.
    piperazine c.
    potassium c.
    sodium c.
    c. synthase
    c. test
citric acid bladder mixture
Citrobacter
    C. amalonaticus
    C. diversus
    C. freundii
Citrotein liquid feeding
Citrucel
    C. sugar-free
citrulline
citrullinemia
c-jun proto-oncogene
C-lactose test
Claforan
Clagett
    C. Barrett esophagogastroscopy
    C. Barrett esophagogastrostomy
clam
    c. enterocystoplasty
    c. ileocystoplasty
clamp
    Adson c.
    Allen anastomosis c.
    Allen intestinal c.
    Allen-Kocher c.
    Allis c.
    approximator c.
    atraumatic c.
    Babcock c.
    Bainbridge intestinal c.
    Baumrucker urinary
      incontinence c.
    Best right-angle colon c.
    Bihrle dorsal c.
    Borge c.
    Buie c.
    Buie pile c.
    bulldog c.
    Carmalt c.
    Cope c.

Crile appendix c.
Crile hemostatic c.
Cunningham c.
Cunningham urinary
 incontinence c.
curved Mayo c.
Daniel colostomy c.
DeBakey c.
DeMartel appendix c.
DeMartel-Wolfson
 anastomosis c.
Dennis c.
Dixon-Thomas-Smith c.
Doyen intestinal c.
Earle hemorrhoid c.
Fehland intestinal c.
Foss intestinal c.
Furniss anastomosis c.
Furniss-Clute c.
Gant c.
Glassman c.
Goldblatt c.
Goldstein Microspike
 approximator c.
Haberer intestinal c.
Harvey Stone c.
Heaney c.
Herrick kidney c.
hilar c.
Hirschmann pile c.
Hurwitz esophageal c.
intestinal c.
Jarvis hemorrhoid c.
Jarvis pile c.
Kelly c.
Kelsey pile c.
kidney pedicle c.
Kleinschmidt appendectomy c.
Kocher c.
Lane intestinal c.
laparoscopic Allis c.
Linnartz intestinal c.
Linton tourniquet c.
Martel c.
Masters intestinal c.
Masters-Schwartz liver c.
Mayo abdominal c.

Mayo-Robson c.
Mayo-Robson intestinal c.
McCleery-Miller intestinal c.
McLean pile c.
Meeker gallbladder c.
Microspike approximator c.
microvascular c.
Mik c.
Mikulicz c.
Mixter c.
Mogen c.
mosquito hemostatic c.
Moynihan c.
noncrushing bowel c.
Nussbaum intestinal c.
occlusive c.
O'Hanlon intestinal c.
partial-occlusion c.
Payr pyloric c.
Péan c.
pedicle c.
Pemberton sigmoid c.
Pennington c.
Petz c.
Rankin c.
Redo intestinal c.
right-angle c.
Roosevelt c.
rubber-shod c.
Satinsky c.
Scudder intestinal c.
serrefine c.
Shoemaker intestinal c.
slotted nerve c.
Stetten intestinal c.
Stone-Holcombe intestinal c.
Stone intestinal c.
straight mosquito c.
Strelinger colon c.
tonsil c.
tubing c.
vascular c.
Wirthlin splenorenal c.
Wolfson intestinal c.
Wylie hypogastric c.
Zachary Cope-DeMartel c.

C

NOTES

clamp *(continued)*
    Zeppelin c.
    Zipser penile c.
clam-shell technique
clandestine intake
clapotage, clapotement
clarithromycin
    c. triple therapy
Clarke-Hadfield syndrome
Clarke-Reich knot pusher
Clark hemoperfusion cartridge
class
    c. I antigen
    c. II antigen
    C. II MHC molecule
    C. I MHC molecule
Classen-Demling papillotome
classic achalasia
classification
    AJCC TNM tumor c.
    Anderson c.
    Ann Arbor c.
    Astler-Coller c. (A, B1, B2, C1, C2)
    Banff c.
    bismuth benign bile duct stricture c.
    Borrmann gastric cancer c.
    Bosniak c.
    Caroli-Sarles c.
    Child c.
    Child esophageal varices c.
    Child hepatic dysfunction c.
    Child liver disease c.
    Child-Pugh c.
    Child-Turcotte c. (CTC)
    Correa c.
    Couinaud c.
    Dagradi esophageal variceal c.
    Dubin-Amelar varicocele c.
    Dukes c. of carcinoma
    gastric mucosal pattern c.
    Japanese cancer c.
    Kasugai c.
    Kelami c.
    Lauren gastric carcinoma c.
    Lukes-Collins c.
    Marseille c.
    Marseille pancreatitis c.
    McNeer c.
    Ming gastric carcinoma c.
    Pugh c.
    Ranson acute pancreatitis c.

    Rappaport c.
    Santiani-Stone c.
    Siurala c.
    Solcia c.
    Sonnenberg c.
    Sydney system gastritis c.
    c. system
    TNM carcinoma c.
    UICC tumor c.
    Visick dysphagia c.
    Whitehead c.
    WHO gastric carcinoma c.
clathrin-coated pit
claudication
Clave needleless system
claw forceps
Clay-Adams
    C.-A. (PE-10, PE-50) catheter
Claybrook sign
clay-colored stool
cleaner
    Endozime AW bacteriostatic enzyme c.
cleaning
    diathermic c.
clean intermittent catheterization (CIC)
cleanser
    Cara-Klenz skin c.
    Rediwash skin c.
    UltraKlenz skin c.
cleansing hypertonic phosphate enema
clear
    c. bile
    c. cell adenocarcinoma
    c. cell carcinoma of kidney
    c. cell hepatocellular carcinoma
    c. cell nonpapillary carcinoma
    c. cell sarcoma
    c. discharge
    enemas until c.
    c. liquid diet
clearance
    aminopyrine c.
    antipyrine c.
    caffeine c.
    cholic acid c.
    creatinine c. (Crcl)
    dextran c.
    fractional c.
    hepatic c.
    ^{125}I iothalamate c.

immunoglobulin G c.
inulin c.
iothalamate c.
kidney c.
lithium c. (CLi)
mucociliary c.
PAH c.
plasma c.
theophylline c.
clearing
esophageal c.
cleavage
bacterial c.
embryonic c.
c. plane
cleaved extracellular domain
cleft palate
Cleocin
Cleveland Clinic weighted scale of endoscopic procedures
CLH
chronic lobular hepatitis
CLi
lithium clearance
click
intermittent c.
prosthetic valve c.
systolic c.
clidinium
CLIM computer program
clindamycin
Clindex
clinical
c. hypergastrinemia
c. monitoring
c. parameter
c. protocol
c. trial
clinicobiological criteria
clinicopathological
clinicopathologic staging
Clinifeed Iso enteral feeding
Clinitest-negative stool
Clinitest-positive stool
Clinitest stool test
Clinoril
Clinoxide

clip
absorbable c.
Heifitz c.
Hulka c.
laparoscopic tie c.
metal c.
silver c.
titanium c.
towel c.
Weck c.
Clipoxide
clitoral recession
clitoris
bifid c.
clitoroplasty
clitorovaginoplasty
cloaca
cloacae
Enterobacter c.
cloacal
c. exstrophy
c. malformation
c. membrane
c. plate
c. remnant
cloacogenic polyp
CLO biopsy
Clomid
clomipramine
clonality
clonazepam
clone
Gliadin-specific T-cell c.
clonic contraction
clonidine
c. suppression test
cloning
molecular c.
clonogenic repopulation
clonorchiasis
biliary c.
clonorchiosis
Clonorchis sinensis
clonus
left-sided c.
right-sided c.

C

NOTES

C-loop
>duodenal C.-l.
>C.-l. of duodenum

Cloquet
>C. hernia
>node of C.

clorazepate dipotassium
clortermine
closed
>c. afferent loop
>c. colon
>c. drainage
>c. duodenum
>c. efferent loop
>c. esophagus
>c. hemorrhoidectomy
>c. injury
>c. pylorus
>c. suction drain
>c. tubule fixation technique

closed-end ostomy pouch
closed-loop intestinal obstruction
close suction drainage system
closing pressure
Clostoban
Clostridium
>C. botulinum
>C. butyricum
>C. cadaveris
>C. difficile (CD)
>C. difficile-associated diarrhea (CDAD)
>C. difficile enterotoxin
>C. difficile toxin assay
>C. fallax
>C. perfringens
>C. ramosum
>C. tertium
>C. welchii

closure
>Beta-Cap catheter c.
>Beta-Cap II c.
>exstrophy c.
>Graham c.
>ileostomy c.
>muscularis tunnel c.
>primary c.
>secondary c.
>Smead-Jones c.
>sutureless colostomy c.
>wound c.

clot
>adherent c.
>black c.
>blood c.
>fresh c.
>intraluminal c.
>non-adherent c.
>overlying c.
>sentinel c.

CLOtest
>*Campylobacter*-like organism test
>*Campylobacter* test

clot-induced urinary tract obstruction
clotrimazole
clotted blood
clotting
>c. abnormality
>c. cascade
>c. factor
>c. parameter
>c. time

cloud
>c. phenomenon
>plasma c.

cloudy
>c. ascites
>c. bile
>c. fluid

cloverleaf
>c. deformity
>C. internal bumper

cloxacillin-induced cholestatic jaundice
CLS
>cisplatinum-Lipiodol-Spongel

clubbed
>c. finger
>c. penis

clubbing
>finger c.

clustered
>c. jejunal waves
>c. waves (CW)

clusterin
>c. mRNA

clysis
clysma
clyster
CM1 polyclonal antibody
c-met
>c.-m. oncogene
>c.-m. receptor

CMG
>cystometrogram

c-mount adapter
CMV
    cisplatin, methotrexate and Velban
    cytomegalovirus
        CMV esophagitis
        CMV inclusion body
        CMV inclusion cyst
        CMV infection
CMV-associated ulceration
CMV-induced esophageal ulceration
CMV-related ulcer
c-myc
    c-m. oncogene
    c-m. proto-oncogene
CNDI
    congenital nephrogenic diabetes
      insipidus
CNNA
    culture-negative neutrocytic ascites
CNS
    central nervous system
CO$_2$
    CO$_2$ breath test
    CO$_2$ electrolyte
    CO$_2$ laser
    CO$_2$ laser probe
CoA
    coenzyme A
coag
    c. waveform
    c. waveform desiccation
coagulase-negative *Staphylococcus*
coagulating
    c. current
    c. electrode
    c. forceps
coagulation
    argon beam c.
    BICAP c.
    bipolar c.
    Bipolar Circumactive Probe c.
    blood c.
    Bovie c.
    disseminated intravascular c.
      (DIC)
    endoscopic microwave c.
    free-beam c.

    heater probe c.
    c. and hemostatic resection of
      the prostate (CHRP)
    infrared c.
    microwave c.
    monopolar c.
    multipolar c.
    c. necrosis
    c. probe
    c. time
    tissue c.
coagulative laser therapy
coagulator
    argon beam c.
    infrared c.
    Redfield infrared c.
coagulopathy
    iatrogenic c.
    c. pancreatitis
coagulum pyelolithotomy
coalesce
coalescence
coalescent ulcer
Coalition
    Digestive Disease National C.
      (DDNC)
coarctation
coarse
    c. granular cast
    c. nodularity
coat
    fibromuscular c.
coaxial
    c. catheter
    c. snare
cobalamin deficiency
cobalt-60
Coban dressing
cobblestone
    c. mucosa
    c. pattern
    c. pattern of hepatocyte
cobblestone-like
    c.-l. appearance
    c.-l. monolayer
cobblestoning
    c. of colon

C

NOTES

cobblestoning *(continued)*
  c. of mucosa
  c. sign
Cobb-Ragbe needle
Cobe
  C. Centrysystem dialyzer 400
  HG
  C. staple gun
  C. stapler
^{57}**Co B**$_{12}$ **excretion**
cobra
  c. catheter
  c. venom factor (CVF)
cocaine
  c. hepatotoxicity
  c. package ingestion
cocarcinogenic
  c. FBA
  c. fecal bile acid
coccidian
  c. body
  c. genus Cyclospora
  c. sporulation
  unsporulated c.
coccidian-like
coccidioidal peritonitis
Coccidioides immitis **peritonitis**
coccidiosis
coccygeal fistula
Cochin China diarrhea
Cochran-Mantel-Haenszel test
CO/CI
  cardiac output/cardiac index
Cockroft method
cocktail
  GI c.
  lytic c.
CO$_2$-CO$_2$ abundance ratio
coculture system
CODAS software
codon
  premature stop c.
coefficient
  glomerular ultrafiltration c.
  prostatic pressure c. (PPC)
  ultrafiltration c.
  c. of variation
coeliac disease
coelioscopy
coenzyme A (CoA)
coffee-grounds
  c.-g. emesis

c.-g. material (CGM)
c.-g. vomitus
Coffey
  C. technique
  C. ureterointestinal anastomosis
Cogentin
cognition
Cohen
  C. antireflux procedure
  C. cross-trigonal reimplantation
  C. cross-trigonal technique
  C. syndrome
  C. test
coherent
  c. bundle
  C. Model 90-K laser
coil
  c. catheter
  coiled c.
  endoprostatic c.
  endorectal-pelvic phased-
  array c.
  Gianturco c.
  Helmholtz double-surface c.
  intraurethral c.
  pelvic phased-array c. (PPA)
  secretory c.
  spring wire c.
  c. stent
Coil-Cath catheter
coiled
  c. coil
  c. coil motif
coincubation
  sperm immunobead c.
coit
  faux pas de c.
COL4A3 gene
COL4A4 gene
COL4A5 gene
colacalize
Colace
colchicine
cold
  c. biopsy
  c. biopsy forceps
  c. cup biopsy
  c. defect
  c. flushing
  c. forceps ablation
  c. ischemia time (CIT)
  c. knife
  c. knife endoureterotomy

c. knife hook
c. scissors
c. snare ablation
c. snare excision
C. Spor disinfectant
c. spot
c. storage
cold-cup resection
cold-stress test
colectasia
colectomy
abdominal c.
laparoscopic c.
subtotal c.
total abdominal c. (TAC)
transverse c.
c. ulcerative colitis
coleoptosis
Cole sign
Coley toxins
coli
Campylobacter c.
enteroadherent *Escherichia c.*
(EAEC)
enteroaggregative *Escherichia c.*
enterohemorrhagic
Escherichia c. (EHEC)
enteroinvasive *Escherichia c.*
(EIEC)
enteropathogenic *Escherichia c.*
(EPEC)
enterotoxigenic *Escherichia c.*
(ETEC)
Escherichia c.
tenia c.
coli
adenomatous polyposis c.
(APC)
aquatosis c.
familial polyposis c. (FPC)
juvenile polyposis c.
melanosis c.
pneumatosis c.
pneumatosis cystoides c.
polyposis c.
colibacillosis

colic
appendicular c.
c. artery
biliary c.
copper c.
Devonshire c.
episodic c.
esophageal c.
gallstone c.
gastric c.
hepatic c.
c. impression
c. impression on the liver
infantile c.
intestinal c.
lead c.
multiple recurrent renal c.
c. omentum
painter's c.
pancreatic c.
c. patch
c. patch esophagoplasty
pseudoesophageal c.
renal c.
saturnine c.
ureteral c.
uterine c.
vermicular c.
zinc c.
colicky
c. abdominal pain
colicoplegia
coliform
c. bacillus
c. bacterium
c. urinary infection
coliforms
colipase
colipuncture
colistimethate
colistin
colitis
acute infectious c.
acute self-limited c. (ASLC)
adenovirus c.
allergic c.
amebic c.

C

NOTES

113

colitis *(continued)*
antibiotic-associated c. (AAC)
bacterial c.
Balantidium coli c.
Behçet c.
Campylobacter c.
Campylobacter fetus c.
caustic c.
chronic ulcerative c. (CUC)
colectomy ulcerative c.
collagenous c.
Crohn c.
c. cystica profunda (CCP)
c. cystica superficialis
cytomegalovirus c.
diabetic c.
diversion c.
familial ulcerative c.
focal c.
fulminant c.
fulminating ulcerative c.
gangrenous ischemic c.
granulomatous transmural c.
c. gravis
hemorrhagic c.
iatrogenic c.
idiopathic c.
infectious c.
inflammatory c.
intractable ulcerative c.
ischemic c.
left-sided c.
lymphocytic c.
microscopic c.
milk-sensitive c.
mucosal ulcerative c. (MUC)
mucous c.
myxomembranous c.
necrotic hemorrhagic c.
nonantibiotic c.
nonspecific c.
pantothenic acid deficiency-
induced c.
c. perineal complication
Peroxynitrite-induced c.
progesterone-associated c.
pseudomembranous c. (PMC)
radiation-induced c.
Salmonella c.
segmental ischemic c.
Shigella c.
single-stripe c. (SSC)
toxic c.

transmural c.
ulcerative c. (UC)
uremic c.
viral c.
Yersinia enterocolitica c.
collagen
alpha-2-beta-1 integrin cell-
surface c. ($\alpha_2\beta_1$)
c. deposition
glutaraldehyde cross-linked c.
(GAX)
c. injection
c. maturation
c. synthesis
c. synthesis inhibitor
type III c.
type IV c.
c. vascular disease
collagenase
collagenous
c. colitis
c. sprue
collapsible tube hydrodynamics
collapsing glomerulopathy
collar
polyglycolic acid c.
preputial c.
collar-button
c.-b. appearance in colon
c.-b. ulceration
collar-button-like ulcer
collateral
c. abdominal circulation
vasodilation of portasystemic c.
collecting
c. duct (CD)
c. duct carcinoma
c. system
c. tubule
c. venule
collection
American type culture c.
duodenal fluid c.
encysted intra-abdominal c.
24-hour urine c.
perinephric fluid c.
pus c.
quantitative stool c.
c. system
collector
Grass force displacement
fluid c.

Misstique female external
urinary c.
Colles fascia
colli
cystitis c.
collimator
high sensitivity c.
Collin
C. abdominal retractor
C. knife
C. mesher
Collings electrosurgery knife
Collins
C. indigo carmine solution
C. intestinal forceps
C. intestinal retractor
C. intracellular electrolyte
solution
C. solution
colliquative diarrhea
Collis
C. antireflux operation
C. gastroplasty
C. repair
colloid
c. osmotic pressure
c. shift on liver-spleen scan
sulfur c. (SC)
^{99m}Tc albumin c.
Tc-sulfur c.
^{99m}Tc tin c.
technetium-99m Tc-99m tin
colloid
technetium-99m sulfur c.
(^{99m}Tc-SC)
technetium-99m Tc-99m tin c.
(^{99m}Tc tin colloid)
colloidal
c. bismuth subcitrate (CBS)
c. bismuth suspension
c. oatmeal
c. thorium
colloid-producing adenocarcinoma
collum glandis
Colly-Seal wafer-type skin barrier
coloanal anastomosis (CAA)
coloboma-heart disease-atresia

**choanae-retarded growth-genital
ear abnormalities (CHARGE)**
colobronchial fistula
colocalization
colocentesis
colocholecystostomy
colocolic
c. intussusception
colocolonic anastomosis
colocolostomy
colocutaneous fistula
colocystoplasty
seromuscular c.
coloenteritis
cologastrocutaneous fistula
Cologel
colohepatopexy
coloileal fistula
cololysis
colon
aganglionic segment of c.
ascending c.
c. cancer
c. cancer screening
c. carcinoma
cathartic c.
closed c.
cobblestoning of c.
collar-button appearance in c.
c. conduit
coned-down appearance of c.
Crohn disease of c. (CDC)
c. cut-off sign
descending c.
distal c.
foreshortening of the c.
giant c.
hepatic flexure of c.
hypoganglionosis of c.
iliac c.
c. impression
c. incarceration
institutional c.
irritable c.
knuckle of c.
lateral reflection of c.
c. lavage cytology

NOTES

colon *(continued)*
    lead-pipe c.
    left c.
    loops of redundant c.
    mesenteric attachments of c.
    mesosigmoid c.
    midsigmoid c.
    c. motility
    c. motility catheter
    pelvic c.
    perforation of c.
    perisigmoid c.
    c. procedure
    rectosigmoid c.
    c. resection
    right c.
    saccular c.
    sigmoid c.
    spastic c.
    spiculations on c.
    spike burst on electromyogram
      of c.
    toxic dilation of c.
    transverse c.
    c. tumor cell lysis
colonalgia
colonic
    c. adenocarcinoma
    c. adenoma
    c. arterial spider
    c. bacterium
    c. dilation
    c. distention
    c. diverticulosis
    c. diverticulum
    c. electromyogram
    c. epithelial proliferation
    c. explosion
    c. fistula
    c. foreign body
    c. gas
    c. hemorrhage
    c. hyperalgesia
    c. ileus
    c. inertia
    c. infiltration
    c. interposition
    c. ischemia
    c. J-pouch
    c. lavage
    c. lavage solution
    c. lesion
    c. lesion identification

    c. lipoma
    c. loop
    c. lymphoid nodule
    c. mass
    c. metastasis
    c. microflora
    c. motility
    c. mucosal line
    c. mucosal pattern
    c. mucosal surface
    c. myenteric plexus
    c. necrosis
    c. neoplasia
    c. nodular lymphoid
      hyperplasia
    c. obstruction
    c. patch
    c. perforation
    c. permeability
    c. pit
    c. pitting
    c. polyp
    c. polyposis
    c. prostaglandins
    c. pseudo-obstruction
    c. pseudo-obstruction syndrome
    c. solitary ulcer syndrome
    c. tattoo
    c. transabdominal sonography
      (CTAS)
    c. transit study
    c. transit test
    c. transit time
    c. tuberculosis
    c. ulcer
    c. varix
    c. vascular lesion
    c. villus
    c. volvulus
    c. wall
colonization
    gut c.
Colonlite
    C. bowel prep
colonofiberscope
    Olympus CG-P-series c.
colonopathy
colonorrhagia
colonorrhea
colonoscope
    ACMI fiberoptic c.
    CF-HM magnifying c.
    CF-LB3R c.

CF-UHM c.
FCS-ML II c.
fiberoptic c.
forward-viewing video c.
Fujinon EC7-CM2 video c.
Fujinon EVC-M video c.
magnifying c.
Olympus CF-HM-series
  magnifying c.
Olympus CF-MB-series c.
Olympus CF-PL-series c.
Olympus CF-TL-series forward-
  viewing video c.
Olympus CF-T-series c.
Olympus CF-TVL-series c.
Olympus CF-UHM-series c.
Olympus CF-UM-series c.
Olympus CF-VL-series c.
Olympus CV-series c.
Olympus EVIS video c.
Olympus PCF-series
  pediatric c.
pediatric c.
Pentax FC-series c.
standard c.
Toshiba TCE-M-series c.
video c.
Welch Allyn video c. 8451
colonoscopic
  c. appendectomy
  c. biopsy
  c. decompression
  c. diagnosis
  c. disimpaction
  c. polypectomy
  c. removal
  c. tattoo
colonoscopy
  cecal c.
  c. complication
  diagnostic c.
  emergency c.
  high-magnification c.
  pediatric c.
  c. screening
  splenic flexure c.
  tandem c. (TC)

  therapeutic c.
  total c.
  upper endoscopy and c.
colonoscopy-related
  c.-r. emphysema
  c.-r. incarceration
colonostomy
colony forming unit (CFU)
colony-stimulating factor-1 (CSF-1)
colopathy
colopexostomy
colopexotomy
colopexy
Colopinto transjugular needle
Coloplast
  C. Flange Mini caps
  C. Flange pouch
  C. mini pouch
  C. ostomy irrigation set
  C. skin barrier
coloplasty pouch
coloplication
coloproctia
coloproctitis
coloproctology
coloproctostomy
coloptosis, coloptosia
colopuncture
color
  c. Doppler ultrasonography
  c. flow Doppler
  stool c.
color-coded
  c.-c. Doppler sonography
  c.-c. duplex sonography
colorectal
  c. adenocarcinoma
  c. biopsy
  c. bleeding
  c. cancer (CRC)
  c. cancer syndrome
  c. carcinogenesis
  c. carcinoma
  c. disease
  c. endometriosis
  c. lymphoma
  c. mucosa

NOTES

colorectal *(continued)*
   c. neoplasm
   c. physiologic dysfunction
   c. physiologic study
   c. polyp
   c. snare
   c. stricture
   c. surgery
   c. trauma
   c. ulcer
   c. villous adenoma
colorectostomy
colorectum
colorrhagia
colorrhaphy
colorrhea
coloscopy
Coloscreen
   C. Self-test
   C. VPI
Coloshield
colosigmoidostomy
colosigmoid resection
colostomy
   c. bag
   c. bridge
   continent c.
   decompression c.
   descending loop c.
   Devine c.
   diverting c.
   diverting loop c.
   divided-stoma c.
   double-barrel c.
   dry c.
   end c.
   end-loop c.
   end-sigmoid c.
   exteriorization c.
   Hartmann c.
   ileoascending c.
   ileosigmoid c.
   ileotransverse c.
   irrigation of c.
   juxta-anal c.
   loop transverse c.
   Mikulicz c.
   permanent end c.
   c. pyloric autotransplantation
   resective c.
   c. rod
   sigmoid-end c.
   sigmoid-loop rod c.

   c. soiling
   takedown of c.
   c. takedown
   temporary end c.
   terminal c.
   transverse-loop rod c.
   Turnbull c.
   wet c.
colosuspension
   Stamey c.
colotomy
colovaginal fistula
colovesical fistula
colpocleisis
   Latzko partial c.
colpocystocele
colpocystotomy
colpocystoureterotomy
colpogram
colporectopexy
colposuspension
   Burch c.
   laparoscopic needle c.
   laparoscopic retropubic c.
colpoureterotomy
column
   anal c.
   butyl-silane extraction c.
   c. chromatography
   C18 Sep-Pack c.
   hemicrypt c.
   c. of Morgagni
   Sepharose 4B-coupled-protein-
     A c.
   variceal c.
columnar
   c. epithelium
   c. metaplasia
columnar-cuboidal adenocarcinoma
  cell
columnar-lined esophagus
Coly-Mycin M
Coly-Mycin S
colypeptic
Colyte
   C. bowel prep
coma
   acute hepatic c.
   electrolyte imbalance c.
   hepatic c.
comatose
combination
   c. biliary brush catheter

c. calculus
prednisone-colchicine c.
combined
c. chemoradiation therapy
c. fat- and carbohydrate-
induced hyperlipidemia
c. hemorrhoids
c. hiatal hernia
c. ureterolysis
comb-like redness sign
Combo Cath wire-guided cytology brush
comet sign
Comfeel
C. skin adhesive
C. skin barrier
Comhaire grading system
co-mitogen
commercial dialysis solution (CDS)
comminution
stone c.
common
c. bile duct (CBD)
c. bile duct exploration
(CBDE)
c. bile duct obstruction
c. bile duct stent
c. bile duct stone
c. bile duct varices
c. cavity phenomenon
c. channel
c. duct cholangiogram
c. duct exploration (CDE)
c. duct sound
c. duct stone
c. hepatic duct
c. pH electrode
c. variable immunodeficiency
(CVI)
communicating hydrocele
communication
anomalous pancreaticobiliary c.
cholangiovenous c.
pseudocyst c.
comorbid condition
comorbidity
Companion feeding pump

compartment
infracolic c.
posterior pararenal c.
supracolic c.
Compat
C. feeding pump
C. feeding tube
Compazine
Compeed Skinprotector dressing
compensated cirrhosis
compensatory testicular hypertrophy
competent
c. ileocecal valve
c. valve
competition
inter-liver c.
competitive protein binding assay
Compleat-B liquid feeding
complement
c. activation
C3a c.
c. fixation test
c. hemolytic activity
c. level
c. regulatory protein
total hemolytic c.
complementary
c. deoxyribonucleic acid
(cDNA)
c. DNA
complement-dependent cytotoxicity (CDC)
complement-independent autologous phase
complement-mediated
c.-m. experimental
glomerulonephritis
c.-m. immune glomerular
disease
complement receptor type I (CR1)
complete
c. blood count (CBC)
c. blood count test
c. bowel obstruction
c. duplication
c. hormonal blockage
c. male epispadias

NOTES

complete *(continued)*
  c. PEG pull
  c. PEG push
  c. replacement PEG
  c. Savary
  c. surgical exploration (CSE)
complex
  adenylate cyclase c.
  AIDS-related c. (ARC)
  anisoylated plasminogen
    streptokinase activator c.
  c. anorectal fistula
  antimajor histocompatibility c.
  avidin-biotin c.
  avidin-biotin-peroxidase c.
  calcium-calmodulin c.
  Carney c.
  CD3-T cell receptor c.
  c. class II expression
  epispadias-exstrophy c.
  Eshmun c.
  exstrophy-epispadias c.
  gastroduodenal artery c.
  Golgi c.
  Heymann nephritis antigenic c.
    (HNAC)
  histocompatibility c.
  interdigestive migrating
    motor c.
  interdigestive myoelectric c.
  major histocompatibility c.
    (MHC)
  membrane-attack c.
  Meyenburg c.
  migrating motor c. (MMC)
  mitochondrial c.
  Mycobacterium avium c.
  nephroblastomatosis c. (NBC)
  OEIS c.
  oligohydramnios c.
  oligometric c.
  c. papillary infolding
  penoscrotal transposition c.
  polysaccharide-iron c.
  refined carbohydrate c.
  sling-ring c.
  c. stone
  streptavidin-biotin peroxidase c.
    (SAB reagent)
  thrombin-antithrombin III c.
  tuberous sclerosis c. (TSC)
  von Meyenburg c. (VMC)

compliance
  bladder c.
  c. of bladder
  rectal c.
  vesical c.
complication
  bacterial c.
  benign pneumatic
    colonoscopy c.
  bowel preparation c.
  cardiopulmonary c.
  cardiorespiratory c.
  cardiovascular c.
  cerebrovascular c.
  colitis perineal c.
  colonoscopy c.
  endoscopy c.
  extraintestinal c.
  feeding c.
  gastrointestinal c.
  hematologic c.
  infectious c.
  metabolic c.
  neurologic c.
  opportunistic c.
  postbiopsy vascular c.
  postoperative c.
  pulmonary c.
  renal c.
  sclerotherapy c.
  vascular c.
component
  lymphoid c.
  secretory c. (SC)
  serum amyloid P c.
compound
  bismuth c.
  c. cyst
  gold c.
compression
  c. button
  c. button gastrojejunostomy
  duodenal c.
  esophageal c.
  extrinsic c.
  gastric c.
  mechanical variceal c.
  spinal cord c.
  c. ultrasound (CUS)
compressor urethrae
compromise
  vascular c.
computed tomography (CT)

computer-aided diagnostic system
computer-controlled sedation
  infusion system
computerization
computerized
    c. electronic endoscopy
    c. image analysis system
    c. tomography (CT)
Compu-void
comutagenic
con A-anti-con A perfusion
concanavalin A
concealed
    c. hemorrhage
    c. penis
    c. umbilical stoma
    c. vomiting
Concentraid Nasal
concentrate
    Maalox Therapeutic C.
    therapeutic c. (TC)
concentrated urine
concentration
    albumin plasma c.
    amylase c.
    calcium c.
    dialysate glucose c.
    endothelin-1 c.
    c. epidermal growth factor
      (cEGF)
    extrapolated plasma caffeine c.
    fasting plasma caffeine c.
    hyaluronic acid c.
    mean corpuscular
      hemoglobin c. (MCHC)
    millimolar c.
    minimal inhibitory c. (MIC)
    plasma caffeine c.
    plasma gastrin c.
    plasma norepinephrine c.
    plasma renin c.
    plasma urea c.
    predialysis plasma phosphate c.
    serum c.
    serum calcium c.
    sodium butyrate c.

    thyroid hormone serum c.
    total protein c.
concentric
    c. hyaline inclusion
    c. needle
concentric-needle electrode
concept
    exudate-transudate c.
    Valsalva leak point pressure c.
conceptus dose
concomitant
    c. antireflux surgery
    c. medication effect
concrement
concretion
    bile c.
    fecal c.
concurrent hepatic laceration
condition
    comorbid c.
    intersex c.
    pathological hypersecretory c.
conditioning
    interceptive c.
    semantic c.
condom
    female c.
    c. urinal
conductance
    urethral electrical c.
conducted current
conduction defect
conductivity
    electrical c.
conduit
    antirefluxing colonic c.
    colon c.
    cutaneous appendiceal c.
    ileal c.
    Mitrofanoff c.
condyloma, pl. condylomata
    c. acuminatum
    anal c.
    flat c.
    c. latum
    perianal c.
Condylox

C

NOTES

cone
    c.-tip catheter
    vaginal c. biopsy
coned cecum
coned-down appearance of colon
cone-shaped cecum
confidence ring
configuration
    bird-beak c.
    golf hole c.
confluence
confluent
conformal radiation therapy
congenital
    c. adrenal hyperplasia (CAH)
    c. aganglionosis
    c. bifid bladder
    c. biliary atresia
    c. biliary cyst
    c. cystic disease
    c. cystosis
    c. diaphragm
    c. diaphragmatic hernia
    c. diverticulosis
    c. duodenal atresia
    c. epispadias
    c. hepatic fibrosis (CHF)
    c. hernia
    c. hydrocele
    c. hypertrophic pyloric stenosis
    c. hypoplasia
    c. lactic acidosis
    c. malrotation of the gut
    c. megacolon
    c. nephrogenic diabetes
      insipidus (CNDI)
    c. penile curvature
    c. penile deviation (CPD)
    c. portacaval shunt
    c. pyloric membrane
    c. pyloric stenosis
    c. renal mass
    c. splenic cyst
    c. splenomegaly
    c. stenosis
    c. urethroperineal fistula
    c. uropathy
congenitally altered anatomy
congested mucosa
congestion
    active c.
    passive c.

congestive
    c. gastropathy
    c. heart failure
    c. hepatomegaly
    c. hypertensive gastropathy
    c. splenomegaly
Congo
    C. red dye
    C. red stain
congophilic material
conical
    c. catheter
    c. centrifuge tube
    c. glans
    c. trocar
conjoined tendon
conjugate
    zenobiotic glutathione c.
conjugated
    c. bile acid
    c. bilirubin
    c. hyperbilirubinemia
conjunctival
    c. erythema
    c. icterus
connective
    c. tissue
    c. tissue disease
    c. tissue disorder
connector
    Luer-Lok c.
    T c.
    Touhy-Borst c.
    Y-port c.
Connell
    C. incision
    C. stitch
    C. suture
conniventes
    valvulae c.
Conn syndrome
conorii
    Rickettsia c.
Conray
    C. (60, 70) contrast material
    C. 280 contrast medium
conscious sedation
Conseal
    C. one-piece continent
      colostomy system
    C. ostomy irrigation set
consensual reflex
consensus interferon

consistency
consortial approach
consortium
    Pediatric Peritoneal Dialysis
    Study c.
constant
    Michaelis c. (Km)
Constene
constipate
constipation
    antepartum c.
    atonic c.
    chronic functional c.
    chronic idiopathic c.
    drug-induced c.
    functional c.
    gastrojejunal c.
    geriatric c.
    idiopathic c.
    intractable c.
    outlet obstruction c.
    postpartum c.
    c. predominant irritable bowel
    syndrome
    proctogenous c.
    psychogenic c.
    slow transit c.
    spastic c.
constitutional hepatic dysfunction
constricting pain
constriction
    mesenteric artery c.
    c. ring
construction
    ileal reservoir c.
    pelvic ileal reservoir c.
    sphincteric c.
    U pouch c.
    vaginal c.
constructional apraxia
consumption
    alcohol c.
    EtOH c.
    salt c.
    whole-cell oxygen c.

contact
    cell-cell c.
    c. dissolution
Contact Laser vaporization
contact-tip laser system
contagiosum
    giant molluscum c.
contamination
    fecal c.
    c. of food
    post-autoclave c.
    c. of water
content
    abdominal c.'s
    bowel c.'s
    gastric c.'s
    hepatic malondialdehyde c.
    intestinal c.'s
    mucosal hexosamine c.
    renal cortical
    malondialdehyde c.
    total glutathione c.
contexture analysis
Contigen
contiguous
    c. loop
Contimed II pelvic floor muscle
monitor
continence
    diurnal c.
    fecal c.
    urinary c.
continent
    c. colostomy
    c. cutaneous
    appendicocystostomy
    c. cutaneous diversion
    c. ileal pouch
    c. ileal reservoir
    c. ileostomy
    c. of stool
    c. urinary diversion
continuity
    bowel c.
continuous
    c. ambulatory peritoneal
    dialysis (CAPD)

C

NOTES

continuous *(continued)*
   c. arteriovenous hemofiltration (CAVH)
   c. arteriovenous hemofiltration with dialysis
   c. arteriovenous ultrafiltration (CAVU)
   c. bladder drainage
   c. bladder irrigation (CBI)
   c. catheter drainage
   c. cycler-assisted peritoneal dialysis
   c. cycling peritoneal dialysis (CCPD)
   c. drip feeding
   c. hypothermic pulsatile perfusion
   c. infusion chemotherapy
   c. murmur
   c. NG suction
   c. prophylaxis
   c. pull-through technique
   c. renal replacement therapy (CRRT)
   c. suture
   c. venovenous hemofiltration (CVVH)

continuous-flow resectoscope
continuously perfused probe
contour
   c. ERCP cannula
   isodose c.
   sawtooth irregularity of bowel c.

contractile
   c. ring dysphagia
   c. stricture

contractility
   normal detrusor c.

contraction
   alcohol-induced extracellular volume c.
   anal sphincter c.
   clonic c.
   fat-induced gallbladder c.
   gallbladder c.
   high-amplitude c. (HAPC)
   isotonic c.
   paradoxical c.
   paradoxical puborectalis c.
   peristaltic c.
   phasic c.
   primary c.

   propagation of c.
   reflex detrusor c.
   ringlike c.'s
   secondary c.
   sliding filament model of c.
   slow phasic c.
   tachyoddia c.'s
   tertiary c.
   tonic c.

contraction-relaxation cycle
Contractubex gel
contracture
   bladder neck c.
   Dupuytren c.
   postinflammatory c.

Contrajet ERCP contrast delivery system
contralateral
   c. reflux

contrast
   c. agent
   barium enema with air c.
   c. chromoscopy using indigo carmine (CCIC)
   Cysto Conray c.
   double c.
   c. enema
   c. enhancement
   c. esophagography
   c. esophagram
   c. fluid
   c. medium
   c. selective cholangiogram
   Solutrast 300 c.

contrast-associated renal failure
contrast-enhanced
   c.-e. computed tomography
   c.-e. fast sequence (CE-FAST)

control
   bleeding c.
   c. bridle
   Centers for Disease C. (CDC)
   endoscopic c.
   EPC pain c.
   fluoroscopic c.
   foot pedal suction c.
   hemorrhage c.
   neural c.
   pain c.
   symptom c.

controlled expansion (CX)
conus medullaris

ConvaTec
- C. Active Life stoma cap
- C. colostomy pouch
- C. Durahesive Wafer ostomy
- C. Little One Sur-Fit pouch
- C. Sur-Fit two-piece pouch

conventional
- c. concentric electromyography
- c. static scanner
- c. stent

Converspaz

convertase
- C3 c.

converter
- sequential video c.

Converzyme

COOH-terminal SH2 domain

Cook
- C. biopsy gun
- C. plastic Luer lock adaptor
- C. rectal speculum
- C. stent
- C. tissue morcellator
- C. TPN catheter
- C. urological trocar

coolant

cooling
- external c.
- homogenous c.
- ice c.
- immersion c.
- perfusion c.
- surface c.
- transarterial perfusion c.
- whole body c.

Coomassie brilliant blue technique

Cooper
- C. hernia
- C. herniotome
- C. ligament

coordination
- R wave c.

Cope
- C. clamp
- C. loop nephrostomy catheter
- C. loop nephrostomy tube

copious irrigation

copolymerized substrate

copper-binding
- c.-b. protein (CBP)
- c.-b. protein test

copper colic

copremesis

coprolith

coproma

coproplanesia

coprostasis

coral calculus

coralgil

cord
- c. bladder
- hepatic c.
- hepatocytic c.
- c. hydrocele
- lipoma of c.
- palpable c.
- spermatic c.
- c. structure
- umbilical c.
- vocal c.

Cordis-Hakim shunt

Cordonnier ureteroileal loop

core
- c. needle biopsy
- c. temperature
- c. of tumor

core-cut system

Corgard

Cori disease

corkscrew esophagus

Corlopam

corneal
- c. foreign body
- c. reflex
- c. ulcer

corner
- c. suture
- C. tampon

cornflake esophageal motility test

cornucopia
- sinusoidal endothelium c.

coronae
- papillomatosis c.

NOTES

coronal
    c. adhesion
    c. epispadias
    c. hypospadias
    c. radiata
    c. sulcus
coronary
    c. azygos
    cafe c.
    c. ligament
    c. sinus
coronavirus gastroenteritis
Corpak
    C. feeding tube
    C. weighted-tip, self-lubricating
        tube
corpora (*pl. of* corpus)
corpora cavernosa, sing. **corpus**
  cavernosum
corporal biopsy
corporeal
    c. aspiration
    c. fibrosis
    c. reconstruction
    c. rotation procedure
    c. venous occlusive dysfunction
corpores (*gen. of* corpus)
corporoplasty
    incisional c.
    modified Essed-Schroeder c.
corporotomy
corpus, gen. **corpores,** pl. **corpora**
    c. callosum agenesis
    c. epididymis
    c. gastric mucosa
    c. gastritis
corpus cavernosum (*sing. of*
  corpora cavernosa)
corpuscle
    pacinian c.
corpus spongiosum
Correa classification
correction
    Yates c.
Correctol
correlation
    Pearson c.
    Spearman rank c.
Corrigan pulse
corrosive
    c. esophageal stricture
    c. esophagitis
    c. gastritis

Corson
    C. needle
    C. needle electrosurgical probe
Cortenema
    C. retention enema
cortex, pl. **cortices**
    adrenal c.
    renal c.
Corticaine
cortical
    c. abscess
    c. adenoma
    c. collecting duct (CCD)
    c. interstitial volume fraction
cortice
    kidney c.
cortices (*pl. of* cortex)
corticoadenoma
    adrenal c.
corticoadrenal
    renal c.
corticomedullary
    c. demarcation
    c. differentiation
corticosteroid
    c. therapy
    c. treatment
corticotropin
Cortifoam
cortisol
cortisone acetate
Cortisporin
corymbifera
    Absidia c.
    Mucor c.
Corynebacterium parvum
cosine curve
cosinor
    c. analysis
    c. rhythmometry
cosmesis
costal margin
cost analysis
COSTART system
costive
costiveness
costochondral tenderness
costocolic fold
costophrenic blunting
costovertebral angle tenderness
    (CVAT)
Cotazym-S

cotransporter
   c. mRNA
   NA+-glucose c.
   taurine c. (TCT)
Cotrim
co-trimoxazole
Cotton
   C. cannulatome
   C. sphincterotome
Cotton-Huibregtse double pigtail stent
Cotton-Leung biliary stent
cottonseed oil
cotton suture
cotton-wool spot
coudé catheter
cough stress test
Couinaud classification
Coulter
   C. EPICS C-flow flow cytometer
   C. EPICS Elite flow cytometer
   C. EPICS 700-series flow cytometer
   C. EPICS V flow cytometer
Coumadin
coumarin
   c. dye laser
   c. green tunable dye laser lithotripsy
coumarin-flash-lamp pumped pulsed dye laser
Councill catheter
Councilman body
count
   CD4 c.
   CD4 lymphocyte c.
   CD8 lymphocyte c.
   CD4+ T-cell c.
   complete blood c. (CBC)
   instrument c.
   mitosis c.
   needle c.
   platelet c.
   red blood cell c.
   sponge c.
   too numerous to c. (TNTC)
   white blood cell c.
counter
   LKB-Wallac scintillation c.
   RackBeta scintillation c.
countercurrent mechanism
countertransporter
   sodium-lithium c. (SLC)
counts per minute (cpm, CPM)
coup de sabre
coupling
   capacitive c.
   electromechanical c.
   excitation-contraction c.
   pharmacomechanical c.
   c. stoichiometry
Courvoisier
   C. gallbladder
   C. gastroenterostomy
   C. law
   C. sign
Courvoisier-Terrier syndrome
couvade syndrome
Couvelaire ileourethral anastomosis
cover
   Foxy Pouch c.
   laparotomy pad c.
   pad c.
   Sur-Fit Pouch c.
covering
   Camwrap plastic c.
Cowan I strain
Cowden
   C. disease
   C. syndrome
Cowper
   C. cyst
   C. gland
cow's milk protein allergy
Coxiella burnetii
Cox-Mantel test
Coxsackievirus
   C. A infection
   C. B infection
   C. infection

NOTES

CP
   chronic pancreatitis
   CP test
CPA
   cyproterone acetate
CPD
   congenital penile deviation
CPH
   chronic persistent hepatitis
CPH-CAH cirrhosis
CPK
   creatine phosphokinase
C-plasty
cpm, CPM
   counts per minute
CPN
   cisplatin nephropathy
CPP
   cerebral perfusion pressure
CR1
   complement receptor type I
cradle
   acoustically transparent c.
cramp
cramping pain
crampy abdominal pain
Cranley phleborrheograph
crater
   ulcer c.
CR Bard Urolase
CRC
   colorectal cancer
Crcl
   creatinine clearance
C-reactive protein
cream
   Dermovate c.
   lidocaine-prilocaine c.
   rectal c.
   Sween C.
   Sween Micro Guard c.
crease
   inguinal c.
   midline abdominal c.
   skin c.
   torso c.
creatine phosphokinase (CPK)
creatinine
   c. clearance (Crcl)
   c. height index (CHI)
   plasma c.
   serum c. (SCr)
   c. test

creation
   Politano-Leadbetter tunnel c.
   tunnel c.
creatorrhea
Crede maneuver
^{51}Cr-EDTA
   51-chromium-labeled
   ethylenediaminetetraacetate
   ^{51}Cr-EDTA excretion
creeping of mesenteric fat
cremasteric
   c. fiber
   c. reflex
cremaster muscle
Cremer-Ikeda papillotome
cremnocele
Creon
   C. 10
   C. 20
crescendo
   c. decrescendo
crescendoing bowel sound
crescent
   c. gastric cardia
   glomerular c.
   c. snare
crescentic
   c. glomerulonephritis
   c. nephritis
Crespo operation
CREST
   calcinosis cutis, Raynaud
   phenomenon, esophageal motility
   disorder, sclerodactyly, and
   telangiectasia
   CREST syndrome
crest
   cupula of ampullary c.
   c. factor
   jejunal c.
Creutzfeldt-Jacob disease
crevicular fluid
CRF
   chronic renal failure
cricoid myotomy
cricomyotomy
cricopharyngeal
   c. achalasia
   c. bar
   c. diverticulum
   c. myotomy
   c. spasm
   c. sphincter

cricopharyngeus
    c. muscle
Cri-du-Chat syndrome
Crigler-Najjar syndrome
Crile
    C. angle retractor
    C. appendix clamp
    C. bile duct forceps
    C. gall duct forceps
    C. hemostat
    C. hemostatic clamp
    C. nerve hook
crinogenic
crisis, pl. crises
    Dietl c.
    gastric c.
cristae
crista urethralis
criteria
    Child c.
    Child-Pugh c.
    clinicobiological c.
    DeMeester c.
    Foley c.
    Geenen c.
    Lown c.
    morphometric c.
    Munich inclusion c.
    Pugh modification of Child c.
    Rome c.
    Savary-Miller c.
    variceal size inclusion c.
criterion, pl. criteria
    Child liver c.
    manometric c.
    Ranson c.
Criticare
    C. HN elemental liquid feeding
    C. HN-Isocal tube feeding set
CRIT-LINE instrument
⁵¹Cr-labeled EDTA
Crohn
    C. colitis
    C. disease (CD)
    C. Disease Activity Index
    C. disease activity index (CDAI)
    C. disease of colon (CDC)
    C. Disease Endoscopic Index of Severity (CDEIS)
    C. duodenal ulcer
    C. ileitis
    C. ileocolitis
    C. regional enteritis
    C. small intestine
Crohns and Colitis Foundation of America (CCFA)
cromoglycate
    disodium c.
    sodium c.
cromolyn
Cronkhite-Canada syndrome
Crosby capsule
Crosby-Kugler capsule for biopsy
cross
    Maltese c.
crossbar
    c. deformity
    inner c.
    outer c.
crossbridge cycle
cross-clamped, crossclamped
crossed renal ectopia
crosshatch marks
crossmatch
    T-cell c.
crossmatched blood
cross-phosphorylation
cross-trigonal repair
CR/OV
    OncoScint C.
        OncoScint colorectal/ovarian carcinoma localization scintigraphy
crowding
    variable nuclear c.
CRRT
    continuous renal replacement therapy
CRS
    cherry-red spot

C

NOTES

CRST
  calcinosis cutis, Raynaud
  phenomenon, sclerodactyly, and
  telangiectasia
  CRST syndrome
cruciate incision
crude drug
crunch
  mediastinal c.
  c. stick anastomosis
crural
  c. fold
  c. venous leakage
crus, pl. **crura**
  c. of diaphragm
crutched stick-type polyurethane
  endoprosthesis
Cruveilhier
  C. sign
  C. ulcer
Cruveilhier-Baumgarten
  C.-B. anomaly
  C.-B. cirrhosis
  C.-B. syndrome
cruzi
  Trypanosoma c.
cryoablation
cryogenic ablation
cryoglobulinemia
  mixed essential c.
  type II c.
cryoprecipitate
cryoprecipitated plasma
cryopreservation
  sperm c.
cryoprostatectomy
cryostat
  c. tissue
  Tissue Tek-II c.
cryosurgery
cryosurgical ablation
cryotherapy
  c. for hemorrhoids
crypt
  c. abscesses
  anal c.
  c. architectural distortion
  c. cell
  c. epithelium
  c. hook
  c. hyperplasia
  ileal c.

  Lieberkühn c.'s
  Morgagni c.
cryptitis
cryptogenic
  c. cirrhosis
  c. liver disease
cryptorchid
  c. testicle
  c. testis
cryptorchidectomy
cryptorchidism
cryptorchidopexy
cryptorchid testicle
cryptorchism
cryptosporidia
Cryptosporidia-**induced diarrhea**
cryptosporidial infection
cryptosporidiosis
Cryptosporidium
  C. muris
  C. oocyst
  C. parvum
  C. species
crypt-villus
  c.-v. site
  c.-v. unit
crystal
  CaC3 c.
  cholesterol monohydrate c.
  cystine c.
  oxalate c.
  phosphate c.
  urate c.
crystallization
crystalloid
crystalluria
crystal-phospholipid interaction
C&S
  culture and sensitivity
  C&S test
CS-9000 densitometer
CSE
  complete surgical exploration
CSF
  CSF glucose
  CSF glutamine
  CSF glutamine test
  CSF protein
CSF-1
  colony-stimulating factor-1
CSG
  chronic superficial gastritis

CSI
    cholesterol saturation index
CT
    computed tomography
    computerized tomography
      helical CT
      CT scan
      CT scan with contrast
       enhancement
      spiral CT
CTAS
    colonic transabdominal sonography
CTC
    Child-Turcotte classification
C-terminal propeptide of type I procollagen
CT-guided
    C.-g. fine-needle aspiration
    C.-g. liver biopsy
    C.-g. needle-aspiration biopsy
    C.-g. pseudocyst drainage
CTL
    cytolytic T lymphocyte
    cytotoxic T lymphocyte
CTL-mediated lysis
CTPV
    cavernous transformation of the portal vein
C-Trak
    C.-T. analyzer
    C.-T. hand-held gamma detector
    C.-T. probe
    C.-T. surgical guidance system
[14]C-triolein breath test
C-type atrial natriuretic peptide (C-ANP)
cub bladder biopsy
cube
    Gelfoam c.
cuboidal epithelia
CUC
    chronic ulcerative colitis
cuff
    c. abscess
    AS 800 c.

    rectal muscle c.
    suprahepatic caval c.
cuffed
    c. endotracheal tube
    c. esophageal endoprosthesis
cul-de-sac
    c.-d.-s. of Douglas
    c.-d.-s. fluid
    c.-d.-s. mass
culdocentesis
culdoplasty
    McCall c.
culdoscope
culdoscopy
Cullen sign
Culp
    C. pyeloplasty
    C. spiral flap pyeloplasty
culture
    aerobic c.
    anaerobic c.
    blood c.
    glomerular cell c.
    c. medium
    mixed growth on c.
    c. and sensitivity (C&S)
    c. and sensitivity test
    shell vial c.
    stool c.
    tissue c.
    urine c.
culture-negative neutrocytic ascites (CNNA)
cumulus
Cunningham
    C. clamp
    C. urinary incontinence clamp
Cunningham-Cotton sleeve coaxial dilator
Cunninghamella
    C. species
cup
    stone c.
    vaginal fistula c.
cup-patch technique
Cuprimine
cupula, pl. **cupulae**

C

NOTES

cupula *(continued)*
    c. of ampullary crest
    gas c.
curative resection
curd
    alum c.
cure
    krebiozen false cancer c.
13C-urea
C-urea breath test (UBT)
curette
    Spratt c.
Curl Cath catheter
Curling ulcer
currant jelly stool
current
    coagulating c.
    conducted c.
    cutting c.
    c. density
    direct c.
    electrocoagulating c.
    membrane c.
curtsy
    Vincent c.
curvature
    congenital penile c.
    penile c.
curvature of stomach
    greater c.o.s.
    lesser c.o.s.
curve
    angulus on the lesser c.
    cosine c.
    gallbladder emptying-refilling c.
    Kaplan-Meier c.'s
    loss of sigmoid c.
    sigmoid c.
    c. of stream
    time-activity c.
    time/concentration c.
    triphasic cystometric c.
curved
    c. bacilli
    c. dissecting forceps
    c. end-to-end anastomosis (CEEA)
    c. flank position
    c. hemostat
    c. Maryland forceps
    c. Mayo clamp
    c. Mayo scissors

    3.5-10 MHz c. array transducer
    c. transjugular needle
curved-needle surgeon's knot
CUS
    compression ultrasound
CUSA
    Cavitron Ultrasonic Surgical Aspirator
    CUSA dissector
Cushing
    C. disease
    C. forceps
    C. suture
    C. syndrome
    C. ulcer
cushingoid facies
cushion
    hemorrhoidal c.
    partial water bath and water c.
    c. sign
    tissue c.
Custom Ultrasonic automatic reprocessor
cut
    blended c.
    electrosurgical c.
    field c.
    c. surface of liver
    c. waveform
    c. waveform desiccation
cutaneobiliary fistula
cutaneous
    c. appendiceal conduit
    c. collateral circulation
    c. diversion
    c. dropsy
    c. electrogastrogram
    c. hyperesthesia
    c. ileocystostomy
    c. lesion
    c. loop ureterostomy
    c. metastasis
    c. ureterostomy
    c. urinary diversion
    c. vesicostomy
cutback
    c. anoplasty
    c. type vaginoplasty
    vaginal c.
cutter
    Endopath endoscopic linear c.

Proximate linear c.
rib c.
suture c.
cutting
c. current
c. electrode
c. LR needle
c. needle
c. wire
CVAT
costovertebral angle tenderness
CVF
cobra venom factor
CVI
common variable immunodeficiency
CVP
central venous pressure
CVVH
continuous venovenous
hemofiltration
CW
clustered waves
CX
controlled expansion
cyanate
urea-derived c.
cyanide
potassium c.
cyanoacrylate
c. glue
cyanobacterium-like body
cyanocobalamin
c. injection
c. radioactive agent
cyanosis
enterogenous c.
cyanotic
cyclase
adenylate c. (AC)
guanylate c.
cycle
contraction-relaxation c.
crossbridge c.
cyclin/PCNA during cell c.
diurnal c.
Krebs c.

cyclic
c. adenosine monophosphate
(cAMP)
c. guanosine monophosphate
(cGMP)
c. urinary disinfectant
c. vomiting
5'-cyclic
-c. adenosine monophosphate
(cAMP)
-c. guanosine monophosphate
(cGMP)
cyclical vomiting
cyclic-GMP
cyclin
cycling
c. dialysis
cyclin/PCNA during cell cycle
cyclizine
cyclobenzaprine
Cyclogyl
cycloheximide
cyclooxygenase
c. inhibition
c. inhibitor
c. pathway
cyclooxygenase-dependent mechanism
cyclopentamine
cyclophosphamide
5-fluorouracil, Adriamycin
and c. (FAC)
vincristine, Adriamycin, and c.
(VAC)
**cyclophosphamide, Velban,
actinomycin-D, bleomycin, and
platinum (VAB-VI)**
Cyclospora
coccidian genus C.
C. species
cyclosporine
c. arteriolopathy
c. nephrotoxicity
c. toxicity
c. tubulopathy
Cyclotrac-SP radioimmunoassay
cycloxygenase
cycrimine

C

NOTES

cylinder
  AMA inflatable c.
  AMS controlled expansion
    penile prosthesis c. (AMS
    700CX penile prosthesis
    cylinder)
  AMS 700CX penile
    prosthesis c.
      AMS controlled expansion
        penile prosthesis cylinder
  banding c.
  suction c.
  Ultrex c.
cylindrical
  c. balloon
  c. confronting cisterna (CCC)
  c. diffuser
**Cymed Micro Skin one-piece
  drainage pouch**
cyprionate
  testosterone c.
cyproheptadine
cyproterone acetate (CPA)
Cys
cyst
  air c.
  allantoic c.
  alveolar hydatid c.
  Bartholin c.
  biliary c.
  branchiogenous c.
  choledochal c.
  chyle c.
  CMV inclusion c.
  compound c.
  congenital biliary c.
  congenital splenic c.
  Cowper c.
  daughter c.
  dermoid c.
  duplication c.
  Echinococcus liver c.
  enteric c.
  enterogenous c.
  epidermoid c.
  esophageal duplication c.
  extraparenchymal renal c.
  fatty c.
  c. fenestration
  gastric duplication c.
  glomerular c.'s
  granddaughter c.
  hepatic c.

  hydatid c.
  ileal duplication c.
  inclusion c.
  intraluminal c.
  junctional c.
  lucent c.
  macroscopic liver c.
  mesenteric c.
  mother c.
  müllerian duct c.
  multilocular c.
  noncommunicating biliary c.
  nonepithelial c.
  nonparasitic splenic c.
  omental c.
  ovarian dermoid c.
  pancreatic c.
  parasitic c.
  parovarian c.
  pilonidal c.
  c. puncture device
  renal c.
  retention c.
  sacrococcygeal c.
  seminal vesical c.
  solitary hepatic c.
  tunic c.
  unilocular c.
  urachal c.
  urinary c.
  vitellointestinal c.
cystadenocarcinoma
  pancreatic mucinous c.
  stage III papillary serous c.
cystadenoma
  ductal c.
  ductectatic mucinous c.
  glycogen-rich c.
  mucinous c.
Cystagon
cystalgia
cystamine
cystathionine
cystatin C
cystauchenitis
cystauchenotomy
cysteamine
  c. bitartrate
cysteamine-induced duodenal ulcer
cystectasia, cystectasy
cystectomy
  partial c.
  pilonidal c.

radical c.
salvage c.
total c.
cysteine
   c. Brucella broth
cysteinyl leukotriene
cystendesis
cystenterostomy
   direct c.
   endoscopic c.
cystgastrostomy
   endoscopic c.
   surgical c.
cystic
   c. artery
   c. dilation
   c. disease of renal medulla
   c. duct
   c. duct angiogram
   c. duct catheterization
   c. duct cholangiocatheter
   c. duct cholangiogram
   c. duct choledochoscopy
   c. duct leakage
   c. duct lumen
   c. duct stone
   c. epithelial proliferation
   c. fibrosis (CF)
   c. fibrosis gene probe
   c. fibrosis transmembrane
     conductance regulator (CFTR)
   c. hamartoma
   c. liver disease
   c. mass
   c. nephroma
   c. plexus
   c. puncture
cystica
   cystitis c.
cystic-choledochal junction
cysticercosis
Cysticercus
   C. cellulosae
cysticercus disease
cysticohepatic junction
cystidoceliotomy
cystidolaparotomy

cystidotrachelotomy
cystifelleotomy
cystine
   c. calculus
   c. crystal
   c. dimethylester (CDE)
   c. lithiasis
   c. stone
cystinosis
cystinuria
cystistaxis
cystitis
   bacterial c.
   c. colli
   c. cystica
   emphysematous c.
   eosinophilic c.
   follicular c.
   gangrenous c.
   c. glandularis
   hemorrhagic c.
   honeymoon c.
   incrusted c.
   interstitial c.
   radiation c.
   viral c.
   xanthogranulomatous c.
cystjejunostomy
Cysto
   C. Conray contrast
   C. Flex stent
   Urovist C.
cystobridge
Cystocath
cystocele
cystochromoscopy
cystocolostomy
cystodiaphanoscopy
cystodiathermy
cystodiverticulum
cystoduodenostomy (CDY)
   endoscopic c.
cystoenterocele
cystoenterostomy
cystoepiplocele
cystofiberscope
   Olympus CYF-series OES c.

NOTES

135

Cystogam
cystogastric fistula
cystogastrostomy (CGY)
· endoscopic c.
cystogastrotome
cystogenic chemical
cystogram
chain c.
micturating c.
static c.
voiding c. (VCG)
cystography
antegrade c.
cystohepatic triangle
Cysto-Hypaque
cystojejunostomy
cystolateral pancreatojejunostomy
cystolith
cystolitholapaxy
cystolithectomy
cystolithiasis
cystolithic
cystolithotomy
cystolysis
cystometer
cystometric bladder capacity
cystometrogram (CMG)
filling c.
cystometrography
voiding c.
cystometry
gas c.
multichannel c.
provoked c.
saline c.
screening c.
simultaneous urethral c.
spontaneous c.
voiding c.
water c.
cystopancreatography
cystopanendoscopy
cystoparalysis
cystopericystectomy
cystopexy
cystophotography
cystoplasty
augmentation c.
Gil-Vernet ileocecal c.
human lyophilized dura c.
nonsecretory sigmoid c.
sigmoid c.
cystoplegia

cystoproctostomy
cystoprostatectomy
cystoprostatourethrectomy
cystoprostatovesiculectomy
cystoptosis, cystoptosia
cystopyelitis
cystopyelonephritis
cystoradiography
cystorectostomy
cystoresectoscope
ALR c.
anterior-posterior c.
Damon-Julian c.
Julian c.
cystorigin
choledochal c.
cystorrhagia
cystorrhaphy
cystorrhea
cystoscope
Albarran laser c.
balloon c.
Braasch direct
catheterization c.
Braasch-Kaplan direct vision c.
Brown-Buerger c.
Broyle retrograde c.
Butterfield c.
French c.
Judd c.
Kelly c.
Kidd c.
Laidley double-catheterizing c.
Lowsley-Peterson c.
McCarthy-Campbell
miniature c.
McCarthy Foroblique
panendoscope c.
McCrea c.
Miller c.
Morganstern c.
National general purpose c.
Nesbit c.
Olympus fiberoptic c.
Storz c.
Surgitek graduated c.
Young c.
cystoscopic
c. electrohydraulic lithotripsy
c. urography
cystoscopy
percutaneous fetal c.
steerable c.

cystosis
 congenital c.
cystospasm
Cystospaz
Cystospaz-M
cystostaxis
cystostomy
 trocar c.
 c. tube
cystotome
 Kelman c.
 Kelman air c.
 Kelman double-bladed c.
 Kelman knife c.
 Kelman knife-cannula c.
 McIntyre reverse c.
 Mendez ultrasonic c.
 reverse c.
cystotomy
 suprapubic c.
cystotrachelotomy
cystoureteritis
cystoureterogram
cystoureterography
cystourethritis
cystourethrocele
cystourethrogram
 micturition c.
 voiding c. (VCUG)
cystourethropexy
 obturator shelf c.
 Pereyra-Raz c.
cystourethroplasty
 Kropp c.
 Leadbetter c.
cystourethroscope
 ACMI c.
 microlens c.
 O'Donoghue c.
 Wappler c.
 Wappler microlens c.
cystourethroscopy
 dynamic c.
cyto-aggression
cytochrome
 b558 membrane-bound c.

c. P450 enzyme
c. P450 system
cytochrome-c-oxidase deficiency
cytochrome P-450
cytogenetic
 c. analysis
cytokeratin
 bile duct type c.
 hepatocyte-type c.
 c. staining
cytokine
 c. antagonist
 fibrogenic c.
 fibrosis-promoting c.
 c. gene expression
 GM-CSF c.
 c. therapy
 c. tumor necrosis factor-α
cytologic
 c. biopsy
 c. diagnosis
 C. software
 c. specimen
cytology
 aspiration biopsy c.
 balloon c.
 brush c.
 c. brush
 colon lavage c.
 endoscopic brush c.
 endoscopic fine-needle
  aspiration c.
 c. examination
 exfoliative c.
 fine-needle aspiration c.
  (FNAC)
 gastric brush c.
 guided-needle aspiration c.
 lavage c.
 salvage c.
 touch c.
cytolysis inhibitor
cytolytic
 c. action
 c. therapy
 c. T lymphocyte (CTL)

NOTES

cytoma
cytomegalovirus (CMV)
  c. colitis
  c. esophagitis
  c. immune globulin
  c. infection (CMV infection)
cytometer
  CAS 200 image c.
  Cell Analysis system 200
    image c.
  Coulter EPICS C-flow flow c.
  Coulter EPICS Elite flow c.
  Coulter EPICS 700-series
    flow c.
  Coulter EPICS V flow c.
  Dickinson FACS 400-series
    flow c.
  FACScan flow c.
cytometric
  c. analysis
  c. pattern
cytometry
  deoxyribonucleic acid flow c.
  DNA flow c.
  flow c.
  fluorescence-activated flow c.
  image c.
  static image DNA c.
cytopenia
cytophotometry
  static c.
cytoplasm
  eosinophilic c.
cytoplasmic
  c. argentaffinity

  c. argyrophilia
  perinuclear antineutrophil c. (p-
    ANC)
  c. protein
cytoprotective
  c. prostaglandin
cytoreductive surgery
cytoskeletal link
cytoskeleton
cytosolic calcium
cytospin collection fluid
Cytotec
cytotoxic
  c. agent
  c. chemotherapy
  c. liver disease
  c. T cell
  c. T-cell response
  c. T lymphocyte (CTL)
cytotoxicity
  antibody-dependent cell-
    mediated c. (ADCC)
  Bartel c.
  complement-dependent c.
    (CDC)
  lymphocyte c.
cytotoxin
  vacuolating c.
Cytoxan
Czerny
  C. rectal speculum
  C. suture
Czerny-Lembert suture

D

D cell

D3

dihydroxyvitamin D3
1,25-dihydroxyvitamin D3
(1,25(OH)2 D3)
25-hydroxyvitamin D3
Iα-hydroxyvitamin D3
1,25(OH)2 D3
1,25-dihydroxyvitamin D3

3-D

3-D computer reconstruction
3-D sonography

D4S231 marker
D4S414 marker
D16S84 marker
D16S283 marker
D16S291 marker
DAB

3,3-diaminobenzidine
tetrahydrochloride solution

dacarbazine
Dacomed

D. Catalyst VCD
D. snap gauge

Dacron

D. graft
D. interposition graft
D. mesh
D. suture

Dacron-impregnated Silastic sheet
DAF

decay-accelerating factor

DAG

diffuse antral gastritis
dimeric acidic glycoprotein

**DaGradi esophageal variceal
classification**
daily

d. intermittent peritoneal
dialysis (DIPD)
d. protein intake (DPI)

Daines-Hodgson anastomosis
Dairy-Ease chewable tablet
Dale

D. abdominal binder
D. Foley catheter holder

DALM

dysplasia-associated lesion or mass

Dalmane

dam

rubber d.

damage

chloroquine-induced d.
chronic tubular d.
drug-induced d.
flucloxacillin-associated liver d.
gastric mucosal d.
Graham scale for drug-induced
gastric d.
histologic d.
hypertensive end-organ d.
indomethacin-induced
mucosal d.
ischemic tubular d.
microsomal d.
oropharyngeal d.
tubular d.

Damon-Julian cystoresectoscope
Danbolt-Closs syndrome
dandy fever
Dane particle
Daniel colostomy clamp
Dansac

D. Karaya Seal one-piece
drainage pouch
D. ostomy irrigation set
D. skin barrier
D. Standard Ileo pouch

dansylcadaverine
Dantec

D. 12-channel Urocolor Video
system
D. Etude system
D. Menuet system
D. rotating disk flowmeter
D. Urodyn 1000 flowmeter
D. Urodyn 1000 uroflowmeter

danthron
Dantrium
dantrolene

d. sodium

**Danubian endemic familial
nephropathy**
dapsone
Darbid
D-arginine

enantiomer D.-a.

Daricon
Daricon PB

D

Darier disease
dark
  d. concentrated urine
  d. stool
  d. urine
darting incision
dartos
  d. fascia
  d. muscle
  d. pouch procedure
Darvocet
Darvocet-N 100
Darvon
data aquisition system
date fever
Datta procedure
daughter
  d. cyst
  d. nodule
Davidoff cell
David rectal speculum
DaVinci handle instrument
Davis
  D. interlocking sound
  D. intubated ureterostomy
  D. intubated ureterotomy
  D. loop
  D. spatula
  D. technique
Davol
  D. sump drain
  D. tunneler
DAWG
  demucosalized augmentation with
    gastric segment
    DAWG procedure
D-cell
  antral D.-c.
  D.-c. density
DC locus allelic
DCP
  des-γ-carboxy prothrombin
DDAVP
  deamino-D-arginine-vasopressin
  desmopressin
    DDAVP nasal spray
DDNC
  Digestive Disease National Coalition
DDS-Acidophilus
DDV ligator
de
  d. novo
  d. novo liver cancer

d. novo malignancy
d. novo needle knife technique
d. novo renal disease
d. Pezzer catheter
dead
  d. bowel
  d. space
DEAE
  diethylaminoethyl
de-air
deaminase
  adenosine d.
1-deamino-8-d-arginine vasopressin
deamino-D-arginine-vasopressin
  (DDAVP)
death
  hepatocellular d.
  ischemic tubular cell d.
Deaver
  D. incision
  D. retractor
  windows of D.
deaza-aminopterin
DeBakey
  D. clamp
  D. forceps
debrancher
  d. deficiency
  d. enzyme
  d. glycogen storage disease
debridement
debris
  purulent d.
  typhlonous d.
debrisoquin
debulking
  percutaneous d.
  d. of tumor
Decadron
decanoate
  naldrolone d.
decapacitation factor
Decapeptyl
decapsulation
  d. of kidney
decarboxylase
  histidine d. (HDC)
  ornithine d. (ODC)
  uroporphyrinogen d. (UROD)
decarboxylation
  amine precursor uptake and d.
  (APUD)
decay-accelerating factor (DAF)

decerebrate posturing
Decholin
decompensated
    d. alcoholic cirrhosis
    d. neobladder
decompression
    balloon d.
    biliary d.
    cardiac d.
    d. catheter
    colonoscopic d.
    d. colostomy
    ductal d.
    endoscopic d.
    endoscopic biliary d.
    gastric d.
    hydrostatic d.
    intestinal d.
    nasogastric d.
    operative d.
    PEG-assisted d.
    percutaneous transhepatic d.
    pericardial d.
    portal d.
    surgical d.
    transduodenal endoscopic d.
    tube d.
    d. tube
    variceal d.
decontamination
    selective intestinal d. (SID)
decorin
    proteoglycan d.
decorticate posturing
decortication
    renal cyst d.
decreased peristalsis
decrescendo
    crescendo d.
decubitus
    d. calculus
    lateral d.
    d. position
    d. ulcer
Deddish-Potts intestinal forceps
dedifferentiate

deep
    d. artery
    d. breathing
    d. dorsal vein
    d. interloop abscess
    d. pain
    d. postanal anorectal space
    d. trigone
de-epithelialization
de-epithelialized flap
deep-seated fungal infection
defecate
    urge to d.
defecating proctogram
defecation
    balloon d.
    fragmentary d.
    infrequent d.
    obstructed d.
    painful d.
    d. syncope
defecatory
    d. difficulty
    d. dyschezia
    d. straining
    d. urgency
defecogram
defecography
defecometry
defect
    acidification d.
    acquired neutrophil
      chemotaxis d.
    amorphous filling d.
    bony d.
    chain-of-lakes filling d.
    cold d.
    conduction d.
    fascial d.
    filling d.
    frondlike filling d.
    hernial d.
    hot d.
    interventricular d.
    intraluminal filling d.
    intrapelvic filling d.
    lobulated filling d.

D

NOTES

defect *(continued)*
    plaque-like linear d.
    renal concentrating d.
deferentectomy
deferentitis
deferoxamine
    d. mesylate infusion test
deficiency
    acquired lactose d.
    amylo-1,6-glucosidase d.
    d. anemia
    antithrombin III d.
    α_1-antitrypsin d.
    arginase d.
    brancher d.
    carbamoyl phosphate
      synthetase d.
    cobalamin d.
    cytochrome-c-oxidase d.
    debrancher d.
    dietary d.
    disaccharidase d.
    d. disease
    essential fatty acid d. (EFAD)
    folate d.
    glucose-6-phosphatase d.
    glucuronyl transferase d.
    hepatic phosphorylase d.
    IgA d.
    immune d.
    intrinsic sphincter d. (ISD)
    iron d.
    lactase d.
    long-chain acyl-CoA
      dehydrogenase d.
    medium-chain acyl-CoA
      dehydrogenase d.
    nutritional d.
    ornithine carbamoyl
      transferase d.
    pancreatic lipase d.
    PiZZ alpha$_1$-antitrypsin d.
    protein C d.
    protein S d.
    pyridoxal 5'-phosphate d.
    thiamine d.
    triglyceride enzyme d.
    vitamin D d.
deficiens
    ejaculatio d.
deficit
    lateralizing sensory d.
    neurologic d.

Deflux system implant
deformans
    peritonitis d.
deformity
    bell clapper d.
    bulb d.
    chain-of-lakes d.
    cloverleaf d.
    crossbar d.
    duodenal bulb d.
    gross d.
    hourglass d.
    keyhole d.
    limb d.
    nasal d.
    penile d.
    phrygian cap d.
    swan-neck d.
    trefoil d.
    Whitehead d.
    Z-type d.
defunctionalization
defunctioning efficiency
degeneration
    acute hepatocellular d.
    Armanni-Ehrlich d.
    feathery d.
    fistulous d.
    hepatocerebral d.
    hepatolenticular d.
    macular d.
degenerative change
degloving
deglutible
deglutition
    d. disorder
    d. mechanism
deglutitive pharyngeal chamber
Degos disease
degradation
    gastric mucosal d.
    proteolytic d.
degranulation
    mast cell d.
0-degree forward optic laparoscope
dehisced
dehiscence
    abdominal incision d.
    d. of cystic stump
    Killian d.
    staple line d.
    suture line d.
    wound d.

dehydrated ethanol
dehydration fever
dehydroemetine
dehydroepiandrosterone (DHA)
    d. sulfate (DHAS)
dehydrogenase
    alcohol d. (ADH)
    aldehyde d.
    glutamate d. (GLDH)
    glyceraldehyde phosphate d.
      (GAPD)
    glyceraldehyde-3-phosphate d.
      (GAPDH)
    β-hydroxyacyl-coenzyme A d.
    ketoglutarate d. (KGDH)
    lactate d. (LDH)
    lactic acid d. (LDH)
    long-chain 3-hydroxyacyl
      coenzyme A d. (LCHAD)
    medium-chain acyl-CoA d.
      (MCAD)
    sorbitol d. (SDH)
deiodinized formamide
Deisting technique
dejecta
dejection
Dejerine-Sottas syndrome
Delaginiere abdominal retractor
Delatestryl
delay
    excretory d.
delayed
    d. capillary refill
    d. gastric emptying
    d. hyperacute transplant
      rejection
    d. nephrogram
    d. primary intention
    d. primary intention healing
    d. upstroke
    d. vesicoureteral reflux
delayed-release tablet
deletion
    d. and mutation detection
      enhancement gel
    somatic allelic d.
Delflex peritoneal dialysis solution

delomorphous cell
Delorme rectal prolapse operation
delta
    d. agent hepatitis
    d. antigen
    d. hepatitis
    d. hepatitis superinfection
    d. over baseline (DOB)
    d. per mil
    d. virus
Delta-Cortef
delta-5-pregnenolone
Deltasone
delusional
Demadex
demarcation
    corticomedullary d.
DeMartel
    D. appendix clamp
    D. appendix forceps
DeMartel-Wolfson anastomosis
    clamp
demeclocycline-induced ascites
DeMeester criteria
dementia
    dialysis d.
Demerol
à demeure catheter
Demling-Classen sphincterotome
DeMorgan spot
demucosalized augmentation with
    gastric segment (DAWG)
Denck esophagoscope
dendritic
    d. calculus
    d. reticular cell
denervation
    sinoaortic d. (SAD)
dengue
    d. fever
    hemorrhagic d.
    d. hemorrhagic fever
    d. hemorrhagic fever infection
    d. virus
Denhardt solution
Denis
    D. Browne abdominal retractor

D

NOTES

143

Denis *(continued)*
D. Browne pouch
D. Browne urethroplsty technique
Dennis
D. clamp
D. forceps
D. intestinal forceps
D. intestinal tube
D. tube
Dennis-Brooke ileostomy
Dennis-Varco pancreaticoduodenostomy
Denonvilliers fascia
densa
lamina d.
macula d.
dense adhesion
densitometer
CS-9000 d.
Hoefer GS 300 laser d.
densitometric unit
densitometry
bone mineral d. (BMD)
video d.
density
bone mineral d.
current d.
D-cell d.
fat d.
filtration slit length d.
gastrin mRNA:G-cell d.
lumbar spine bone mineral d. (LSMB)
prostate-specific antigen d. (PSAD)
radiopaque d.
slit pore length d.
Dent
D. sleeve
D. sleeve catheter
D. sleeve device
D. supplement
dentate
d. line
d. margin
denticulatum
pentastomum d.
denuded mucosa
denutrition
Denver
D. peritoneovenous shunt
D. shunt

Denys-Drash syndrome
deodorized tincture of opium (DTO)
deoxycholate
sodium d.
deoxycholic acid
deoxydoxorubicin
deoxyepinephrine
5'-deoxy-5-fluorouridine (5'-DFUR)
deoxyribonucleic
d. acid (DNA)
d. acid flow cytometry
d. acid synthesizer
deoxyspergualin (DSP)
Depage-Janeway gastrostomy
Depakene
deparaffinization
Depen
dependent rubor
depletion
mucous d.
plasma volume d.
protein d.
depolarization
Depo-Provera
deposit
C3 d.
electron-dense mesangial d.
hemato-oxyphilic d.
hemosiderin d.
mesangial d.
deposition
collagen d.
ion beam-assisted d.
matrix d.
microdroplet fat d.
perisinusoidal fibrin d.
Depostat
Depot
Lupron D.
DEPO-Testosterone
depot injection
depressed adenoma
depression
orbital d.
pterygoid d.
respiratory d.
deprivation
androgen d.
neoadjuvant hormonal d.
deranged hemostatic mechanism
derivative
hematoporphyrin d. (HpD)

Photofrin d.
photosensitizing
hemoporphyrin d.
sialylated d.
derma
dermacate
dermal suture
dermatitis herpetiformis (DH)
dermatolymphatic invasion
dermatomyositis
dermatosis of hemodialysis
dermoid cyst
Dermovate cream
DeRoyal Surgical grab bag
DES
diethylstilbestrol
diffuse esophageal spasm
desaturation
arterial oxygen d.
oxygen d.
des-γ-carboxy
d.-c. prothrombin (DCP)
d.-c. prothrombin level
des-carboxy-prothrombin
descending
d. colon
d. diaphragm
d. duodenum
d. inhibitory reflex
d. loop colostomy
d. perineum syndrome
descensus
d. aberrans testis
bladder d.
d. paradoxus testis
d. uteri
descent
open renal d.
perineal d.
testicular d.
Deschamps ligature carrier
DESD
detrusor external sphincter
dyssynergia
deserpidine
Desferal Mesylate challenge for hemochromatosis

Desican test
desiccation
blend waveform d.
coag waveform d.
cut waveform d.
electrosurgical d.
desipramine
d. hydrochloride
Desjardins
D. gallbladder forceps
D. gallbladder probe
D. gallbladder scoop
D. gallstone forceps
D. gallstone probe
D. point
Desmarres paracentesis knife
desmoid tumor
desmoplastic reaction
desmopressin (DDAVP)
d. acetate
d. response
Desmoreaux lamp
desmosomal
d. junction
desoximetasone
desquamation
tubular cell d.
dessusception
destruens
adenoma d.
Desyrel
detection
anti-liver microsomal
antibody d.
breath isotope bacterial
urease d.
gastroenteropathy d.
hepatitis B DNA d. (HBV DNA)
hepatitis C RNA d. (HCV RNA)
immunohistochemical d.
detection-system
stone-tissue d.-s. (STDS)
detector
C-Trak hand-held gamma d.
The Early D.

NOTES

D

determinant
    antigenic d.
    mAb IOT2-recognizing
      monomorphic DR d.
determination
    IHA d.
    indirect hemagglutination d.
detorsion
detrusodetrusor facilitative reflex
detrusor
    acontractile d.
    d. activity index
    d. areflexia
    d. external sphincter
      dyssynergia (DESD)
    d. hyperactivity
    d. hyperreflexia
    d. instability (DI)
    d. pressure
    d. sphincter dyssynergia (DSD)
    d. stability
    d. underactivity
    d. urethral dyssynergia
detrusosphincteric inhibitory reflex
detrusourethral inhibitory reflex
detubularization
detubularized right colon reservoir
detumescence
Deucher abdominal retractor
deuterium oxide
devascularization
    paraesophagogastric d.
devastated urethra
developer
    Hemoccult Sensa d.
development
    embryologic d.
deviated septum
deviation
    axis d.
    congenital penile d. (CPD)
    tongue d.
    tracheal d.
    ulnar d.
    uvular d.
device
    Accutorr oscillometric d.
    ACMI ulcer measuring d.
    Aerochamber pediatric
      spacer d.
    angled delivery d. (ADD)
    autostapling d.

    BAS-300 transurethral
      thermotherapy d.
    bioartificial liver support d.
    broken stent retrieval d.
    charge-coupled d. (CCD)
    circular stapling d.
    cyst puncture d.
    Dent sleeve d.
    Digiflator digital inflation d.
    Dilamezinsert d.
    double-headed PI90 stapling d.
    EEA stapling d.
    endoscopically deliverable
      tissue-transfixing d.
    endoscopic hemoclip d.
    ErecAid vacuum erection d.
    Erlangen magnetic
      colostomy d.
    extracorporeal liver assist d.
      (ELAD)
    fingerstick d.
    flexible delivery d.
    flexible Olympus GF-eUM3 d.
    fog reduction elimination d.
      (FRED)
    Gastro-Port II feeding d.
    GIA autosuture d.
    Gould polygraph gastric
      motility measuring d.
    implantable penile venous
      compression d.
    indwelling stomal d.
    IntraSonix TULIP laser d.
    ligation d.
    linear stapling d.
    Makler insemination d.
    Makler sperm counting d.
    Menuet Compact urodynamic
      testing d.
    Microgyn II urinary
      incontinence d.
    miniature ultrasound suction d.
    Nachlas-Linton esophagogastric
      balloon tamponade d.
    needlescope d.
    Nottingham Key-Med
      introducing d.
    Olympus clip-fixing d.
    Olympus UES-series snare
      cautery d.
    OraSure salivary collection d.
    pneumatic compression d.
    PortSaver PercLoop d.

Pos-T-Vac vacuum erection d.
Prostatron transurethral
  thermotherapy d.
pyxigraphic d.
Q-Maxx side-firing laser d.
Quantum inflation d. (QID)
Rigiflator hand-held
  inflation/deflation d.
RigiScan d.
"ring-type" rigidity
  measuring d.
robotic-automated assist d.
silicone pressure sensor d.
Soehendra stent retrieval d.
SofTouch vacuum erection d.
Sonoblate ablation d.
Sony Promavica still
  capture d.
Synergist vacuum erection d.
Thermex-II transurethral
  prostate heating d.
thread-locking d.
transparent elastic band
  ligating d.
Trimedyne Optilase 1000 d.
Turapy d.
UV-Flash ultraviolet germicidal
  exchange d.
vacuum constriction d. (VCD)
vacuum entrapment d.
vacuum erection d. (VED)
vacuum extraction d.
vacuum tumescence d.
VTU-1 vacuum erection d.
Wallstent delivery d.
wire-guided metal spiral
  retrieval d.
Wolf Piezolith 2300
  lithotripsy d.
Devine
  D. colostomy
  D. exclusion
  D. hypospadias repair
Devine-Devine procedure
devitalization
devolvulization
  endoscopic d.

Devonshire colic
DEXA
  dual-energy x-ray absorption
dexamethasone
  d. sodium phosphate
  d. suppression test
  vincristine, doxorubicin and d.
    (VAD)
Dexatrim
dexbrompheniramine
Dexedrine
Dexol 300
Dexon
  D. polyglycolic acid mesh
  D. suture
dexpanthenol
dextran
  d. clearance
  iron d.
  d. sieving
dextran 40, 70, 75
dextrinizing time
dextrinosis
  limit d.
dextroamphetamine
dextropropoxyphene
dextrose
DF
  discriminant function
DFT
  Doppler flow test
5'-DFUR
  5'-deoxy-5-fluorouridine
d-galactosamine
DGER
  duodenogastroesophageal reflux
DGR
  duodenogastric reflux
DH
  dermatitis herpetiformis
DHA
  dehydroepiandrosterone
DHAS
  dehydroepiandrosterone sulfate
DHFK
  Dow Hollow Fiber kidney

D

NOTES

DHPG
dihydroxypropoxymethyl guanine
DI
detrusor instability
DiaBeta
diabetes
alimentary d.
fibrocalculous pancreatic d.
(FCPD)
gestational d.
d. home screening test
d. insipidus
insulin-dependent d.
d. mellitus
diabetic
d. colitis
d. diet
d. enteropathy
d. gastroparesis
d. gastropathy
d. impotence
insulin-treated d.
d. ketoacidosis
d. microangiopathy
d. nephropathy
d. neuropathy
d. patient
diabetica
balanitis d.
diabeticorum
gastroparesis d.
Diabinese
diacetate
2',7'-dichlorofluoresin d.
diacylglycerol
Diacyte
D. DNA ploidy analysis
Diafen
diagnosis
colonoscopic d.
cytologic d.
differential d.
endoscopic d.
endoscopic ultrasonographic d.
endoscopic ultrasound d.
enteroscopy d.
histologic d.
needle biopsy d.
noninvasive d.
pancreatic tumor d.
prenatal d.
scintigraphic d.
serologic d.

ultrasonic d.
wastebasket d.
diagnostic
d. angiography
d. colonoscopy
d. duodenoscope
d. fiberoptic stomatoscopy
d. imaging evaluation
d. laparoscope
d. paracentesis
Dialyflex dialysis fluid
dialysate
bicarbonate d.
calcium-free d.
d. glucose concentration
high-calcium d.
low-calcium d.
peritoneal d.
dialysate-to-plasma ratio
dialysis
d. access surgery
chronic ambulatory
peritoneal d. (CAPD)
continuous ambulatory
peritoneal d. (CAPD)
continuous arteriovenous
hemofiltration with d.
continuous cycler-assisted
peritoneal d.
continuous cycling
peritoneal d. (CCPD)
cycling d.
daily intermittent peritoneal d.
(DIPD)
d. dementia
d. disequilibrium syndrome
d. encephalopathy syndrome
extracorporeal d.
high-flux d.
d. modality
nightly intermittent
peritoneal d. (NIPD)
peritoneal d. (PD)
d. to plasma (D-P)
renal d.
terminal anuria vesical d.
dialysis-associated hypotension
dialysis-related ascites
**dialysis-to-plasma urea ratio (D-P
urea ratio)**
dialytic
d. treatment
d. ultrafiltration (DU)

dialyzer
    AN69 membrane d.
    CA110 d.
    CA cellulose acetate membrane
      hollow-fiber d.
    Fresenius AG d.
    Gambro d.
    HD-secura d.
    high flux d.
    d. membrane
    760 polysulfone d.
    Renaflo hollow fiber d.
    Renalin d.
    Renal systems d.
    Renatron d.
    Terumo d.
diameter
    inner d. (ID)
    maximum d.
    outer d. (OD)
    unequal calf d.
diaminedichloroplatinum
diaminobenzidine
3,3-diaminobenzidine
  tetrahydrochloride solution (DAB)
diamond jaw needle holder
diamorphine
Dianeal
    D. K-141
dianhydrogalactiol
diaphoresis
diaphoretic
diaphragm
    congenital d.
    crus of d.
    descending d.
    d. disease
    duodenal d.
    leaves of d.
    mucosal ileal d.
    pelvic d.
    urogenital d.
diaphragmatic
    d. abscess
    d. breathing
    d. hernia
    d. hernial trauma

    d. hiatus
    d. pinch
    d. pinchcock
    d. surface of liver
diaphragmatocele
diaphragm-like stricture
Diaqua
diarrhea
    acute infectious d.
    Aeromonas d.
    antibiotic-associated d.
    antibiotic-induced d.
    anxiety-related d.
    beta-lactam-associated d.
    bile salt d.
    bilious d.
    bloody d.
    choleraic d.
    cholera toxin-induced d.
    chronic d.
    Clostridium difficile-
      associated d. (CDAD)
    Cochin China d.
    colliquative d.
    Cryptosporidia-induced d.
    dysenteric d.
    enteral d.
    enterotoxin d.
    explosive d.
    familial chloride d.
    fatty d.
    flagellate d.
    functional d.
    gastrogenous d.
    gluten-sensitive d.
    hemorrhagic d.
    ileostomy d.
    infantile d.
    infectious d.
    inflammatory d.
    intermittent d.
    intractable d.
    irritative d.
    lactose-associated d.
    lienteric d.
    liquid d.
    malabsorptive d.

D

NOTES

diarrhea *(continued)*
    maldigestive d.
    mechanical d.
    morning d.
    mucous d.
    nocturnal d.
    osmotic d.
    d. pancreatica
    pancreatogenous d.
    postvagotomy d.
    raw milk-associated d.
    rotavirus d.
    secretory d.
    serous d.
    stercoral d.
    d. stool
    summer d.
    toxic d.
    travelers' d.
    tropical d.
    unrelenting d.
    viral d.
    virulent d.
    watery d.
diarrheal, diarrheic
diary
    voiding d.
Diasonics DRF ultrasound unit
Diasonic Therasonic lithotriptor
Diasorb
diastase
    d. digestion
    d. predigestion
diastasis
    palpable rib d.
    pubic d.
    d. recti abdominis
    rectus d.
diastatic serosal tear
diastematomyelia
diastolic murmur
diathermal snare
diathermic
    d. cleaning
    d. fistulotomy
    d. loop
    d. loop biopsy
    d. precut needle
    d. resection
diathermocoagulation
diathermy
    BICAP bipolar d.

    d. hemorrhoidectomy
    d. wire
diathesis, pl. **diatheses**
diatrizoate
    meglumine d.
    d. meglumine
    post-dilation meglumine d.
    sodium methylglucamine d.
Diazemuls
diazepam
    d. emulsified injection
diaziquone (AZQ)
DIB
    duodenoileal bypass
dibasic aminoacidopathy
Dibenzyline
dibucaine
DIC
    disseminated intravascular
      coagulation
    drip infusion cholangiography
    DIC parameter
dichlorofluorescein
2',7'-dichlorofluoresin diacetate
dichotomization
dichroism
    circular d.
Dickinson FACS 400-series flow
   cytometer
diclofenac
    d. analgesic therapy
    d. sodium
dicloxacillin
dicyclomine
Didrex
didronel
didymalgia
didymitis
diencephalic syndrome
diet
    absolute d.
    acid-ash d.
    ADA d.
    advance to regular d.
    alkaline-ash d.
    balanced d.
    basal d.
    basic d.
    bland d.
    blenderized d.
    BRAT d.
    BRATT d.
    CAPS-free d.

challenge d.
chemically defined d.
clear liquid d.
diabetic d.
elemental d.
elimination d.
exclusion d.
fasting d.
fiber-deficient d.
fractionated d.
full liquid d.
gastric d.
Giordano-Giovannetti d.
gluten-free d.
grapefruit d.
high bulk, low fat d.
high calorie d.
high carbohydrate d.
high fat d.
high fiber d.
high protein d.
high roughage d.
hypercaloric d.
hyperprotidic d.
lactose-free d.
liquid d.
liver d.
low calorie d.
low fat d.
low fiber d.
low residue d.
low roughage d.
low sodium d.
Meulengracht d.
milk d.
modified liver d.
Moro-Heisler d.
Portagen d.
progressive d.
reducing d.
regular d.
rice-fruit d.
Schmidt d.
semielemental d.
Sippy d.
smooth d.
soft d.

soft bland d.
steroid-dependent d.
steroid-refractory d.
Travasorb Hepatic D.
Travasorb Renal D.
vegetarian d.
very-low-calorie d. (VLCD)
Weight Watchers d.
Western d.
dietary
    d. cholesterol
    d. deficiency
    d. energy intake
    d. fat
    d. fiber
    d. gluten
    d. habit
    d. protein restriction
    d. purine
    d. supplementation
dietetic
    d. regimen
dietetics
diethylaminoethyl (DEAE)
diethylenetriamine pentaacetic acid (DTPA)
diethylenetriamine pentaacetic acid renography (DTPA renography)
diethylpropion
diethylstilbestrol (DES)
dieting plateau
dietitian
Dietl crisis
dietogenetics
Dietrol
Dieulafoy
    D. cirsoid aneurysm
    D. disease
    D. gastric erosion
    D. lesion
    D. triad
    D. ulcer
    D. vascular malformation
    D. vascular malformation of the stomach
Dieulafoy-like lesion

D

NOTES

diff
  differential
difference
  potential d. (PD)
  transmembrane electrical
    potential d.
differential (diff)
  d. diagnosis
  d. renal function test
  d. ureteral catheterization test
  WBC d.
differentiation
  cellular d.
  chondrogenic d.
  corticomedullary d.
  endothelial cell d.
  genital d.
  gonadal d.
  impaired cell d.
  leiomyosarcomatoid d.
  osteogenic d.
  rhabdomyoblastic d.
  sexual d.
difficile
  Clostridium d. (CD)
difficulty
  defecatory d.
Diff-Quik stain
diffractometry
  x-ray d.
Diffu-K
diffuse
  d. angiodysplasia
  d. antral gastritis (DAG)
  d. diabetic glomerulosclerosis
  d. esophageal spasm (DES)
  d. lobular fibrosis
  d. malignant mesothelioma
    (DMM)
  d. mesangial proliferation
  d. metastasis
  d. mucosal polyposis
  d. nodular hyperplasia (DNH)
  d. pain
  d. pancreatitis
  d. patchy nephrogram
  d. proliferative
    glomerulonephritis
  d. redness (DR)
  d. tenderness
  d. varioliform gastritis
  d. vasculitis of polyarteritis
    nodosa type

diffusely tender abdomen
diffuser
  cylindrical d.
diffusion
  interstitial d.
  pericapillary d.
  transcapillary d.
Diflucan
diflunisal
DIF-test
  direct immunofluorescence test
digastric
  d. impression
  d. triangle
Di-Gel
DiGeorge syndrome
Digepepsin
digestant
digestion
  brush-border d.
  diastase d.
  proteolytic d.
  RNAse d.
  solid food d.
digestive
  d. apparatus
  D. Disease National Coalition
    (DDNC)
  d. enzyme
  d. fever
  d. glycosuria
  d. system
  d. tract
digestorius
  apparatus d.
  tubus d.
Digiflator digital inflation device
digital
  d. rectal evacuation
  d. rectal examination (DRE)
  d. subtraction angiography
digitalis
digitally-guided biopsy
digitonin
Digitrapper
  D. Mark II pH monitoring
    system
  D. MKIII
digitrapper
  Synthetics dual-channel, solid
    state d.
digits
  sausage d.

Dignity incontinence pants
digoxin
dihydroergotoxine
dihydropyridine
dihydrotestosterone
dihydroxyphenylalanine (DOPA)
dihydroxypropoxymethyl guanine
  (DHPG)
dihydroxy salt
1,25-dihydroxyvitamin D
dihydroxyvitamin D3
    1,25-d. D. (1,25(OH)2 D3)
diiodohydroxyquin
diisopropyl iminodiacetic acid
  (DISIDA)
Dilamezinsert
    D. device
    D. instrument
Dilantin
dilatation (*var. of* dilation)
dilated
    d. bile duct
    d. duct
    d. gallbladder
    d. loops of bowel
    d. pupil
    d. vein
dilating
    d. catheter
    d. catheter-gastrostomy tube
    assembly
    d. set
dilation, dilatation
    achalasia balloon d.
    anal d.
    aneurysmal d.
    balloon d.
    biliary d.
    bowel d.
    Brown-McHardy pneumatic
    mercury bougie d.
    capillary d.
    colonic d.
    cystic d.
    ductal d.
    Eder-Puestow d.
    endoscopic d.

endoscopic papillary balloon d.
  (EPD)
esophageal d.
d. of esophagus
extrahepatic biliary cystic d.
gastric d.
Grüntzig balloon d.
d. of hemorrhoids
hepatic web d.
hydrostatic balloon d.
inadequate d.
intrahepatic biliary cystic d.
intrahepatic ductal d.
mechanical ureteral d.
medical d.
mucosal vascular d.
percutaneous balloon d.
periportal sinusoidal d.
peroral esophageal d.
pneumatic bag d.
pneumatic bag esophageal d.
pneumatic balloon catheter d.
pneumostatic d.
pyloric d.
d. range
rectal d.
submucosal vascular d.
d. therapy
through-the-scope d.
through-the-scope balloon d.
tract d.
transurethral balloon d.
TTS balloon d.
urethral d.
Uromat d.
dilator
    achalasia d.
    Achiever balloon d.
    American Dilation System d.
    American Endoscopy d.
    Amplatz fascial d.
    anal d.
    Bakes common duct d.
    balloon d.
    biliary balloon d.
    bougie d.
    Brown-McHardy pneumatic d.

D

NOTES

dilator *(continued)*
    Celestin graduated d.
    Cunningham-Cotton sleeve
      coaxial d.
    Dotter d.
    Eder-Puestow metal olive d.
    Einhorn d.
    ELIMINATOR PET biliary
      balloon d.
    ERCP d.
    esophageal d.
    esophageal balloon d.
    Ferris biliary duct d.
    fluoroscopy-guided balloon d.
    French d.
    Grüntzig d.
    Hegar rectal d.
    high diameter d.
    Hurst d.
    Hurst bullet-tip d.
    Hurst mercury-filled d.
    Hurst-Tucker pneumatic d.
    Key-Med advanced d.
    Kollmann d.
    Kron bile duct d.
    Kron gall duct d.
    Maloney mercury-filled
      esophageal d.
    Maloney tapered-tip d.
    mercury-filled d.
    mercury-weighted d.
    Microvasive Rigiflex balloon d.
    modified polyethylene d.
    Murphy common duct d.
    Nottingham One-Step
      tapered d.
    Nottingham ureteral d.
    Olbert balloon d.
    Optilume prostate balloon d.
    d. placement
    d. placement failure
    Plummer d.
    pneumatic balloon d.
    polyethylene balloon d.
    polyvinyl d.
    probe d.
    prostate balloon d.
    Quantum TTC balloon d.
    rectal d.
    Rigiflex achalasia d.
    Rigiflex balloon d.
    Rigiflex TTS balloon d.
    Russell peel-away sheath d.
    Savary d.
    Savary-Gilliard over-the-wire d.
    Savary tapered thermoplastic d.
    Sippy esophageal d.
    Soehendra catheter d.
    Starck d.
    Stucker bile duct d.
    through-the-scope d.
    TTS d.
    Tucker spindle-shaped d.
    vessel d.
    Walther d.
Dilaudid
dilaurate
    fluorescein d. (FDL)
dildo, dildoe
diltiazem
    d. therapy
**dilute Russell viper venom test
(DRVVT)**
dilution
    agar d.
dilutional hyponatremia
dilutions
    serial d.
dimenhydrinate
dimercaptosuccinic
    d. acid (DMSA)
    d. acid renal scan
    d. acid scintigraphy (DMSA
      scintigraphy)
dimeric
    d. acidic glycoprotein (DAG)
    d. IgA
dimethyl
    d. iminodiacetic acid scan
    d. sulfoxide (DMSO)
dimethylester
    cystine d. (CDE)
**dimethyl-4-phenylpiperazinium
(DMPP)**
dimethylsulfoxide
**dimethyltriazenoimidazolecarboxamide
(DTIC)**
diminished
    d. bowel sounds
    d. branching abnormality
    d. gag reflex
diminutive
    d. adenomatous polyp
    d. colonic polyp
    d. hyperplastic polyp
dimorphic

dimpling
  focal d.
  postanal d.
  skin d.
Dinamap Plus monitor
dinitrate
  isosorbide d.
  d. and mononitrate ester
dinner
  d. pad
  test d.
dinucleotide
  flavin adenine d.
Diodrast
DIONEX 2000 system
dioxethedrin
dioxide
  thorium d.
DiPAS-positive granule
DIPD
  daily intermittent peritoneal dialysis
Dipentum
diphallia
diphallus
diphemanil
diphenoxylate
diphenylthiazole
diphosphatase
  adenosine d. (ADPase)
diphosphate
  adenosine d. (ADP)
  d. buffer solution
5'-diphosphate
  uridine 5'-d. (UDP)
diphosphonate
  ^{99m}Tc labeled stannous
    methylene d.
diphtheria
diphtheritic enteritis
Diphyllobothrium lata
diploid tumor
diploidy
dipotassium
  clorazepate d.
Diprospan
dipstick
  d. protein

  urinalysis d.
  urine d.
dipyridamole
direct
  d. bilirubin
  d. cautery puncture
  d. cholangiography
  d. current
  d. current electrocoagulation
  d. current electrotherapy trial
  d. cystenterostomy
  d. immunobead test
  d. immunofluorescence test
    (DIF-test)
  d. inguinal hernia
  d. laryngoscopy
  d. manipulation
  d. tubular toxicity
  d. vesicoureteral scintigraphy
    (DVS)
  d. vision
  d. vision internal urethrotomy
    (DVIU)
  d. vision liver biopsy
direct-beam coupler for TURP
director
  grooved d.
Direx Tripter X-1 lithotriptor
Disa
  D. electromyography
  D. needle electrode
  D. 5500 urograph
disaccharidase
  d. deficiency
  d. enzyme activity
disaggregation
disappearing phenomenon
discharge
  anal d.
  bloody d.
  cervical d.
  clear d.
  nasal d.
  nipple d.
  purulent d.
  vaginal d.
discoloration

D

NOTES

discomfort
 epigastric d.
disconnection
 ureteral endoscopic d.
discontinuity
 pelvic d.
discrete
 d. bleeding source
 d. mass
discriminant function (DF)
discriminator
 EMI APED amplifier d.
disease
 acalculous gallbladder d.
 acid-peptic d.
 acquired cystic kidney d.
  (ACKD)
 actinomycotic esophageal d.
 acute abdominal vascular d.
 acute graft-vs-host d.
 acute idiopathic inflammatory
  bowel d.
 acute polycystic d.
 Addison d.
 adrenal d.
 adult familial hyaline
  membrane d.
 adult polycystic d. (APCD)
 adult polycystic kidney d.
  (APKD)
 adult polycystic liver d.
  (APLD)
 alcoholic liver d. (ALD)
 alpha-chain d.
 alpha heavy-chain d.
 Alstrom d.
 Andersen d.
 anorectal d.
 anti-GBM d.
 antiglomerular basement
  membrane d.
 α_1-antitrypsin d. (AATD)
 α_1-antitrypsin deficiency d.
 aplastic bone d.
 atheroembolic renal d. (AERD)
 atherosclerotic renovascular d.
 atypical gallbladder d.
 autoimmune d.
 autoimmune thyroid d.
 autosomal dominant polycystic
  kidney d. (ADPKD)
 autosomally recessively
  inherited d.

 autosomal recessive kidney d.
  (ARKD)
 Banti d.
 Barrett d.
 Behçet d.
 benign anorectal d. (BAD)
 Berger d.
 Besnier-Boeck-Schaumann d.
 Biermer d.
 biliary tract d.
 black liver d.
 bleeding acid-peptic d.
 Blount d.
 Botkin d.
 Bouchard d.
 Bourneville d.
 bowel d.
 Bowen d.
 Bradley d.
 brancher glycogen storage d.
 branch renal artery d.
 Bright d.
 Bruton d.
 Budd d.
 Byler d.
 calculous gallbladder d.
 calculus d.
 Caroli d.
 Castleman d.
 celiac sprue d.
 Chagas d.
 Chagas-Cruz d.
 Cherchevski d.
 Chiari d.
 Child classification of liver d.
 cholestatic liver d.
 cholesterol ester storage d.
  (CESD)
 choline deficiency liver d.
 chronic active liver d.
 chronic cholestatic liver d.
 chronic glomerular d.
 chronic graft-versus-host d. (c-
  GVHD)
 chronic inflammatory d.
 chronic liver d.
 chronic parenchymal liver d.
 chronic progressive
  tubulointerstitial d.
 chylomicron retention d.
 chylopoietic d.
 coeliac d.
 collagen vascular d.

colorectal d.
complement-mediated immune
  glomerular d.
congenital cystic d.
connective tissue d.
Cori d.
Cowden d.
Creutzfeldt-Jacob d.
Crohn d. (CD)
cryptogenic liver d.
Cushing d.
cysticercus d.
cystic liver d.
cystic d. of renal medulla
cytotoxic liver d.
Darier d.
debrancher glycogen storage d.
deficiency d.
Degos d.
de novo renal d.
diaphragm d.
Dieulafoy d.
diverticular d.
drug-related liver d.
Dubin-Sprinz d.
duodenal ulcer d.
Dupuytren d.
early-onset graft-vs-host d.
echinococcal cyst d.
end-stage d.
end-stage renal d. (ESRD)
estrogen-induced liver d.
extra-abdominal d.
extracapsular d.
extramammary Paget d.
  (EMPD)
Fabry d.
familial Crohn d.
fatty liver d.
Fenwick d.
fibrocystic d. of the pancreas
Forbes d.
fulminant Crohn d.
gamma heavy-chain d.
Gamna d.
gastric mucosal d.

gastritis-associated peptic
  ulcer d.
gastroduodenal Crohn d.
gastroesophageal reflux d.
  (GERD)
Gaucher d.
Gee-Herter-Heubner d.
Gee-Thaysen d.
Gierke d.
Gilbert d.
glomerular basement
  membrane d.
glycogen storage d.
gonococcal perihepatis pelvic
  inflammatory d.
Goodpasture d.
Gordon d.
graft-versus-host d. (GVHD)
granulomatous d.
Graves d.
Grey Turner d.
Gross d.
H d.
Hartnup d.
Hebra d.
hepatic cystic d.
hepatic Hodgkin d.
hepatic metastatic d.
hepatic veno-occlusive d.
hepatic venous web d.
hepatobiliary d.
hepatobiliary fibropolycystic d.
hepatocellular d.
hepatolenticular d.
herring-worm d.
Hers d.
Herter-Heubner d.
Hirschsprung d.
Hodgkin d.
Hoehn and Yahr stage (0-1-2-
  3-4-5) for Parkinson d.
homologous protein-overload d.
hookworm d.
Hutinel d.
hydatid cyst d.
hyperacute graft-vs-host d.

D

NOTES

disease *(continued)*
    hypertensive autosomal
      dominant polycystic kidney d.
    idiopathic inflammatory
      bowel d.
    ileocolic d.
    ileocolonic Crohn d.
    immunodeficiency d.
    immunoproliferative small
      intestinal d. (IPSID)
    infantile polycystic d. (IPCD)
    infiltrative d.
    inflammatory bowel d. (IBD)
    intramural atheromatous d.
    iron storage d.
    ischemic bowel d.
    Johne d.
    Katayama d.
    kidney d.
    Kinnier Wilson d.
    Klemperer d.
    Köhlmeier-Degos d.
    Kyasanur Forest d.
    Lane d.
    Leigh d.
    Leiner d.
    Leyden d.
    light chain deposition d.
    liver d.
    macrovascular d.
    malabsorption d.
    malignant biliary obstructive d.
    Marie-Strumpell d.
    Marion d.
    Ménétrier d.
    Ménière d.
    mesenteric inflammatory d.
    mesenteric vascular d.
    metabolic liver d.
    metabolic stone d.
    metastatic d.
    microcystic d. of renal
      medulla
    Milroy d.
    minimal-change d.
    mixed connective tissue d.
      (MCTD)
    mucosal d.
    muscle layer d.
    mycobacterial d.
    myeloproliferative d.
    neoplastic d.
    neurohumoral d.

    Niemann-Pick d.
    nil d.
    noncalculous d.
    nonobstructive hepatic
      parenchymal d.
    nonorgan confined d.
    oasthouse urine d.
    obstructive gastroduodenal
      Crohn d.
    oral d.
    organic neurologic d.
    Ormond d.
    Osler-Weber-Rendu d.
    ovarian d.
    Paget d.
    Paget extramammary d.
    Paget perianal d.
    panacinar d.
    pancreatic d.
    pancreaticobiliary d.
    parasitic d.
    parasitic liver d.
    parathyroid d.
    parenchymal liver d.
    paroxysmal motor d.
    patella d.
    pelvic inflammatory d. (PID)
    peptic reflux d.
    peptic ulcer d. (PUD)
    perforated ulcer d.
    perianal d.
    Peyronie d.
    pilonidal d.
    pilonidal sinus d.
    polycystic kidney d.
    polycystic liver d. (PCLD,
      PLD)
    Pompe d.
    post-jejunoileal-bypass
      hepatic d.
    pre-eclamptic liver d.
    primary glomerular d.
    pseudoalcoholic liver d.
    radiation-induced d.
    Rayer d.
    reactive airway d. (RAD)
    recessive polycystic kidney d.
    Recklinghausen d.
    rectal d.
    reflux d.
    renal d.
    renal arterial occlusive d.
    renal bone d.

renal cystic d.
renal hydatid d.
Rendu-Osler-Weber d.
rheumatic d.
Rokitansky d.
Ruysch d.
Saunders d.
schistosomal liver d.
scleroderma bowel d.
sexually related intestinal d.
sexually transmitted d. (STD)
sickle cell d.
sigmoid d.
skeletal muscle d.
small intestinal Crohn d.
space-occupying d.
Spencer d.
Steinert d.
steroid-dependent Crohn d.
steroid-refractory Crohn d.
stone d.
subserosal d.
suprahilar d.
systemic mast cell d.
Takayasu d.
Tangier d.
terminal ileal d.
thin basement membrane d.
  (TBMD)
thromboembolic d.
thyroid d.
transfusion-related chronic
  liver d.
tubulointerstitial d.
tunnel d.
ulcero-erosive d.
upper tract d.
urinary tract d.
valvular heart d.
Van Bogaert d.
van Buren d.
vascular d.
venereal d.
veno-occlusive d. (VOD)
veno-occlusive liver d.
venous outflow obstructive d.

venous web d.
von Gierke d.
von Hippel-Lindau d.
von Recklinghausen d.
von Rokitansky d.
von Willebrand's d.
Weber-Christian d.
Werdnig-Hoffman d.
Westphal-Strümpell d.
Whipple d. (WD)
Wilkie d.
Wilson d. (WD)
Wolman d.
disialosyl Lea
DISIDA
  diisopropyl iminodiacetic acid
  DISIDA scan
disimpaction
  colonoscopic d.
disinfectant
  Abocide d.
  Actril d.
  Asepti-steryl d.
  Burnishine d.
  Calgocide d.
  Cold Spor d.
  cyclic urinary d.
  Endospore d.
  Enzol d.
  Metricide d.
  Omnicide d.
  ProCide d.
  Sporacidin d.
  Vespore d.
  Wavicide d.
disinfection
  high level d. (HLD)
disintegration
  endoscopic stone d.
DisIntek reagent strip
disjoined pyeloplasty
disk
  anal d.
  bilaminar embryonic d.
  laser d.
  d. margin

D

NOTES

disk *(continued)*
  Marlen double-faced
    adhesive d.
  Molnar d.
dislodgement
dismembered
  d. anastomosis
  d. pyeloplasty
  d. reimplanted
    appendicocystostomy
dismutase
  superoxide d. (SOD)
disobliteration
disodium
  Cefotetan d.
  d. cromoglycate
  d. edetate
Disonate
disopropyliminodiacetic acid
disorder
  autoimmune connective
    tissue d.
  autosomal dominant d.
  blood coagulation d.
  cardiovascular d.
  connective tissue d.
  deglutition d.
  esophageal motility d.
  evacuation d.
  fat storage d.
  feeding d.
  functional bowel d. (FBD)
  gastric motility d.
  humoral immunodeficiency d.
  intestinal motility d.
  iron overload d.
  lower motor neuron bladder d.
  lymphoproliferative d.
  metabolic d.
  mixed connective tissue d.
  motility d.
  myeloproliferative d.
  neurodegenerative d.
  neurologic d.
  nonspecific esophageal
    motility d. (NEMD)
  nonspecific motility d.
  pelvic floor d.
  posttransplant
    lymphoproliferative d. (PTLD)
  psychological d.
  psychosomatic d.
  pulmonary d.

  seizure d.
  spastic motor d.
  urachal d.
  vasomotor d.
  vesiculobullous d.
disordered acrosome reaction of
  spermatozoa
Disorders
  National Association of
    Anorexia Nervosa and
    Associated D.
Di-Spaz
Dispenstirs
displacement
  bowel d.
  fiber lock d.
disposable
  d. forceps
  d. sheathed flexible
    sigmoidoscope
disruption
  pancreatic duct d.
Disse
  space of D.
  D. space
dissecting
  d. abdominal aneurysm
  d. balloon
dissection
  aortic d.
  blunt d.
  blunt and sharp d.
  circumferential mucosal d.
  en bloc d.
  extended obturator node and
    iliopsoas node d.
  extraperitoneal endoscopic
    pelvic lymph node d.
    (EEPLND)
  finger fracture d.
  intracapsular d.
  intramural air d.
  laparoscopic pelvic lymph
    node d. (LPLND)
  limited obturator node d.
  lymph node d.
  d. margin
  nerve sparing d.
  node d.
  partial zonal d. (PZD)
  plane of d.
  preadventitial d.
  scissors d.

d. scissors
sharp d.
spontaneous d.
submucosal d.
dissector
CUSA d.
Mixter d.
Niblitt d.
sponge d.
ultrasonic d.
ultrasonic aspirator and d.
disseminated
d. CMV infection
d. histoplasmosis
d. intravascular coagulation
(DIC)
dissemination
metastatic d.
dissimilatory sulfate reduction
dissociated medium
dissolution
contact d.
d. of gallstone
methyl tertbutyl ether stone d.
MTBE gallstone d.
distal
d. bile duct
d. blind stomach
d. colon
d. convoluted tubule
d. duodenum
d. esophageal ring
d. esophageal stenosis
d. esophageal stricture
d. esophagus
d. gastrectomy
d. ileitis
d. pancreatectomy
d. renal tubular acidosis
(dRTA)
d. renal tubular necrosis
d. shave section
d. splenorenal shunt (DSRS)
d. tubular acting agent
d. tubule (DT)
d. ureterectomy
d. venous plexus

distant heart sound
distasonis
Bacteroides d.
distended
d. abdomen
d. bladder
distensibility
distensible hydrodynamics
distention, distension
abdominal d.
colonic d.
esophageal balloon d.
gaseous d.
gastric d.
intraesophageal balloon d.
(IEBD)
postprandial d.
rectal d.
d. ulcer
visible abdominal d.
distortion
crypt architectural d.
distress
epigastric d.
functional bowel d. (FBD)
mild d.
moderate d.
respiratory d.
distribution
geographic d.
liver d.
node d.
vasoactive intestinal peptide d.
volume of d. (Vd)
disturbance
acid-base d.
gait d.
disulfide cross-linked fibril
disulfiram-like effect
dithiothreitol (DTT)
Ditropan
Diucardin
Diupres
diuresis
post-obstructive d.
diuretic
high-ceiling d.

D

NOTES

diuretic *(continued)*
  loop d.
  d. nuclear renography
  osmotic d.
  d. renal quantitative camera
    study
  thiazide d.
Diurigen
diurnal
  d. continence
  d. cycle
  d. enuresis
  d. incontinence
  d. urine osmolality
Diutensen-R
divalent mineral
diversion
  biliopancreatic d.
  Bricker urinary d.
  Camey enterocystoplasty
    urinary d.
  d. colitis
  continent cutaneous d.
  continent urinary d.
  cutaneous d.
  cutaneous urinary d.
  Duke pouch cutaneous
    urinary d.
  fecal d.
  Gil-Vernet ileocecal cystoplasty
    urinary d.
  hemi-Kock urinary d.
  ileal conduit urinary d.
  ileocolic urinary d.
  Khafagy modified ileocecal
    cystoplasty urinary d.
  Kock pouch cutaneous
    urinary d.
  Mainz pouch cutaneous
    urinary d.
  primary urinary d.
  d. proctitis
  Studer reservoir urinary d.
  subcutaneous urinary d.
  supravesical urinary d.
  transductal cystodigestive d.
  urinary d.
diversionary ileostomy
diversus
  Citrobacter d.
diverticula (*pl. of* diverticulum)
diverticular
  d. bleeding

  d. disease
  d. hemorrhage
diverticulectomy
  bladder d.
  endocavitary bladder d.
  Harrington esophageal d.
  pharyngoesophageal d.
  urethral d.
  vesical d.
diverticulitis
  acute d.
  chronic d.
  duodenal d.
  d. evaluation
  Meckel d.
  sigmoid d.
diverticuloma
diverticulopexy
diverticulosis
  acquired d.
  colonic d.
  congenital d.
  gastric d.
diverticulum, pl. diverticula
  d. of Akerlund
  biliary d.
  caliceal d.
  colonic d.
  cricopharyngeal d.
  duodenal d.
  epiphrenic d.
  esophageal d.
  false d.
  Ganser d.
  giant d.
  Graser d.
  hepatic d.
  Hutch d.
  hypopharyngeal d.
  intestinal d.
  intraluminal duodenal d. (IDD)
  intramural d.
  inverted sigmoid d.
  juxtapapillary duodenal d.
  Kirchner d.
  Meckel d.
  midesophageal d.
  mucosal d.
  noncommunicating d.
  d. of Nuck
  pancreatic d.
  perforated d.
  periampullary duodenal d.

peripapillary d.
pharyngeal d.
pharyngoesophageal d.
Rokitansky d.
ruptured sigmoid d.
sigmoid d.
traction d.
urachal d.
urethral d.
vesical d.
Zenker d.
diverting
 d. colostomy
 d. loop colostomy
 d. loop ileostomy
 d. stoma
divided-stoma colostomy
divisum
 pancreas d. (PD)
Dixon-Thomas-Smith clamp
Dizac
DMM
 diffuse malignant mesothelioma
DMPP
 dimethyl-4-phenylpiperazinium
DMSA
 dimercaptosuccinic acid
 DMSA scintigraphy
 ^{99m}Tc DMSA
DMSO
 dimethyl sulfoxide
DNA
 deoxyribonucleic acid
 DNA aneuploidy
 branched chain DNA (bDNA)
 complementary DNA
 DNA flow cytometry
 genomic DNA
 DNA haploid cell
 HBV DNA
  hepatitis B DNA detection
 HBV genomic DNA
 hepatitis B-like DNA
 DNA hypomethylation
 DNA labeling kit
 DNA laddering
 DNA ploidy pattern

DNA polymerase
DNA polymorphism
DNA proliferation
DNA Sequencing System
single-parameter DNA
DNA stemline
DNA synthesis
DNCB immunological study
DNH
 diffuse nodular hyperplasia
DOB
 delta over baseline
Dobbhoff
 D. biofeedback monitor
 D. bipolar coagulation probe
 D. feeding tube
 D. gastric decompression tube
 D. PEG tube
docusate
 d. sodium
dodecylsulfate
 sodium d.
dog ear
dog-ear of anastomosis
Dogiel type (I, II) morphology
DO2-haplotype
Dohlman esophagoscope
dolantin
dolasetron
dolichocolon
Dolobid
dolphin grasping forceps
dolphin-type atraumatic forceps
domain
 alternative cell attachment d.
 carboxy-terminal
  noncollagenous d.
 cleaved extracellular d.
 COOH-terminal SH2 d.
 Kringle d.
 membrane-spanning d. (MDS)
 NH2-terminal SH2 d.
 nucleotide-binding d. (NBD)
 SH2-binding d.
 src-homology 2 d.
dome
 d. of liver

D

NOTES

Domeboro solution
dome-shaped internal bumper
dome-tip electrode
domperidone
donation
organ d.
Donnagel
Donnagel-PG
Donnamar
Donnapine
Donnatal
Donnazyme
donor
artificial insemination d. (AID)
d. hepatectomy
living-related d.
living unrelated d. (LURD)
d. of nitric oxide
sulphydryl d.
donor-specific transfusion (DST)
donor-type microchimerism
Donovan body
donovani
Leishmania d.
donovanosis
Donphen
DOPA
dihydroxyphenylalanine
dopamine
d. agonist
d. b-hydroxylase
dopaminergic medication
Dopar
Doppler
color flow D.
endoscopic color D.
D. flow test (DFT)
Intradop intraoperative D.
D. probe
pulsed D.
D. QAD-1
D. Quantum color flow system
D. ultrasonography
D. ultrasound intestinal blood
flow measurement
d'orange
peau d.
Dorbane
Dorbantyl Forte
Dormia
D. stone basket
D. stone basket catheter

Dornier
D. compact lithotriptor
D. electrohydraulic watertank
lithotriptor (HM3, HM4)
D. extracorporeal shock wave
lithotripsy
D. gallstone lithotriptor
D. HM4 lithotriptor
D. HM3 waterbath lithotriptor
D. MFL 5000 urological
workstation
D. MPL 9000 gallstone
lithotripsy
D. Urotract cysto table
dorsal
d. bud
d. lithotomy
d. lithotomy position
d. lumbotomy incision
d. nerve of penis
d. pancreatic duct
d. point
d. position
d. slit
d. tunical tuck
d. vein patch graft
dorsosacral position
dosage
sclerosant d.
dose
breakthrough d.
conceptus d.
Dosepak
Hytrin D.
dose-response
dosimeter
single-channel in vivo light d.
dot-blot hybridization
dot-plotted probe
Dotter dilator
Doubilet sphincterotomy
double
d. bladder
d. chamber hemodiafiltration
d. contrast
d. contrast barium meal
d. contrast radiography
d. duct sign
d. enterostomy
d. gallbladder
d. incontinence
d. J-shaped reservoir
d. loop pouch

d. loop tourniquet
d. penis
d. pigtail stent
d. pyloroplasty
d. pylorus
d. reverse alpha-sigmoid loop
d. tracking of barium
d. uterus
double-antibody sandwich system
double-balloon technique
double-barrel
  d.-b. colostomy
  d.-b. ileostomy
  d.-b. reservoir
double-bubble duodenal sign
double-channel
  d.-c. endoscope
  d.-c. fistulotome
  d.-c. sphincterotome
  d.-c. videoendoscope
double-contrast
  d.-c. air barium enema
  d.-c. barium enema
    examination
double-cuff urinary sphincter
double-dose I.V. Timentin
double-folded cup-patch technique
double-headed
  d.-h. PI90 stapling device
  d.-h. P190 stapler
double-J
  d.-J. catheter
  d.-J. stent
  d.-J. Surgitek catheter stent
  d.-J. ureteral stent
double-lumen
  d.-l. balloon catheter
  d.-l. endoprosthesis
  d.-l. irrigation cannula
  d.-l. tapered-tip papillotome
  d.-l. tube
double-pigtail
  d.-p. endoprosthesis
  d.-p. prosthesis
double-puncture laparoscopy
double-spoon forceps
double-stapled ileal reservoir

double-staple technique
doubling time
doubly ligated
doughnut-shaped balloon
doughy abdomen
Douglas
  D. abscess
  cul-de-sac of D.
  D. fold
  D. pouch
  D. rectal snare
Dow-Corning ileal pouch catheter
Dowd, Dowd II prostatic balloon
  dilatation catheter
Dow Hollow Fiber kidney (DHFK)
down
  tacked d.
downhill esophageal varix
down-regulation
downscatter
downstaging
  hormonal d.
downstream
  d. signaling protein
  d. signal transduction
Down syndrome
doxazosin
  d. mesylate
doxepin
Doxinate
doxorubicin
doxycycline
  d. monohydrate
doxycycline-metronidazole-bismuth
  subcitrate triple therapy
Doyen
  D. abdominal retractor
  D. abdominal scissors
  D. forceps
  D. gallbladder forceps
  D. intestinal clamp
  D. intestinal forceps
  D. retractor
  D. rib elevator
D-P
  dialysis to plasma
  D-P urea ratio

D

NOTES

DPEG
dual percutaneous endoscopic gastrostomy
D-penicillamine
DPI
daily protein intake
DQ2 haplotype
DR
diffuse redness
HLA DR
DR1 HLA-DRB tissue type
DR2
DR2 HLA-DRB tissue type
DR2 1501 HLA-DRB tissue type
DR2 1502 HLA-DRB tissue type
DR2 1601 HLA-DRB tissue type
DR2 1602 HLA-DRB tissue type
DR3
HLA DR3
DR3 HLA-DRB tissue type
DR4
HLA DR4
DR4 HLA-DRB tissue type
DR5
heterozygous DR5
DR7
DR7 haplotype
DR7 HLA-DRB tissue type
DR9 HLA-DRB tissue type
drain
Blair silicone d.
Chaffin-Pratt d.
cigarette d.
closed suction d.
Davol sump d.
ERCP nasobiliary d.
fluted J-Vac d.
four-wing Malecot d.
Hemovac d.
Hollister irrigator d.
Jackson-Pratt d.
J-Vac d.
Mikulicz d.
nasobiliary d.
nasocystic d.
Nélaton rubber tube d.
Penrose d.
Penrose sump d.
perineal d.

Pezzer d.
Quad-Lumen d.
Redivac suction d.
Redon d.
Relia-Vac d.
stab-wound d.
suction d.
sump d.
surgical d.
Synder d.
Teflon nasobiliary d.
transnasal pancreatico-biliary d.
transpapillary d.
T-tube d.
two-wing Malecot d.
van Sonnenberg d.
van Sonnenberg sump d.
d. volume
Wangensteen d.
drainable ostomy pouch
drainage
biliary d.
button d.
closed d.
continuous bladder d.
continuous catheter d.
CT-guided pseudocyst d.
endoscopic d.
endoscopic biliary d.
endoscopic nasobiliary catheter d.
endoscopic pancreatic d.
endoscopic transpapillary cyst d. (ETCD)
external d.
gravity-dependent d.
incision and d. (I&D)
J-Vac closed wound d.
lymphocele d.
nasobiliary d.
nasogastric d.
nasopancreatic d.
open d.
percutaneous abscess d.
percutaneous antegrade biliary d.
percutaneous biliary d. (PBD)
percutaneous transhepatic d. (PTD)
percutaneous transhepatic biliary d. (PTBD)
postoperative irrigation-suction d.

sanguineous d.
serosanguineous d.
suction d.
tidal d.
transduodenal d.
transgastric d.
transhepatic biliary d.
transmural d.
transpapillary d.
T-tube d.
d. tube
Wangensteen d.
wound d.
drainage-resistant pseudocyst
Drake Uroflometer
Drake-Willock
D.-W. delivery system
D.-W. peritoneal dialysis
    system
Dramamine
Drapanas shunt
drape
fenestrated d.
Lingeman 3 in 1 procedure d.
Lingeman TUR d.
O'Connor d.
surgical d.
Drash syndrome
DRB gene
DRE
digital rectal examination
Dreiling tube
dressing
Adaptic d.
adhesive d.
antiseptic d.
bio-occlusive d.
bolus d.
bulky d.
Coban d.
Compeed Skinprotector d.
dry sterile d.
Elastoplast d.
d. forceps
gauze d.
Kling d.
LYOfoam d.

Montgomery strap d.
nonadhesive d.
occlusive d.
occlusive collodion d.
OpSite d.
pressure d.
sterile d.
Tegaderm d.
Telfa d.
tie-over d.
dribble
postmicturition d.
dribbling
drift
pronator d.
drinking habit
drip
alkaline milk d.
d. infusion cholangiography
    (DIC)
intravenous d.
Murphy d.
postnasal d.
driver
automatic needle d.
Haney needle d.
laparoscopic needle d.
needle d.
dromedary hump
dronabinol
drooling
drooping
droperidol
dropped bladder
dropsy
abdominal d.
cutaneous d.
nutritional d.
peritoneal d.
Drosophila melanogaster
dRTA
distal renal tubular acidosis
drug
anorectic d.
antagonistic d.
anticholinergic d.
antiemetic d.

D

NOTES

drug *(continued)*
  antilipemic d.
  antimotility d.
  antimycobacterial d.
  antisecretory d.
  antispasmodic d.
  d. carrier system
  crude d.
  d. hepatotoxicity
  H2 receptor-blocking d.
  hydrochloretic d.
  lipid-lowering d.
  d. metabolism
  neurolytic d.
  neuropsychotropic d.
  non-nephrotoxic d.
  nonsteroidal anti-
    inflammatory d. (NSAID)
  parasympatholytic d.'s
  parasympathomimetic d.'s
  prokinetic d.
  psychotropic d.
  d. reaction
  recreational d.
  d. resistance
  second-line d.
  d. therapy
  vasoactive d.
drug-induced
  d.-i. acute hepatic injury
  d.-i. cholestasis
  d.-i. cirrhosis
  d.-i. constipation
  d.-i. damage
  d.-i. esophagitis
  d.-i. gastritis
  d.-i. hepatitis
  d.-i. pain
  d.-i. pancreatitis
  d.-i. priapism
  d.-i. renal failure
  d.-i. steatosis
  d.-i. ulcer
drug-related liver disease
DRVVT
  dilute Russell viper venom test
DRw8 HLA-DRB tissue type
DRw10 HLA-DRB tissue type
DRw11 HLA-DRB tissue type
DRw12 HLA-DRB tissue type
DRw13 HLA-DRB tissue type
DRw14 HLA-DRB tissue type

dry
  d. colostomy
  d. ejaculation
  d. heaves
  d. mucous membrane
  d. skin
  d. sterile dressing
  d. swallow
  d. swallow on esophageal
    manometry
  d. vomiting
  d. weight
DS
  Bactrim DS
  Septra DS
  Sulfatrim DS
  trimethoprim-sulfamethoxazole
    DS
  Uroplus DS
DSD
  detrusor sphincter dyssynergia
DSP
  deoxyspergualin
DSRS
  distal splenorenal shunt
DST
  donor-specific transfusion
  duodenal secretin test
DT
  distal tubule
DTIC
  dimethyltriazenoimidazolecarbox-
    amide
DTO
  deodorized tincture of opium
DTPA
  diethylenetriamine pentaacetic acid
    indium-111 DTPA
    DTPA renography
DTT
  dithiothreitol
DU
  dialytic ultrafiltration
  duodenal ulcer
dual
  d.-energy x-ray absorptiometry
  d.-energy x-ray absorption
    (DEXA)
  d. percutaneous endoscopic
    gastrostomy (DPEG)
  d. percutaneous gastrostomy
    tube
dual-energy CT scan

dual-lumen
    d.-l. catheter
    d.-l. papillotome
dual-photon absorptiometry
Dual-Port system
Dubin-Amelar varicocele
   classification
Dubin-Johnson syndrome
Dubin-Sprinz
    D.-S. disease
    D.-S. syndrome
Dubrof shaker
Duchenne-type muscular dystrophy
duck-bill forceps
Duckett
    D. meatal advancement
    D. procedure
ducreyi
    Haemophilus d.
duct
    accessory pancreatic d.
    anomalous pancreaticobiliary d.
    (APBD)
    arborization of d.'s
    beaded hepatic d.
    bifurcation of common bile d.
    bile d.
    collecting d. (CD)
    common bile d. (CBD)
    common hepatic d.
    cortical collecting d. (CCD)
    cystic d.
    dilated d.
    dilated bile d.
    distal bile d.
    dorsal pancreatic d.
    ductal d.
    excretory d.
    extrahepatic bile d.
    fusiform widening of d.
    gall d.
    Gartner d.
    genu of pancreatic d.
    hepatic d.
    impacted cystic d.
    infected bile d.
    infundibulum of bile d.

    inner medullary collecting d.
    (IMCD)
    interlobular bile d.
    intrahepatic d.
    intrahepatic bile d.
    intrahepatic biliary d.
    intrapancreatic bile d.
    left hepatic d.
    d. lumen
    Luschka d.
    main pancreatic d. (MBD,
    MPD)
    medullary collecting d.
    mesonephric d.
    middle extrahepatic bile d.
    müllerian d.
    narrow-caliber d.
    non-transected pancreatic d.
    normal caliber d.
    pancreatic d.
    papillomatosis of intrahepatic
    bile d.
    perilobular d.
    preampullary portion of bile d.
    prepapillary bile d.
    proximal bile d.
    Rathke d.
    right hepatic d.
    d. of Santorini
    serpiginous microcystic d.
    Skene d.
    subvesical d.
    tear d.
    terminal bile d.
    terminal inner medullary
    collecting d.
    upstream pancreatic d.
    vitelline d.
    Wharton d.
    d. of Wirsung
    wolffian d.
ductal
    d. cystadenoma
    d. decompression
    d. dilation
    d. duct
    d. epithelial hyperplasia

D

NOTES

ductal *(continued)*
    d. hypertension
    d. stricture
    d. system
    d. system perforation
ductectatic
    d. mucinous cystadenoma
    d. tumor
ductography
    post-sphincterotomy d.
ductopenia
ductopenic rejection
ductular structure
ductule
    d. efferentes
Duecollement
    D. hemicolectomy
    D. maneuver
Duette double lumen ERCP instrument
dufourmentel technique
Duhamel
    D. colon operation
    D. pull-through
Duke
    D. pouch
    D. pouch cutaneous urinary diversion
Dukes
    D. A, B, C, signet cell
    D. B-1
    D. classification of carcinoma
    D. stage
    D. staging system
Dul45 cell line
Dulbecco modified Eagle medium
Dulcolax
    D. bowel prep
dull
    d. pain
    d. to percussion abdomen
dullness
    hepatic d.
    liver d.
    d. to percussion
    shifting d.
    splenic d.
    tympanitic d.
dumbbell-shaped
    d.-s. calyceal extension
    d.-s. shadow
dumdum fever

Dumon-Gilliard
    D.-G. endoprosthesis system
    D.-G. prosthesis introducer
    D.-G. prosthesis pushing tube
dumping
    late d.
    d. stomach
    d. syndrome
duocrinin
duodenal
    d. adenocarcinoma
    d. adenoma
    d. atresia
    d. bleeding
    d. bulb
    d. bulb deformity
    d. cancer
    d. cap
    d. carcinoid
    d. C-loop
    d. compression
    d. diaphragm
    d. diverticulitis
    d. diverticulum
    d. effect
    d. endoscopic polypectomy
    d. erosion
    d. fistula
    d. fluid collection
    d. foreign body
    d. gastrinoma
    d. hemangiomatosis
    d. hematoma
    d. impression
    d. impression on liver
    d. injury
    d. juice
    d. leiomyoma
    d. lesion
    d. loop
    d. lumen
    d. lymphoma
    d. mass
    d. metastasis
    d. mucosa
    d. neurofibroma
    d. obstruction
    d. orifice
    d. papilla
    d. perforation
    d. polyp
    d. polyposis
    d. reflux

d. secretin test (DST)
d. stenosis
d. stump
d. sweep
d. switch
d. telangiectasia
d. terminus
d. trauma
d. tuberculosis
d. tumor
d. ulcer (DU)
d. ulceration
d. ulcer disease
d. varices
d. varix
d. villus
d. wall hamartoma
d. web
duodenale
　Ancylostoma d.
duodenalis
　Giardia d.
duodenectomy
duodenitis
　chronic atrophic d.
　erosive d.
duodenobiliary
　d. pressure gradient
　d. reflux
duodenocaval fistula
duodenocholecystostomy
duodenocholedochotomy
duodenocolic fistula
duodenocystostomy
duodenoenterocutaneous fistula
duodenoenterostomy
duodenogastric reflux (DGR)
duodenogastroesophageal reflux (DGER)
duodenogastroscopy
　retrograde d. (RDG)
duodenography
　hypotonic d.
duodenoileal bypass (DIB)
duodenoileitis
duodenojejunal
　d. flexure

d. fold
d. hernia
d. junction
duodenojejunostomy
　suprapapillary Roux-en-Y d.
duodenolysis
duodenomesocolic fold
duodenopancreaticocholedochal rupture
duodenopancreatic reflux
duodenorrhaphy
duodenoscope
　diagnostic d.
　Fujinon EVD-XL video d.
　large-channel therapeutic d.
　master d.
　Olympus EW-series
　　fiberoptic d.
　Olympus JF-series video d.
　Olympus JF-V-series video d.
　Olympus JT-series video d.
　Olympus PJF-series pediatric d.
　side-viewing fiberoptic or
　　video d.
　standard d.
　therapeutic d.
　therapeutic side-viewing d.
　video d.
duodenoscopy
duodenostomy
　Witzel d.
duodenotomy
　transverse d.
duodenum
　Brunner gland of d.
　brunneroma of d.
　button of d.
　C-loop of d.
　closed d.
　descending d.
　distal d.
　obstruction d.
　scarified d.
　supravaterian d.
　ulcer d.
Duo-Flow catheter
DUPAN 2 tumor marker

D

NOTES

duplicate uterus
duplication
   alimentary tract d.
   d. anomaly
   complete d.
   d. cyst
   gastric d.
   incomplete d.
   renal d.
   tubular d.
   tubular colonic d.
Dupuytren
   D. contracture
   D. disease
   D. hydrocele
   D. suture
   D. tourniquet
durable healing
Duracep biopsy forceps
Dura-II positionable penile prosthesis
dural patch reconstruction
Duraphase inflatable penile prosthesis
duration
   d. time
Duricef
Duroziez sign
Durrani
   D. dorsal vein complex ligation needle
   D. needle
duskiness
   stomal d.
dusky stoma
Duval
   D. pancreaticojejunostomy
   D. procedure
Duvoid
DVIU
   direct vision internal urethrotomy
DVS
   direct vesicoureteral scintigraphy
dwell period
D-xylose
   D.-x. absorption test
   D.-x. malabsorption
dyad
   mother-infant d.
dyadic relationship
Dyazide
Dyclone

dye
   Alcian blue d.
   basic d.
   cationic d.
   Congo red d.
   Evans blue d.
   indigo carmine d.
   indocyanine green d. (ICG)
   iodine d.
   Kiton red d.
   d. laser
   metachromatic d.
   methylene blue d.
   orthochromatic d.
   radiopaque d.
   rapid emptying of d.
   rhodamine 6G d.
   d. scattering method
   d. sham intrarenal lesion
   d. spraying
DynaCell motility morphometry measurement workstation
DynaCirc
Dynaflex
   D. penile implant
   D. penile prosthesis
DYNAFLUVE
   dynamic fluorescence video endoscopy
dynamic
   d. closure pressure
   d. cystourethroscopy
   d. fluorescein angiography
   d. fluorescence video endoscopy (DYNAFLUVE)
   d. graciloplasty
   d. ileus
   d. infusion cavernosometry
   d. infusion cavernosometry and cavernosonography
dynograph
dynorphin
dysarthric
dysautonomia
   Riley-Day syndrome of familial d.
dysautonomy
dyschezia
   defecatory d.
dys-coordinate hyoid movement
dysdiadochokinesia
dysenteriae
   Shigella d.

dysenteric
d. algid malaria
d. diarrhea
dysentery
amebic d.
bacillary d.
balantidial d.
bilharzial d.
fulminating d.
helminthic d.
Japanese d.
malignant d.
Shigella d.
Sonne d.
spirillar d.
spirochetal d.
viral d.
dysesthesia
dysfunction
anal sphincter d.
anorectal sensorimotor d.
autonomic d.
cardiopulmonary baroreflex d.
cavernous autonomic nerve d.
colorectal physiologic d.
constitutional hepatic d.
corporeal venous occlusive d.
ejaculatory d.
erectile d.
esophageal body motor d.
gastric d.
geriatric voiding d.
hindgut d.
human erectile d.
intrinsic sphincter d. (ISD)
late graft d.
neurogenic erectile d.
neuropathic d.
neutrophil d.
nondiabetic neurogenic
  erectile d.
outlet d.
pelvic floor d.
platelet d.
postgastrectomy d.
posttransplant renal d.

psychogenic erectile d.
psychologic d.
puborectalis d.
sphincter d.
sphincter of Oddi d. (SOD)
transfer d.
traumatic corporeal veno-
  occlusive d.
urodynamic d.
veno-occlusive d.
visceral d.
dysfunctional
d. bleeding
d. voiding
dysgenesis
anorectal d.
gonadal d.
dysgenetic
d. fibrous band
d. gonad
dysgerminoma
dyskeratosis follicularis
dyskinesia
bile duct d.
biliary d.
dyskinetic puborectalis
dyslipidemia
dyslipidosis
dysmorphic vessel
dysmorphy
extrarenal d.
dysmotility
chronic intestinal d. (CID)
esophageal d.
gallbladder d.
dysorexia
dyspareunia
dyspepsia
acid d.
adhesion d.
atonic d.
biliary d.
cholelithic d.
fermentative d.
flatulent d.
functional d.

D

NOTES

dyspepsia *(continued)*
    gastric d.
    gastroduodenal d.
    mononuclear d.
    nervous d.
    nonorganic d.
    non-ulcer d., nonulcer d.
        (NUD)
    postcholecystectomy flatulent d.
    reflex d.
dyspeptic
dysphagia
    d. aortica
    Atkinson scoring system for d.
    contractile ring d.
    esophageal d.
    liquid food d.
    d. lusoria
    d. nervosa
    oropharyngeal d.
    postvagotomy d.
    pre-esophageal d.
    progressive d.
    sideropenic d.
    soft food d.
    solid food d.
    transfer d.
    vallecular d.
dysphonia
dysphoria
dysplasia
    arteriohepatic d.
    Barrett d.
    epithelial d.
    fibrous d.
    genital d.
    high-grade d. (HGD)
    low-grade d. (LGD)
    malignant d.
    mucosal d.
    multicystic renal d.
    non-ulcer d., nonulcer d.
    polypoid d.
    renal d.
    renal duplication with
        segmental renal d.
    urothelial d.
dysplasia-associated lesion or mass
    (DALM)

dysplasia-to-carcinoma sequence
dysplastic kidney
dyspnea
dysraphic malformation
dysraphism
    bony d.
    occult spinal d.
    spinal d.
dysreflexia
    autonomic d.
dysrhythmia
    ESWL related d.
    gastric d.
    glucagon-evoked gastric d.
dysspermatogenic sterility
dyssynergia
    detrusor external sphincter d.
        (DESD)
    detrusor sphincter d. (DSD)
    detrusor urethral d.
    pelvic floor d.
    rectoanal d.
    vesical external sphincter d.
        (VSD)
    vesicosphincteric d.
dystonia
dystonic phenomenon
dystopia
    d. transversa externa testis
    d. transversa interna testis
dystrophica
    epidermolysis bullosa d.
dystrophic calcification
dystrophy
    Duchenne-type muscular d.
    muscular d.
    myotonic d.
    myotonic muscular d.
dysuria
dysuric

E
    erythrocyte
E1, E₁
        prostaglandin E.
        E. protein
E2
        prostaglandin E. (PGE2)
        E. protein
E-1023
        enzyme immunoassay E.
E₁ (*var. of* E1)
e10 electrosurgery system
E1b protein
Eadie-Hofstee
        E.-H. plot
        E.-H. transformation
EAEC
        enteroadherent *Escherichia coli*
Eagle-Barrett syndrome
Eagle minimal essential medium
EAL
        endoscopic aspiration lumpectomy
ear
        dog e.
Earle
        E. hemorrhoid clamp
        E. medium
        E. rectal probe
        E. solution
early
        The E. Detector
early-onset graft-vs-host disease
early satiety
earth-eating
EAS
        external anal sphincter
Easi-Lav lavage
easily reducible hernia
Eastern Cooperative Oncology Group
easy bruisability
eater
        liver e.
eating habit
EBA
        extrahepatic biliary atresia
Ebbehoj procedure
EBL
        estimated blood loss
Ebola hemorrhagic fever

ebrotidine
EBS
        estrogen binding site
EBV
        Epstein-Barr virus
EC
        epithelial cell
        esophageal candidiasis
            thymic EC
ECA
        enterobacterial common antigen
EC-cell
        antral E.-c.
ECF
        extracellular fluid
echinococcal
        e. abscess
        e. cyst disease
        e. liver abscess
echinococciasis
echinococcosis
        biliary e.
        hepatic e.
        hepatic-alveolar e.
Echinococcus
        E. granulosus
        life cycle of E.
        E. liver cyst
        E. multilocularis
echocolonoscope
        CF-UM3 e.
echo-Doppler
echoduodenoscope
        Olympus XJF-UM20 e.
echoduodenoscopy
echoendoscope
        linear-type e.
        Olympus CF-UM-series e.
        Olympus GF-UM-series e.
        Olympus GIF-EUM-series e.
        Olympus GIF-series e.
        Olympus JF-UM-series e.
        Olympus UM-series e.
        Olympus VU-M-series e.
        Olympus XIF-UM-series e.
        radial sector scanning e.
echoendoscopy (EUS)
echogastroscope
echogenic
        e. liver

E

echogenicity
central e.
echographic
homogeneous e.
echolucent
echomorphologic
echo pattern
echo-poor layer
echoprobe
Olympus XMP-U2 catheter e.
echorich
echovirus
e. infection
ECI automatic reprocessor
Eckhout vertical gastroplasty
ECL
enterochromaffin-like
ECL cell
ECL cell hyperplasia
ECL Western blotting
ECLoma
ECLP
extracorporeal liver perfusion
ECM
extracellular matrix
ECOG performance status scale
Ecotrin
ECPL
endocavitary pelvic
lymphadenectomy
ectasia
antral vascular e.
cecal vascular e.
gastric antral vascular e.
(GAVE)
mucinous ductal e.
tortuous venous e.
vascular e.
ectatic
e. vascular lesion
e. vessel
ectoderm
ectopia
crossed renal e.
intra-abdominal transverse
testicular e.
e. testis
testis e.
transverse testicular e.
ureteral e.
e. vesicae
ectopic
e. adrenal rest

e. anus
e. gastric mucosa
e. gestation
e. kidney
e. pancreas
e. pregnancy
e. sigmoid pregnancy
e. testis
e. ureter
e. ureterocele
e. varices
ectopy
acquired gastric e.
gastric mucosal e.
ectoscopy
ECU
extracorporeal ultrafiltration
ED1
monoclonal antibody E.
EDA+
extradomain A positive
EDAP LT.01 lithotriptor
edema
angioneurotic e.
antral e.
bullous e.
bullous e. vesicae
focal e.
idiopathic e.
laryngeal e.
nephrotic e.
pedal e.
perianal e.
pericholecystic e.
peripheral e.
peripheral extremity e.
pitting e.
pulmonary e.
sacral e.
edematous
e. gallbladder
e. hyperemic mucosa
e. pancreatitis
e. tag
edentulous
Eder-Bernstein gastroscope
Eder-Chamberlin gastroscope
Eder gastroscope
Eder-Hufford
E.-H. gastroscope
E.-H. rigid esophagoscope

Eder-Palmer
    E.-P. semiflexible fiberoptic
      endoscope
    E.-P. semiflexible gastroscope
Eder-Puestow
    E.-P. dilation
    E.-P. dilator shaft
    E.-P. guidewire
    E.-P. metal olive dilator
    E.-P. olive
edetate
    disodium e.
edge
    e. enhancement
    heaped up e.'s
    hepatic e.
    ligament reflecting e.
    liver e.
    Poupart ligament shelving e.
    ulcer with heaped up e.'s
EdGr
    Edmondson grading
    EdGr system
Edlich gastric lavage tube
Edmondson
    E. grading (EdGr)
    E. grading system
    E. grading system for
      hepatocellular carcinoma
EDNO
    endothelium-derived nitric oxide
EDRF
    endothelium-derived relaxing factor
edrophonium
    e. test
ED-SPAZ
EDTA
    ethylenediaminetetraacetic acid
    ^{51}Cr-EDTA excretion
    ^{51}Cr-labeled EDTA
Edwards syndrome
EEA
    end-to-end anastomosis
    EEA AutoSuture stapler
    EEA stapler
    EEA stapler gun

    EEA stapling device
    EEA stapling of varices
EEG
    electroencephalography
EEGF
    esophageal epidermal growth factor
EEJ
    electroejaculation
EEPLND
    extraperitoneal endoscopic pelvic
      lymph node dissection
EES
    expandable esophageal stent
E.E.S.
EFAD
    essential fatty acid deficiency
effect
    antinociceptive e.
    banana peel e.
    blooming e.
    choleretic e.
    concomitant medication e.
    disulfiram-like e.
    duodenal e.
    esophageal e.
    first-pass e.
    gastric e.
    gender e.
    halo e.
    hypothermic e.
    intracellular flush e.
    irradiation e.
    local alcohol instillation e.
    metabolic e.
    mitrogenic e.
    mutagenic e.
    normothermic e.
    octreotide e.
    physiological trophic e.
    placebo e.
    preservation times e.
    prokinetic e.
    sieving e.
    systemic e.
    topic e.
    tubulotoxic e.

E

NOTES

effective
    e. dose equivalent radiation
    e. renal plasma flow (ERPF)
EFFERdose
    Zantac E.
efferent
    e. arteriole
    e. limb
    e. loop
    e. renal sympathetic nerve
      activity (ERSNA)
efferentes
    ductule e.
Effer-Syllium
efficiency
    defunctioning e.
effluent
    anal e.
    ileostomy e.
    peritoneal dialysis e. (PDE)
    transverse colostomy e.
efflux
EG
    esophagogastric
EGBT
    esophagogastric balloon tamponade
EGD
    esophagogastroduodenoscopy
EGE
    eosinophilic gastroenteritis
egesta
EGF
    epidermal growth factor
    ^{125}I-h-EGF
    intragastric EGF
    luminal EGF
    subcutaneous EGF
EGFR
    epidermal growth factor receptor
EGG
    electrogastrography
eggerthii
    Bacteroides e.
egophony
EGS
    electrogalvanic stimulation
    EGS Model 100
      electrogalvanic stimulator
EGTA
    ethylene glycol tetraacetic acid
Egyptian splenomegaly
EHEC
    enterohemorrhagic *Escherichia coli*

EHL
    electrohydraulic lithotripsy
    EHL probe
Ehlers-Danlos syndrome
EHM
    extrahepatic metastasis
EHPVO
    extrahepatic portal vein obstruction
Ehrlich reagent
EHT
    electro-hydro-thermal
    EHT electrode
EIA
    enzyme immunoassay
    enzyme-linked immunosorbent assay
    EIA kit
EIA-2
    second-generation enzyme
      immunoassay
eicosanoid
eicosapentaenoic acid (EPA)
EIEC
    enteroinvasive *Escherichia coli*
eight-lumen esophageal manometry catheter
Einhorn
    E. dilator
    E. string test
EIS
    endoscopic injection sclerotherapy
Eisenberger technique
Eitest MONO P-II test
ejaculatio
    e. deficiens
    e. praecox
    e. retardata
ejaculation
    antegrade e.
    dry e.
    premature e.
    retrograde e.
ejaculatory
    e. duct obstruction
    e. duct reflux
    e. dysfunction
    e. impotence
ejecta
ejection
EJP
    excitatory junction potential
ekiri
Ektachem slide test
EL2-LS2 flexible video laparoscope

ELAD
extracorporeal liver assist device
ELAM-1
endothelial leukocyte adhesion
molecule-1
ligand for E.
elastalloy
e. esophageal endoprosthesis
E. esophageal stent
elastase
neutrophil e.
serum e. 1
elastic
e. band ligation
e. bougie
e. ligature
e. O ring
e. silicone membrane
elastica interna
elasticum
pseudoxanthoma e.
Elastoplast dressing
Elavil
ELBF
estimated liver blood flow
ELBNS
extraperitoneal laparoscopic bladder
neck suspension
elbowed
e. bougie
e. catheter
electrical
e. conductivity
single potential analysis of
cavernous e.
e. waveform
electric tissue morcellator
electroblotting
electrocautery
bipolar e.
Bovie e.
Bugbee e.
e. knife
light e.
monopolar e.
Neomed e.

e. pencil
e. resection
electrocholecystectomy
electrocholecystocausis
electrocoagulating
e. biopsy forceps
e. current
electrocoagulation
bipolar e. (BPEC)
direct current e.
endoscopic e.
monopolar e.
multipolar e.
e. necrosis
snare e.
transendoscopic e.
electrocystography
electrode
abdominal patch e.
ACMI monopolar e.
antimony pH e.
ASSI laparoscopic e.
ball e.
bio potential skin e.
bipolar glass e.
Bugbee e.
button e.
Cameron-Miller e.
coagulating e.
common pH e.
concentric-needle e.
cutting e.
Disa needle e.
dome-tip e.
EHT e.
electro-hydro-thermal e.
E. Electrolyte
Eppendorf needle e.
flat spatula e.
glass pH e.
Greenwald Control Tip
cystoscopic e.
hook tip laparoscopic e.
indifferent e.
intraluminal reference e.
ion-specific e.
e. jelly

NOTES

E

electrode *(continued)*
  J-hook tip laparoscopic e.
  knife e.
  Lletz-Leep active loop e.
  loop-tipped e.
  Microelectrode MI-506 small-caliber pH e.
  Microglass pH e.
  midgastric e.
  model 440 M1.5, M4 e.
  needle e.
  needle-tip laparoscopic e.
  pencil-tipped e.
  e. placement
  e. probe
  renal sympathetic nerve activity recording e.
  reusable laparoscopic e.
  right-angle e.
  single-fiber EMG e.
  spatula tip laparoscopic e.
  spoon tip laparoscopic e.
  St. Mark pudendal e.
  surface e.
  three-quarter circle e.
  unipolar glass e.
  VaporTrode e.
electroejaculation (EEJ)
  rectal probe e.
electroejaculator
  G&S E.
electroencephalography (EEG)
electrogalvanic
  e. stimulation (EGS)
  e. stimulator
electrogastrogram
  cutaneous e.
electrogastrograph
electrogastrography (EGG)
electrohemostasis
electrohydraulic
  e. lithotripsy (EHL)
  e. lithotripsy probe
  e. lithotriptor
  e. lithotriptor probe
  percutaneous transhepatic choledochoscopic e.
  e. shock wave lithotripsy (ESWL)
electro-hydro-thermal (EHT)
  e.-h.-t. electrode
electroimmunodiffusion assay
electroincision

electrolyte
  e. abnormality
  e. balance
  bicarbonate e.
  calcium e.
  chloride e.
  CO_2 e.
  Electrode E.
  e. flush solution
  e. imbalance coma
  e. loss
  potassium e.
  e. preparation
  sodium e.
  stool e.
electrolyte-polyethylene glycol lavage solution
electromagnetic
  e. flow transducer
  e. lithotriptor
electromechanical
  e. coupling
  epinephrine-induced gastroduodenal e.
  e. impactor (EMI)
electromicroscopy
electromyogram (EMG)
  colonic e.
electromyography
  conventional concentric e.
  Disa e.
  intra-anal e.
  needle electrode e.
  noninvasive intra-anal e.
  pelvic floor e.
  rhabdosphincter e.
  single-fiber needle e.
  video pressure flow e.
electron
  e. immunoperoxidase observation
  e. microscopy
electron-dense mesangial deposit
electronic
  e. endoscope
  e. recording nappies
electrophoresis
  agarose gel e.
  horizontal e.
  e. immunoblot analysis
  immunofixation e.
  polyacrylamide gel e. (PAGE)
  pulsed field gel e. (PFGE)

serum e.
urine e.
electrophoretic mobility
electrophysiology of the gastric
musculature
electroresection
electrostimulation
electrosurgery
electrosurgical
e. curved scissors
e. cut
e. cutting knife
e. desiccation
e. fulguration
e. generator
e. monopolar spatula probe
e. needle
e. scissors
e. snare
e. snare polypectomy
e. spatula
e. unit (ESU)
electrotherapy
Elema-Siemens AB pressure
transducer
element
hepatic subcellular e.
elemental
e. diet
e. diet treatment
e. phosphate
elephantiasis
e. scroti
elevated WBC count
elevator
Alexander e.
Doyen rib e.
Stille e.
eleventh
e. rib flank incision
e. rib transperitoneal incision
elimination
e. diet
spontaneous partial e.
stool e.
ELIMINATOR
E. biliary stent

E. nasal biliary catheter set
E. pancreatic stent
E. PET biliary balloon dilator
E. stone extraction basket
Eliminator
Fecal Odor E. (FOE)
ELISA
enzyme-linked immunoassay
first-generation ELISA
ELISA-I
enzyme-linked
immunosorbent assay I
ELISA-II
ELISA-III test, ELISA-3 test
ELISA-II test, ELISA-2 test
ELISA-I test, ELISA-1 test
sensitive and specific ELISA
ELISA test
ELISA titer
Ellik evacuator
Elliot position
Elliott gallbladder forceps
ellipsoid
e. method
elliptical incision
Ellsner gastroscope
Elmiron
ELMISKOP 101 electron
microscope
elongated
e., pseudostratified nucleus
eluate
acetonitrile e.
ELUS
endoluminal rectal ultrasonography
elusive
e. polyp
e. ulcer
eluted antibody
elutriation
T-cell depletion by e.
EM
erythema multiforme
EMA
antiendomysial antibody
antibody to EMA
emaciation

E

NOTES

emasculation
embarrassment
    circulatory e.
    respiratory e.
emboli (*pl. of* embolus)
embolic agent
embolism
    bile pulmonary e.
    cholesterol e.
    mesenteric arterial e.
    pulmonary e.
embolization
    angiographic e.
    angiographic variceal e.
    arterial e.
    bilateral pudendal artery e.
    cholesterol crystal e. (CCE)
    Gelfoam e.
    splenic arterial e.
    transarterial e.
    transcatheter arterial e. (TAE)
    transcatheter hepatic arterial e.
    transcatheter splenic arterial e.
    (TSAE)
    transcatheter variceal e.
    transhepatic e. (THE)
embolotherapy
    transcatheter e.
embolus, pl. **emboli**
    metallic e.
    pulmonary e.
    talc e.
embryologic development
embryology
embryoma
    e. of the kidney
embryonal
    e. adenoma
    e. testicular carcinoma
    e. tumor
embryonic cleavage
Emcyt
emepronium
    e. bromide
emergency
    e. appendectomy
    e. colonoscopy
    e. laparotomy
emergent appendectomy
emesis
    bilious e.
    coffee-grounds e.
Emete-con

emetic
    e. reflex
emetine
emetocathartic
Emetrol
EMG
    electromyogram
    sphincter EMG
EMI
    electromechanical impactor
    EMI APED amplifier
    discriminator
    EMI 9813B photomultiplier
eminence
    hypothenar e.
    thenar e.
emission
    gamma e.
    nocturnal e.
emitter
    light e.
EMLA anesthetic
emobolization
emollient laxative
emotional support
EMPD
    extramammary Paget disease
emphysema
    AATD-related e.
    α_1-antitrypsin disease-related e.
    colonoscopy-related e.
    endoscopy-related e.
    panacinar e.
    panlobular e.
    subcutaneous e.
    unilateral periorbital e.
emphysematous
    e. cholecystitis
    e. cystitis
    e. gastritis
    e. pyelonephritis
emptying
    delayed gastric e.
    e. delta volume
    gastric e. (GE)
    liquid e.
    neorectal e.
    rectal e.
    Roux limb e.
    solid e.
    T-half e.
empyema
    e. of gallbladder

empyocele
EMS
  esophageal manometric sequence
emulsion
  Calogen LCT e.
  intralipid fat e.
  intravenous lipid e.
  lipid e.
Emulsoil
  E. bowel prep
E-Mycin
EN
  enteral nutrition
en
  e. bloc dissection
  e. bloc distal pancreatectomy
  e. bloc resection
  e. bloc technique
  e. coup de sabre
  e. face
  e. face view
ENA
  extracted nuclear antigen
  ENA screen
enalapril
ENANB
  enterically transmitted non-A, non-B
  ENANB hepatitis
enanthate
  testosterone e.
enantiomer D-arginine
enbobabcock
encapsulated
  e. carcinoid tumor
  e. plasmodium
  e. renal cell carcinoma
encapsulation
  peritoneal e.
  tumor e.
encasement
  ureteral e.
encephaloid gastric carcinoma
encephalopathy
  bilirubin e.
  hepatic e. (HE)
  portal-systemic e. (PSE)

  postshunt e.
  Wernicke e.
encephalotrigeminal syndrome
encircle
encirclement
  anal e.
encopresis
encroachment
  scrotal e.
encrustation
  e. of stent
encysted
  e. calculus
  e. intra-abdominal collection
end
  advanced glycation e. (AGE)
  e. colostomy
  e. expiratory
  e. ileostomy
  e. stoma
endarterectomy
  e. knife
endemic
  e. deep mycosis
  e. nonbacterial infantile
    gastroenteritis
end-end stapler
Endep
end-expiratory intragastric pressure
end-fire transrectal probe
end-hole ureteral catheter
end-loop
  e.-l. colostomy
  e.-l. ileocolostomy
  e.-l. ileostomy
  e.-l. stoma
Endo
  E. pants
endoanal mucosectomy
Endo-Assist
  E.-A. disposable atraumatic
    grasping forceps
  E.-A. disposable hemostat
  E.-A. disposable ligature carrier
  E.-A. disposable needle holder
  E.-A. reusable knot pusher
endoauscultation

E

NOTES

Endo-Avitene
  E.-A. MCH
  E.-A. microfibrillar collagen
    hemostat
Endo-Babcock stapler
endobag
EndoBib
endobiliary ascariasis
endobrachyesophagus
endobronchial fistula
Endocam
endocamera
  Polaroid e. EC-3
endocarditis
  enterococcal e.
  marantic e.
  native valve bacterial e.
  Streptococcus bovis e.
endocast
endocavitary
  e. bladder diverticulectomy
  e. pelvic lymphadenectomy
    (ECPL)
Endoclip, Endo Clip
Endocoil esophageal stent
endocolitis
endocrine
  e. cell
  e. screening
  e. system
  e. therapy
endocystitis
endocytosis
  fluid-phase e.
endocytotic vesicle
endodermic cell
Endodynamics suction polyp trap
endoenteritis
endogastritis
Endo-gauge
endogenous
  e. biotin
  e. lipophilic antioxidant
  e. mutation
  e. obesity
  e. opioid
  e. peroxidase
  e. peroxidase activity
  e. pyrogen
  e. renal antigen
EndoGIA (30, 60) stapler

Endolav
  E. lavage pump
  Meditron EL-100 E.
endoligature
endoloop
endoluminal
  e. rectal ultrasonography
    (ELUS)
  e. ultrasonography
  e. ultrasound
EndoMate grab bag
endometrial carcinoma
endometrioma
  ovarian e.
endometriosis
  colorectal e.
endometrium
endomysial IgA
EndoNet
  Pentax E.
Endopath
  E. endoscopic linear cutter
  E. Optiview laparoscopic
    obturator
  E. (30, 60) stapler
endoperoxide
  PGG2 e.
  PGH2 e.
endophlebitis hepatica obliterans
endophotography
endophytic
endoplasmic
  e. reticulum (ER)
  e. reticulum-bound polysome
endoprostatic coil
endoprosthesis
  biliary e.
  Celestin e.
  crutched stick-type
    polyurethane e.
  cuffed esophageal e.
  double-lumen e.
  double-pigtail e.
  elastalloy esophageal e.
  esophageal e.
  exchange of e.
  expandable biliary e.
  expandable metal mesh e.
  Key-Med Atkinson e.
  large-bore biliary e.
  Medoc-Celestin e.
  pancreatic e.
  peroral e.

pigtail e.
plastic e.
Procter-Livingstone e.
self-expandable stainless steel
    braided e.
Titan e.
transpapillary endoscopic e.
Wallstent e.
Wilson-Cook e.
endopyelotomy
endopyeloureterotomy
    percutaneous e.
endorectal
    e. coil magnetic resonance
        imaging
    e. ileal pouch
    e. ileal pull-through
    e. probe
    e. pull-through
    e. surface coil MRI
    e. ultrasound (ERUS)
endorectal-pelvic phased-array coil
β-endorphin
endosac
endo-scissors
    rotating e.-s.
endoscope
    AccuSharp e.
    ACMI e.
    battery-powered e.
    CF-HM e.
    Cho/Dyonics two-portal e.
    double-channel e.
    Eder-Palmer semiflexible
        fiberoptic e.
    electronic e.
    end-viewing e.
    FCS two-channel ultra high-
        magnification e.
    FG-series two-channel e.
    FGS-ML-series two-channel e.
    FGS-series two-channel e.
    FGS-SML-series two-channel e.
    fiberoptic e.
    flexible e.
    flexible fiberoptic e.
    forward-viewing e.

Fujinon EG-FP-series e.
Fujinon EVE-series e.
Fujinon EVG-CT-series e.
Fujinon EVG-FP-series e.
Fujinon EVG-F-series e.
Fujinon FP-series e.
Fujinon UGI-FP-series video e.
Hirschowitz e.
e. impaction
JFB III e.
J-shaped e.
Karl Storz e.
Kussmaul e.
LoPresti e.
magnifying e.
Messerklinger e.
mother/daughter e.
near-infrared electronic e.
oblique-viewing e.
Olympus Aloka GF-EU-
    series e.
Olympus CV-series e.
Olympus DES-series e.
Olympus EUS-series e.
Olympus EVIS Q-series e.
Olympus GF-UM-series e.
Olympus GIF-HM-series e.
Olympus GIF-J-series e.
Olympus GIF-Q-series e.
Olympus GIF-T-series e.
Olympus GIF-XP-series e.
Olympus GIF-XV-series e.
Olympus JF-T-series e.
Olympus JF-TV-series e.
Olympus JF-V-series e.
Olympus PJF-series pediatric e.
Olympus P-series e.
Olympus TJF-series e.
Olympus UM-series e.
Olympus V-series e.
Olympus XCF-XK-series e.
Olympus XP-series e.
Olympus XQ-series e.
pediatric e.
Pentax EC-series video e.
Pentax EG-series video e.
Pentax FD-series video e.

E

NOTES

endoscope *(continued)*
Pentax FG-series video e.
rigid e.
semiflexible e.
semirigid e.
side-viewing e.
Simpson e.
Surgenomic e.
Toshiba video e.
transcutaneous sonogram e.
two-channel e.
UGI e.
ultrasound e.
upper GI e.
video e.
Visicath e.
Weerda e.
Welch Allyn video e.
endoscope-body position relationship
endoscopic
e. alligator forceps
e. aspiration lumpectomy (EAL)
e. assessment
e. atrophic gastritis
e. band ligation
e. band ligation of varices
e. BICAP probe
e. biliary decompression
e. biliary drainage
e. biliary stent
e. biliary stent placement
e. biopsy
e. biopsy forceps
e. biopsy site
e. brush cytology
e. camera
e. cholangiography
e. color Doppler
e. color Doppler assessment
e. color Doppler ultrasonography
e. control
e. cystenterostomy
e. cystgastrostomy
e. cystoduodenostomy
e. cystogastrostomy
e. decompression
e. devolvulization
e. diagnosis
e. dilation
e. Doppler probe
e. Doppler ultrasonography

e. drainage
e. duct stone
e. electrocoagulation
e. electrohydraulic lithotripsy
e. enterogastric reflux gastritis
e. erythematous/exudative gastritis
e. esophagitis
e. esophagogastric variceal ligation
e. evaluation
e. examination
e. extirpation cicatricial obliteration
e. extraction pancreatic duct stone
e. finding
e. fine-needle aspiration cytology
e. fine needle puncture
e. fistulotomy
e. flowprobe
e. four-quadrant tattoo
e. fulguration
e. gastritis
e. gastrostomy
e. gastrostomy tube
e. grasping forceps
e. heat probe
e. hemoclip device
e. hemorrhagic gastritis
e. hemostasis
e. hemostatic therapy
e. incision
e. India ink injection
e. injection
e. injection sclerosis
e. injection sclerotherapy (EIS)
e. injection therapy
e. jejunostomy
e. laser
e. laser cautery
e. laser therapy
e. light source
e. magnetic extractor
e. management
e. manometry
e. microwave
e. microwave coagulation
e. mucosal resection
e. nasobiliary catheter drainage
e. optical urethrotomy
e. pancreatic drainage

e. pancreatic duct
sphincterotomy
e. pancreatic stenting (EPS)
e. pancreatic therapy
e. pancreatography
e. papillary balloon dilation
(EPD)
e. papillotomy (EPT)
e. papillotomy and stenting
e. photography
e. polypectomy
e. procedure
e. pulsed dye laser
e. pulsed dye laser lithotripsy
e. raised erosive gastritis
e. reflectance
e. reflectance spectrophotometry
e. removal
e. retroflexion
e. retrograde biliary stenting
e. retrograde cannulation
e. retrograde cholangiogram
e. retrograde cholangiography
(ERC)
e. retrograde
cholangiopancreatography
(ERCP)
e. retrograde
cholangiopancreatography
catheter
e. retrograde
cholecystoendoprosthesis
(ERCCE)
e. retrograde ileography
e. retrograde pancreatogram
(ERP)
e. retrograde pancreatography
(ERP)
e. retrograde parenchymography
(ERP)
e. retrograde parenchymography
of pancreas (ERPP)
e. retrograde sclerotherapy
e. rugal hyperplastic gastritis
e. scissors
e. sclerosis
e. sclerotherapy

e. sessile
e. sessile polypectomy
e. sewing machine
e. sigmoidopexy
e. small bowel biopsy
e. snare
e. snare resection
e. sphincterectomy
e. sphincter of Oddi
manometry
e. sphincterotomy (ES)
e. sphincterotomy-induced
duodenal perforation
e. sphincterotomy-induced
pancreatitis
e. stent
e. stent exchange
e. stenting
e. stigmata of hemorrhage
e. stone disintegration
e. stricturotomy
e. surveillance
e. suture-cutting forceps
e. system
e. tattoo
e. technology
e. therapy
e. thermo-disinfector
e. transesophageal fine-needle
aspiration
e. transpapillary cannulation
e. transpapillary catheter of the
gallbladder
e. transpapillary cyst drainage
(ETCD)
e. treatment
e. tube
e. ultrasonographic diagnosis
e. ultrasonographic imaging
e. ultrasonography (EUS)
e. ultrasound
e. ultrasound diagnosis
e. ultrasound evaluation
e. variceal ligation (EVL)
e. variceal sclerotherapy
e. washing pipe
e. Water Pik

E

NOTES

endoscopically
   e. deliverable tissue-transfixing
     device
   e. normal patient
endoscopic-controlled lithotripsy
endoscopist
endoscopy
   advanced therapeutic e.
   American Society for
     Gastrointestinal E. (ASGE)
   anal e.
   e. complication
   computerized electronic e.
   dynamic fluorescence video e.
     (DYNAFLUVE)
   fiberoptic e.
   flexible e.
   fluorescent electronic e.
   gastrointestinal e.
   high-altitude e.
   high-magnification e.
   intestinal e.
   intraoperative e.
   intraoperative biliary e.
   outpatient e.
   pancreaticobiliary e.
   pediatric e.
   peripartum e.
   peroral e.
   postsurgical e.
   primary diagnostic e.
   e. procedure
   e. suite
   TEM transanal e.
   therapeutic upper e.
   transesophageal e.
   transnasal e.
   UGI e.
   ultra high-magnification e.
   upper alimentary e.
   upper gastrointestinal e.
   video e.
endoscopy-related emphysema
Endoshears
EndoSheath
   Vision System E.
endosnare
endosonography
   e. instrument
endosonography-guided drainage of
  pancreatic pseudocyst
EndoSound endoscopic ultrasound
  catheter

EndoSpeak
Endospore disinfectant
Endostapler
Endostat II bipolar/monopolar
  electrosurgical generator
endostethoscope
Endotek machine
Endotek-Ultra
endothelial
   e. cell
   e. cell differentiation
   e. leukocyte adhesion
     molecule-1 (ELAM-1)
   e. tube
endothelial-dependent relaxation
endothelin (ET)
   e. A (EtA)
   e. A receptor
endothelin-1
   e.-1 concentration
endothelin-3
endotheliosis
   glomerular e.
endothelium
   gastrointestinal e.
   sinusoidal e.
endothelium-dependent
   e.-d. fibrinolysis
   e.-d. vasodilation
endothelium-derived
   e.-d. nitric oxide (EDNO)
   e.-d. relaxing factor (EDRF)
   e.-d. relaxing hormone
Endotorque
   Greenen E.
endotoxemia
   systemic e.
endotoxin
   bacterial e.
endotracheal
   e. intubation
   e. tube
   e. tube placement
ENDO-Tube nasal jejunal feeding
  tube
endoureteral ultrasound sonography
endoureterotomy
   cold knife e.
endourologic
endourological cold-knife incision
endourology
Endovations disposable cytology
  brush

endovenous
Endozime
    E. AW bacteriostatic enzyme
      cleaner
    E. sponge
end-point dilution titer
Endrate
end-sigmoid colostomy
end-stage
    e.-s. cirrhosis
    e.-s. disease
    e.-s. renal disease (ESRD)
    e.-s. renal failure
end-to-end
    e.-t.-e. anastomosis (EEA)
    e.-t.-e. branch reanastomosis
    e.-t.-e. enterostomy
end-to-side
    e.-t.-s. anastomosis
    e.-t.-s. arteriotomy
    e.-t.-s. choledochojejunostomy
    e.-t.-s. portacaval shunt
    e.-t.-s. reimplantation
    e.-t.-s. vasoepididymostomy
      technique
Enduron
Enduronyl
end-viewing
    e.-v. endoscope
    e.-v. gastroscope
enema
    air contrast barium e. (ACBE)
    5-aminosalicylic acid e.
    analeptic e.
    antegrade e.
    5-ASA e.
    barium e. (BE)
    blind e.
    cleansing hypertonic
      phosphate e.
    contrast e.
    Cortenema retention e.
    double-contrast air barium e.
    flatus e.
    Fleet e.
    Fleet Babylax e.
    flexible barium e.

    flocculation on barium e.
    full-column barium e.
    Gastrografin e.
    high e.
    hydrocortisone e.
    hydrogen peroxide e.
    Kayexalate e.
    lactulose e.
    Malone antegrade continence e.
    mesalamine e.
    methylene blue e.
    nuclear e.
    NuLytely e.
    nutrient e.
    oil retention e.
    phosphate e.
    Phospho-Soda e.
    prednisolone e.
    puddling on barium e.
    retention e.
    retrograde flow on barium e.
    Rowasa e.
    saline cleansing e.
    single-contrast barium e.
    small-bowel e.
    soapsuds e. (SSE)
    steroid foam e.
    sucralfate retention e.
    sulfasalazine e.
    tap water e.
    theophylline olamine e.
    turpentine e.
    water soluble contrast e.
enemas until clear
enemator
enemiasis
energy dispersive x-ray analysis
Enfamil with iron formula
enflurane
Engerix-B
    HBV E.-B.
engorgement
    liver e.
engraftment
enhanced
    e. chemiluminescence Western
      blotting (ECL Western blotting)

E

NOTES

enhanced *(continued)*
    e. reverse transcriptase
      polymerase chain reaction
      assay
enhancement
    contrast e.
    CT scan with contrast e.
    edge e.
ENK
    enkephalin
1-ENK
    leucine-enkephalin
enkephalin (ENK)
enlarged
    e. prostate
    e. uterine size
enlargement
    ovarian e.
    parotid gland e.
    salivary gland e.
    tonsillar e.
    tube e.
    uterine e.
enolase
    neuron-specific e. (NSE)
Enovil
enoxacin
Enrich feeding
ENS
    enteric nervous system
ensheathing trocar
ensnarement
Ensure
    E. Plus
    E. Plus formula
    E. Plus liquid feeding
    E. pudding
entactin
entamebiasis
Entamoeba
    E. histolytica
    E. histolytica abscess
enteral
    e. alimentation
    e. diarrhea
    e. feeding
    e. nutrition (EN)
enteralgia
enterectasis
enterectomy
enterelcosis
enteric
    e. adenovirus

    e. cyst
    e. excitatory motoneuron
    e. fever
    e. fistula
    e. ganglia
    e. ganglion cell
    e. hormone
    e. hyperoxaluria
    e. immunogen
    e. infection
    e. inhibitory motoneuron
    e. nervous system (ENS)
    e. neuron
    e. neuronal circuit
    e. neuronal reflex
    e. oxaluria
enterically transmitted non-A, non-B (ENANB)
enterically transmitted non-A, non-B hepatitis (ET-NANBH)
enteric-coated
    e.-c. aspirin
    e.-c. capsule
enteritidis
    Salmonella e.
enteritis
    Campylobacter e.
    Campylobacter fetus e.
    chronic cicatrizing e.
    Crohn regional e.
    diphtheritic e.
    eosinophilic e.
    granulomatous e.
    idiopathic diffuse ulcerative
      nongranulomatous e.
    leishmanial e.
    mucomembranous e.
    mucous e.
    e. necroticans
    phlegmonous e.
    e. polyposa
    pseudomembranous e.
    radiation e.
    regional e.
    segmental e.
    tuberculous e.
    ulcerative e.
    viral e.
enteroadherent *Escherichia coli* (EAEC)
enteroaggregative *Escherichia coli*
enteroanastomosis
enteroanthelone

enteroapocleisis
Enterobacter
   E. aerogenes
   E. cloacae
   E. hafniae
   E. liquefaciens
enterobacterial common antigen
  (ECA)
enterobiliary
Enterobius vermicularis
enterobrosis, enterobrosia
enterocele
   partial e.
   e. sac
enterocentesis
enterocholecystostomy
enterocholecystotomy
enterochromaffin cell
enterochromaffin-like (ECL)
   e.-l. cell
enterocleisis
   omental e.
enteroclysis
   small-bowel e.
   e. tube
enterococcal endocarditis
enterococci
Enterococcus
   E. faecalis
enterococcus
enterocolitica
   Yersinia e.
enterocolitis
   Aeromonas-associated e.
   antibiotic-induced e.
   bacterial e.
   gangrenous ischemic e.
   granulomatous e.
   hemorrhagic e.
   Hirschsprung-associated e.
    (HAEC)
   necrotizing e. (NEC)
   pseudomembranous e.
   radiation e.
   regional e.
   Salmonella typhimurium e.
enterocolostomy

enterocutaneous fistula
enterocyst
enterocystocele
enterocystoma
enterocystoplasty
   Camey e.
   clam e.
   sigmoid e.
enterocyte
   CD23 e.
Enterocytozoon bieneusi
enterodynia
enteroenteral fistula
enteroenteric fistula
enteroenterostomy
   Parker-Kerr e.
   two-layer e.
enterogastritis
enterogastrone
enterogenous
   e. cyanosis
   e. cyst
enteroglucagon
enterography
enterohemorrhagic *Escherichia coli*
  (EHEC)
enterohepatocele
enteroidea
enteroinsular axis
enteroinvasive
   e. *Escherichia coli* (EIEC)
enterokinase
enterolith
   calcified e.
enterolithiasis
enterolithotomy
enterology
enterolysis
enteromenia
enterometer
enteromycosis
enteronitis
enteroparesis
enteropathica
enteropathic organism
enteropathogenic *Escherichia coli*
  (EPEC)

NOTES

E

enteropathy
allergic e.
bile salt-losing e.
chronic bacterial e.
diabetic e.
food-sensitive e.
gluten-sensitive e.
idiopathic e.
protein-losing e.
radiation e.
soya-induced e.
enteroperitoneal abscess
enteropexy
enteroplasty
enteroplegia
enteroplex
enteroplexy
Enteroport feeding pump
enteroproctia
enterorrhagia
enterorrhaphy
enterorrhexis
enteroscope
magnifying e.
Olympus SIF-M-series video e.
Olympus SIF-series video e.
Olympus SIF-SW-series
video e.
Olympus SSIF-series video e.
Olympus XSIF-series video e.
Pentax VSB-P-series e.
sonde e.
temporary e.
tube e.
video push e.
enteroscopy
e. diagnosis
intraoperative e.
push e.
push-type e.
Roux-en-Y limb e.
small bowel e. (SBE)
transgastrostomic e. (TGE)
video small bowel e.
enterospasm
enterostasis
enterostaxis
enterostenosis
enterostomal therapy (ET)
enterostomy
double e.
end-to-end e.
enterotome

enterotomy
antimesenteric e.
inadvertent e.
longitudinal e.
enterotoxication
enterotoxigenic *Escherichia coli*
(ETEC)
enterotoxin
Clostridium difficile e.
e. diarrhea
enterotoxism
enterotropic
enterourethral fistula
enterourethrostomy
enterovaginal fistula
enterovesical fistula
enterovesicoplasty
enthesis
enthetic
entocele
entoderm
Entolase
Entozyme
Entract
E. catheter
E. stent
E. stone retriever
entrapment
e. of bowel
e. sack
e. sack introducer
EntriStar
E. feeding tube
E. polyurethane PEG tube
Entrition Entri-Pak feeding
entropion
eversion e.
entry site
enucleation
enuresis
e. alarm
e. alarm technique
diurnal e.
monosymptomatic e.
nocturnal e.
environment
bactericidal stomach e.
enzimoimmunoassay MEIA Abbott
Enzol disinfectant
Enzygnost antiHIV 1+2 test
**enzymatic spectrophotometric
analysis**

enzyme
angiotensin converting e.
(ACE)
AP marker e.
brancher e.
brush-border marker e.
carboxypeptidase B-like e.
cellular e.
e. change
circulating e.
cytochrome P450 e.
debrancher e.
digestive e.
gluconeogenesis-associated e.
glycolytic e.
glycosaminoglycan-degrading e.
HK e.
e. immunoassay (EIA)
e. immunoassay E-1023
lactase e.
LDH e.
lipase e.
lipolytic e.
liver e.
lysosomal e.
NAG lysosomal marker e.
pancreatic e.
plasma e.
proteinase e.
proteolytic e.
SDH e.
enzyme-conjugated anti-IgA antibody
enzyme-linked
e.-l. immunoassay (ELISA)
e.-l. immunosorbent assay
(EIA)
e.-l. immunosorbent assay II
(ELISA-II)
enzyme-linked immunosorbent assay I (ELISA-I)
enzymic protein
Enzymun test
eo
eosinophil

EORTC
European Organization for Research
and Treatment of Cancer
eosin
hematoxylin and e. (H&E)
e. stain
eosinophil (eo)
eosinophilia
eosinophilic
e. ascites
e. ballooning
e. cholangiopathy
e. cystitis
e. cytoplasm
e. enteritis
e. esophagitis
e. gastritis
e. gastroenteritis (EGE)
e. gastroenteritis syndrome
e. gastroenteropathy
e. granuloma
e. ileal perforation
eosinophiluria
EPA
eicosapentaenoic acid
EPC pain control
EPD
endoscopic papillary balloon dilation
EPEC
enteropathogenic *Escherichia coli*
ephedrine
EpHM
intraesophageal pH monitoring
EPI
exocrine pancreatic insufficiency
epicritic pain
epicystotomy
epidemic
e. gangrenous proctitis
e. gastritis
e. gastroenteritis
e. hemorrhagic fever
e. hepatitis
e. nausea
e. nephropathy
e. nonbacterial gastroenteritis
e. vomiting

E

NOTES

epidemica
 nephropathia e.
epidemiological
epidemiology
epidermal
 e. growth factor (EGF)
 e. growth factor receptor
  (EGFR)
epidermidis
 Staphylococcus e.
epidermoanal canal
epidermoid
 e. carcinoma
 e. cyst
epidermolysis
 e. bullosa
 e. bullosa acquisita
 e. bullosa dystrophica
epididymal
 e. sarcoidosis
 e. sperm aspiration (ESA)
 e. tubule
 e. tunic
epididymectomy
epididymidectomy
epididymis, pl. **epididymides**
 appendix e.
 caput e.
 cauda e.
 corpus e.
 microsurgical extraction of
  sperm from e. (MASE)
epididymisoplasty
epididymitis
 mumps e.
epididymo-orchitis
epididymoplasty
epididymotomy
epididymovasectomy
epididymovasostomy
epidural catheter
epigastralgia
epigastric
 e. angle
 e. discomfort
 e. distress
 e. fold
 e. hernia
 e. incision
 e. pain
 e. spot
epigastrium

epigastrocele
epiglottis
epi-illumination
epimer
 7β-e. of chenodeoxycholic acid
epinephrine
epinephrine-induced gastroduodenal
  electromechanical
epiphenomenon
epiphrenic diverticulum
epiplocele
epiploic
 e. appendage
 e. appendix
 e. foramen
epiplopexy
epipodophyllotoxin
epirubicin
episcleritis
episiotomy
 e. scar
episodic
 e. colic
 e. vomiting
epispadia
epispadiac orifice
epispadial
epispadias
 balanitic e.
 complete male e.
 congenital e.
 coronal e.
 incontinent e.
 penile e.
 penopubic e.
 subsymphyseal e.
epispadias-exstrophy complex
epistaxis
 renal e.
epitaxial nucleation
epithelia
 CF e.
 cuboidal e.
 nontumorous and tumorous e.
 oviduct e.
epithelial
 e. cell (EC)
 e. dysplasia
 e. endocrine cell
 e. inclusion body
 e. restitution and renewal
 e. tumor

epithelioid
    e. granuloma
    e. leiomyoma
epithelium
    adenomatous e.
    airway e.
    Barrett e.
    celomic e.
    columnar e.
    crypt e.
    flattening of ileal e.
    follicle-associated e.
    gastric e.
    gastric foveolar e.
    gastric-type surface e.
    germinal e.
    hyperplastic foveolar e.
    metaplastic e.
    nonkeratinizing squamous e.
    parietal e.
    proliferation of the gastric e.
    specialized columnar e.
    squamous e.
    surface e.
    transitional e.
    villous e.
epithelium-lined tubule
epitope
    antibody to GOR e.
    B-cell e.
    Goodpasture e.
    HLA class II-restricted T
      cell e.
    immunodominant T cell e.
    Lewis Y carbohydrate e.
    nephritogenic e.
    T-cell e.
epitrochlear
EPL
    extracorporeal piezoelectric
    lithotripsy
      Piezolith EPL
EPO
Epodyl
epoetin alfa
Epogen
Epon 812 resin

epoophoron
epoprostenol sodium
EPP
    erythropoietic proporphyria
Eppendorf
    E. needle electrode
    E. tube
EPS
    endoscopic pancreatic stenting
    expressed prostatic secretions
epsilon-aminocaproic acid
Epstein-Barr
    E.-B. viral infection
    E.-B. virus (EBV)
EPT
    endoscopic papillotomy
Equalactin
equal fluid balance
equation
    Harris-Benedict energy
      requirement e.
equilibrium
    acid-base e.
    solute e.
equina
    cauda e.
equipment
    ERCP e.
equivalent
    meconium ileus e. (MIE)
equivocal
ER
    endoplasmic reticulum
eradication
Erbotom F2 electrocoagulation unit
ERC
    endoscopic retrograde
    cholangiography
ERCCE
    endoscopic retrograde
    cholecystoendoprosthesis
ERCP
    endoscopic retrograde
    cholangiopancreatography
    ERCP balloon extractor
    ERCP cannula
    ERCP cannulation

E

NOTES

ERCP *(continued)*
ERCP catheter
ERCP conventional prosthesis
ERCP dilator
ERCP equipment
ERCP guidewire
ERCP manometry
ERCP nasobiliary drain
ERCP sphincterotome
ERCP-guided biopsy
ERCP-induced splenic rupture
ErecAid
E. vacuum erection device
E. vacuum system
erectile
e. dysfunction
e. potency
e. sinusoid
erection
artificial e.
artificial e. test
intraoperative penile e.
nocturnal e.
nonbuckling e.
penile e.
pharmacologically induced e.
reflex e.
reflexogenic e.
vacuum constriction e.
ERF
esophagorespiratory fistula
ergot alkaloids
ergotamine
Erlangen
E. magnetic colostomy device
E. papillotome
E. pull-type sphincterotomy
Erlangen-type papillotome
eroded polyp
E-rosetted
erosion
cancerous e.
cervical e.
chronic e.
Dieulafoy gastric e.
duodenal e.
gastric antral e.
gastric mucosal e.
idiopathic chronic e.
implant e.
limiting plate e.
linear e.

salt and pepper duodenal e.
stress e.
erosive
e. duodenitis
e. esophagitis
e. gastritis
e. gastropathy
e. prepyloric change
erosive/hemorrhagic gastritis
erotic vomiting
ERP
endoscopic retrograde
pancreatogram
endoscopic retrograde
pancreatography
endoscopic retrograde
parenchymography
ERPF
effective renal plasma flow
ERPP
endoscopic retrograde
parenchymography of pancreas
ERSNA
efferent renal sympathetic nerve
activity
eructation
ERUS
endorectal ultrasound
Eryc
Ery-Tab
erythema
conjunctival e.
joint e.
e. multiforme (EM)
e. nodosum
palmar e.
e. toxicum
erythematosus
lupus e.
procainamide-induced systemic
lupus e.
systemic lupus e. (SLE)
erythematous
e. gastropathy
e. streak
Erythrocin
erythrocyte (E)
e. aggregation
neuraminidase-treated sheep e.
e. sedimentation rate (ESR)
e. sedimentation rate test
e. sickling

erythrocytosis
    absolute e.
    stress e.
erythroid colony formation
erythromycin
    e. base
    e. estolate hepatotoxicity
    e. ethylsuccinate
    e. lactobionate
erythromycin-induced cholecystitis
erythroplasia
    e. of Queyrat
    Zoon e.
erythropoetin
erythropoiesis
    ineffective e.
erythropoietic
    e. proporphyria (EPP)
    e. protoporphyria
erythropoietin
    human recombinant e.
    recombinant e.
    recombinant human e. (rh-
      EPO)
    e. therapy
ES
    endoscopic sphincterotomy
ESA
    epididymal sperm aspiration
Esca Buess + fistula funnel
Escherichia coli
escutcheon
    female e.
    male e.
E-selectin expression
Eshmun complex
Esidrix
Esimil
ESKA-Buess esophageal tube
esmolol
esogastritis
EsophaCoil self-expanding
    esophageal stent
esophagalgia
esophageal
    e. achalasia
    e. acid infusion test

    e. adenocarcinoma
    e. A ring
    e. atresia
    e. balloon
    e. balloon dilator
    e. balloon distention
    e. balloon tamponade
    e. banding
    e. banding technique
    e. band ligation
    e. biopsy
    e. body motor dysfunction
    e. bougienage
    e. B ring
    e. cancer
    e. candidiasis (EC)
    e. carcinoma
    e. cast
    e. clearing
    e. colic
    e. compression
    e. condyloma acuminatum
    e. condyloma virus
    e. contractile ring
    e. dilation
    e. dilation treatment
    e. dilator
    e. diverticulum
    e. duplication cyst
    e. dysmotility
    e. dysphagia
    e. ectopic sebaceous gland
    e. effect
    e. endoprosthesis
    e. epidermal growth factor
      (EEGF)
    e. fistula
    e. foreign body
    e. function test
    e. fungal infection
    e. globus sensation
    e. groove
    e. hematoma
    e. hyperkeratosis
    e. hyperkinesia
    e. impression
    e. infection

E

NOTES

esophageal *(continued)*
  e. inlet
  e. intramural hematoma
  e. intubation
  e. leiomyoma
  e. Lewy body
  e. lumen
  e. malignancy
  e. manometric sequence (EMS)
  e. manometry
  e. mass
  e. motility
  e. motility disorder
  e. motility perfused catheter
  e. mucosa
  e. mucosal ring
  e. muscular ring
  e. myotomy
  e. obstruction
  e. osteophyte
  e. perforation
  e. perfusate
  e. perfusion catheter
  e. peristalsis
  e. peristaltic pressure
  e. pH monitoring
  e. photodynamic therapy
  e. plexus
  e. polyp
  e. prosthesis
  e. reflux
  e. resection
  e. ring
  e. rupture
  e. scleroderma
  e. shunt
  e. single balloon
  e. sound
  e. spasm
  e. sphincter
  e. sphincter relaxation
  e. squamous cell carcinoma
  e. squamous papilloma
  e. stenosis
  e. stent
  e. Strecker stent
  e. stricture
  e. tear
  e. transection
  e. transit scan
  e. transit time
  e. trauma
  e. tube
  e. tuberculosis
  e. tumor
  e. ulcer
  e. ulceration
  e. variceal bleeding
  e. variceal sclerosant
  e. variceal sclerosis
  e. variceal sclerotherapy
  e. varices
  e. varix
  e. wall
  e. wall thickness (EWT)
  e. web

esophagectasis, esophagectasia
esophagectomy
  Ivor Lewis two-stage
  subtotal e.
  transhiatal blunt e.
  transthoracic e.
  e. with thoracotomy
esophagi *(pl. of* esophagus)
esophagitis
  acid-pepsin reflux e.
  acid-peptic e.
  alkaline reflux e.
  aspergillosis e.
  bacterial e.
  Barrett e.
  Candida e.
  candidal e.
  caustic e.
  chemical-induced e.
  chronic peptic e.
  CMV e.
  corrosive e.
  cytomegalovirus e.
  drug-induced e.
  endoscopic e.
  eosinophilic e.
  erosive e.
  herpes simplex e.
  herpetic e.
  herpetiform e.
  histological e.
  infectious e.
  Leishmania e.
  monilial e.
  mucormycosis e.
  nonreflux e.
  nonspecific e.
  peptic e.
  pill e.
  polycystic chronic e.

radiation e.
reflux e. (RE)
refractory e.
retention e.
severe erosive e.
severe reflux e.
stasis e.
streptococcal e.
tuberculous e.
tuberculous infectious e.
ulcerative e.
esophagobronchial fistula
esophagocardial malignancy
esophagocardioplasty
esophagocele
esophagocolic anastomosis
esophagoduodenostomy
esophagodynia
esophagoenterostomy
esophagofiberscope
esophagogastrectomy
Ivor Lewis e.
thoracoabdominal e.
esophagogastric (EG)
e. balloon tamponade (EGBT)
e. fat pad
e. intubation
e. junction
e. pH-metry
e. tamponade
e. variceal bleeding
e. varix
esophagogastroanastomosis
esophagogastroduodenoscopy (EGD)
pediatric e.
esophagogastromyotomy
esophagogastroplasty
Grondahl-Finney e.
esophagogastroscopy
Abbott e.
Clagett Barrett e.
intrathoracic e.
Johnson e.
Thal e.
Woodward e.
esophagogastrostomy
Abbott e.

Clagett Barrett e.
intrathoracic e.
Johnson e.
Thal e.
Woodward e.
esophagography
contrast e.
esophagojejunostomy
loop e.
Roux-en-Y e.
Roux-Y e.
esophagomediastinal fistula
esophagomycosis
esophagomyotomy
esophagoplasty
colic patch e.
esophagoplication
esophagoprobe
Olympus ultrasonic e.
esophagoproximal gastrectomy
esophagopulmonary fistula
esophagorespiratory fistula (ERF)
esophago-Roux-en-Y-jejunostomy
esophagosalivary reflex
esophagoscope
ACMI fiberoptic e.
ballooning e.
Blom-Singer e.
Boros e.
Broyle e.
Bruening e.
Brunings e.
Chevalier Jackson e.
child e.
Denck e.
Dohlman e.
Eder-Hufford rigid e.
Eutaw-Hoffman e.
fiberoptic e.
Foregger rigid e.
Foroblique fiberoptic e.
full-lumen e.
Haslinger e.
Holinger e.
Hufford e.
infant e.
Jackson e.

E

NOTES

esophagoscope *(continued)*
Jasbee e.
Jesberg e.
J-scope e.
Kalk e.
large-bore rigid e.
Lell e.
LoPresti fiberoptic e.
Moersch e.
Mosher e.
Moure e.
Negus rigid e.
Olympus EF-series e.
optical e.
oval e.
oval-open e.
Roberts e.
Roberts folding e.
Roberts-Jesberg e.
Roberts oval e.
Sam Roberts e.
Schindler e.
Storz e.
Tesberg e.
Tucker e.
Universal e.
Yankauer e.
esophagoscopy
video e.
esophagospasm
esophagostenosis
esophagostomy
esophagotomy
esophagram
barium e.
contrast e.
esophagus, pl. **esophagi**
abdominal e.
achalasia-like e.
aperistaltic e.
A ring of e.
atonic e.
Barrett e. (BE)
B ring of e.
cervical e.
closed e.
columnar-lined e.
corkscrew e.
dilation of e.
distal e.
nutcracker e.
pneumatic bag dilation of e.
scleroderma of e.

spastic e.
strictured e.
thoracic e.
tortuous e.
variceal sclerotherapy in e.
ESR
erythrocyte sedimentation rate
ESR immunological study
immunological study
ESRD
end-stage renal disease
essential
e. amino acid
e. fatty acid
e. fatty acid deficiency
(EFAD)
e. hematuria
ester
cholesterol e.
dinitrate and mononitrate e.
NG-nitro-L-arginine methyl e.
(L-NAME)
esterase
leukocyte e.
e. stain
esterified fecal acid
esthesioneuroblastoma
estimated
e. blood loss (EBL)
e. liver blood flow (ELBF)
Estracyt
estradiol transderm patch
estramustine
e. phosphate
e. phosphate sodium
estrogen binding site (EBS)
estrogen-induced
e.-i. cholestasis
e.-i. liver disease
ESU
electrosurgical unit
ESWL
electrohydraulic shock wave
lithotripsy
extracorporeal shock wave
lithotripsy
Modulith SL20 device for
ESWL
ESWL related dysrhythmia
ET
endothelin
enterostomal therapy

EtA
>endothelin A
>EtA antagonist
>EtA receptor

EtB
>EtB antagonist
>EtB receptor

ETCD
>endoscopic transpapillary cyst
>drainage

ETEC
>enterotoxigenic *Escherichia coli*

ethacrynic acid

ethanol (EtOH, ETOH)
>e. abuse
>dehydrated e.
>gastric first-pass metabolism
>of e. (GFPM)
>e. injection
>e. injection therapy

ethanolamine
>e. oleate
>e. oleate sclerosant

ethanolamine oleate

ethanol-induced tumor necrosis (ETN)

ethanolism

ethanol-specific impairment

Ethaquin

ethaverine

ether
>methyl tert-butyl e., methyl
>tertiary butyl ether (MTBE)
>trimethylsilyl e.

Ethibond suture

Ethicon trocar

ethidium
>e. bromide
>e. bromide staining

Ethiflex suture

ethmoid

ethopropazine

ethoxysclerol

ethyl alcohol

ethylcellulose

ethylchlorformate polymerized antigen

ethylene
>e. glycol
>e. glycol tetraacetic acid
>(EGTA)
>e. oxide
>e. oxide gas (ETO)

ethylenediamine
>theophylline e.

ethylenediaminetetraacetate
>51-chromium-labeled e. (^{51}Cr-
>EDTA)

ethylenediaminetetraacetic acid (EDTA)

ethylene oxide gas (ETO)

ethylsuccinate
>erythromycin e.

etiology

etiopathogenesis

ETN
>ethanol-induced tumor necrosis

ET-NANBH
>enterically transmitted non-A, non-B
>hepatitis

ETO
>ethylene oxide gas
>ETO sterilization

EtOH, ETOH
>ethanol
>EtOH consumption

etoposide

Etude cystometer uroflowmeter

EU
>excretory urography

eubacterial strain

Eubacterium
>*E. lentum*
>*E. limosum*

Eucestoda

euchlorhydria

euglycemic hyperinsulinemia

Eulexin

Euro-Collins
>E.-C. fluid
>E.-C. solution

European Organization for Research and Treatment of Cancer (EORTC)

E

NOTES

EUS
echoendoscopy
endoscopic ultrasonography
Eutaw-Hoffman esophagoscope
eutectic mixture
Eutonyl
euvolemic
Evac-Q-Kit
E.-Q.-K. bowel prep
Evac-Q-Kwik
E.-Q.-K. bowel prep
evacuation
digital rectal e.
e. disorder
hematobilia e.
e. pouchography
e. proctography
rectal e.
stool e.
evacuator
Ellik e.
Urovac bladder e.
Evac-U-Gen
Evac-U-Lac
evagination
evaluation
diagnostic imaging e.
diverticulitis e.
endoscopic e.
endoscopic ultrasound e.
follow-up e.
manometric e.
medical e.
metabolic e.
presurgical medical e.
pretransplant e.
sexual e.
status e.
videourodynamic e.
evanescent
Evans blue dye
EVE Fujinon videocolonoscope
event
thromboembolic e.
eventration
eversion
e. entropion
e. normal
e. operation
e. orchiopexy
vaginal e.
evert
everted umbilicus

everting suture
eviration
evisceration
total abdominal e. (TAE)
EVL
endoscopic variceal ligation
evoked potential
Ewald
E. breakfast
E. gastroscope
E. test meal
E. tube
Ewing sarcoma
EWT
esophageal wall thickness
ex
e. vivo
e. vivo cannulation
e. vivo perfusion
exacerbation of pain
examination, exam
arterioportographical e.
cytology e.
digital rectal e. (DRE)
double-contrast barium
enema e.
endoscopic e.
follow-up e.
merthiolate fresh stool e.
microscopic urine e.
rectal e.
tomodensitometric e.
exanthesis
e. arthrosia
excavated gastric carcinoma
excavatio rectouterina
excavatum
pectus e.
excess
base e.
e. mucus
excessive
e. bleeding
e. straining
exchange
cation e.
e. of endoprosthesis
endoscopic stent e.
plasma e.
short-dwell hypertonic e.
sodium e.
wire-guided balloon-assisted
endoscopic biliary stent e.

exchanger
    cation e.
    heat e.
    thymocyte NA+/H+ e.
excision
    abdominoperineal e.
    cold snare e.
    laser hemorrhoid e.
excitation-contraction coupling
excitatory junction potential (EJP)
exclusion
    Devine e.
    e. diet
    subtotal gastric e.
excoriation
excrement
excrementitious
excreta
excrete
excretion
    basal renal e.
    biliary e.
    ^{57}Co B$_{12}$ e.
    ^{51}Cr-EDTA e.
    24-hour fecal fat e.
    pulmonary methane e.
    quantified protein e.
    renal acid e.
    urinary e.
    urinary chloride e.
    urinary kallikrein e.
    urinary protein e.
    urinary sodium e. (UNaV)
    urinary urea nitrogen e.
      (UUN)
    waste nitrogen e.
    whole-kidney fractional e.
excretor
    methane (CH4) e.
    non-CH4 e.
excretory
    e. azoospermia
    e. delay
    e. duct
    e. function
    e. urogram
    e. urography (EU, EXU)

excursion
    respiratory e.
excystation
exdwelling ureteral occlusion
    balloon catheter
exenteration
    anterior e.
    anterior pelvic e.
    pelvic e.
    posterior pelvic e.
    supralevator pelvic e.
    total pelvic e.
exercise
    Kegel pelvic muscle e.
    pelvic floor e. (PFE)
exercise-associated acute renal
    failure
exeresis
    palliative e.
exertional rhabdomyolysis
exfoliative
    e. cytology
    e. gastritis
exit
    e. site
    e. site of catheter
    e. site infection
Ex-Lax
Exna
exocrine
    e. function
    e. insufficiency
    e. pancreatic insufficiency
      (EPI)
exocytosis
exogenous
    e. calcium
    e. cholecystokinin or cerulein
    e. IGF-1
    e. obesity
    e. PGE2
    e. thiol
exomphalos
exon 1, 2, 3, 4, 5
exophytic
    e. adenocarcinoma

E

NOTES

203

exophytic *(continued)*
    e. mass
    e. wart
exotoxin
    Pseudomonas e. A
expandable
    e. biliary endoprosthesis
    e. esophageal stent (EES)
    e. intrahepatic portacaval shunt
       stent
    e. metallic stent
    e. metal mesh endoprosthesis
    e. olive
expanding retroperitoneal hematoma
expansile abdominal mass
expansion
    controlled e. (CX)
    intravascular volume e.
    mesangial matrix e.
    volume e.
expenditure
    resting energy e. (REE)
expiratory
    end e.
exploration
    common bile duct e. (CBDE)
    common duct e. (CDE)
    complete surgical e. (CSE)
    laparoscopically guided
       transcystic e.
exploratory
    e. celiotomy
    e. laparotomy
explosion
    colonic e.
explosive
    e. diarrhea
    e. doubling time
exposure
    occupational toxin e.
    toxin e.
expressed prostatic secretions (EPS)
expression
    breast cancer-associated protein
      pS2 e.
    carbohydrate antigen 19-9
      immunohistochemical e.
    complex class II e.
    cytokine gene e.
    E-selectin e.
    fibronectin e.
    p53 e.
    tissue-specific gene e.

exquisite
    e. pain
    e. tenderness
exquisitely tender abdomen
exsanguinated
exsanguinating hemorrhage
exsanguination
exsiccation fever
exstrophic bladder plate
exstrophy
    bladder e.
    cloacal e.
    e. closure
    vesical e.
exstrophy-epispadias complex
extended
    e. left subcostal incision
    e. obturator node and iliopsoas
      node dissection
    e. pelvic lymphadenectomy
    e. pyelotomy
extensibility
    penile e.
extension
    caliceal e.
    dumbbell-shaped calyceal e.
    e. fiber
    full e.
exteriorization
    e. colostomy
externa
    lamina rara e. (LRE)
external
    e. anal sphincter (EAS)
    e. anal sphincter muscle
    e. appliance
    e. beam radiation therapy
    e. biliary fistula
    e. biliary lavage
    e. cooling
    e. cooling appliance
    e. drainage
    e. fistula
    e. hemorrhoid
    e. inguinal ring
    e. ligament
    e. oblique
    e. oblique aponeurosis
    e. oblique fascia
    e. rectal sphincter
    e. ring
    e. rotation
    e. shock wave lithotripsy

e. skin tag
e. spermatic vein
e. sphincterotomy
e. stimulus
e. swelling
e. trauma
e. ureteral catheter
e. urethrotomy
e. vacuum therapy
external-beam irradiation
externally releasable knot
extirpation
surgical e.
extra
e. heart sound
extra-abdominal disease
extra-anatomical renal
revascularization technique
extracapillary crescent formation
extracapsular
e. disease
e. tumor
extracellular
e. calcium
e. fluid (ECF)
e. fluid volume
e. hyperosmolarity
e. matrix (ECM)
extracolonic
extracorporeal
e. cardiopulmonary circuit
e. dialysis
e. liver assist device (ELAD)
e. liver perfusion (ECLP)
e. partial nephrectomy
e. piezoelectric lithotripsy
(EPL)
e. piezoelectric shockwave
lithotripsy
e. renal preservation
e. repair
e. shock wave
e. shock wave lithotripsy
(ESWL)
e. shock wave lithotriptor
e. surgery
e. ultrafiltration (ECU)

extracted
e. ductal sperm
e. nuclear antigen (ENA)
extraction
e. balloon
e. balloon technique
e. bile duct stone
foreign body e.
harpoon e.
e. pancreatic stone
stone e.
extractor
Applied Biosystems 340A
nucleic acid e.
endoscopic magnetic e.
ERCP balloon e.
Soehendra stent e.
E. three-lumen retrieval balloon
catheter
E. XL triple lumen retrieval
balloon
extractum senna
extradomain A positive (EDA+)
extraglandular endocrine cell
proliferation
extrahepatic
e. bile duct
e. bile duct cancer
e. bile duct obstruction
e. biliary atresia (EBA)
e. biliary cystic dilation
e. biliary obstruction
e. biliary stricture
e. cancer
e. cholestasis
e. metastasis (EHM)
e. obstruction
e. portal vein
e. portal vein obstruction
(EHPVO)
e. portal venous hypertension
e. shunt
extraintestinal
e. complication
extralymphatic metastasis
extramammary Paget disease
(EMPD)

E

NOTES

extramedullary plasmacytoma
extramucosal mass
extramural
  e. lesion
  e. pseudocyst
extrapancreatic
  e. nerve plexus
  e. pseudocyst
extraparenchymal renal cyst
extraperitoneal
  e. endoscopic pelvic lymph
    node dissection (EEPLND)
  e. laparoscopic bladder neck
    suspension (ELBNS)
  e. laparoscopic nephrectomy
  e. tissue
extrapolated plasma caffeine
  concentration
extraprostatitis
extrapulmonary *Pneumocystis carinii*
  infection
extrapyramidal function assessment
extrarenal
  e. antigen
  e. dysmorphy
  e. mass
  e. vasculitis
extrasphincteric anal fistula
Extra Stiff Amplatz wire
extravaginal torsion
extravasated iodinated contrast
  material

extravasation
  e. of contrast medium
  peripelvic e.
  red blood cell e.
  urinary e.
extravascular space
extraversion
  urinary e.
extravesical
  e. anastomosis
  e. seromuscular tunnel
  e. ureteral reimplantation
    technique
  e. ureterolysis
extremity weakness
extrinsic
  e. compression
  e. mass
extrude
extubate
EXU
  excretory urography
exuberant granulation tissue
exudate
  pharyngeal e.
exudate-transudate concept
exudative
  e. ascites
  e. peritonitis
exulceratio simplex
E-Z Paque

F2α
  prostaglandin F. (PGF2α)
F2 focal point
F9 cell
F60S polysulphone
fabianii
  Hansenula f.
FABP
  fatty acid binding protein
Fabricius
  bursa of F.
Fabry disease
FAC
  5-fluorouracil, Adriamycin and
    cyclophosphamide
face
  en f.
  linear streaks en f.
  stable f.
face-a-face venacavaplasty
faceplate
  Marlen Neoprene All-
    Flexible f.
  Torbot f.
  United Surgical Hypalon f.
faceted gallstone
facial tenderness
facies
  cushingoid f.
  moon f.
  Potter f.
FACS, FACScan
  fluorescence-activated cell sorter
factitial proctitis
factor-α
  cytokine tumor necrosis f.
factor
  acidic fibroblast growth f.
  adverse prognostic f.
  alcoholic prognostic f.
  atrial natriuretic f. (ANF)
  autocrine motility f. (AMF)
  bacterial f.
  B-cell differentiation f.
  binary f.
  chemotactic f.
  clotting f.
  cobra venom f. (CVF)
  concentration epidermal
    growth f. (cEGF)

crest f.
decapacitation f.
decay-accelerating f. (DAF)
endothelium-derived relaxing f.
  (EDRF)
epidermal growth f. (EGF)
esophageal epidermal growth f.
  (EEGF)
fibroblast-derived f.
granulocyte colony-
  stimulating f. (G-CSF)
granulocyte macrophage colony-
  stimulating f. (GM-CSF)
growth f.
guanine nucleotide-releasing f.
  (GNRF)
heparin-binding epidermal
  growth f. (HB-EGF)
hepatocyte growth f. (HGF,
  HPG)
host f.
human epidermal growth f. (h-
  EGF)
human growth f. (HGF)
insulin-like growth f. (IGF)
insulin-like growth f.-2 (IGF-2)
intrinsic f. (IF)
f. IXa
müllerian inhibiting f.
new differentiation f. (NDF)
nuclear roundness f.
oxidase cytosolic f.
paracrine f.
pathogenetic f.
platelet activating f. (PAF)
platelet-derived growth f.
  (PDGF)
polypeptide growth f.
prognostic f.
progression f.
psychological f.
salivary epidermal growth f.
  (sEGF)
transforming growth f. (TGF)
tumor necrosis f. (TNF)
urethral resistance f. (URA)
vascular permeability f. (VPF)
von Willebrand f.
washout f.
f. Xa

F

factor *(continued)*
   f. XIa
   f. XIIa
factor-β1
   transforming growth f. (TGF-β1)
factor-1
   colony-stimulating f. (CSF-1)
   heparin-binding growth f.
   insulin-like growth f. (IGF-1)
   salivary epidermal growth f.
factor-β2
   transforming growth f. (TGF-β2)
factor-β3
   transforming growth f. (TGF-β3)
Fader
   F. Tip stent
   F. Tip ureteral stent
faecalis
   Enterococcus f.
   Streptococcus f.
FAG
   fundic atrophic gastritis
Fahrenheit thermometer
failed nipple valve
failure *(var. of* multiple organ failure)
   acute hepatic f.
   acute intrinsic renal f.
   acute renal f. (ARF)
   anemia of chronic renal f.
   chronic renal f. (CRF)
   congestive heart f.
   contrast-associated renal f.
   dilator placement f.
   drug-induced renal f.
   end-stage renal f.
   exercise-associated acute renal f.
   fulminant hepatic f. (FHF)
   fulminant hepatocellular f.
   fulminant liver f.
   intubation f.
   irradiation f.
   kidney f.
   late-onset hepatic f.
   liver f.
   multiorgan system f.
   multiple organ f., failure (MOF)
   multiple system organ f. (MSOF)

   nephrotoxic acute renal f.
   nonoliguric acute renal f.
   oliguric renal f.
   parenchymatous acute renal f.
   postischemic acute renal f.
   radiocontrast-induced acute renal f.
   renal f.
   respiratory f.
   subfulminant liver f.
   f. to thrive
   treatment f.
   vascular access f.
falciform ligament
falciparum malaria
fallax
   Clostridium f.
fallopian tube
Fallot tetralogy
false
   f. colonic obstruction
   f. diverticulum
   f. tympanites
"false channel" formation
false-negative (FN)
false-positive (FP)
   f.-p. scintiscan
familial
   f. adenomatous polyposis (FAP)
   f. aggregation
   f. chloride diarrhea
   f. cholemia
   f. cholestasis
   f. chronic idiopathic jaundice
   f. colonic varices
   f. colorectal polyposis
   f. Crohn disease
   f. fat-induced hyperlipidemia
   f. gastrointestinal polyposis
   f. hamartomatous polyposis
   f. hepatitis
   f. hyperbetalipoproteinemia and hyperprebetalipoproteinemia
   f. hypercholesteremic xanthomatosis
   f. hypercholesterolemia
   f. hypercholesterolemia with hyperlipemia
   f. hyperchylomicronemia
   f. hyperchylomicronemia with hyperprebetalipoproteinemia
   f. hyperlipoproteinemia

f. hyperprebetalipoproteinemia
f. hypertriglyceridemia
f. intestinal polyposis
f. intestinal pseudo-obstruction
f. juvenile nephrophthiasis
f. juvenile nephrophthisis
f. juvenile polyposis
f. Mediterranean fever (FMF)
f. nephritis serum
f. nephrosis
f. nonhemolytic jaundice
f. pancreatitis
f. paroxysmal polyserositis (FPP)
f. pheochromocytoma
f. polyposis coli (FPC)
f. polyposis syndrome
f. recurrent polyserositis
f. ulcerative colitis
f. unconjugated hyperbilirubinemia
f. visceral myopathy

family
Caliciviridae virus f.
secretin-glucagon-vasoactive intestinal peptide f.
tachykinin-bombesin f.

famotidine
f. maintenance treatment
f. pharmacokinetics

fan
f. elevator retractor
f. retractor

FANA
fluorescent antinuclear antibody
Fancon-De Toni-Debre syndrome
Fanconi syndrome
fan-type laparoscopic retractor
FAP
familial adenomatous polyposis
Farabeuf retractor
fascia, fascias, pl. **fasciae**
anterior rectus f.
anterior renal f.
Buck f.
Colles f.
dartos f.

Denonvilliers f.
external oblique f.
fusion f.
Gerota f.
internal oblique f.
f. lata buttress
lateral oblique f.
lumbosacral f.
posterior renal f.
prevertebral f.
rectal f.
renal f.
rim of f.
Scarpa f.
transversalis f.
Waldeyer f.
fascial
f. defect
f. layer
f. sling approach
f. stranding
fasciculate bladder
fasciculation
fasciitis
necrotizing f.
Fasciola
F. hepatica
F. hepatica infestation
fascioliasis
hepatic f.
fasciolopsiasis
Fasciolopsis buski
Fas gene
fashion
helical f.
retrograde f.
fastener
Brown-Mueller T-bar f.
fastidium cibi
fasting
f. diet
f. plasma caffeine concentration
f. serum gastrin
f. serum gastrin level
FasTrac hydrophilic-coated guidewire

F

NOTES

fast twitch striated muscle fiber
fat
  abdominal f.
  f. cell
  creeping of mesenteric f.
  f. density
  dietary f.
  herniated preperitoneal f.
  f. indigestion
  macrovesicular f.
  microvesicular f.
  f. pad
  paratesticular f.
  pericolonic f.
  perivesical f.
  preperitoneal f.
  properitoneal f.
  protruding f.
  f. storage disorder
  subcutaneous f.
fatigue
  structural f.
  suture f.
fat-induced gallbladder contraction
fat-soluble
  f.-s. bilirubin
  f.-s. vitamin
fat-storing liver cell
fatty
  f. acid
  f. acid binding protein (FABP)
  f. acid-free bovine serum
    albumin
  f. ascites
  f. cirrhosis
  f. cyst
  f. diarrhea
  f. food
  f. food intolerance
  f. infiltration of liver
  f. liver
  f. liver disease
  f. liver hepatitis
  f. liver of pregnancy
  f. meal
  f. meal sonogram (FMS)
  f. metamorphosis
  f. micromedionodular cirrhosis
  f. necrosis
  f. omental apron
  f. stool
  f. tissue
faux pas de coit

favored gait
FB-25K jumbo biopsy forceps
FBA
  fecal bile acid
  cocarcinogenic FBA
FBD
  functional bowel disorder
  functional bowel distress
FBV
  fiber bundle volume
FCC-COCA1 gene
FCPD
  fibrocalculous pancreatic diabetes
FCS-ML
  FCS-ML II colonoscope
  FCS-ML II fiberscope
  FCS-ML II gastroscope
FCS two-channel ultra high-
magnification endoscope
FDI
  frequency-duration index
FDL
  fluorescein dilaurate
  FDL test
Fe
  Slow Fe
feathery degeneration
feature
  AESOP ReView f.
  manometric f.
  pathognomonic f.
febrile
  f. morbidity
  f. pleomorphic anemia
fecal
  f. abscess
  f. alpha$_1$antitrypsin test
  f. analysis
  f. bile acid (FBA)
  f. concretion
  f. contamination
  f. contamination of food
  f. contamination of water
  f. continence
  f. diversion
  f. fat test
  f. fistula
  f. flora
  f. fluid
  f. homogenate
  72-hour f. fat test
  f. impaction
  f. incontinence

f. leukocyte
f. leukocyte count test
f. marker
f. material
f. obstruction
f. occult blood test (FOBT)
F. Odor Eliminator (FOE)
f. paradoxical puborectalis
  spasm
f. peritonitis
f. PMN-elastase
f. reservoir
f. residue
f. spillage
f. stasis
f. transmission
f. tumor
f. urobilinogen
f. vomiting
fecalith
fecaloid
fecaloma
fecal-oral
  f.-o. route
  f.-o. transmission
fecaluria
Fecatest
feces
  impacted f.
  inspissated f.
  retained f.
feculence
feculent
  f. vomitus
fecundity
Federici sign
fed response
feedback
  tubuloglomerular f. (TGF)
feeding
  Amin-Aid powdered f.
  bolus f.
  Build Up enteral f.
  Citrotein liquid f.
  Clinifeed Iso enteral f.
  Compleat-B liquid f.
  f. complication

continuous drip f.
Criticare HN elemental
  liquid f.
f. disorder
Enrich f.
Ensure Plus liquid f.
enteral f.
Entrition Entri-Pak f.
Finkelstein f.
Flexical enteral f.
forced f., forcible f.
Fortison enteral f.
gastric f.
gastrostomy f.
f. gastrostomy
f. gastrostomy tube
gavage f.
half-strength f.
Hepatic-Aid powdered f.
HN f.
hyperosmotic f.
intermittent drip f.
intravenous f.
Isocal HCN liquid f.
Isotein HN f.
isotonic f.
jejunostomy elemental diet f.
jejunostomy tube f.
lactose-free f.
Lonalac f.
low-residue f.
Magnacal liquid f.
Meritene liquid f.
modified sham f.
nasal f.
nasojejunal f.
Osmolite HN enteral f.
parenteral f.
Portagen f.
Precision Isotein HN
  powdered f.
Precision Isotonic powdered f.
Precision LR powdered f.
Renu enteral f.
Resource enteral f.
semielemental enteral f.
Stresstein liquid f.

F

NOTES

feeding *(continued)*
    Sustacal HC liquid f.
    Sustagen liquid f.
    TraumaCal enteral f.
    Traum-Aid HBC enteral f.
    Travasorb HN powdered f.
    Travasorb MCT liquid f.
    Travasorb STD liquid f.
    tube f.
    f. tube
    f. tube placement
    Vital f.
    Vitaneed f.
    Vivonex HN powdered f.
    Vivonex TEN f.
Feen-A-Mint
FEFEK
    fractional excretion of potassium
Fehland intestinal clamp
Feldene
FELI
    fractional excretion of lithium
felodipine
Felty syndrome
female
    f. catheter
    f. condom
    f. escutcheon
    f. urethral syndrome
Femina vaginal weight
feminizing genitoplasty
femoral
    f. bruits
    f. canal
    f. hemodialysis catheter
    f. hernia
    f. ligament
    f. triangle
FENa
    fractional excretion of sodium
fenbufen
fencing reflex
fenestrated
    f. cup biopsy forceps
    f. drape
fenestration
    cyst f.
fenfluramine
Fenger gallbladder probe
fenoldopam
fentanyl
Fenwick disease
Fenwick-Hunner ulcer

Feosol
Ferguson gallstone scoop
fermentative dyspepsia
ferricytochrome-C
Ferris biliary duct dilator
ferritin
    anionic f.
    cationized f.
    serum f.
ferromagnetic tamponade
ferrous
    f. salts poisoning
    f. sulfate
ferryl-free radical
fertility
    f. status
fertilization
    in vitro f.
Festalan
Festal II
fetal
    f. calf serum
    f. liver-derived B cell
    f. sulfoglycoprotein antigen (FSA)
fetid
fetoprotein
    α-f., alpha fetoprotein (AFP)
    α_1-f.
    β-f.
    fucosylated α-f.
    fucosylation index of α-f.
    γ-f.
    α-f. level
fetor
    fetor f.
fetus
    Campylobacter f.
Feulgen
    F. reaction
    F. staining
fever
    Aden f.
    Assam f.
    bilious remittent f.
    bouquet f.
    breakbone f.
    Burdwan f.
    cachectic f.
    Charcot intermittent f.
    dandy f.
    date f.
    dehydration f.

dengue f., dengue
hemorrhagic f.
digestive f.
dumdum f.
Ebola hemorrhagic f.
enteric f.
epidemic hemorrhagic f.
exsiccation f.
familial Mediterranean f.
(FMF)
food f.
hemorrhagic f.
hemorrhagic f. with renal
syndrome
hepatic f.
hepatic intermittent f.
inanition f.
Kinkiang f.
Korean hemorrhagic f.
Lassa hemorrhagic f.
low-grade f.
Manchurian hemorrhagic f.
Mediterranean f.
polka f.
Q f.
solar f.
spiking f.
thirst f.
typhoid f.
urticarial f.
viral hemorrhagic f.
Yangtze Valley f.
FF
follicular fluid
FFP
fresh frozen plasma
FG-110 Fuginon camera
FG-series two-channel endoscope
FGS-ML II gastroscope
FGS-ML-series two-channel
endoscope
FGS-series two-channel endoscope
FGS-SML-series two-channel
endoscope
FG-32UA
Pentax/Hitachi F.

FHF
fulminant hepatic failure
FHVP
free hepatic venous pressure
fialuridine
fiber
afferent f.
f. bundle
f. bundle volume (FBV)
circular muscle f.'s
cremasteric f.
dietary f.
extension f.
fast twitch striated muscle f.
GBM collagen f.
f. lock displacement
optical f.
f. optics
oxidative-glycolytic f.
sling muscle f.
slow twitch striated muscle f.
Urolase neodymium:YAG
laser f.
viscoelastic collagen f.
Fiberall
FiberCon
fiber-deficient diet
fiberduodenoscope
fiberendoscope
fibergastroscope
fluorescence f.
FiberOptic
F. sensor
fiberoptic
f. bundle
f. catheter
f. colonoscope
f. endoscope
f. endoscopy
f. esophagoscope
f. gastroscope
f. injection sclerotherapy (FIS)
f. instrument technology
f. light cable
f. panendoscopy
f. sigmoidoscope
f. sigmoidoscopy

F

NOTES

fiberoptics
fibers
    ragged-red f.
fiberscope
    CF-HM f.
    FCS-ML II f.
    GIF-HM f.
    Hirschowitz gastroduodenal f.
    Olympus Aloka EU-MI
      ultrasound gastrointestinal f.
    Olympus GF-EU-series
      ultrasound gastrointestinal f.
    Olympus OES f.
    Olympus XK-series oblique-
      viewing flexible f.
    Pentax f.
    side-viewing f.
    ultrasound gastrointestinal f.
fiberTome system
fibril
    disulfide cross-linked f.
    twisted β-pleated sheet f.
fibrillary glomerulonephritis
fibrin
    f. glue
    f. score
    f. seal
    f. sponge
    f. strand
    f. tissue adhesive
fibrinogen
    f. degradation product
fibrinolysis
    endothelium-dependent f.
fibrinolytic activity
fibrinopeptide-A
fibroadenoma
fibroadenomatosis
    biliary f.
fibroadipose tissue
fibroblast
    HE9 f.
    interstitial f.
    perivascular f.
    quiescent human f.
    3T3 murine f.
fibroblast-derived factor
fibrocalculous pancreatic diabetes
  (FCPD)
fibrocongestive splenomegaly
fibrocystic
    f. change
    f. disease of the pancreas

fibrodysplastic
fibroelastic
    f. connective tissue stroma
    f. tissue
fibroelastosis
fibrofatty adventitia
fibrogenesis
fibrogenic
    f. cascade
    f. cytokine
fibroid
    f. polyp
    uterine f.
fibrolamellar
    f. carcinoma
    f. hepatocarcinoma
    f. hepatocellular carcinoma
      (FL-HCC)
    f. hepatoma
fibroma
    ovarian f.
fibromatosis
    mesenteric f.
    penile f.
fibromuscular
    f. coat
    f. hyperplasia
fibromyoma
fibromyxoma
fibronectin
    f. expression
    f. monoclonal antibody
    plasma f.
fibronectin-binding protein
fibroplasia
    intimal f.
    medial f.
    perimedial f.
fibropurulent perisplenitis
fibrosa
    appendix f.
fibrosarcoma
fibrosing piecemeal necrosis
fibrosis
    alcoholic f.
    arachnoid f.
    cavernous f.
    chronic sclerosing hyaline f.
    congenital hepatic f. (CHF)
    corporeal f.
    cystic f. (CF)
    diffuse lobular f.
    hepatic f.

idiopathic retroperitoneal f.
interstitial f.
intralobular f.
mixed intralobular f.
noncirrhotic portal f. (NCPF)
pancreatic f.
paravariceal f.
pentastomum denticulatum f.
periductal f.
perilobular f.
peripancreatic f.
periportal f.
perisinusoidal f.
periureteral f.
perivenular f.
portal-to-portal f.
portal tract f.
progressive perivenular
  alcoholic f. (PPAF)
retroperitoneal f.
secondary biliary f.
sinusoidal f.
stripe interstitial f.
transmural f.
tubulointerstitial f.
vesical f.
fibrosis-promoting cytokine
fibrotic
fibrous
  f. cavernitis
  f. dysplasia
  f. histiocytoma
  f. obliterative cholangitis
  f. sheath
  f. stroma
  f. tissue
fibrovascular polyp
Ficoll-Hypaque
  F.-H. gradient centrifugation
  F.-H. gradient sedimentation
FIDUS probe
field cut
field-of-view camera
figure-of-eight suture
filament
  actin f.

filarial
  f. hydrocele
  f. lymphedema
filariasis
filiform
  f. bougie
  f. polyp
  f. polyposis
  f. stricture
  f. tip
filling
  f. cystometrogram
  f. defect
film
  high-abdominal plain f.
  plain f.
  postevacuation f.
  soft x-ray f.
filmy adhesion
filter
  Amicon D-20 f.
  Baermann stool f.
  Baxter CA-210 f.
  charcoal f.
  fluorescence excitation f.
  Fresenius F-40 f.
  Gambro FH88H f.
  Gene Screen nylon
    membrane f.
  Greenfield f.
  Hospal Biospal f.
  interference barrier f.
  Millex-GS 0.22 mm pore-
    size f.
  Millex-GV 0.22-mm f.
  Millipore f.
  Percoll f.
  Renal System HF250 f.
  suprarenal Greenfield f.
  Zeta probe nylon f.
filtered glucose
filtering
  high-pass f.
filtration
  f. fraction
  glomerular f.

F

NOTES

filtration *(continued)*
  f. slit length density
  spontaneous ascites f.
filtration-slit membrane
fimbriae
final
  f. motor neuron
  f. position
finasteride
finding
  cholangiographic f.
  endoscopic f.
  focal f.
  manometric f.
  roentgen f.
  sensory f.
  spinal fluid f.
  ultrasonographic f.
fine
  f. gastric mucosal pattern
  f. granular cast
  f. needle
  f. reticular pattern
  f. tissue forceps
finely fatty foamy liver
fine-needle
  f.-n. aspiration (FNA)
  f.-n. aspiration cytology
    (FNAC)
  f.-n. biopsy
  f.-n. percutaneous
    cholangiogram
  f.-n. transhepatic cholangiogram
  f.-n. transhepatic
    cholangiography
fine-toothed forceps
finger
  clubbed f.
  f. clubbing
  f. fracture dissection
  f. fracture technique
  f. intrinsic
finger-like
  f.-l. epithelial process
  f.-l. villus
fingerprick latex agglutination test
fingerstick device
fingertip lesion
Finkelstein feeding
Finney
  F. Flexirod penile prosthesis
  F. gastroenterostomy
  F. operation

  F. pyloroplasty
  F. strictureplasty
Finochietto retractor
FiO$_2$
  fractional percentage of inspired
  oxygen
Fioricet
Fiorinal
Firlit-Kluge stent
first-generation ELISA
first-line screening technique
first-order kinetics
first-pass
  f.-p. effect
  f.-p. metabolism
first-stage repair
FIS
  fiberoptic injection sclerotherapy
FISH
  fluorescence in-situ hybridization
fish
  f. bone ingestion
  f. oil supplementation
  f. tapeworm
Fisher
  F. Accumet pH meter
  F. Capillary System
  F. exact probability test
  F. two-tailed exact test
Fishman-Doubilet test
fish-mouth incision
fish-scale gallbladder
fissure
  anal f.
  cecal f.
  portal f.
  umbilical f.
fissured tongue
fist fornication
fistula, pl. **fistulae, fistulas**
  abdominal f.
  amphibolic f., amphibolous f.
  anal f.
  anorectal f.
  antecubital arteriovenous f.
  aortoduodenal f. (ADF)
  aortoenteric f.
  aortoesophageal f.
  aortogastric f.
  aortograft duodenal f.
  aortosigmoid f.
  arterial-enteric f.
  arterioportal f.

arteriovenous f.
AV f.
benign duodenocolic f.
biliary f.
biliary-bronchial f.
biliary-cutaneous f.
biliary-duodenal f.
biliary-enteric f.
bilioenteric f.
bladder f.
Blom-Singer
   tracheoesophageal f.
brachioaxillary bridge graft f.
   (BAGF)
brachiosubclavian bridge
   graft f. (BSGF)
bronchoesophageal f.
calyceal f.
cholecystenteric f.
cholecystocholedochal f.
cholecystocolonic f.
cholecystoduodenal f.
cholecystoduodenocolic f.
choledochocolonic f.
choledochoduodenal f.
choledochoenteric f.
coccygeal f.
colobronchial f.
colocutaneous f.
cologastrocutaneous f.
coloileal f.
colonic f.
colovaginal f.
colovesical f.
complex anorectal f.
congenital urethroperineal f.
cutaneobiliary f.
cystogastric f.
duodenal f.
duodenocaval f.
duodenocolic f.
duodenoenterocutaneous f.
endobronchial f.
enteric f.
enterocutaneous f.
enteroenteral f.
enteroenteric f.

enterourethral f.
enterovaginal f.
enterovesical f.
esophageal f.
esophagobronchial f.
esophagomediastinal f.
esophagopulmonary f.
esophagorespiratory f. (ERF)
external f.
external biliary f.
extrasphincteric anal f.
fecal f.
forearm graft arteriovenous f.
gastric f.
gastrocolic f.
gastrocutaneous f.
gastroduodenal f.
gastroenteric f.
gastrointestinal f.
gastrojejunocolic f.
genitourinary f.
graft-enteric f.
hepatic f.
hepatopleural f.
horseshoe f.
H-type f.
ileosigmoid f.
ileovesical f.
intersphincteric anal f.
intestinal f.
intrahepatic AV f.
intrahepatic spontaneous
   arterioportal f.
jejunocolic f.
Mann-Bollman f.
mesenteric f.
mesenteric arteriovenous f.
mucous f.
pancreatic f.
pancreatic cutaneous f.
pancreaticopleural f.
pararectal f.
parietal f.
perianal f.
perineal f.
perineal urinary f.
pleurobiliary f.

F

NOTES

217

fistula *(continued)*
    postbiopsy f.
    postoperative f.
    postoperative pleurobiliary f.
    posttraumatic pancreatic-
      cutaneous f.
    f. probe
    pseudocystobiliary f.
    rectal f.
    rectolabial f.
    rectourethral f.
    rectourinary f.
    rectovaginal f.
    rectovesical f.
    rectovestibular f.
    rectovulvar f.
    renogastric f.
    respiratory-esophageal f.
    retroperitoneal f.
    Seton treatment of high
      anal f.
    sigmoidovesical f.
    spermatic f.
    splanchnic AV f.
    splenic AV f.
    splenobronchial f.
    stercoral f.
    suprasphincteric f.
    sylvian f.
    thigh graft arteriovenous f.
    Thiry f.
    Thiry-Vella f. (TVF)
    thoracic f.
    tracheoesophageal f. (TEF)
    transsphincteric anal f.
    ulcerogenic f.
    umbilical f.
    urachal f.
    ureterocolic f.
    ureterocutaneous f.
    ureterouterine f.
    ureterovaginal f.
    urethrocavernous f.
    urethrorectal f.
    urethrovaginal f.
    urinary f.
    urinary umbilical f.
    urogenital f.
    vaginal f.
    vasocutaneous f.
    Vella f.
    vesical f.
    vesico-acetabular f.

    vesicocolic f.
    vesicocutaneous f.
    vesicoenteric f.
    vesicointestinal f.
    vesico-ovarian f.
    vesicorectal f.
    vesicosalpingovaginal f.
    vesicouterine f.
    vesicovaginal f.
    vesicovaginorectal f.
fistulation
    spreading f.
fistulectomy
fistulization
fistuloenterostomy
fistulogram
fistulography
fistulotome
    double-channel f.
    needle-knife f.
fistulotomy
    choledochoduodenal f.
    diathermic f.
    endoscopic f.
    laying-open f.
    Parks method of anal f.
    Parks staged f.
fistulous
    f. degeneration
    f. orifice
    f. tract
FITC
    fluorescein isothiocyanate
Fite stain
Fitz-Hugh and Curtis syndrome
five-port "fan" placement
fixation
    f. anomaly
    intestinal f.
    pubic f.
    sacrospinalis ligament
      vaginal f.
    sacrospinous ligament
      vaginal f.
fixative
    ice-cold buffered
      picroformaldehyde f.
    Saccomanno f.
    Zamboni f.
fixed
    f. drain pipe urethra
    f. ring retractor
    f. segment of bowel

FK-506
flabby abdomen
flagella
    polar sheathed f.
flagellate
    f. diarrhea
Flagyl
flail chest
flame photometry
flammeus
    nevus f.
flank
    f. approach
    bulging f.
    f. incision
    f. mass
    f. position
    f. roll positioning
flap
    abdominal fasciocutaneous f.
    advancement of rectal f.
    Bakamjian f.
    Boari bladder f.
    Boari-Ockerblad f.
    Byars f.
    de-epithelialized f.
    foreskin f.
    gracilis muscle f.
    island pedicle f.
    liver f.
    Martius f.
    Mathieu island onlay f.
    myocutaneous f.
    Ockerblad-Boari f.
    onlay island f.
    para-exstrophy skin f.
    penile island f.
    Scardino f.
    surgical f.
    f. technique
    tubed groin f.
    tubularized cecal f.
    u-shaped skin f.
    ventrum penis f.
flapping tremor sign
flap-valve mechanism
flare cell

flare-up (adj.)
FLASH
    flat low-angle shot
    FLASH pulse sequence
flat
    f. abdomen
    f. adenoma
    f. carcinoma
    f. condyloma
    f. depressed lesion
    f. elevated lesion
    f. low-angle shot (FLASH)
    f. plate of abdomen
    f. spatula electrode
flattened duodenal fold
flattening
    histogram f.
    f. of ileal epithelium
flatulence
flatulent
    f. dyspepsia
Flatulex
flatus
    f. enema
    f. tube insertion
flavin
    f. adenine dinucleotide
    f. mononucleotide
Flavobacterium meningosepticum
flavoxate hydrochloride
flavus
    Aspergillus f.
Fleet
    F. Babylax enema
    F. bowel prep
    F. enema
    F. Phospho-Soda
    F. Phospho-Soda buffered
        saline laxative
fleroxacin
flexed
Flexeril
flexible
    f. aspiration needle
    f. barium enema
    f. delivery device
    f. dental suction

F

NOTES

flexible *(continued)*
- f. endoscope
- f. endoscopic overtube
- f. endoscopy
- f. fiberoptic choledochoscope
- f. fiberoptic endoscope
- f. forward-viewing panendoscope
- f. gastroscope
- f. laparoscopy
- f. nephroscope
- f. nephroscopy
- f. Olympus GF-eUM3 device
- f. sigmoidoscope
- f. sigmoidoscopy
- f.-tip guidewire
- f. ureteropyeloscopy
- f. ureteroscope
- f. video laparoscope (FVL)

flexible-tip Bentsen guidewire
Flexical enteral feeding
Flexicath silicone subclavian cannula
Flexi-Flate
- F.-F. (I, II) penile prosthesis
- F.-F. penile implant

Flexiflo
- F. feeding pump
- F. Inverta-PEG gastrostomy kit
- F. Inverta-Peg tube
- F. kit
- F. Lap-J laparoscopic jejunostomy kit
- F. over-the-guidewire gastrostomy kit
- F. stoma creator tube
- F. tungsten-weighted feeding tube
- F. Versa-PEG tube

Flexirod penile prosthesis
flexneri
   Shigella f.
FlexSure HP test
flexure
- duodenojejunal f.
- hepatic f.
- left colonic f.
- right colonic f.
- sigmoid f.
- splenic f.

Flexxicon II PC internal jugular catheter

FL-HCC
   fibrolamellar hepatocellular carcinoma
FLI
   fluorescent light intensity
flip-flap
   Mathieu-Horton-Devine f.-f.
   f.-f. procedure
   f.-f. technique
flipped T-wave
floating
- f. gallbladder
- f. gallstone
- f. stool
- f. table

Flocare 500 feeding pump
flocculation on barium enema
Flo-Gard pump
Flolan
Flood syndrome
floor
   inguinal f.
   f. of inguinal region
   pelvic f.
floppy type of Nissen fundoplication
flora
   bacterial f.
   fecal f.
   GI tract f.
   gut f.
   intestinal f.
   normal f.
   proximal human colonic f.
florid
   f. duct lesion
   f. polyposis
Florida urinary pouch
Floropryl
flow
   azygos blood f. (AzBF)
   blood f.
   f. cytometric analysis
   f. cytometric study
   f. cytometry
   effective renal plasma f. (ERPF)
   estimated liver blood f. (ELBF)
   forearm blood f.
   hepatofugal f.
   hepatopetal f.
   high-velocity f.

light f.
f. microsphere florescent
  immunoassay technique
nephron plasma f.
noninvasive assessment of
  urinary f.
obstruction of bile f.
outer cortical blood f. (OCBF)
petal-fugal f.
plasma f.
f. rate
renal plasma f. (RPF)
splanchnic blood f.
splenic venous blood f.
turbulent f.
flowmeter
Dantec rotating disk f.
Dantec Urodyn 1000 f.
laser Doppler f.
Life-Tech f.
Model 500F electromagnetic f.
flowprobe
endoscopic f.
Floxin
floxuridine
flucloxacillin-associated liver damage
**flucloxacillin-induced delayed
  cholestatic hepatitis**
fluconazole
bistriazole f.
fluctuant
f. mass
fluctuation
GB vol+ f.
GB vol- f.
flucytosine
fluffs
Fluhrer rectal probe
fluid
f. absorptive capacity
f. analysis
ascitic f.
BiCart dialysis f.
bile-stained f.
bile-tinged f.
bloody peritoneal f.
chylous ascitic f.

cloudy f.
contrast f.
crevicular f.
cul-de-sac f.
cytospin collection f.
Dialyflex dialysis f.
Euro-Collins f.
extracellular f. (ECF)
fecal f.
follicular f. (FF)
free f.
intraglandular f.
irrigating f.
IV f.'s
LDH level of ascitic f.
LKB Optiphase 2
  scintillation f.
f. loss
malodorous f.
milky f.
motor oil peritoneal f.
nonmalodorous f.
oviductal f.
peripancreatic f.
peritoneal f.
peritubular f.
f. phase marker
prune juice peritoneal f.
renal tubular f.
f. replacement therapy
f. restriction
f. resuscitation
sanguineous f.
f. sequestration
serosanguineous f.
f. shift
straw-colored f.
synovial f.
f. transport
turbid peritoneal f.
University of Wisconsin f.
f. wave
fluid-air interface
fluid-filled
f.-f. sac
f.-f. small bowel

F

NOTES

fluidity
    hepatocellular basolateral
    plasma membrane f.
fluid-phase
    f.-p. endocytosis
    f.-p. pinocytosis
fluke
    giant intestinal f.
    liver f.
flu-like syndrome
flumazenil
flumecinol
flunisolide
fluocinolone
fluorescein
    f. dilaurate (FDL)
    f. dilaurate test
    f. isothiocyanate (FITC)
    f. isothiocyanate-conjugated
    antibody
    f. isothiocyanate-labeled
    monoclonal antibody
    linear f.
    scattered f.
    sodium f. (NaF)
    f. string test
    superficial f.
fluorescence
    f. angiography
    f. excitation filter
    f. fibergastroscope
    f. in-situ hybridization (FISH)
    pericentral pyridine
        nucleotide f.
    periportal pyridine nucleotide f.
fluorescence-activated
    f.-a. cell sorter (FACS,
    FACScan)
    f.-a. flow cytometry
fluorescent
    f. antinuclear antibody (FANA)
    f. electronic endoscopy
    f. gene scanning
    f. light intensity (FLI)
fluoride
    phenyl-methane-sulfonyl f.
5-fluorocytosine
fluorodeoxyuridine (FUDR)
fluoroquinolone
fluoroscope
    C-arm f.
fluoroscopic
    f. control

    f. guidance
    f. monitoring
fluoroscopy
fluoroscopy-guided balloon dilator
Fluoro Tip ERCP cannula
Fluorotome double-lumen
    sphincterotome
fluorouracil
5-fluorouracil (5-FU)
5-fluorouracil,
    -f. Adriamycin and
    cyclophosphamide (FAC)
    -f. mitomycin C radiation
    (FUMIR)
fluorourodynamics
fluoxetine hydrochloride
fluoxymesterone
fluphenazine
flurbiprofen
flush
    carcinoid f.
    saline f.
flushing
    cold f.
flutamide
    f. therapy
fluted J-Vac drain
fluvastatin
flux
    lumen-to-bath sodium f.
    proton f.
    sodium f.
FMF
    familial Mediterranean fever
fMLP chemoattractant receptor
fMLP-stimulated O2
FMS
    fatty meal sonogram
FN
    false-negative
FNA
    fine-needle aspiration
FNAC
    fine-needle aspiration cytology
FNH
    focal nodular hyperplasia
foam
    f. cell
    hydrocortisone f.
foamy
    f. liver
    f. stool

FOBT
  fecal occult blood test
  FOBT-positive
focal
  f. accumulation of tracer
  f. biliary cirrhosis
  f. colitis
  f. collagen synthesis
  f. colonic mucosal ulcer
  f. dimpling
  f. edema
  f. fatty infiltration
  f. fatty infiltration of liver
  f. finding
  f. glomerulosclerosis
  f. ileus
  f. necrotizing glomerulonephritis
  f. nodular hyperplasia (FNH)
  f. nonfatty infiltration of liver
  f. pancreatitis
  f. sclerosis
  f. segmental glomerulosclerosis
    (FSGS)
  f. tenderness
  f. tumor
foci of tumor
focused shock wave
FOE
  Fecal Odor Eliminator
Foerster
  F. abdominal ring retractor
  F. sponge forceps
Fogarty
  F. balloon
  F. balloon biliary catheter
  F. biliary probe
  F. catheter
  F. irrigation catheter
fog reduction elimination device
  (FRED)
folate
  f. anemia
  f. deficiency
  f. malabsorption
  polyglutamate f.
fold
  aryepiglottic f.

  cecal f.
  cholecystoduodenocolic f.
  costocolic f.
  crural f.
  Douglas f.
  duodenojejunal f.
  duodenomesocolic f.
  epigastric f.
  flattened duodenal f.
  gastric f.
  gastropancreatic f.
  giant gastric f.
  gluteal f.
  haustral f.
  hepatopancreatic f.
  ileocolic f.
  inguinal f.
  interhaustral f.
  Kerckring f.
  mucosal f.
  Nélaton f.
  palatopharyngeal f.
  f. pattern
  rectal f.
  rugal f.
  semilunar-shaped f.
  sentinel f.
  sigmoid f.
  tri-radiate cecal f.
folded fundus
Foley
  F. catheter
  F. criteria
  F. operation
  F. Y-plasty pyeloplasty
  F. Y-V plasty
folic acid
folinic acid
Folin phenol reagent
follicle
  lymphoid f.
  mucosal lymphoid f.
follicle-associated epithelium
follicle-stimulating hormone (FSH)
follicular
  f. atresia
  f. cholecystitis

F

NOTES

223

follicular *(continued)*
  f. cystitis
  f. fluid (FF)
  f. gastritis
  f. lymphoid hyperplasia
follicularis
  dyskeratosis f.
  keratosis f.
folliculitis
followers
following bougie
follow-through
  small-bowel f.-t. (SBFT)
follow-up (adj.)
  f.-u. evaluation
  f.-u. examination
Fontana-Masson stain
food
  f. allergen
  f. allergy
  bland f.
  f. bolus
  f. bolus impaction
  f. bolus obstruction
  f. chain
  f. challenge
  cholecystokinetic f.
  contamination of f.
  fatty f.
  fecal contamination of f.
  f. fever
  gas-producing f.
  greasy f.
  f. particle
  f. poisoning
  f. residue
  sieving of solid f.
  solid f.
  f. supplement
food-sensitive enteropathy
foot
  f. pedal suction control
  f. process (FP)
footprint
  thermobaric f.
foramen
  f. of Bochdalek
  epiploic f.
  greater sciatic f.
  f. of Winslow
Forbes disease
force
  isometric f.

forced
  f. alimentation
  f. feeding
forceps
  ACMI Martin endoscopy f.
  Adair-Allis f.
  Adson f.
  Adson-Brown tissue f.
  Adson tissue f.
  Allen intestinal f.
  alligator jaws f.
  alligator-type grasping f.
  Allis f.
  atraumatic locking/grasping f.
  Babcock f.
  Babcock intestinal f.
  Backhaus towel f.
  Ballenger f.
  Barracuda flexible cystoscopic
    hot biopsy f.
  Barrett intestinal f.
  basket f.
  basket-type crushing f.
  bayonet-type f.
  Beasley-Babcock f.
  Behrend cystic duct f.
  Best gallstone f.
  Bevan gallbladder f.
  Billroth f.
  biopsy f.
  bite biopsy f.
  Blake gallstone f.
  bowel f.
  Brunner intestinal f.
  Buie f.
  Buie pile f.
  bulldog f.
  Carmalt f.
  Child intestinal f.
  Children's Hospital intestinal f.
  claw f.
  coagulating f.
  cold biopsy f.
  Collins intestinal f.
  Crile bile duct f.
  Crile gall duct f.
  curved dissecting f.
  curved Maryland f.
  Cushing f.
  DeBakey f.
  Deddish-Potts intestinal f.
  DeMartel appendix f.
  Dennis f.

Dennis intestinal f.
Desjardins gallbladder f.
Desjardins gallstone f.
disposable f.
dolphin grasping f.
dolphin-type atraumatic f.
double-spoon f.
Doyen f.
Doyen gallbladder f.
Doyen intestinal f.
dressing f.
duck-bill f.
Duracep biopsy f.
electrocoagulating biopsy f.
Elliott gallbladder f.
Endo-Assist disposable
  atraumatic grasping f.
endoscopic alligator f.
endoscopic biopsy f.
endoscopic grasping f.
endoscopic suture-cutting f.
FB-25K jumbo biopsy f.
fenestrated cup biopsy f.
fine tissue f.
fine-toothed f.
Foerster sponge f.
foreign body f.
foreign body-retrieving f.
Fujinon biopsy f.
gallstone f.
Gavin-Miller intestinal f.
Gemini gall duct f.
Gerald f.
Gilbert cystic duct f.
Glassman-Allis intestinal f.
Glenn diverticulum f.
grasping f.
grasp tripod f.
Gray cystic duct f.
Haberer intestinal f.
Halsted f.
Hasson bullet-tip f.
Hasson needle-nose f.
Hasson ring f.
Hasson spike-tooth f.
Healy intestinal f.
hook f.

Hosemann f.
hot biopsy f.
hot flexible f.
Jarvis hemorrhoid f.
jeweler's f.
Johns Hopkins gallbladder f.
Judd-Allis intestinal f.
Judd-DeMartel gallbladder f.
Julian splenorenal f.
jumbo biopsy f.
Keen Edge disposable
  biopsy f.
Kelly f.
Kleppinger f.
Kocher f.
Koerte gallstone f.
Lahey gall duct f.
Lalonde hook f.
lancet-shaped biopsy f.
Lane intestinal f.
Laplace f.
Lillie intestinal f.
Lockwood-Allis intestinal f.
long-jaw disposable f.
loop-type snare f.
loop-type stone-crushing f.
Lovelace f.
Lower gall duct f.
Luer hemorrhoid f.
Maxum reusable f.
Mayo-Blake gallstone f.
Mayo-Pean f.
Mayo-Robson intestinal f.
Mazzariello-Caprini f.
McGill f.
McGivney hemorrhoid f.
McNealey-Glassman-Mixter f.
Medicon-Jackson rectal f.
Mikulicz peritoneal f.
Miller rectal f.
Millin f.
Mill-Rose RiteBite biopsy f.
Mixter f.
Mixter gallstone f.
mosquito f.
Moynihan gall duct f.
Muir hemorrhoid f.

F

NOTES

forceps *(continued)*
Nelson f.
Nissen gall duct f.
Nussbaum intestinal f.
Ochsner f.
O'Hara f.
Olympus alligator-jaw
  endoscopic f.
Olympus basket-type
  endoscopic f.
Olympus Endo-Therapy
  disposable biopsy f.
Olympus FB-series f.
Olympus FG-series f.
Olympus FS-K-series
  endoscopic suture-cutting f.
Olympus grasping rat-tooth f.
Olympus hot biopsy f.
Olympus magnetic extractor f.
Olympus mini-snare f.
Olympus pelican-type
  endoscopic f.
Olympus rat-tooth
  endoscopic f.
Olympus rubber-tip
  endoscopic f.
Olympus shark-tooth
  endoscopic f.
Olympus tripod-type
  endoscopic f.
Olympus W-shaped
  endoscopic f.
Ombredanne f.
Orr gall duct f.
packing f.
Payr pyloric f.
Péan f.
pelican biopsy f.
Pennington f.
Percy intestinal f.
perforating f.
pinch f.
Porter duodenal f.
Positrap three prong non-
  retracting grasping f.
Potts f.
Potts-Smith f.
Precisor disposable biopsy f.
radial jaw biopsy f.
radial jaw bladder biopsy f.
radial jaw hot biopsy f.
radial jaw 3 single-use
  biopsy f.

Randall stone f.
Ratliff-Blake gallstone f.
Ratliff-Mayo f.
rat-tooth f.
Reich-Nechtow f.
f. removal
ring f.
RiteBite biopsy f.
Robbers f.
Robson intestinal f.
Rochester-Carmalt f.
Rochester gallstone f.
Rochester-Mixter f.
Rochester-Ochsner f.
Rochester-Péan f.
Rudd-Clinic hemorrhoidal f.
Russian tissue f.
Schindler peritoneal f.
Schnidt gall duct f.
Schnidt thoracic f.
Schoenberg intestinal f.
Scudder intestinal f.
Seitzinger tripolar cutting f.
Semken tissue f.
shark tooth f.
Singley intestinal f.
smooth tissue f.
sponge f.
spoon f.
Steinmann intestinal f.
Stille-Barraya intestinal f.
Stille gallstone f.
stone f.
stone-grasping f.
stone-holding basket f.
straight Maryland f.
SureBite biopsy f.
Therma Jaw disposable hot
  biopsy f.
Thorek gallbladder f.
Thorek-Mixter gallbladder f.
three-armed basket f.
three-pronged grasping f.
tissue f.
tonsil f.
toothed tissue f.
traumatic grasping f.
tripod grasping f.
Troutman rectus f.
Turrell-Wittner rectal f.
Varco gallbladder f.
Westphal gall duct f.
Williams intestinal f.

W-shaped f.
Yeoman rectal biopsy f.
Yeoman-Wittner rectal f.
Young intestinal f.
forcible feeding
Forder retractor
Fordyce
    F. granule
    F. spot
forearm
    f. blood flow
    f. graft arteriovenous fistula
Foregger rigid esophagoscope
foregut
foreign
    f. body
    f. body extraction
    f. body forceps
    f. body ingestion
    f. body management
    f. body reaction
    f. body removal
    f. body-retrieving forceps
    f. body sensation
    f. body trauma
    f. object
foreshortening of the colon
foreskin
    f. flap
    f. restoration
Forest
    F. (I, II) lesion
forestomach
fork
    stimulation f.
form
    band f.
    wax-matrix slow-release f.
    WBC immature f.'s
formaldehyde solution
formalin-fixed
    f.-f. tissue
formamide
    deiodinized f.
formation
    abscess f.
    adhesion f.

branching tubule f.
calculous f.
erythroid colony f.
extracapillary crescent f.
"false channel" f.
gallstone f.
germinal center f.
Gothic arch f.
kerion f.
median bar f.
micelle f.
physicochemical basis of
  gallstone f.
pseudoaneurysm f.
scar f.
stone granuloma f.
struvite crystal f.
formatio reticularis
forme
    f. fruste
    f. tardive
formed stool
formers
    stone f.
forms
formula
    Advance f.
    Enfamil with iron f.
    Ensure Plus f.
    Isomil SF f.
    I-Soyalac f.
    Lofenalac f.
    Lonalac f.
    Nursoy f.
    Nutramigen f.
    Portagen f.
    predigested protein f.
    Pregestimil f.
    ProSobee f.
    ProSobee liquid f.
    RCF f.
    Similac PM 60/40 low-iron f.
    SMA f.
    Soyalac f.
    soy-based f.
formyl peptide receptor

F

NOTES

fornication
    fist f.
fornix
    caliceal f.
    gastric f.
Foroblique
    50-degree F. optic laparoscope
    F. fiberoptic esophagoscope
    F. lens
    F. resectoscope
Fortaz
Forte
    Dorbantyl F.
    Robinul F.
Fortison enteral feeding
Fortuna syringe
forward-viewing
    f.-v. endoscope
    f.-v. telescope
    f.-v. video colonoscope
foscarnet
    f. therapy
    f. treatment
Foss
    F. bifid gallbladder retractor
    F. biliary duct retractor
    F. intestinal clamp
fossa, pl. **fossae**
    hypochondriac f.
    f. navicularis
    prostatic f.
    pyriform f.
Fouchet test
foul
    f. smelling
foul-smelling
    f.-s. odor
    f.-s. stool
Fourier transform infrared spectroscopy (FTIR)
four-lumen
    f.-l. polyvinyl manometric catheter
    f.-l. tube
Fournier gangrene
four phases of swallowing
four-port "diamond" placement
four-pronged polyp grasper
four-quadrant tattooing
four-wing Malecot drain
foveola, pl. **foveolae**
    gastric f.
foveola-gland ratio

foveolar
    f. gastric mucosa
    f. hyperplasia
foveolosulciolar gastric mucosa
Fowler position
Fowler-Stephens
    F.-S. maneuver
    F.-S. orchiopexy
    F.-S. procedure
Foxy Pouch cover
FP
    false-positive
    foot process
FPC
    familial polyposis coli
FPP
    familial paroxysmal polyserositis
fraction
    alpha-gliadin f.
    anionic IgG 4 f.
    cortical interstitial volume f.
    filtration f.
    gallbladder ejection f. (GBEF)
    globulin f.
    mesangial volume f.
    non-T-cell f.
    packing f.
    plasma protein f.
fractional
    f. clearance
    f. excretion of lithium (FELI)
    f. excretion of potassium (FEFEK)
    f. excretion of sodium (FENa)
    f. percentage of inspired oxygen (FiO$_2$)
    f. proximal reabsorption
    f. weight change
fractional percentage of inspired oxygen (FiO$_2$)
fractionated
    f. diet
    f. voiding
fractionation of bilirubin
fracture
    trabecular bone f.
fragilis
    Bacteroides f.
fragment
    anucleate f.
    autotransplantation of splenic f.
    N-terminal f.

nuclear f.
residual f.
fragmentary defecation
fragmentation
laser-induced f.
stone f.
ultrasonic f.
Fraley
F. sign
F. syndrome
Francis test
frank
f. blood
f. blood in stool
f. cirrhosis
f. pus
Frankfeldt rectal snare
Franklin-Silverman biopsy cannula
Franz abdominal retractor
Frazier
F. suction tip
F. suction tube
FreAmine amino acid solution
FRED
fog reduction elimination device
Frederick-Miller tube
Fredet-Ramstedt operation
free
f. acetate
f. air
f. band of colon
f. fatty acid
f. fecal bile acid
f. fluid
f. hepatic venous pressure (FHVP)
f. jejunal graft
f. radical
f. radical scavenger
f. reflux
f. ribosome
f. subphrenic gas
f. thyroxine (FT4)
f. tie
free-beam
f.-b. coagulation
f.-b. laser system

freeing up of adhesions
free-standing ambulatory surgical center
free-to-total PSA ratio
freezing
gastric f.
Freiburg biopsy set
fremitus
French
F. bougie
F. Cope loop nephrostomy catheter
F. cystoscope
F. dilator
F. double-J ureteral stent
F. eye needle
F. introducer set
F. mushroom tip catheter
F. Pharmacovigilance system
F. pigtail nephrostomy catheter
F. stent
F. Swan-Ganz balloon
F. Teflon pyeloureteral catheter
F. T-tube
Frenta
F. Mat feeding pump
F. System II feeding pump
frenulum
frequency
pulse repetition f. (PRF)
f. of stool
urinary f.
frequency-duration index (FDI)
frequency-urgency-pain syndrome
Fresenius
F. AG dialyzer
F. F-40 filter
F. volumetric dialysate balancing system
fresh
f. clot
f. frozen plasma (FFP)
Freund adjuvant
freundii
Citrobacter f.
friability
cervical f.

F

NOTES

friable
> f. mucosa

friction
> f. knot
> f. rub

friction-fit
> f.-f. adapter
> f.-f. adaptor

Friedländer bacillus
Friedman perineal retractor
Frimberger-Karpiel 12 o'clock papillotome
frondlike filling defect
frontal tenderness
frothy
frozen section
fructose
> f. intolerance

fructose-1,6-bisphosphatase
fruity odor
fruste
> forme f.

FSA
> fetal sulfoglycoprotein antigen

FSGS
> focal segmental glomerulosclerosis

FSH
> follicle-stimulating hormone

FT4
> free thyroxine

FTIR
> Fourier transform infrared spectroscopy

5-FU
> 5-fluorouracil

5-FU-cisplatinum
fucosylated
> f. α-fetoprotein

fucosylation index of α-fetoprotein
FUDR
> fluorodeoxyuridine

fugax
> proctalgia f.

Fujinon
> F. biopsy forceps
> F. CEG-FP-series videoelectroscope
> F. EC7-CM2 video colonoscope
> F. EG-FP-series endoscope
> F. EVC-M video colonoscope
> F. EVD-XL video duodenoscope

> F. EVE-series endoscope
> F. EVG-CT-series endoscope
> F. EVG-FP-series endoscope
> F. EVG-F-series endoscope
> F. FG-series endoscopic camera
> F. FP-series endoscope
> F. PRO-PC flexible fiberoptic sigmoidoscope
> F. SIG-EK-series flexible fiberoptic sigmoidoscope
> F. SIG-E-series flexible fiberoptic sigmoidoscope
> F. SIG-ET-series flexible fiberoptic sigmoidoscope
> F. sigmoidoscope
> F. SP-501 sonoprobe system
> F. UGI-FP-series video endoscope
> F. video endoscopy cart
> F. video endoscopy system

fulguration
> electrosurgical f.
> endoscopic f.

full
> f. extension
> f. liquid diet
> f. range of motion

full-column barium enema
Fuller rectal shield
full-length viral genome
full-lumen esophagoscope
fullness
> abdominal f.
> adnexal f.
> postprandial f.
> pyloric f.

full-surface micro mesh teeth
fulminant
> f. colitis
> f. Crohn disease
> f. hepatic failure (FHF)
> f. hepatitis A
> f. hepatitis B
> f. hepatitis C
> f. hepatitis D
> f. hepatitis E
> f. hepatocellular failure
> f. liver failure
> f. viral hepatitis (FVH)

fulminating
> f. appendicitis
> f. dysentery

f. pancreatitis
f. ulcerative colitis
fumigatus
    Aspergillus f.
FUMIR
    5-fluorouracil, mitomycin C
    radiation
function
    anal sphincter f.
    bowel f.
    cardiopulmonary baroreflex f.
    discriminant f. (DF)
    excretory f.
    exocrine f.
    gallbladder f.
    gastrin cell f.
    impaired colonic motor f.
    kidney f.
    Leydig cell secretory f.
    Maddrey discriminant f.
    P450 f.
    pharyngoesophageal f.
    puborectalis muscle f.
    pudendal nerve f.
    rectoanal f.
    rectosigmoid f.
    renal f.
    Sertoli cell secretory f.
    sexual f.
    sieving f.
    sphincter f.
    splenic f.
    split renal f.
functional
    f. bladder capacity
    f. bleeding
    f. bowel disorder (FBD)
    f. bowel distress (FBD)
    f. bowel syndrome
    f. castration
    f. constipation
    f. cystic duct obstruction
    f. diarrhea
    f. disorder stomach
    f. dyspepsia
    f. pain
    f. profile length

fundal
    f. gastritis
    f. plication
    f. varix
fundectomy
fundi (*pl. of* fundus)
fundic
    f. atrophic gastritis (FAG)
    f. gland atrophy
    f. gland gastritis
    f. gland heterotopia
    f. gland polyp
    f. mucosa
fundic-antral junction
fundoplasty
    Gomez f.
    Thal f.
fundoplication
    Belsey Mark IV 240-degree f.
    Belsey partial f.
    Belsey two-thirds wrap f.
    floppy type of Nissen f.
    intrathoracic Nissen f.
    Nissen f.
    Nissen 360-degree wrap f.
    Rossetti modification of
      Nissen f.
    slipped Nissen f.
fundopyloric mucosal border
fundus, pl. **fundi**
    bald gastric f.
    folded f.
    gallbladder f.
    gastric f.
fundusectomy
fungal
    f. abscess
    f. ball
    f. bezoar
    f. infection
    f. liver abscess
    f. peritonitis
    f. spore
fungating
fungemia
fungi
    ovoid f.

F

NOTES

Fungizone
funguria
funicular
    f. hydrocele
    f. inguinal hernia
    f. stump
funiculopexy
funis
funisitis
funnel
    Esca Buess + fistula f.
Furacin
Furadantin
furamide
Furantoin
fura pentapotassium salt
furazolidone
Furlow cylinder inserter
Furlow-Fisher modification of Virag 1 operation
furnace
Furniss anastomosis clamp

Furniss-Clute clamp
furor medicus
furosemide
furrier suture
furuncle
fusible calculus
fusiform
    f. widening of duct
fusion
    f. fascia
    tissue f.
    urethrohymenal f.
    viral membrane f.
Fusobacterium
F value
FVH
    fulminant viral hepatitis
FVL
    flexible video laparoscope
Fx1A antibody
fyn protein

G

G cell
G protein
gabexate mesilate
GAG
glycosaminoglycan
gag
Millard mouth g.
mouth g.
g. reflex
g. response
gagging
GAGUA
glycosaminoglycans uronate
gain
symptomatic fluid g.
weight g.
gait
antalgic g.
ataxic g.
broad-based g.
g. disturbance
favored g.
parkinsonian g.
spastic g.
steppage g.
Trendelenburg g.
unsteady g.
Galacto-light assay
β-galactose
galactose-1-phosphate
uridyltransferase
galactose elimination capacity
(GEC)
galactosemia
β-galactosidase activity
galactosyltransferase
g. isoenzyme II
galanin
g. antiserum
Galant reflex
Galeati gland
galenic preparation
gall
g. duct
g. duct spoon
gallbladder
adenomyoma of g.
g. bag positioner
g. bed

bilobed g.
g. calculus
g. carcinoma
cholesterolosis of g.
chronically inflamed g.
g. contraction
Courvoisier g.
dilated g.
double g.
g. dysmotility
edematous g.
g. ejection fraction (GBEF)
g. ejection rate (GBER)
g. emptying-refilling curve
empyema of g.
endoscopic transpapillary
catheter of the g.
fish-scale g.
floating g.
g. function
g. fundus
gangrene of g.
hourglass constriction of g.
g. hydrops
g. ileus
inflamed g.
infundibulum of g.
g. lift
mobile g.
mucocele of g.
multiseptate g.
nonvisualization of g.
palpable g.
perforation of g.
porcelain g.
g. scan
g. scoop
g. sludge
stasis g.
g. stasis
g. stone
strawberry g.
thick-walled g.
thin-walled g.
g. torsion
torsion of g.
g. trauma
trauma of g.
g. trocar
g. varices

G

233

gallbladder *(continued)*
    g. wall
    g. wall abscess
    wandering g.
gallium 67
gallium scan
gallop rhythm
gallows-type retractor
gallstone
    asymptomatic g.
    bilirubin pigment g.
    black pigment g.
    brown pigment g.
    calcified g.
    cholesterol-containing g.
    g. colic
    dissolution of g.
    faceted g.
    floating g.
    g. forceps
    g. formation
    g. ileus
    g. incidence
    innocent g.
    intragastric g.
    g. migration
    mixed-cholesterol g.
    mulberry g.
    g. pancreatitis
    g. pattern
    pigment g.
    pigmented g.
    g. probe
    radiolucent g.
    retained g.
    silent g.
    symptomatic g.
GALT
    gastrointestinal-associated lymphoid
      tissue
    gut-associated lymphoid tissue
galvanic probe
Gambee suture
Gambro
    G. AK10 machine
    G. dialyzer
    G. FH88H filter
gamete
    g. intrafallopian transfer
      (GIFT)
    g. micromanipulation

gamma
    g. aminobutyric acidergic
      neuron
    g. camera
    g. emission
    g. globulin
    g. globulin therapy
    g. heavy-chain disease
    interferon g.
    g. interferon
    g. transverse colon loop
gamma-1a
    interferon g.-1a
gamma-aminobutyric
    g.-a. acid
    g.-a. acid accumulation
gamma-1b
    interferon g.-1b
gamma-globulin
    antithymocyte g.-g. (ATGAM)
gamma-glutamyl
    g.-g. transferase (GGT)
    g.-g. transpeptidase (GGTP)
gamma-glutamyl-transpeptidase
gamma-interferon
Gamna disease
ganciclovir
ganglia
    enteric g.
    intramural g.
ganglion cell loss
ganglioneuroma
ganglioneuromatosis
ganglion-free muscle strip
ganglioside
    GM3 g.
gangliosides
gangrene
    Fournier g.
    g. of gallbladder
    gas g.
gangrenosum
    pyoderma g. (PG)
gangrenous
    g. appendicitis
    g. appendix
    g. bowel
    g. cholecystitis
    g. cystitis
    g. ischemic colitis
    g. ischemic enterocolitis
Ganser diverticulum

Gantanol
    Azo G.
Gant clamp
Gantrisin
    Azo G.
gantry
gap
    anion g.
    g. junction
    stool osmotic g.
    underwater spark g.
GAPD
    glyceraldehyde phosphate
    dehydrogenase
GAPDH
    glyceraldehyde-3-phosphate
    dehydrogenase
GAP test
Garamycin
garbled speech
Gardnerella vaginalis
Gardner syndrome (GS)
gargle
    viscous Xylocaine g.
Garren
    G. balloon
    G. gastric bubble
Garren-Edwards
    G.-E. balloon
    G.-E. gastric (GEG)
    G.-E. gastric bubble
Gartner duct
gas
    g. abscess
    arterial blood g. (ABG)
    bowel g.
    g. chromatography
    g. chromatography/mass
     spectroscopy (GC/MS)
    colonic g.
    g. cupula
    g. cystometry
    g. density line
    ethylene oxide g. (ETO)
    free subphrenic g.
    g. gangrene
    hydrogen g.

    g. isotope ratio mass
     spectrometry
    g. pattern
    g. sterilization
    g. thermometer
gas-bloat syndrome
gaseous
    g. cholecystitis
    g. distention
gas-forming pyogenic liver infection
gasket
    United Surgical Seal Tite g.
gasless
    g. laparoscopic approach
    g. laparoscopy
GASP
    gastric augment and single pedicle
    tube
gas-producing food
gassiness
gassy
gastralgia
gastrectasis, gastrectasia
gastrectomized patient
gastrectomy
    Billroth I g.
    Billroth II g.
    distal g.
    esophagoproximal g.
    high subtotal g.
    Horsley g.
    partial g.
    Pólya g.
    proximal g.
    subtotal g.
    total g.
gastreen as histamine
gastric
    g. accommodation test
    g. achlorhydria
    g. acid
    g. acidity
    g. acidity reduction
    g. acid pump inhibitor
    g. acid rebound
    g. actinomycosis
    g. adenocarcinoma

G

NOTES

gastric *(continued)*
- g. adenopapillomatosis
- g. air bubble
- g. analysis
- g. angioma
- g. angiomyolipoma
- g. anisakiasis
- g. anoxia
- g. antral erosion
- g. antral sessile polyp
- g. antral vascular ectasia (GAVE)
- g. antrum
- g. arteriovenous malformation
- g. aspirate
- g. aspiration
- g. aspiration tube
- g. atony
- g. atresia
- g. atrophy
- g. augment and single pedicle tube (GASP)
- g. bacterial overgrowth (GBO)
- g. balloon
- g. balloon implantation
- g. bezoar
- g. bleeding
- g. bleeding time (GBT)
- g. brush cytology
- g. bypass (GBP)
- g. bypass surgery
- g. calculus
- g. cancer
- g. capacity
- g. carcinoid
- g. carcinoid tumor
- g. carcinoma
- g. carcinosarcoma
- g. cardia
- g. cell kinetics
- g. channel
- g. chloroma
- g. coin removal
- g. colic
- g. compression
- g. contents
- g. crisis
- g. decompression
- g. diet
- g. dilation
- g. distention
- g. diverticulosis
- g. duplication
- g. duplication cyst
- g. dysfunction
- g. dyspepsia
- g. dysrhythmia
- g. effect
- g. electrical stimulation
- g. emptying (GE)
- g. emptying scan
- g. emptying test
- g. emptying time
- g. epithelial cell infiltration
- g. epithelial cell replication
- g. epithelium
- g. feeding
- g. first-pass metabolism of ethanol (GFPM)
- g. fistula
- g. fold
- g. foreign body
- g. fornix
- g. foveola
- g. foveolar epithelium
- g. freezing
- g. fundus
- g. fundus wrap
- Garren-Edwards g. (GEG)
- g. gland
- g. hemorrhage
- g. heterotopia
- g. hyperacidity
- g. hyperemia
- g. hyperplastic polyp
- g. hypersecretion
- g. hypothermia
- g. hypothermia machine
- g. ileus
- g. impression
- g. impression on liver
- g. indigestion
- g. inflammatory fibroid polyp
- g. inhibitory polypeptide (GIP)
- g. juice
- g. Kaposi sarcoma
- g. lavage
- g. lavage tube
- g. leiomyoma
- g. leiomyosarcoma
- g. lesion
- g. lipoma
- g. luminal pH
- g. lymphoma
- g. malaria
- g. mass

g. metaplasia
g. microenvironment
g. motility disorder
g. mucormycosis
g. mucosa
g. mucosal barrier
g. mucosal damage
g. mucosal degradation
g. mucosal disease
g. mucosal ectopia in rectum
  (GMER)
g. mucosal ectopy
g. mucosal erosion
g. mucosal injury
g. mucosal laminin receptor
g. mucosal pattern
  classification
g. mucosal prolapse
g. mucus
g. muscularis mucosa
g. mycosis
g. myoelectrical activity
g. neobladder
g. neurasthenia
g. omentum
g. outlet
g. outlet obstruction (GOO)
g. outline
g. oxyntic cell receptor
g. pacemaker cell
g. pacemaker region
g. partition
g. perforation
g. petechia
g. pH monitor
g. pigment
g. pit
g. pitting
g. plasma
g. plasmacytoma
g. plexus
g. pneumocystosis
g. polyp
g. polypectomy
g. polyposis
g. pool
g. pouch

g. pseudolymphoma
g. rebound
g. red spot
g. remnant
g. retention
g. rupture
g. sarcoma
g. sclerosis
g. secretion
g. secretory test
g. serosa
g. stapling
g. stasis
g. stump
g. syphilis
g. tear
g. teratoma
g. tetany
g. transit time
g. transposition
g. trauma
g. tuberculosis
g. ulcer
g. ulceration
g. urease activity
g. variceal bleeding
g. varices
g. varix
g. vein
g. venacaval shunt
g. vertigo
g. volume
g. volvulus
g. window
g. xanthoma
gastrica, gen. **gastricae**
  achylia g.
  area g.
gastric inhibitory peptide (GIP)
gastric-type surface epithelium
^{125}**I-gastrin**
gastrin
  antral g.
  g. cell
  g. cell function
  g. cell hyperfunction
  fasting serum g.

G

NOTES

gastrin *(continued)*
^{125}I-g.
g. gene
g. mRNA
g. mRNA:G-cell density
g. mRNA level
g. mRNA species
g. receptor
G. RIA kit II
serum g.
g. stimulation test
gastrin-17
gastrinoma
duodenal g.
gastrin-releasing
g.-r. peptide (GRP)
g.-r. peptide/bombesin
gastrin-secreting
g.-s. cell
g.-s. non-beta islet cell tumor
gastritis
acute erosive g. (AEG)
acute hemorrhagic g.
alcoholic hemorrhagic g.
alkaline reflux g.
antral g.
antral atrophic g. (AAG)
antral-predominant g.
antrum g.
aspirin-induced g.
atrophic g.
bile reflux g.
bleeding g.
Campylobacter pyloridis g.
catarrhal g.
chemical g.
chronic g.
chronic active g.
chronic atrophic g. (CAG)
chronic cystic g.
chronic erosive g.
chronic follicular g.
chronic superficial g. (CSG)
cirrhotic g.
corpus g.
corrosive g.
g. cystica polyposa
g. cystic profunda
diffuse antral g. (DAG)
diffuse varioliform g.
drug-induced g.
emphysematous g.
endoscopic g.

endoscopic atrophic g.
endoscopic enterogastric
reflux g.
endoscopic
erythematous/exudative g.
endoscopic hemorrhagic g.
endoscopic raised erosive g.
endoscopic rugal
hyperplastic g.
eosinophilic g.
epidemic g.
erosive g.
erosive/hemorrhagic g.
exfoliative g.
follicular g.
fundal g.
fundic atrophic g. (FAG)
fundic gland g.
giant hypertrophic g.
granulomatous g.
Helicobacter pylori-induced g.
hemorrhagic g.
histological chronic active g.
hypertrophic g.
hypertrophic lymphocytic g.
(HLG)
idiopathic g.
idiopathic chronic erosive g.
interstitial g.
isolated granulomatous g.
lymphocytic g. (LG)
multifocal atrophic g. (MAG)
nonerosive g.
nonerosive nonspecific g.
nonspecific g.
nonspecific erosive g.
phlegmonous g.
polypous g.
postgastrectomy g.
postoperative g.
proliferative hypertrophic g.
pseudomembranous g.
radiation g.
reflux g.
reflux bile g.
severe g.
specific g.
stress g.
superficial g.
Sydney classification of g.
syphilitic g.
toxic g.
tuberculous g.

type A g.
type B g.
type B antral g.
ulcerative g.
varioliform g.
g. varioliformis
verrucous g.
viral g.
zonal g.
**gastritis-associated peptic ulcer
disease**
gastroalbumorrhea
gastroanastomosis
gastroatonia
gastroblennorrhea
gastrocalcinin
gastrocamera
Olympus GTF-A g.
Gastroccult
G. test
gastrocele
gastrochronorrhea
gastrocolic
g. fistula
g. ligament
g. omentum
g. reflex
gastrocolitis
gastrocolostomy
gastrocutaneous fistula
gastrocystoplasty
gastroduodenal
g. artery (GDA)
g. artery complex
g. carcinoid
g. Crohn disease
g. double ulcer
g. dyspepsia
g. fistula
g. lumen
g. misperfusion
g. mucosa
g. mucosal injury
g. mucosal protection
gastroduodenitis
neutrophilic g.
gastroduodenopancreatectomy

gastroduodenoscopy
gastroduodenostomy
Billroth I g.
Jaboulay g.
vagotomy and antrectomy
with g.
gastrodynia
gastroenteric
g. fistula
gastroenteritis
acute g. (AGE)
acute infectious g.
acute infectious nonbacterial g.
astrovirus g.
calicivirus g.
coronavirus g.
endemic nonbacterial
infantile g.
eosinophilic g. (EGE)
epidemic g.
epidemic nonbacterial g.
infantile g.
infectious g.
nonbacterial g.
Norwalk g.
rotavirus g.
viral g.
winter g.
gastroenteroanastomosis
gastroenterocolitis
gastroenterocolostomy
gastroenterologist
Gastroenterology
American College of G.
(ACG)
gastroenterology
gastroenteropancreatic tumor
gastroenteropathy
g. detection
eosinophilic g.
protein-losing g.
gastroenteroplasty
gastroenteroptosis
gastroenterostomy
Balfour g.
Billroth I g.
Billroth II g.

NOTES

239

gastroenterostomy *(continued)*
  Braun-Jaboulay g.
  Courvoisier g.
  Finney g.
  Heineke-Mikulicz g.
  Hofmeister g.
  Pólya g.
  Roux-en-Y g.
  Schoemaker g.
  truncal vagotomy and g.
  Von Haberer g.
  Wolfler g.
gastroenterotomy
gastroepiploic
  g. arcade
  g. artery (GEA)
  g. blood vessel
gastroesophageal (GE)
  g. hernia
  g. incompetence
  g. junction
  g. reflux (GER)
  g. reflux disease (GERD)
  g. reflux scan
  g. scintigraphy
  g. scintiscan
  g. sphincter
  g. variceal plexus
gastroesophagitis
gastroesophagostomy
gastrogastrostomy
gastrogavage
gastrogenic
gastrogenous diarrhea
Gastrografin
  G. contrast medium
  G. enema
  G. GI series
  G. swallow
GastrograpH ambulatory pH monitoring system
gastrohepatic
  g. bare area
  g. ligament
  g. omentum
gastrohydrorrhea
gastroileac augmentation
gastroileal reflex
gastroileostomy
gastrointestinal (GI)
  g. absorption
  g. assistant (GIA)
  g. bleed

  g. bleeding (GIB)
  g. cancer
  g. cancer-associated antigen (GICA)
  g. complication
  g. endoscopy
  g. endothelium
  g. eosinophilic granuloma
  g. fistula
  g. histoplasmosis
  g. immunodeficiency syndrome
  g. Kaposi sarcoma
  g. lavage
  g. lesion
  g. motility
  g. myenteric plexus
  g. needle
  g. neuroendocrinology
  g. neurofibroma
  g. peptide hormone
  g. polyposis
  g. reflux
  g. regularity peptide
  g. smooth muscle
  g. stoma
  g. telangiectasia
  g. tract (GIT)
  g. tract hemorrhage
  g. transit
  upper g. (UGI)
gastrointestinal-associated lymphoid tissue (GALT)
gastrojejunal
  g. constipation
  g. loop obstruction syndrome
gastrojejunocolic fistula
gastrojejunostomy
  antecolic long-loop isoperistaltic g.
  Billroth II g.
  compression button g.
  loop g.
  Roux-en-Y g.
  Roux-Y g.
gastrolavage
gastrolienal ligament
gastrolithiasis
gastrologist
gastrology
gastrolysis
Gastrolyte oral solution
gastromegaly
gastromyxorrhea

gastronesteostomy
gastropancreatic
    g. fold
    g. ligament
    g. reflex
gastroparesis
    diabetic g.
    g. diabeticorum
    idiopathic g.
    nondiabetic g.
    postvagotomy g.
    transient g.
gastropathic
gastropathy
    aphthous g.
    benign hyperplastic g.
    cardiofundic g.
    congestive g.
    congestive hypertensive g.
    diabetic g.
    erosive g.
    erythematous g.
    hemorrhagic g.
    hypertrophic g.
    idiopathic g.
    idiopathic hypertrophic g.
    papulous g.
    portal hypertensive g. (PHG)
    prolapse g.
    protein-losing g.
    varioliform gastritis or g.
gastropexy
    Boerema anterior g.
    Hill posterior g.
gastrophrenic ligament
gastroplasty (GP)
    Collis g.
    Eckhout vertical g.
    Gomez horizontal g.
    greater curvature banded g.
    horizontal g.
    Laws g.
    Mason vertical banded g.
    O'Leary lesser curvature g.
    silicone elastomer ring
      vertical g. (SRVG)
    Stamm g.

    tubular vertical g.
    unbanded g.
    vertical banded g. (VBG)
    vertical ring g. (VRG)
    vertical Silastic ring g.
gastroplication
Gastro-Port II feeding device
gastroptyxis
gastropylorectomy
Gastroreflex ambulatory pH
    monitor/recorder
gastrorenal shunt
gastrorrhagia
gastrorrhaphy
gastrorrhea
gastrorrhexis
gastroschisis
    Silastic silo reduction of g.
    Silon tent for g.
gastroscope
    ACMI g.
    Benedict g.
    Bernstein g.
    Cameron g.
    Cameron omni-angle g.
    Chevalier Jackson g.
    Eder g.
    Eder-Bernstein g.
    Eder-Chamberlin g.
    Eder-Hufford g.
    Eder-Palmer semiflexible g.
    Ellsner g.
    end-viewing g.
    Ewald g.
    FCS-ML II g.
    FGS-ML II g.
    fiberoptic g.
    flexible g.
    GFC g.
    GFT Olympus g.
    Herman-Taylor g.
    Hirschowitz g.
    Housset-Debray g.
    Janeway g.
    Jenning-Streifeneder g.
    Kelling g.
    Krentz g.

G

NOTES

gastroscope *(continued)*
    Mancke flex-rigid g.
    Mikulicz g.
    Olympus GIF-K-series g.
    pediatric g.
    Pentax g.
    peroral g.
    Schindler semiflexible g.
    Sielaff g.
    Taylor g.
    Tomenius g.
    Universal g.
    Wolf-Henning g.
    Wolf-Knittlingen g.
    Wolf-Schindler semiflexible g.
gastroscopic
gastroscopy
    high-magnification g.
    infrared transillumination g.
Gastrosed
gastrospasm
gastrosphincteric pressure gradient
gastrosplenic
    g. ligament
    g. omentum
gastrostaxis
gastrostenosis
gastrostogavage
gastrostolavage
gastrostomy
    Beck g.
    g. bumper
    g. button
    button g.
    Depage-Janeway g.
    dual percutaneous
      endoscopic g. (DPEG)
    endoscopic g.
    feeding g.
    g. feeding
    Glassman g.
    Kader g.
    Olympus g.
    Partipilo g.
    percutaneous endoscopic g.
      (PEG)
    Russell percutaneous
      endoscopic g.
    g. scarring
    Ssabanejew-Frank g.
    Stamm g.
    Surgitek One-Step percutaneous
      endoscopic g.

    g. tube
    g. tube migration
    ultrasound-assisted percutaneous
      endoscopic g.
    venting percutaneous g. (VPG)
    Witzel g.
gastrotome
gastrotomy
gastrotonometer
gastrotonometry
gastrotoxic
gastrotropic
Gastrovist
    G. contrast medium
gastroxia
gastroxynsis
Gastrozepine
Gas-X
gate
    sampling g.
Gates
    method of G.
Gaucher
    G. cell
    G. disease
    G. splenomegaly
Gauderer-Ponsky PEG operation
Gauder Silicon PEG catheter
Gau gastric balloon
gauge
    Dacomed snap g.
    intra-abdominal pressure g.
    LeVeen inflator with
      pressure g.
    snap g.
    Statham P23 strain g.
Gaur balloon distension technique
gauze
    g. dressing
    iodoform g.
    g. pack
    g. sponge
    Surgicel g.
    Vaseline g.
gavage
    g. feeding
GAVE
    gastric antral vascular ectasia
    GAVE syndrome
Gavin-Miller intestinal forceps
Gaviscon
Gaviscon-2

GAX
glutaraldehyde cross-linked collagen
GAX-collagen
gay bowel syndrome
Gaymar water-circulating blanket
Gazayerli
G. knot pusher
GB
GB vol- fluctuation
GB vol+ fluctuation
GBEF
gallbladder ejection fraction
GBER
gallbladder ejection rate
GBM
glomerular basement membrane
GBM collagen fiber
perimesangial GBM
GBM polyanion
GBO
gastric bacterial overgrowth
GBP
gastric bypass
GBS
group B streptococcus
GBT
gastric bleeding time
GC-16
Surgitek graduated
cystocope G.
G-cell
G.-c. hyperplasia
GC/MS
gas chromatography/mass
spectroscopy
G-CSF
granulocyte colony-stimulating
factor
GCT
giant cell transformation
granular cell tumor
GCW
glomerular capillary wall
GDA
gastroduodenal artery
G:D-cell ratio

GE
gastric emptying
gastroesophageal
GE junction
GE reflux
GE RT 3200 Advantage II
GEA
gastroepiploic artery
GEA graft
GEC
galactose elimination capacity
Gee-Herter-Heubner
G.-H.-H. disease
G.-H.-H. syndrome
Geenen
G. criteria
G. cytology brush
G. Endotorque guide
G. Endotorque guidewire
G. sphincterotomy
Gee-Thaysen disease
GEG
Garren-Edwards gastric
GEG bubble
gel
agar g.
agarose g.
Betadine g.
boronate g.
Contractubex g.
deletion and mutation detection
enhancement g.
g. filtration chromatography
polyacrylamide g.
Sephacryl S-300 HR g.
viscoelastic g.
gelatine Hank buffered solution
(GHBSS)
gelatinous ascites
gelatin sponge
gelatin-subbed slide
GELdose
Zantac G.
Gelfoam
G. cube
G. embolization

G

NOTES

Gelfoam *(continued)*
G. particles transarterial embolization treatment
Gelpi self-retaining retractor
gelsolin
recombinant human g.
Gelusil
Gelusil-II
Gelusil-M
Gély suture
gemfibrozil
Gemini
G. gall duct forceps
G. paired wire helical basket
gender
g. effect
g. reassignment
gene
adenomatous polyposis coli g.
ADPKD1 g.
ADPKD2 g.
Break-cluster homology g.
Cβ g.
cagA g.
g. carrier
c-Ha-ras g.
G. Clean II kit
COL4A3 g.
COL4A4 g.
COL4A5 g.
DRB g.
Fas g.
FCC-COCA1 g.
gastrin g.
HDA-DR3 g.
HLA g.
HLA class II g.
HLA-DQw2 g.
HLA-DR3 g.
hMLH1 g.
immunogenic g.
kallikrein-like g.
Ki-ras g.
K-ras g.
LMP g.
MCH g.
g. MutL
MutS g.
p53 g.
PKD1 g.
polymorphic g.
prodynorphin g.
proenkephalin g.

proopiomelanocortin g.
G. Screen nylon membrane filter
TAP g.
tap 2 peptide transporter g.
TGF-β1 g.
tumor suppressor g.
uromodulin g.
Vα g.
Vβ g.
α-gene
TNF α-g.
gene A
gene-blotting study
gene-linkage analysis (GLA)
GeneraBloc
general
g. anesthesia
g. endotracheal anesthesia (GETA)
g. peptic ulcer
generalized
g. glycogenosis
g. peritonitis
generation
Chiron RIBA HCV test system second g.
Ortho HCV ELISA test system second g.
generator
banana plug dipolar g.
electrosurgical g.
Endostat II bipolar/monopolar electrosurgical g.
isolated g.
spark-gap shock wave g.
Symmetry endo-bipolar g.
Valleylab SSE2L g.
genetic
g. alteration
g. hemochromatosis (GH)
g. heterogeneity
g. marker
g. predisposition
Genetics Systems microplate reader spectrophotometer
gene-transfer therapy
genital
g. differentiation
g. dysplasia
g. end bulb
g. rash

g. reconstruction
g. wart
genitalia
ambiguous external g.
anomalous g.
genitofemoral nerve
genitography
retrograde g.
genitoplasty
feminizing g.
masculinizing g.
genitourinary
g. carcinoma
g. fistula
g. neoplasm
g. prolapse
g. tract
genodermatosis
genome
full-length viral g.
genome/ml
genomic
g. deoxyribonucleic acid
g. DNA
g. DNA probe
g. sequence
g. site
genotype
ADPKD1 g.
ADPKD2 g.
g. II
g. III
g. III 2a
g. IV 2b
g. V 3
gentamicin
g. sulfate
Genta stain
gentian violet
genu
g. of pancreatic duct
genuine stress urinary incontinence (GSUI)
Geocillin
geographic
g. distribution
g. tongue

geophagia, geophagism, geophagy
GER
gastroesophageal reflux
Gerald forceps
GERD
gastroesophageal reflux disease
Gerhardt table
geriatric
g. constipation
g. voiding dysfunction
geriatrics
Geridium
Geriplex-FS
germ
g. cell carcinoma
g. cell hypoplasia
g. cell tumor
germicide
liquid chemical g. (LCG)
germinal
g. center formation
g. epithelium
germline mutation
Gerota
G. capsule
G. fascia
gestation
ectopic g.
gestational diabetes
GETA
general endotracheal anesthesia
GFC gastroscope
GFPM
gastric first-pass metabolism of ethanol
GFR
glomerular filtration rate
AmB-induced reduction GFR
amphotericin B-induced reduction glomerular filtration rate
single-nephron GFR
GFS Mark II inflatable penile prosthesis
GFT Olympus gastroscope

G

NOTES

245

GGT
gamma-glutamyl transferase
GGT test
GGTP
gamma-glutamyl transpeptidase
GH
genetic hemochromatosis
GHBSS
gelatine Hank buffered solution
Ghedini-Weinberg serologic test
GHP
^{99m}Tc GHP
GI
gastrointestinal
Gingival Index
GI bleeding scan
GI cancer
GI cocktail
GI tract
GI tract flora
GIA
gastrointestinal assistant
GIA autosuture apparatus
GIA autosuture device
GIA instrument
GIA stapler
Gianotti-Crosti syndrome
giant
g. cell
g. cell adenocarcinoma
g. cell hepatitis
g. cell transformation (GCT)
g. colon
g. diverticulum
g. fibrous mesothelioma
g. gastric fold
g. hypertrophic gastritis
g. intestinal fluke
g. mitochondria
g. molluscum contagiosum
g. peptic ulcer
Gianturco
G. coil
G. metal urethral stent
G. stent
G. Z-stent
Gianturco-Rosch
G.-R. biliary Z-stent
G.-R. self-expandable Z-stent
stent
Giardia
G. duodenalis

G. intestinalis
G. lamblia
giardiasis
GIB
gastrointestinal bleeding
Gibbon indwelling ureteral stent
Gibson-Balfour abdominal retractor
Gibson incision
Gibson-type incision
GICA
gastrointestinal cancer-associated
antigen
Giemsa stain
Giemsa-stained section
Gierke disease
GIF-HM
G.-H. fiberscope
GIFT
gamete intrafallopian transfer
Gigasept
Gilbert
G. cholemia
G. cystic duct forceps
G. disease
G. sign
G. syndrome
Gilchrist
G. ileocecal bladder
G. procedure
Gill renal tourniquet
Gil-Vernet
G.-V. ileocecal cystoplasty
G.-V. ileocecal cystoplasty
urinary diversion
G.-V. operation
G.-V. procedure
G.-V. retractor
G.-V. technique
Gingival Index (GI)
gingivostomatitis
herpetic g.
Giordano-Giovannetti diet
Giordano sphincter
GIP
gastric inhibitory peptide
gastric inhibitory polypeptide
GIP/Medi-Globe prototype needle
girdle
Neptune g.
shoulder g.
Gironcoli hernia
girth
abdominal g.

GIT
  gastrointestinal tract
Gittes
  G. procedure
  G. technique
  G. urethropexy
Gittes-Loughlin
  G.-L. bladder neck suspension
  G.-L. procedure
GL
  glucagon
GLA
  gene-linkage analysis
glabella reflex
glabrata
    Candida g.
    Torulopsis g.
glabrous cirrhosis
Glahn test
gland
  anal g.
  anal intramuscular g.
  Brunner g.
  cardiac-type g.
  Cowper g.
  esophageal ectopic
    sebaceous g.
  Galeati g.
  gastric g.
  Lieberkühn g.'s
  Littré g.
  misplaced g.
  mucus-secreting g.
  oxyntic g.
  periductal g.
  pyloric g.
glandis
  collum g.
glandular
  g. hypospadias
glandularis
  cystitis g.
glandular structure
glandulectomy
glandulopexy
glans

conical g.
  g. wings
glansplasty
  meatal advancement and g.
    (MAGPI)
glanuloplasty
Glasgow coma scale
glass
  g. penile prosthesis
  g. pH electrode
Glasser gastrostomy tube
Glassman
  G. clamp
  G. gastrostomy
Glassman-Allis intestinal forceps
Glaxo stain
Glazyme APF-EIA-TEST test
GLDH
  glutamate dehydrogenase
Gleason
  G. cancer grade
  G. score
  G. staging system
gleet
gleety
Glenn-Anderson
  G.-A. advancement
  G.-A. technique
Glenn diverticulum forceps
gliadin
  g. IgA
Gliadin-specific T-cell clone
Glidewire
  G. Gold surgical guidewire
  G. guidewire
  Microvasive G.
  Terumo G.
glide wire
Glidex coated Percuflex catheter
glimepride
glioma-polyposis
glipizide
Glisson
  G. capsule
  G. cirrhosis
globular hyalin
γ-globulin

G

NOTES

globulin
α_2 g.
alpha-2 g.
antilymphocyte g.
antithymocyte g. (ATG)
α_1-antitrypsin g.
Aza-antilymphocyte g.
cytomegalovirus immune g.
g. fraction
gamma g.
hepatitis B hyperimmune g.
immune serum g.
intravenous immune g. (IVIg)
Minnesota antilymphocyte g.
prophylactic gamma g.
sex hormone binding g.
(SHBG)
tetanus g.
globus
g. hystericus
g. pharyngis
glomerular
g. basement membrane (GBM)
g. basement membrane disease
g. capillary
g. capillary hypertension
g. capillary pressure
g. capillary wall (GCW)
g. cell culture
g. cell proliferation
g. contractile cell
g. crescent
g. cysts
g. endothelial myxovirus-like
microtubular inclusion
g. endotheliosis
g. epithelial cell
g. epithelial cell toxin
puromycin aminonucleoside
g. extracellular matrix
g. fibronectin mRNA
g. filtration
g. filtration rate (GFR)
g. hyperfiltration
g. hypertrophy
g. injury
g. macrophage infiltration
g. mesangium
g. metabolism
g. microvascular thrombosis
g. neutrophil infiltration
g. proteinuria
g. tip lesion (GTL)

g. tuft
g. ultrafiltrate
g. ultrafiltration
g. ultrafiltration coefficient
glomerulation
glomeruli (*pl. of* glomerulus)
atubular g.
obsolescent g.
glomerulitis
glomerulonephritides
glomerulonephritis (GN)
acute g.
antiglomerular basement
membrane g.
biopsy-verified chronic g.
chronic g. (CGN)
complement-mediated
experimental g.
crescentic g.
diffuse proliferative g.
fibrillary g.
focal necrotizing g.
idiopathic crescentic g.
idiopathic membranous g.
idiopathic rapidly
progressive g. (IRPGN)
IgA g.
immune complex g. (IC-GN)
immunotactoid g.
membranoproliferative g.
(MPGN)
membranous g. (MGN)
mesangial proliferative g.
mesangiocapillary g.
mesangioproliferative g.
pauciimmune crescentic g.
poststreptococcal g. (PSGN)
poststreptococcal acute g.
rapidly progressive g. (RPGN)
recurrent focal sclerosing g.
type I mesangiocapillary g.
glomerulopathy
Adriamycin g.
amyloid-like g.
collapsing g.
immunotactoid g. (ITGP)
inflammatory g.
nonamyloid g.
toxic g.
glomerulosa
zona g.
glomerulosclerosis
diffuse diabetic g.

focal g.
focal segmental g. (FSGS)
segmental g.
glomerulus, pl. **glomeruli**
amyloidotic g.
human g.
glomus tumor
glossitis
Rider-Moeller g.
glossodynia
glove
Tactyl 1 g.
GLPT
glutamate pyruvate transaminase
glucagon (GL)
g. precipitation
glucagon-evoked gastric dysrhythmia
glucagonoma
g. syndrome
glucocorticoid
g. treatment
glucocorticoids
gluconate
calcium g.
quinidine g.
gluconeogenesis
gluconeogenesis-associated enzyme
gluconeogenic-competent human
proximal tubule cell
gluconeogenic pathway
glucoreceptor
glucose
G. analyzer II test
CSF g.
filtered g.
g. intolerance
luminal g.
g. test
g. tolerance
g. transporter
g. uptake
glucose-6-phosphatase deficiency
glucose-6-phosphate isomerase
glucose-galactose malabsorption
glucosuria
Glucotrol
glucuronides

glucuronosyltransferase
glucuronyl
g. transferase
g. transferase deficiency
glue
cyanoacrylate g.
fibrin g.
tissue g.
glutamate
g. dehydrogenase (GLDH)
g. pyruvate transaminase (GLPT)
glutamic
g. acid
g. acid hydrochloride
glutamic-oxaloacetic transaminase (GOT)
glutamic-pyruvic transaminase (GPT)
glutaminase
mitochondrial phosphate-dependent g.
phosphate-dependent g. (PDG)
glutamine
g. aminotransferase pathway
CSF g.
g. nitrogen
g. test
γ-glutamyl transferase
γ-g. t. level
serum γ-g. t.
glutamyl transpeptidase (GTP)
glutaral
glutaraldehyde
activated alkaline g.
g. alarm
g. cross-linked collagen (GAX)
glutaraldehyde-induced proctitis
glutathione
g. metabolism
g. transferase
glutathione-S-transferase (GST)
gluteal fold
gluten
g. challenge
dietary g.

NOTES

gluten *(continued)*
    g. sensitivity
    wheat g.
gluten-dependent population
gluten-free diet
gluten-sensitive
    g.-s. diarrhea
    g.-s. enteropathy
gluteus
    g. maximus
    g. maximus transposition
Gluzinski test
glyburide
glycated albumin
glyceraldehyde-3-phosphate
    dehydrogenase (GAPDH)
glyceraldehyde phosphate
    dehydrogenase (GAPD)
glycerol
Glycerol-T
glyceryl trinitrate (GTN)
glycine
glycocalyx
    podocyte g.
glycochenodeoxycholate
^{14}C-glycocholate breath test
glycogen
    g. phosphorylase
    g. storage disease
glycogenic acanthosis
glycogenosis
    brancher deficiency g.
    generalized g.
    hepatophosphorylase
      deficiency g.
    hepatorenal g.
    Type III g.
glycogen-rich cystadenoma
glycol
    ethylene g.
    polyethylene g. (PEG)
glycolate
glycolipid
    mucin-type g.
glycolysis
    aerobic g.
    anaerobic g.
glycolytic
    g. enzyme
    g. inhibition
glycoprotein
    g. accumulation
    dimeric acidic g. (DAG)

heterodimeric g.
    g. III
    microfil-associated g. (MAGP)
    N-linked g.
    TAG-72 g.
glycoprotein-2
    sulfated g. (SGP-2)
glycopyrrolate
    g. test
glycosaminoglycan (GAG)
    g. heparin
    g.'s layer
    g.'s uronate (GAGUA)
glycosaminoglycan-degrading enzyme
glycosidase
glycoside
glycosuria
    alimentary g.
    digestive g.
glycosylation
    nonenzymatic g.
glycyltryptophan test
Glynazan
Glypressin
GM3 ganglioside
GM-CSF
    granulocyte macrophage colony-
      stimulating factor
      GM-CSF cytokine
Gmelin test
GMER
    gastric mucosal ectopia in rectum
GMP
    guanosine 5'-monophosphate
GN
    glomerulonephritis
gnawing pain
GNRF
    guanine nucleotide-releasing factor
GnRH
    gonadotropin-releasing hormone
goblet
    g. cell
    g. cell hyperplasia
    g. cell metaplasia
Goelet retractor
gold
    cationic colloidal g. (CCG)
    g. compound
    G. probe
    g. Probe Direct bipolar
      hemostasis catheter

G. Probe electrohemostasis
   catheter
g. salt
g. seed implant
g. seed implantation technique
gold-198
Goldberg Anorectic Attitude scale
Goldblatt
   G. clamp
   G. hypertension
   G. kidney phenomenon
Goldman classification operative
   risk
Goldschmiedt technique
Goldstein Microspike approximator
   clamp
Goldwasser suture carrier
golf hole configuration
Golgi
   G. apparatus
   G. complex
Goligher
   G. extraperitoneal ileostomy
   G. retractor
GoLYTELY
   G. bowel prep
   G. solution
Gomco
   G. suction
   G. suction tube
Gomez
   G. fundoplasty
   G. horizontal gastroplasty
   G. horizontal gastroplasty with
      reinforced stoma
Gompertzian tumor kinetics
gonad
   dysgenetic g.
   intersex g.
   streak g.
   vanishing g.
gonadal
   g. differentiation
   g. dysgenesis
   g. vein
gonadectomy
gonadoblastoma

gonadoliberin
gonadopathy
gonadotoxic
gonadotroph
gonadotrophin
gonadotropin
   human chorionic g. (HCG)
   human menopausal g.
gonadotropin-releasing hormone
   (GnRH)
gonangiectomy
gondii
   Toxoplasma g.
gonecystolith
gonococcal
   g. perihepatis pelvic
      inflammatory disease
   g. proctitis
gonocyte
gonodoblastoma
gonorrhea
   rectal g.
gonorrheal proctitis
gonorrhoeae
   Neisseria g.
GOO
   gastric outlet obstruction
Goodpasture
   G. disease
   G. epitope
   G. reactivity
   G. syndrome
Goodsall rule
Goodwin
   G. cup-patch principle
   G. technique
Goodwin-Hohenfellner technique
Goodwin-Scott technique
Gopalan syndrome
GOR
   antibody to G. (anti-GOR)
Gordon disease
Gore-Tex
   G.-T. catheter
   G.-T. graft
   G.-T. soft tissue patch
gorge

G

NOTES

gorget
    probe g.
Gorlin
    G. basal cell nevus syndrome
    G. syndrome
goserelin
    g. acetate
Gosset appendectomy retractor
GOT
    glutamic-oxaloacetic transaminase
Gothic arch formation
Gott
    G. shunt
    G. tube
Gould
    G. polygraph gastric motility
      measuring device
    G. pressure monitor
    G. pressure transducer
Goulding procedure
Gouley catheter
Gowers sign
GP
    gastroplasty
gp330 receptor
G3PDH
    G. CDNA probe
    G. mRNA species
GPL unit
GPT
    glutamic-pyruvic transaminase
Grabstald (Memorial) staging
  system
gracilis
    g. muscle
    g. muscle flap
    g. myocutaneous neovagina
    g. neosphincter
graciloplasty
    dynamic g.
grade
    Gleason cancer g.
    hemorrhoid g.
    mucosal PMN g.
    Savary-Miller II g.
graded
    g. alcohol
    g. esophageal balloon
      distention test
gradient
    acinar g.
    albumin g.
    biliary-duodenal pressure g.

    duodenobiliary pressure g.
    gastrosphincteric pressure g.
    hepatic venous pressure g.
    (HVPG)
    serum-ascites albumin g.
    (SAAG)
    transcapillary hydrostatic
      pressure g.
    transmural hydrostatic
      pressure g.
gradient-echo
    magnetization prepared-rapid g.-
      e. (MP-RAGE)
gradient-recalled acquisition in a
  steady state (GRASS)
grading
    Edmondson g. (EdGr)
    histologic g.
    tumor g.
graft
    aortic g.
    aortoenteric g.
    aortohepatic arterial g.
    autogenous tunica vaginalis g.
    g. bed
    bovine g.
    branched vascular g.
    buccal mucosal patch g.
    bypass g.
    C g.
    Dacron g.
    Dacron interposition g.
    dorsal vein patch g.
    free jejunal g.
    GEA g.
    Gore-Tex g.
    HLA identical kidney g.
    Horton-Devine dermal g.
    Impra g.
    interposition Dacron g.
    loop forearm g.
    Marlex g.
    mucosal g.
    murine g.
    omental pedicle flap g.
    patch g.
    g. placement
    prosthetic arterial g.
    reduced-size g.
    renal artery g.
    "scotty dog" g.
    segmental liver g.
    seromuscular intestinal patch g.

g. spatulation
split-thickness skin g.
g. survival
synthetic vascular g.
Thiersch-Duplay tube g.
tube g.
tubed free skin g.
graft-enteric fistula
graft-versus-host disease (GVHD)
Graham
G. catheter
G. closure
G. closure with omental pouch
G. plication
G. scale for drug-induced gastric damage
G. test
Gram
G. stain
G. stain of stool
G. stain of stool test
Gram-negative, gram-negative
G.-n. bacterium
G.-n. rod
G.-n. sepsis
Gram-positive, gram-positive
G.-p. bacterium
G.-p. sepsis
Gram-stain morphology
granddaughter cyst
granny knot
Grant gallbladder retractor
granular
g. cast
g. cell myoblastoma
g. cell tumor (GCT)
granularity
granule
acidophilic PAS-positive g.
carcinoid secretory g.
DiPAS-positive g.
Fordyce g.
hemosiderin g.
Weibel-Palade g.
zymogen g.

granulocyte
g. colony-stimulating factor (G-CSF)
g. macrophage colony-stimulating factor (GM-CSF)
granulocytopenia
granuloma
amebic g.
barium g.
eosinophilic g.
epithelioid g.
gastrointestinal eosinophilic g.
hepatic g.
g. inguinale
noncaseating tubercle-like g.
plasma cell g.
portal zone g.
stone g.
suture g.
umbilical g.
granulomatosa
Miescher cheilitis g.
granulomatosis
lipophagic intestinal g.
Wegener g.
granulomatous
g. cholangitis
g. disease
g. enteritis
g. enterocolitis
g. gastritis
g. hepatitis
g. ileitis
g. peritonitis
g. prostatitis
g. transmural colitis
granulosa cell tumor
granulosus
Echinococcus g.
grapefruit diet
Graser diverticulum
grasp
palmar g.
plantar g.
g. tripod forceps
grasper
Allis tooth g.

G

NOTES

grasper *(continued)*
  atraumatic g.
  bowel g.
  four-pronged polyp g.
  laparoscopic g.
  Polaris g.
  three-pronged g.
  traumatic locking g.
  umbilical port g.
grasping forceps
GRASS
  gradient-recalled acquisition in a
    steady state
Grass
  G. force displacement fluid
    collector
  G. Model SIU5A stimulation
    isolation unit
  G. Model S9 stimulator
Grassi test
gravel
Graves
  G. disease
  G. technique
gravidarum
  hyperemesis g.
  icterus g.
gravimetric
  g. technique
  g. weighing
gravis
  colitis g.
  icterus g.
  myasthenia g.
gravity
gravity-dependent drainage
Grawitz tumor
gray
  G. cystic duct forceps
  g. scale
  g. scale imaging
  g. scale sonography
  g. scale ultrasonography
  g. scale ultrasound
greasy food
greater
  g. curvature banded
    gastroplasty
  g. curvature of stomach
  g. curvature ulcer
  g. curve position
  g. omentum

  g. peritoneal sac
  g. sciatic foramen
green
  indocyanine g.
  g. sputum
  g. stool
Greenen
  G. Endotorque
  G. pancreatic stent
Greene retractor
Greenfield
  G. caval catheter
  G. filter
Greenville gastric bypass
Greenwald
  G. Control Tip cystoscopic
    electrode
  G. needle
  G. Roth Grip-Tip suture guide
  G. sound
Greer EZ Access drainage pouch
Gregoir-Lich procedure
Greishaber self-retaining retractor
Grey
  G. Turner disease
  G. Turner sign
  G. Turner sign of
    retroperitoneal hemorrhage
Grice suture needle
gridiron incision
Griffen Roux-en-Y bypass
Grimelius
  G. silver stain
  G. staining
  G. technique
Grimelius-positive cell
grip
  hook g.
  power g.
  precision g.
  three-finger g.
  two-finger g.
Grip-Tip suture guide
gritty
  g. tumor
Grocco sign
Grocott methenamine silver stain
groin
  g. incision
Grondahl-Finney
  esophagogastroplasty
groove
  esophageal g.

Liebermeister g.
oval-form colonic g.
g. pancreatitis
radial g.
spindle colonic g.
grooved director
gross
g. deformity
G. disease
g. hematuria
G. test
ground-glass
g.-g. appearance
g.-g. body of Hadziyannis
g.-g. cell
group
Astra/Merck G.
Benelux Multicentre Trial
Study G.
g. B streptococcus (GBS)
Eastern Cooperative
Oncology G.
hydroxyl g.
Lewis blood g.
phytyl g.
growth
g. factor
g. factor beta
g. factor isoform
g. regulation
somatic g.
GRP
gastrin-releasing peptide
Grüntzig, Gruentzig
G. balloon
G. balloon catheter
G. balloon catheter
G. balloon dilation
G. dilator
Grynfeltt triangle
GS
Gardner syndrome
G&S Electroejaculator
GST
glutathione-S-transferase
GSUI
genuine stress urinary incontinence

GTF-A
GTL
glomerular tip lesion
GTL-16 gastric carcinoma cell
GTN
glyceryl trinitrate
GTP
glutamyl transpeptidase
guanosine triphosphate
GTPase activating protein
GTP-dependent signaling protein
GTP-regulatory protein
G-tube
button-type G.-t.
Moss G.-t.
G.U.
Neosporin G.
guaiac
g. gum
g. test
guaiac-impregnated slide
guaiac-negative stool
guaiac-positive stool
guanadrel
guanethidine
parenteral g.
guanfacine
guanidine thiocyanate
guanidinium thiocyanate buffer
guanine
dihydroxypropoxymethyl g.
(DHPG)
g. nucleotide
g. nucleotide-releasing factor
(GNRF)
guanoclor
guanosine
g. monophosphate
g. 5′-monophosphate (GMP)
g. monophosphate pathway
g. triphosphate (GTP)
guanoxan
guanylate cyclase
guard
mouth g.
guarding
abdominal g.

G

NOTES

guarding *(continued)*
  involuntary g.
  muscle g.
  g. sign
  voluntary g.
guard-ring tocodynamometer
guar gum
gubernacular vein
gubernaculum
Guenzberg test
Guerin
  valve of G.
guidance
  choledochoscopic g.
  fluoroscopic g.
guide
  catheter g.
  Geenen Endotorque g.
  Greenwald Roth Grip-Tip
    suture g.
  Grip-Tip suture g.
  image guide (IG)
  J-wire g.
  light g. (LG)
  Lunderquist-Ring torque g.
  master image g.
  g. and mini-snare technique
  g. passage
  Roth Grip-Tip suture g.
  soft-tipped wire g.
  suture g.
guided-needle aspiration cytology
guided transcutaneous biopsy
guide-eye instrument
guideline
  string g.
guidewire *(See also* wire)
  Amplatz Super Stiff g.
  Bentson g.
  Bentson floppy-tipped g.
  Bentson-type Glidewire g.
  cannula with pre-loaded 0.35-
    inch g.
  Eder-Puestow g.
  ERCP g.
  FasTrac hydrophilic coated g.
  flexible-tip g.
  flexible-tip Bentsen g.
  Geenen Endotorque g.
  Glidewire g.
  Glidewire Gold surgical g.
  HPC g.
    hydrophilic-coated guidewire

  hydrophilic-coated g. (HPC
    guidewire)
  hydrophilic polymer-coated
    steerable g.
  Hydro Plus coated g.
  Lubriglide-coated g.
  Lumenator injectable g.
  Lumina g.
  Lunderquist g.
  Microvasive Geenen
    Endotorque g.
  Microvasive Glidewire g.
  nonconductive g.
  olive over g.
  Pathfinder exchange g.
  Placer g.
  slipper-tipped g.
  Teflon-coated g.
  Terumo g.
  Terumo hydrophilic g.
  Terumo/Meditech g.
  Terumo-Radiofocus hydrophilic
    polymer-coated g.
  Wilson-Cook Protector g.
  Wilson-Cook THSF-series g.
  Wilson-Cook Tracer g.
  Zebra exchange g.
guiding catheter
Guillain-Barré syndrome
guillotine needle biopsy
gullet
gum
  guaiac g.
  guar g.
  Karaya g.
gumma
gun
  Bard Biopty g.
  biopsy g.
  Biopty g.
  Cobe staple g.
  Cook biopsy g.
  EEA stapler g.
  intruducer g.
  Mentor g.
  modified caulking g.
  Moss T-anchor introducer g.
  spring-loaded biopsy g.
gunpowder lesion
gurgle
gurgling bowel sounds
Gussenbauer suture
gustatory sweating

gut
artificial g.
caffeine g.
g. colonization
congenital malrotation of
the g.
g. flora
nervous g.
plain g.
g. rest
Gutaform
gut-associated lymphoid tissue
(GALT)

gutter
lateral g.
left g.
paracolic g.
right g.
guttered T tube
Guyon sign
GVHD
graft-versus-host disease
gynecologic
g. laparoscopy
gynecomastia

NOTES

G

H
    H disease
H2
    histamine 2
    H2 blocker
    H2 breath test
    H2 receptor antagonist (H2RA)
    H2 receptor-blocker
    H2 receptor-blocking drug
    H2 receptors
H2-antagonist therapy
H2O2-induced injury
H2-receptor antagonist therapy
H3 histone
H-600 normothermic irrigation
Haberer
    H. abdominal spatula
    H. intestinal clamp
    H. intestinal forceps
habit
    bowel h.
    dietary h.
    drinking h.
    eating h.
habitus
    body h.
Hadefield-Clarke syndrome
Hadju-Cheney acroosteolysis syndrome
Hadziyannis
    ground-glass body of H.
HAE
    hereditary angioedema
HAEC
    Hirschsprung-associated enterocolitis
haematobium
    Schistosoma h.
Haemophilus
    H. ducreyi
    H. influenzae
haemostasis
Hafnia alvei
hafniae
    Enterobacter h.
Hafter diet trick
HAI
    histological activity index
hair ball

hairy
    h. leukoplakia
    h. tongue
Halban procedure
Halcion
Haldane-Priestly tube
Haldol
Hale
    H. colloidal iron stain
    H. colloidal iron technique
Haley M-O
half-body irradiation
half-hitch knot
half-life
half-normal saline
half-strength feeding
haliphagia
halitosis
Hallberg biliointestinal bypass
halo effect
haloperidol
halothane
    h. hepatotoxicity
halothane-induced hepatitis
Halsted
    H. forceps
    H. hemostat
    H. inguinal herniorrhaphy
    H. suture
Halsted-Bassini
    H.-B. hernia repair
    H.-B. herniorrhaphy
Ham
    H. F12 medium
    H. test
hamartoma
    ampullary h.
    angiomatous lymphoid h.
    Brunner gland h.
    cystic h.
    duodenal wall h.
    mesenchymal h.
    pancreatic h.
    Peutz-Jeghers h.
hamartomatous
    h. gastric polyp
    h. lesion
    h. polyp
    h. polyposis
Hamel test

H

Hamilton-Thorn motility analyzer
hammock
Hampton
    H. line
    H. sign
hand-held retractor
Handi-Cath catheter kit
handling
    renal tubular sodium h.
hand temperature
Haney needle driver
Hanger test
hanging panniculus
Hank
    H. balanced salt solution
      (HBSS)
    H. buffer solution
Hanley rectal bladder procedure
Hanot-Chauffard syndrome
Hanot cirrhosis
Hansel stain
Hansenula fabianii
Hanta virus
HAPC
    high-amplitude contraction
haplotype
    DQ2 h.
    DR7 h.
    histocompatibility h.
    HLA h.
    HLA-DQ2 h.
    HLA DR17 h.
haptoglobin
    serum h.
haptotoxic range
Hara classification of gallbladder
  inflammation
hard
    h. adhesion
    h. stool
Har-el pharyngeal tube
Harewood suspension procedure
harmonic scalpel
harpoon extraction
Harrington
    H. Deaver retractor
    H. esophageal diverticulectomy
    H. splanchnic retractor
Harris
    H. band
    H. hematoxylin
    H. tube

Harris-Benedict energy requirement
  equation
Harrison spot test
Hartmann
    H. closure of rectum
    H. colostomy
    H. operation
    H. point
    H. pouch
    H. procedure
    H. reconstruction technique
Hartnup
    H. disease
    H. syndrome
Harvard pump
harvester
    Arandel cell h
    Brandel cell h
harvesting
    h. en bloc
Harvey Stone clamp
Hashimoto
    H. struma
    H. thyroiditis
Hashizume endoscopic ligator kit
Hashmat shunt
Hashmat-Waterhouse shunt
Haslinger esophagoscope
Hasson
    H. bullet-tip forceps
    H. cannula
    H. needle-nose forceps
    H. open laparoscopy cannula
    H. ring forceps
    H. spike-tooth forceps
hatching
    blastocyst h.
    h. test
H+-ATPase
    vacuolar H.-A.
Hauri technique
Hausted all purpose chair
haustral
    h. blunting
    h. fold
    h. indentation
    h. marking
    h. pattern
    h. pouch
haustrum, pl. haustra
HAV
    hepatitis A virus
Havrix

Hawaii virus
Hay test
HB
 Tagamet H.
HBAg
 hepatitis B antigen
HBcAg
 hepatitis B core antigen
  recombinant HBcAg (rHBcAg)
HBeAg
 hepatitis Be antigen
  HBeAg immunological study
  purified HBeAg
HBeAg-positive
HBe antibody
HB-EGF
 heparin-binding epidermal growth
  factor
HBIG
 hepatitis B immunoglobulin
HBsAg
 hepatitis B surface antigen
  HBsAg immunological study
  HBsAg subtype
HBSS
 Hank balanced salt solution
HBV
 hepatitis B virus
  HBV DNA
  HBV Engerix-B
  HBV genomic DNA
HBV-associated DNA polymerase
HBV-specific T cell
HBVV
 hepatitis B virus vaccine
HC
 hemochromatosis
 high calorie
  ProctoCream HC
HC-1
 Anusol-HC-1
HCA
 hepatocellular adenoma
HCC
 hepatocellular carcinoma
HCG
 human chorionic gonadotropin

HCl
 hydrochloric acid
  benazepril HCl
  lomefloxacin HCl
  meperidine HCl
  midazolam HCl
  tetracycline HCl
  Tris HCl
  Vancocin HCl
  yohimbine HCl
HCN
 high calorie and nitrogen
  Isocal HCN
HCS
 hematocystic spot
HCTZ-TA
 hydrochlorothiazide-triamterene
HCV
 hepatitis C virus
  HCV antibody
  HCV EIA II
  HCV EIA 20 test
  HCV ELISA test
  HCV protein
  HCV RNA
HD
 hemodialysis
HDA-DR3 gene
HDAg
 hepatitis D antigen
HDC
 histidine decarboxylase
HDL
 high-density lipoprotein
HDL-C
 high-density lipoprotein cholesterol
HDP
 ^{99m}Tc HDP
HD-secura dialyzer
HDV
 hepatitis delta virus
 hepatitis D virus
HE
 hepatic encephalopathy
H&E
 hematoxylin and eosin
  H&E stain

NOTES

H

HE9 fibroblast
head
    Medusa h.
    h. of pancreas
    h. symptom
headlamp
    Keeler Magnalite h.
healed ulcer
healing
    delayed primary intention h.
    durable h.
    h. by primary intention
    h. by secondary intention
    wound h.
Healy intestinal forceps
Heaney clamp
heaped up edges
heart
    h. rate monitoring
    h. transplant
    h. transplantation
heartburn
    nocturnal h.
    h. of pregnancy
heart-kidney transplant
heart-lung machine
heat
    h. exchanger
    h. probe
    h. probe thermocoagulation
    h. shock protein (HSP)
heater
    h. probe
    h. probe coagulation
    h. probe therapy
    telescope h.
heat-inactivated fetal calf serum
HeatProbe lavage
heat-sterilized by autoclave
heave
    dry h.'s
heavy silk suture
Hebra disease
hedrocele
Hegar
    H. bougie
    H. rectal dilator
^{125}I-h-EGF
h-EGF
    human epidermal growth factor
Heidenhain cell
Heifitz clip

heilmanii
    Helicobacter h.
Heimlich
    H. maneuver
    H. maneuver for choking
Heineke-Mikulicz
    H.-M. gastroenterostomy
    H.-M. incision
    H.-M. principle
    H.-M. pyloroplasty
Heiss loop
HeLa cells
helical
    h. CT
    h. fashion
helical-ridged ureteral stent
Helicobacter
    H. heilmanii
    H. pylori (HP)
    H. pylori-induced gastritis
Helicobacter-**induced gastric injury**
helium insufflation
helium-neon laser
Heller
    H. cardiomyotomy
    H. myotomy
    H. operation
HELLP
    hemolysis, elevated liver enzymes,
      and low platelet count
    HELLP syndrome
Helmholtz double-surface coil
helminth
    h. infection
helminthemesis
helminthiasis
helminthic
    h. appendicitis
    h. dysentery
    h. pseudotumor
helminthism
Helmstein balloon
helper T cell
Hemaccel
hemagglutination
    indirect h. (IHA)
hemangioblastoma
    cerebral h.
    spinal h.
hemangioblastomatosis
    cerebelloretinal h.
    von Hippel-Lindau
    cerebellar h.

hemangioendothelial sarcoma
hemangioepithelioma
hemangioma
    cavernous h.
    hepatic h.
    strawberry h.
    vascular h.
hemangiomatosis
    duodenal h.
    splenic capillary h.
hemangiopericytoma
hemangiosarcoma
hematemesis
Hematest
    H. test
hematin cast
hematobilia
    h. evacuation
hematocele
hematocelia
hematochezia
hematochyluria
hematocrit
    hemoglobin and h. (H&H)
hematocystic spot (HCS)
hematocystis
hematocyturia
hematogenous
    h. micrometastasis
    h. spread of infection
hematologic
    h. abnormality
    h. complication
    h. study
hematoma
    duodenal h.
    esophageal h.
    esophageal intramural h.
    expanding retroperitoneal h.
    intrahepatic h.
    intramural h.
    mesenteric h.
    parenchymal h.
    perianal h.
    perirenal h.
    pulsatile h.
    rectus sheath h.

    renal h.
    septal h.
    subcapsular h.
    warfarin-associated
        subcapsular h.
hematomphalocele
hemato-oxyphilic deposit
hematopathology
hematopoiesis
    hepatic extramedullary h.
hematopoietic
    h. cell
    h. lineage
hematoporphyrin
    h. derivative (HpD)
hematospermatocele
hematospermia
hematoxylin
    h. and eosin (H&E)
    h. and eosin stain
    Harris h.
    h. stain
hematoxylin and eosin (H&E)
hematuresis
hematuria
    angioneurotic h.
    benign familial h.
    essential h.
    gross h.
    idiopathic h.
    initial h.
    macroscopic h.
    microscopic h.
    painful h.
    painless h.
    renal h.
    terminal h.
    total h.
    urethral h.
    vesical h.
hematuria-dysuria syndrome
HemaWipe
    H. test
heme-albumin
    intravenous h.-a.
heme-negative stool

NOTES

H

heme-positive
    h.-p. NG aspirate
    h.-p. stool
HemeSelect
hemiacidrin
    h. irrigation
hemianopsia
hemiballismus
hemiblock
    anterior h.
hemicolectomy
    Duecollement h.
    laparoscopic-assisted h.
hemicolon
hemicrypt column
hemigastrectomy
hemihepatectomy
hemihypertrophy
hemi-Kock
    h.-K. procedure
    h.-K. system
    h.-K. urinary diversion
heminephroureterectomy
hemi-orchiectomy
hemiparesis
hemiplegia
hemipyonephrosis
hemiscrotectomy
hemi-scrotectomy
hemiscrotum
hemobilia
Hemoccult
    H. II
    H. II test
    H. Sensa
    H. Sensa developer
    H. Sensa slide
    H. Sensa test
    H. test
hemocholecyst
hemochromatosis (HC)
    African h.
    Desferal Mesylate challenge
      for h.
    genetic h. (GH)
    idiopathic h.
    perinatal h.
    precirrhotic h.
hemochromatotic cirrhosis
hemoconcentration
hemoculture
hemocyanin
    keyhole limpet h. (KLH)

hemocytometer
hemodiafiltration
    double chamber h.
hemodialysis (HD)
    A2008 ABGII h. machine
    dermatosis of h.
    simplified nocturnal home h.
      (SNHHD)
    venovenous h.
    venovenous continuous h.
hemodialysis-associated ascites
hemodialyzer
    ALTRA-FLUX h.
    1550 Baxter h.
    2008E h.
    ultrafiltration h.
hemoductal pancreatitis
hemodynamics
    intraglomerular h.
    intrarenal h.
    renal h.
hemofilter
hemofiltration
    arteriovenous h.
    continuous arteriovenous h.
      (CAVH)
    continuous venovenous h.
      (CVVH)
    h. therapy (HFT)
hemoglobin
    h. content indices (IHb)
    h. and hematocrit (H&H)
    mean corpuscular h. (MCH)
    mucosal blood h.
hemoglobinemia
    paroxysmal nocturnal h.
hemoglobin and hematocrit (H&H)
hemoglobinuria
    paroxysmal nocturnal h. (PNH)
Hemoject
    H. injection catheter
    H. needle
hemolysis
hemolysis, elevated liver enzymes, and low platelet count (HELLP)
hemolytic
    h. anemia
    h. jaundice
    h. splenomegaly
    h. strep
hemolytic-uremic syndrome (HUS)
hemonephrosis

hemoperfusion
    albumin-coated resin h.
    charcoal h.
    h. with charcoal
hemopericardium
hemoperitoneum
HEMOPHAN membrane
hemophilia
    renal h.
hemoptysis
hemopyelectasis, hemopyelectasia
HemoQuant
    H. assay
    H. fecal blood test
hemorrhage
    acute nonvariceal upper
      gastrointestinal h.
    colonic h.
    concealed h.
    h. control
    diverticular h.
    endoscopic stigmata of h.
    exsanguinating h.
    gastric h.
    gastrointestinal tract h.
    Grey Turner sign of
      retroperitoneal h.
    hepatic h.
    internal h.
    intestinal h.
    intra-abdominal h.
    intramural intestinal h.
    intraperitoneal h.
    lower gastrointestinal h.
    nonvariceal upper GI h.
    pancreatitis-related h.
    postgastrectomy h.
    postpolypectomy h.
    refractory variceal h.
    renal h.
    renal cyst h.
    stigmata of recent h. (SRH)
    stress ulcer h.
    subcapsular h.
    subconjunctival h.
    subepithelial h.
    submucosal gastric h.

    torrential h.
    upper GI h.
    variceal h.
hemorrhagic
    h. ascites
    h. colitis
    h. cystitis
    h. dengue
    h. diarrhea
    h. enterocolitis
    h. fever
    h. fever with renal syndrome
    h. gastritis
    h. gastropathy
    h. necrotizing pancreatitis
    h. nephritis
    h. pancreatitis
    h. radiation injury
    h. speck
hemorrhoid
    h. banding
    bleeding h.
    combined h.'s
    cryotherapy for h.'s
    dilation of h.'s
    external h.
    h. grade
    internal h.
    ligation of h.'s
    Lord dilation of h.'s
    mixed h.'s
    mucocutaneous h.'s
    necrotic h.'s
    prolapsed h.'s
    prolapsing internal h.'s
    rubber band ligation of h.
    strangulated h.
    thrombosed external h.
    thrombosed internal and
      external h.
hemorrhoidal
    h. banding
    h. cushion
    h. plexus
    h. prolapse
    h. sclerotherapy
    h. tag

NOTES

H

hemorrhoidectomy
ambulatory h.
closed h.
diathermy h.
laser h.
Lord h.
modified Whitehead h.
open h.
radical h.
semi-open h.
HemoSelect test
hemosiderin
h. deposit
h. granule
hemosiderin-laden macrophage
hemosiderosis
hemospermia
h. spuria
h. vera
hemostasis
endoscopic h.
hemostat
Carmalt h.
Crile h.
curved h.
Endo-Assist disposable h.
Endo-Avitene microfibrillar
collagen h.
Halsted h.
Kelly h.
Kocher h.
microfibrillar collagen h.
(MCH)
Mixter h.
mosquito h.
Ochsner h.
Rochester-Péan h.
Westphal h.
hemostatic
h. agent
h. bond strength
h. suture
hemothorax
hemotympanum
Hemovac drain
hemuresis
Henke triangle
Henle
H. band
loop of H. (LH)
H. loop
Henning sign
Henoch-Schönlein purpura

Hepa
Amino Mel H.
hepadialysis
Hepaplastin test
heparan sulfate proteoglycan
(HSPG)
heparin
glycosaminoglycan h.
low-molecular weight h.
(LMWH)
heparin-binding
h.-b. epidermal growth factor
(HB-EGF)
h.-b. growth factor-1
heparin-induced
h.-i. lipolysis
h.-i. thrombocytopenia (HIT)
heparinization
heparinized saline
hepatalgia
HepatAmine amino acid solution
hepatectomy
donor h.
partial h.
recipient h.
triple lobe h.
hepatic
h. abnormality
h. abscess
h. adenoma
h. adhesion
h. allograft
h. amebiasis
h. amyloidosis
h. angiosarcoma
h. architecture
h. arteriogram
h. arteriography
h. artery
h. artery aneurysm
h. artery infusion pump
h. artery ligation
h. bed
h. blood pool scan
h. calculus
h. candidal infection
h. capsule
h. circulation
h. cirrhosis
h. clearance
h. colic
h. coma
h. copper overload

h. cord
h. cyst
h. cystic disease
h. diverticulum
h. duct
h. dullness
h. echinococcosis
h. edge
h. encephalopathy (HE)
h. extramedullary hematopoiesis
h. fascioliasis
h. fever
h. fibrosis
h. fistula
h. flexure
h. flexure of colon
h. glycogen store
h. granuloma
h. hemangioma
h. hemorrhage
h. hilar region
h. hilum
h. Hodgkin disease
h. insufficiency
h. intermittent fever
h. iron index (HII)
h. lectin
h. leiomyosarcoma
h. ligament
h. lipase (HL)
h. lobectomy
h. malignancy
h. malondialdehyde content
h. mass lesion
h. metabolism
h. metastatic disease
h. 3-methylglutaryl coenzyme
    A reductase (HMG-CoA)
h. osteodystrophy
h. outflow tract
h. parenchyma
h. peliosis
h. perfusion index (HPI)
h. phosphorylase deficiency
h. porphyria
h. resection
h. rupture

h. sarcoidosis
h. schistosomiasis
h. sclerosis
h. sinusoids
h. span
h. steatosis
h. stimulatory substance (HSS)
h. subcellular element
h. subsegmentectomy
h. telangiectasia
h. toxemia
h. trauma
h. triad
h. triglyceride lipase (HTGL)
h. tumor
h. uptake
h. urea
h. vein
h. vein injury
h. vein thrombosis
h. vein wedge pressure
h. venogram
h. venography
h. veno-occlusive disease
h. venous outflow
h. venous outflow obstruction
    (HVOO)
h. venous pressure
h. venous pressure gradient
    (HVPG)
h. venous pressure gradient
    reduction
h. venous web disease
h. venule
h. web
h. web dilation
h. wedge pressure
hepatica
    Fasciola h.
Hepatic-Aid
    H.-A. powdered feeding
hepatic-alveolar echinococcosis
hepatico-cystic junction
hepaticodochotomy
hepaticoduodenostomy
hepaticoenterostomy
hepaticogastrostomy

NOTES

hepaticojejunostomy
   Roux-en-Y h.
hepaticolithotomy
hepaticolithotripsy
hepaticostomy
hepaticotomy
hepaticus
   peliosis h.
hepatis
   incisura vesicae felleae h.
   peliosis h.
   porta h.
hepatitic
hepatitis, pl. **hepatitides**
   h. A
   active chronic h.
   acute h. (AH)
   acute alcoholic h.
   acute mononucleosis-like h.
   acute parenchymatous h.
   acute self-limited h.
   acute viral h. (AVH)
   h. A infection
   alcoholic h.
   amebic h.
   anesthetic h.
   anicteric h.
   anicteric viral h.
   autoimmune h.
   h. A vaccine
   h. A virus (HAV)
   h. B
   h. B antigen (HBAg)
   h. B core antigen (HBcAg)
   h. B DNA detection (HBV DNA)
   h. Be antigen (HBeAg)
   h. B hyperimmune globulin
   h. B immunoglobulin (HBIG)
   h. B infection
   h. B-like DNA
   h. B-like DNA virus
   blood-borne non-A, non-B h.
   h. B surface antigen (HBsAg)
   h. B surface antigen subdeterminant
   h. B vaccine
   h. B virus (HBV)
   h. B virus-encoded antigen
   h. B virus vaccine (HBVV)
   h. C
   h. carrier
   cholangiolitic h.

   cholestatic h.
   cholestatic viral h.
   chronic h. (CH)
   chronic active h. (CAH)
   chronic active viral h. (CAVH)
   chronic active viral h., non-A, non-B (CAVH-NAB)
   chronic active viral h., type B (CAVH-B)
   chronic aggressive h. (CAH)
   chronic autoimmune h.
   chronic fibrosing h.
   chronic interstitial h.
   chronic lobular h. (CLH)
   chronic persistent h. (CPH)
   chronic progressive h.
   chronic type B h.
   chronic viral h.
   h. C infection
   h. C RNA detection (HCV RNA)
   h. C viremia
   h. C virus (HCV)
   h. C virus enzyme immunoassay (HCV EIA 20 test)
   h. C virus RNA (HCV RNA)
   h. D
   h. D antigen (HDAg)
   delta h.
   delta agent h.
   h. delta virus (HDV)
   h. D infection
   drug-induced h.
   h. D superinfection
   h. D virus (HDV)
   h. E
   h. E infection
   ENANB h.
   enterically transmitted non-A, non-B h. (ET-NANBH)
   epidemic h.
   h. E virus (HEV)
   familial h.
   fatty liver h.
   flucloxacillin-induced delayed cholestatic h.
   fulminant viral h. (FVH)
   giant cell h.
   granulomatous h.
   halothane-induced h.
   herpetic h.

hyperglobulinemic h.
idiopathic autoimmune
  chronic h.
infectious h.
intrahepatic h.
ischemic h.
isoniazid-induced h.
lobular h.
long incubation h.
lupoid h.
malarial h.
MS-1 h.
MS-2 h.
murine h.
NANB h.
neonatal h.
newborn h.
non-A, non-B h.
non-A, non-B
  posttransfusion h.
nonspecific reactive h.
normal carrier h.
occult h.
oxacillin-associated anicteric h.
persistent chronic h.
persistent viral h. (PVH)
persistent viral h., non-A, non-
  B (PVH-NANB)
persistent viral h., type B
  (PVH-B)
plasma cell h.
posttransfusion h.
quiescent h.
h. serologic markers
serum h.
short incubation h.
subacute h.
subclinical h.
superimposed alcoholic h.
syphilitic h.
terbutaline h.
toxic h.
transfusion-associated h.
h. type 1
Type 1 autoimmune h.
type 2 autoimmune h.
viral h., virus h.

viral h. type A
viral h. type B
hepatization
hepatobiliary
  h. disease
  h. fibropolycystic disease
  h. malignancy
  h. manifestation
  h. scan
  h. scintigraphy
  h. tree
hepatoblastoma
hepatocanalicular cholestasis
hepatocarcinogenesis
hepatocarcinoma
  fibrolamellar h.
hepatocele
hepatocellular
  h. adenoma (HCA)
  h. atypia
  h. ballooning
  h. basolateral plasma
    membrane fluidity
  h. carcinoma (HCC)
  h. cholestasis
  h. death
  h. disease
  h. jaundice
  h. necrosis
  h. protein
hepatocerebral degeneration
hepatocholangioenterostomy
hepatocholangiojejunostomy
hepatocholangiostomy
hepatocolic ligament
hepatocystic
hepatocystocolic ligament
hepatocyte
  ballooning degeneration of h.
  cobblestone pattern of h.
  h. growth factor (HGF, HPG)
  lipid-laden h.
  h. lysosome
  h. necrosis
  periportal h.
  polygonal h.
  h. proliferation inhibitor (HPI)

NOTES

H

hepatocyte *(continued)*
 h. protein synthesis
  pseudoductular transformation
  of h.'s
 h. transplantation
hepatocyte-type cytokeratin
hepatocytic cord
hepatoduodenal
 h. ligament
 h. reflection
hepatoduodenal-peritoneal reflection
hepatoduodenostomy
hepatodynia
hepatodysentery
hepatofugal
 h. arterioportal shunt
 h. flow
 h. porto-systemic venous shunt
hepatogastric ligament
hepatogastroduodenal ligament
hepatogastroenterology
hepatogenic, hepatogenous
hepatography
hepatohemia
hepatoid adenocarcinoma
hepato-iminodiacetic acid (HIDA)
hepatojugular reflux
hepatolenticular
 h. degeneration
 h. disease
hepatolith
hepatolithectomy
hepatolithiasis
hepatologist
hepatology
hepatoma
 fibrolamellar h.
hepatomegaly
 congestive h.
hepatomphalocele
hepatomphalos
hepatonephoric syndrome
hepatonephromegaly
hepatopancreatic fold
hepatopathic
hepatopathy
 radiation h.
hepatopetal
 h. flow
hepatopexy
hepatophosphorylase deficiency
 glycogenosis
hepatophrenic ligament

hepatopleural fistula
hepatoportal sclerosis
hepatoportoenterostomy
 Kasai-type h.
hepatoptosis
hepatorenal
 h. angle
 h. bypass
 h. glycogenosis
 h. ligament
 h. syndrome (HRS)
hepatorrhagia
hepatorrhaphy
hepatorrhea
hepatorrhexis
hepatoscopy
hepatosplenomegaly
hepatosplenopathy
hepatostomy
hepatotherapy
hepatotomy
hepatotoxemia
hepatotoxic
hepatotoxicity
 acetaminophen h.
 Amanita mushroom h.
 anesthetic h.
 anticonvulsant agent h.
 antidepressant drug h.
 antidiabetic agent h.
 antineoplastic drug h.
 antipsychotic drug h.
 antithyroid drug h.
 carbamazepine h.
 cardiovascular drug h.
 chemotherapeutic agent h.
 cocaine h.
 drug h.
 erythromycin estolate h.
 halothane h.
 hydrazide h.
 nitrofurantoin h.
 2-nitropropane h.
 phenylbutazone h.
 potentiation of drug h.
 yellow phosphorus h.
hepatotoxin
hepatoumbilical ligament
Hep-B-Gammagee
HEPES
 H. buffer
 H. solution
Heptavax-B

Her-2/neu oncogene
herald
    h. bleed
    h. patch
hereditary
    h. angioedema (HAE)
    h. flat adenoma syndrome
      (HFAS)
    h. fructose intolerance
    h. hemorrhagic telangiectasia
      (HHT)
    h. internal anal sphincter
      myopathy
    h. nephritis
    h. nonpolyposis colorectal
      cancer (HNPCC)
    h. nonpolyposis colorectal
      carcinoma
    h. pancreatitis (HP)
    h. tyrosinemia
Hering
    canal of H.
Hermansky-Pudlak syndrome
Herman-Taylor gastroscope
hermetically
hernia, pl. **herniae**
    abdominal wall h.
    antevesical h.
    axial hiatal h.
    Barth h.
    Béclard h.
    bladder h.
    Bochdalek h.
    cecal h.
    Cheatle-Henry h.
    Cloquet h.
    combined hiatal h.
    congenital h.
    congenital diaphragmatic h.
    Cooper h.
    diaphragmatic h.
    direct inguinal h.
    duodenojejunal h.
    easily reducible h.
    epigastric h.
    femoral h.
    funicular inguinal h.

    gastroesophageal h.
    Gironcoli h.
    hiatal h., hiatus h.
    Holthouse h.
    incarcerated h.
    h. incarceration
    incisional h.
    incomplete h.
    indirect inguinal h.
    inguinal h.
    inguinofemoral h.
    inguinoscrotal h.
    inguinosuperficial h.
    interstitial h.
    intraepiploic h.
    intrailiac h.
    irreducible h.
    h. knife
    Krönlein h.
    lateral ventral h.
    Laugier h.
    Lesgaft h.
    Littré h.
    Madden repair of incisional h.
    Maydl h.
    mesenteric h.
    mesocolic h.
    Morgagni h.
    multiorgan h.
    pantaloon h.
    paraesophageal diaphragmatic h.
    paraesophageal hiatal h.
    parahiatal h.
    paraileostomal h.
    parapubic h.
    parastomal h.
    parietal h.
    h. pouch
    properitoneal h.
    reducible h.
    h. repair
    retrograde h.
    retroperitoneal h.
    retrosternal h.
    Richter h.
    Rieux h.
    Rokitansky h.

NOTES

H

hernia *(continued)*
  rolling hiatal h.
  h. sac
  sciatic h.
  scrotal h.
  sliding esophageal hiatal h.
  sliding hiatal h.
  spigelian h.
  h. stapler
  strangulated h.
  traumatic diaphragmatic h.
  Treitz h.
  umbilical h.
  h. uteri inguinale
  h. uteri inguinalis
  Velpeau h.
  ventral h.
  vesicle h.
  voluminous hiatus h.
  "w" h.
hernial
  h. defect
  h. repair
  h. sac
herniated preperitoneal fat
herniation
  ureteroneocystostomy h.
hernioenterotomy
herniolaparotomy
hernioplasty
herniorrhaphy
  Bassini inguinal h.
  Halsted-Bassini h.
  Halsted inguinal h.
  Hill-type hiatus h.
  Lichtenstein h.
  Macewen h.
  Madden incisional h.
  McVay h.
  pants-over-vest h.
  Ponka h.
  Shouldice inguinal h.
  ventral h.
  vest-over-pants h.
herniotome
  Cooper h.
herniotomy
heroin
herpangina
herpes
  h. infection
  h. labialis
  h. pharyngitis

  h. simplex
  h. simplex esophagitis
  h. simplex infection
  h. simplex virus (HSV)
  h. zoster
herpesvirus
  h. simplex (HVS)
herpetic
  h. esophagitis
  h. gingivostomatitis
  h. hepatitis
  h. stomatitis
  h. ulcer
herpetiform esophagitis
herpetiformis
  dermatitis h. (DH)
herpkinetic circulation
Herrick kidney clamp
herring-worm disease
Hers disease
Herter-Heubner disease
Herzberg test
Hesselbach
  H. ligament
  H. triangle
HETE
  hydroxyeicosatetraenoic acid
heterochromatin
heteroconjugate
  antilymphocyte h.
heterodimer
heterodimeric
  h. glycoprotein
  h. protein
heteroduplex analysis
heterogeneity
  genetic h.
  intratumoral h.
heterogeneous texture
heterogenous pseudocyst
heterologous
  h. anti-GBM antibody
  h. liver perfusion
heterotopia
  fundic gland h.
  gastric h.
heterotopic
  h. gastric mucosa
  h. pancreas
heterotrimer
heterozygosity
heterozygote

heterozygous
    h. DR5
    h. ornithine transcarbamylase
      (HOTC)
HEV
    hepatitis E virus
Hexabrix
hexagon snare
hexamethonium
    h. bromide
hexocyclium
hexokinase (HK)
Heyde syndrome
Heyer-Schulte
    H.-S. Small-Carrion sizing set
    H.-S. stent
Heyman antibody
Heymann nephritis antigenic
  complex (HNAC)
HFAS
    hereditary flat adenoma syndrome
HFT
    hemofiltration therapy
HG
    Cobe Centrysystem dialyzer
      400 H.
HgCl2
    mercury chloride
HGD
    high-grade dysplasia
HGF
    hepatocyte growth factor
    human growth factor
HGF-stimulated renal epithelial cell
H&H
    hemoglobin and hematocrit
HHM
    humoral hypercalcemia of
      malignancy
HHT
    hereditary hemorrhagic
      telangiectasia
hiatal hernia
hiatus
    diaphragmatic h.
    h. hernia
    patulous h.

Hibiclens
Hibistat
Hibond N+ nylon membrane
hiccup, hiccough, pl. **hiccups**
Hickman
    H. catheter
    H. percutaneous introducer
HIDA
    hepato-iminodiacetic acid
    HIDA scan
    ^{99m}Tc HIDA
hidden antigen
hidradenitis suppurativa
Higgins
    H. India ink
    H. technique
high
    h. anion-gap metabolic acidosis
    h. bulk, low fat diet
    h. calorie (HC)
    h. calorie diet
    h. calorie and nitrogen (HCN)
    h. carbohydrate diet
    h. diameter dilator
    h. enema
    h. fat diet
    h. fiber diet
    h. flow priapism
    h. flux dialyzer
    h. frequency sonography
    h. intermuscular abscess
    h. intraluminal pressure
    h. level disinfection (HLD)
    h. ligation
    h. ligation of hernia sac
    h. lithotomy
    h. neurological lesion
    h. nitrogen (HN)
    h. pressure zone (HPZ)
    h. protein diet
    h. rectal washout
    h. resolution endoluminal
      sonography (HRES)
    h. roughage diet
    h. sensitivity collimator
    h. small-bowel obstruction

NOTES

H

high *(continued)*
  h. subtotal gastrectomy
  h. testis
high-abdominal plain film
high-affinity,
  h.-a. low-capacity system
  h.-a. sodium-dependent
    phosphate transport system
high-altitude endoscopy
high-amplitude contraction (HAPC)
high-calcium dialysate
high-ceiling diuretic
high-compliance latex balloon
high-density
  h.-d. lipoprotein (HDL)
  h.-d. lipoprotein cholesterol
    (HDL-C)
high-dose pulse steroid
high-echoic area
high-ending vagina
high-flux
  h.-f. dialysis
  h.-f. dialysis membrane
  h.-f. polysulphone
high-grade
  h.-g. cholestasis
  h.-g. dysplasia (HGD)
  h.-g. obstruction
high-loop cutaneous ureterostomy
highly selective vagotomy
high-magnification
  h.-m. colonoscopy
  h.-m. endoscopy
  h.-m. gastroscopy
high-pass filtering
high-performance liquid
  chromatography (HPLC)
high-pitched bowel sounds
high-power field (hpf)
high-power photomicrograph
high-pressure
  h.-p. arterial baroreceptor
  h.-p. liquid chromatography
    (HPLC)
high-resolution
  h.-r. 25-megahertz
    ultrasonography
  h.-r. real-time scanner
high-speed electrical tissue
  morcellator
high-velocity flow
HII
  hepatic iron index

hilar
  h. carcinoma
  h. clamp
  h. mass
  h. plate
  h. structure scar tissue
Hill
  H. antireflux operation
  H. hiatus hernia repair
  H. median arcuate repair
  H. posterior gastropexy
  H. rectal retractor
  H. repair
Hill-Ferguson rectal retractor
Hill-type hiatus herniorrhaphy
hilum
  hepatic h.
  splenic h.
  h. stimulation
hilus
  liver h.
hindgut
  h. carcinoid
  h. dysfunction
  h. pattern
Hinkle-James rectal speculum
Hinman
  H. procedure
  H. syndrome
Hinman-Allen syndrome
hipoplastic
hippocratic succussion
Hippuran
hippuran clearance technique
hipran
Hiprex
Hirschmann
  H. anoscope
  H. pile clamp
  H. speculum
Hirschowitz
  H. endoscope
  H. gastroduodenal fiberscope
  H. gastroscope
Hirschsprung-associated enterocolitis
  (HAEC)
Hirschsprung disease
hirsuitoid papilloma
hirsutism
  adrenal h.
His
  angle of H.
  bundle of H.

Hismanal
Histalog stimulation test
histamine
    gastreen as h.
    h. test
histamine 2 (H2)
histamine-producing mast cell
histamine₂ receptor antagonist
    (H2RA)
histamine-resistant achlorhydria
histaminergic type 2 receptor
histidine
    h. decarboxylase (HDC)
histiocyte
    pigmented h.
histiocytic lymphoma
histiocytoma
    fibrous h.
histiocytosis
    malignant h.
Histoacryl
histochemical pattern
histochemical-ultrastructural analysis
histochemistry
histocompatibility
    h. antigen
    h. complex
    h. haplotype
    h. testing
histocytochemical technique
Histofine SAB kit
histogram flattening
histologic
    h. cirrhosis
    h. damage
    h. diagnosis
    h. grading
histological
    h. activity index (HAI)
    h. chronic active gastritis
    h. esophagitis
histology
histolytica
    Entamoeba h.
histometry
histomorphometric

histone
    H3 h.
histopathology
    renal h.
Histoplasma capsulatum
histoplasmosis
    disseminated h.
    gastrointestinal h.
    intestinal h.
    mediastinal h.
    recurrent colonic h.
histrionic personality
HIT
    heparin-induced thrombocytopenia
Hitachi
    H. 717 analyzer
    H. 737 autoanalyzer
    H. F-2000 fluorescence
        spectrophotometer
hitch
    psoas h.
HIV
    human immunodeficiency virus
    HIV infection
    HIV P24 antigen
HIVAN
    HIV-associated nephropathy
HIV-associated nephropathy
    (HIVAN)
hive
Hi-Vegi-Lip
HK
    hexokinase
    HK enzyme
H+,K+-ATPase acid pump inhibitor
H+/K+ ATPase enzyme system
HL
    hepatic lipase
HLA
    human leukocyte antigen
    human lymphocyte antigen
        HLA class II antigen
        HLA class II gene
        HLA class II phenotype
        HLA class II restricted
        HLA class II-restricted
        interferon-gamma

NOTES

H

HLA *(continued)*
    HLA class II-restricted T cell
      epitope
    HLA DR
    HLA DR3
    HLA DR4
    HLA DR17 haplotype
    HLA gene
    HLA haplotype
    HLA identical kidney graft
    HLA mismatch
    HLA typing
    HLA typing immunological
      study
HLA-A
HLA-B
HLA-B8
HLA-DP allele
HLA-DQ2
    H.-D. haplotype
    H.-D. molecule
HLA-DQw2 gene
HLA-DR
    H.-D. antigen
    H.-D. DNA typing
    H.-D. matching
    H.-D. typing
HLA-DR+
HLA-DR2 subtyping
HLA-DR3 gene
HLA-identical sibling
HLD
    high level disinfection
HLG
    hypertrophic lymphocytic gastritis
HM4
    Dornier electrohydraulic
      watertank lithotriptor (HM3,
      HM4)
    HM4 lithotriptor
HMB-45 monoclonal antibody
  marker
HMG-CoA
    hepatic 3-methylglutaryl coenzyme
      A reductase
hMLH1 gene
HN
    high nitrogen
    hypertensive nephrosclerosis
    HN feeding
HNAC
    Heymann nephritis antigenic
      complex

HNPCC
    hereditary nonpolyposis colorectal
      cancer
hobnailed cell
hobnail liver
hockey-stick incision
Hodge intestinal decompression tube
Hodgkin disease
Hodgson technique of modified
  Lich procedure
hoe
    Joe h.
Hoefer GS 300 laser densitometer
Hoehn
    H. and Yahr stage
    H. and Yahr stage (0-1-2-3-4-
      5) for Parkinson disease
Hofmeister
    H. anastomosis
    H. gastroenterostomy
    H. operation
    H. procedure
    H. technique
Hofmeister-Pólya anastomosis
Hoguet maneuver
holder
    Bihrle dorsal clamp-T-C
      needle h.
    Bookler swivel-ball
      laparoscope h.
    Bovie h.
    Capillary System slide h.
    Cath-Secure catheter h.
    Dale Foley catheter h.
    diamond jaw needle h.
    Endo-Assist disposable
      needle h.
    Jacobson needle h.
    Lloyd-Davis knee and leg h.
    Mayo-Hegar needle h.
    microneedle h.
    microvascular needle h.
    needle h.
    T-C needle h.
    Young needle h.
Holihesive Skin Barrier
Holinger esophagoscope
Hollander test
Hollande solution
Hollenhorst plaque
Hollister
    H. Convex insert
    H. First Choice pouch

H. Guardian F skin barrier
H. Holligard pouch
H. irrigator drain
H. Karaya 5 ostomy pouch
H. Karaya Seal pouch
H. Premium paste
H. Premium pouch
H. urostomy bag
hollow viscus
holmium:YAG laser
holodiastolic
holosystolic
Holter
H. valve
vesicovaginal H.
Holthouse hernia
Holyoke
H. briefs
H. pants
homatropine methylbromide
home
h. parenteral nutrition (HPN)
h. screening test
h. uroflowmetry
homeostasis
sodium h.
Homer Wright rosette
HomeSelect test
hominis
Blastocystis h.
Mycoplasma h.
homocladic anastomoses
homocysteine
protein-bound h.
homocystinuria
homodimerization
ligand-dependent receptor h.
homogenate
cecal h.
fecal h.
mucosal h.
sphincter of Oddi h.
homogeneity
homogeneous
h. ablation
h. echographic
h. texture

homogenous
h. cooling
h. radioimmunoassay
homologous
h. protein-overload disease
h. serum jaundice
homosexual rectal trauma
homovanillic acid (HVA)
homozygote
homozygous sickle cell anemia
honeymoon cystitis
hood
latex h.
hooded prepuce
hook
Barr fistula h.
cold knife h.
Crile nerve h.
crypt h.
h. forceps
h. grip
Joseph h.
h. knife
Neivert polyp h.
nerve h.
Pratt crypt h.
Pratt rectal h.
Pucci-Seed h.
Rosser crypt h.
h. scissors
Shambaugh fistula h.
Stewart crypt h.
h. tip laparoscopic electrode
Whitaker h.
hookworm
h. disease
Hopkins
H. II rod lens
H. rod-lens system for rigid
choledochoscope
H. symptom checklist
H. telescope
hordein
hordeolum
horizontal
h. electrophoresis
h. gastroplasty

NOTES

H

horizontal *(continued)*
  h. mattress suture
  h. transmission
hormonal
  h. downstaging
  h. therapy
hormone
  adrenocorticotropic h. (ACTH)
  h. antagonist
  antidiuretic h. (ADH)
  endothelium-derived relaxing h.
  enteric h.
  follicle-stimulating h. (FSH)
  gastrointestinal peptide h.
  gonadotropin-releasing h.
    (GnRH)
  human menopausal h.
  LH-FSH releasing h.
  luteinizing h. (LH)
  luteinizing hormone-releasing h.
    (LHRH)
  parathyroid h. (PTH)
  peptide h.
  plasma parathyroid h. (PTH)
  secosteroid h.
  thyroid h.
  thyrotropin-releasing h.
hormone-stimulated cAMP synthesis
Horner syndrome
Horn sign
horseradish peroxidase-conjugated
  anti-rabbit IgG
horseshoe
  h. abscess
  h. fistula
  h. kidney
Horsley
  H. anastomosis
  H. gastrectomy
  H. suture
Horton-Devine dermal graft
Hosemann forceps
hose-pipe appearance of terminal
  ileum
Hospal Biospal filter
host
  h. factor
  immunocompetent h.
  immunocompromised h.
Hostaform
  plastic cylinder H.
hostility
  h. score

hot
  h. appendix
  h. biopsy
  h. biopsy forceps
  h. biopsy technique
  h. defect
  h. flexible forceps
  h. spot
  h. squeeze
HOTC
  heterozygous ornithine
    transcarbamylase
Hounsfield unit
24-hour
  24-h. ambulatory esophageal
    pH monitoring
  24-h. ambulatory gastric pH
    monitor
  24-h. ambulatory pH-metry
  24-h. ambulatory pH test
  24-h. esophageal pH probe
  24-h. fecal fat excretion
  24-h. gastric acidity test
  24-h. home pH-metry
  24-h. urine collection
hourglass
  h. constriction of gallbladder
  h. deformity
  h. narrowing
  h. stomach
  h. stricture
house advancement anoplasty
houseflap anoplasty
Housset-Debray gastroscope
Houston
  valve of H.
Howard test
Howel-Evans syndrome
Howell-Jolly body
Howell Rotatable BII papillotome
Howship-Romberg sign
HP
  Helicobacter pylori
  hereditary pancreatitis
  hyperplastic polyp
    Ku-Zyme HP
HPA
  hypothalamic-pituitary-adrenal
  hypothalamic-pituitary axis
HPC guidewire
HpD
  hematoporphyrin derivative

HpD dye
low-dose HpD
hpf
high-power field
hpfast rapid urease test
HPG
hepatocyte growth factor
HPI
hepatic perfusion index
hepatocyte proliferation inhibitor
HPLC
high-performance liquid
chromatography
high-pressure liquid chromatography
HPLO
H. pylori-like organism
HPN
home parenteral nutrition
HPT
human proximal tubule
hyperparathyroidism
HPV
human papillomavirus
HPV 16
human papillomavirus 16
H. pylori-like organism (HPLO)
HPZ
high pressure zone
H2RA
histamine$_2$ receptor antagonist
H2 receptor antagonist
HRES
high resolution endoluminal
sonography
HRS
hepatorenal syndrome
HSE
hypertonic saline-epinephrine
solution
HSE solution
H-shaped
H.-s. ileal pouch-anal
anastomosis
H.-s. tilt tag
HSP
heat shock protein

HSP-70
H. cDNA
H. messenger ribonucleoprotein
acid level
H. mRNA
HSPG
heparan sulfate proteoglycan
HSS
hepatic stimulatory substance
HSV
herpes simplex virus
5-HT
5-hydroxytryptamine
serotonin
5-HT test
HTGL
hepatic triglyceride lipase
H-thymidine
3H-thymidine
HTLV-I
human T-cell leukemia virus of type
I
antibody to HTLV-I (anti-
HTLV-I)
HTLV-I-associated myelopathy
H-type fistula
Hueter maneuver
Hufford esophagoscope
Huggins operation
Huibregtse biliary stent
Huibregtse-Katon papillotome
Hulbert
H. electrosurgical knife
H. endo-electrode set
Hulka clip
hum
venous h.
human
h. adenovirus 12
h. albumin
h. apo A-I DNA probe
h. chorionic gonadotropin
(HCG)
h. chromosome 6
h. cytochrome P-450 enzyme
system
h. cytotoxic T cell

NOTES

H

human *(continued)*
  h. epidermal growth factor (h-EGF)
  h. erectile dysfunction
  h. fibronectin cDNA probe
  h. gastrin probe
  h. glomerulus
  h. growth factor (HGF)
  h. gut bacterium
  h. immunodeficiency virus (HIV)
  h. insulin
  h. intestinal epithelial cell
  h. leukocyte antigen (HLA)
  h. lymphocyte antigen (HLA)
  h. lymphocyte chromosomal aberration test
  h. lyophilized dura cystoplasty
  h. menopausal gonadotropin
  h. menopausal hormone
  h. papillomavirus (HPV)
  h. papillomavirus 16 (HPV 16)
  h. PDGF receptor
  h. proximal tubule (HPT)
  h. recombinant erythropoietin
  h. recombinant TGF
  h. serum albumin
  h. T-cell leukemia virus of type I (HTLV-I)
humeral neck
humoral
  h. arm
  h. hypercalcemia of malignancy (HHM)
  h. immunity
  h. immunodeficiency disorder
hump
  dromedary h.
hunger pain
Hunner
  H. stricture
  H. ulcer
Hunt-Lawrence pouch
Hunt test
Huppert test
Hurst
  H. bougienage
  H. bullet-tip dilator
  H. dilator
  H. mercury bougie
  H. mercury-filled dilator
Hurst-Tucker pneumatic dilator
Hurst-type bougie

Hurwitz esophageal clamp
HUS
  hemolytic-uremic syndrome
husband
  artificial insemination h. (AIH)
Huschke ligament
husk
  ispaghula h.
Hutch diverticulum
Hutinel disease
HVA
  homovanillic acid
HVOO
  hepatic venous outflow obstruction
HVPG
  hepatic venous pressure gradient
HVR1
  hypervariable region 1
HVS
  herpesvirus simplex
hyalin
  alcoholic h.
  globular h.
  Mallory h.
hyaline
  h. cast
hyalinized stroma
hyalinosis
  arteriolar h.
hyaluronic
  h. acid
  h. acid concentration
hybridization
  dot-blot h.
  fluorescence in-situ h. (FISH)
  nucleic acid h.
  quantitative liquid h.
  reverse-dot h.
  sequence-sequence oligonucleotide h.
  Southern blot h.
hybridoma-derived monoclonal antibody
Hybritech
  H. PSA scan
  H. Tandem prostate specific antigen assay
  H. Tandem-R assay kit
  H. Tandem-R PSA assay
Hycamtin
hydatid
  h. cyst
  h. cyst disease

h. cyst intra-hepatic rupture
h. sand
hydatidiform mole
hydatidocele
hydatidosis
renal h.
Hydergine
Hyde shunt
HydraClense sitz bath
hydralazine
hydramnios
acute h.
hydrargyria, hydrargyrism
hydrated
hydration
intravenous h.
hydraulic capillary infusion system
Hydra Vision IV urology system
hydrazide hepatotoxicity
hydremic ascites
hydrindantin
hydrobromide
hydrocalycosis
hydrocele
abdominoscrotal h.
communicating h.
congenital h.
cord h.
Dupuytren h.
h. feminae
filarial h.
funicular h.
h. muliebris
noncommunicating h.
Nuck h.
postoperative h.
hydrocelectomy
hydrochloretic drug
hydrochloric
h. acid (HCl)
h. acid secretion
h. acid test
hydrochloride
amiloride h.
amitriptyline h.
bethanechol h.
bupivacaine h.

buspirone h.
ciprofloxacin h.
desipramine h.
flavoxate h.
fluoxetine h.
glutamic acid h.
lomefloxacin h.
meperidine h.
oxyphencyclimine h.
papaverine h.
phenazopyridine h.
pramoxine h.
procaine h.
propoxyphene h.
ranitidine h.
thioridazine h.
tolazoline h.
vancomycin h.
yohimbine h.
hydrochlorothiazide
h. and reserpine
h. and spironolactone
h. and triamterene
hydrochlorothiazide-triamterene
(HCTZ-TA)
hydrocholecystis
Hydrocil
hydrocirsocele
hydrocodone
hydrocolpos
hydrocortisone
h. acetate
h. enema
h. foam
hydrodistention
Hydrodiuril
HydroDIURIL
hydrodynamics
collapsible tube h.
distensible h.
Hydroflex
H. penile implant
H. penile prosthesis
H. sphincter
hydroflumethiazide
hydrogen
h. breath test

NOTES

H

hydrogen *(continued)*
h. gas
h. ion
h. peroxide
h. peroxide enema
hydrolysis
intragastric h.
urea h.
Hydromer
H. coated polyurethane stent
H. grafted catheter
hydrometrocolpos
hydromorphone
Hydromox
Hydromox-R
hydronephrosis
bilateral h.
prenatal fetal h.
h. in utero
hydronephrotic
Hydro-Par
hydroperitoneum, hydroperitonia
hydroperoxide
lipid h.
hydrophila
Aeromonas h.
hydrophilic
h. polymer-coated steerable
guidewire
**hydrophilic-coated guidewire (HPC
guidewire)**
hydrophilicity
hydrophobic binding region
hydrophone
Imotec needle h.
needle h.
Hydro Plus
H. P. coated guidewire
H. P. stent
hydropneumoperitoneum
hydropneumothorax
Hydropres
Hydropres-25
Hydropres-50
hydrops
gallbladder h.
hydrorchis
Hydro-Serp
Hydroserpine
hydrostatic
h. balloon
h. balloon catheter
h. balloon dilation

h. decompression
h. pressure
Hydro-T
hydrothorax
cirrhotic h.
hydroureter
hydroureteronephrosis
hydroxide
aluminum h.
ammonium h.
magnesium h.
potassium h. (KOH)
**β-hydroxyacyl-coenzyme A
dehydrogenase**
hydroxyapatite
6-hydroxybenzoate
hydroxyeicosatetraenoic acid (HETE)
hydroxyindoleacetic
5-h. acid
hydroxyl
h. group
h. radical
h. radical scavenger
hydroxylamine
hydroxylated vitamin D
hydroxyl-free radical
hydroxyquinoline
hydroxystilbamidine
5-hydroxytryptamine (5-HT)
hydroxyurea
25-hydroxyvitamin
25-h. D (25-OH-D3)
25-h. D3
25-h. D level
hydroxyzine
hydruria
hydruric
hygiene
perianal h.
Hygroton
Hymenolepis nana
hymenoplasty
hymenotomy
hyointestinalis
Campylobacter h.
Hyoscine-N-Butylbromide
hyoscyamine
h. sulfate
Hyosophen
hypanakinesia, hypanakinesis
Hypaque
H. contrast medium
H. swallow

hyperabduction
hyperacidity
    gastric h.
hyperactive
    h. bowel sounds
    h. rectosigmoid junction
hyperactivity
    detrusor h.
hyperacute
    h. graft-vs-host disease
    h. rejection
hyperal
hyperaldosteronism
hyperalgesia
    colonic h.
    visceral h.
hyperalimentation
    central h.
    intravenous h.
    parenteral h.
    peripheral h.
hyperammonemia
hyperamylasemia
hyperbetalipoproteinemia
    familial h. and
        hyperprebetalipoproteinemia
hyperbilirubinemia
    conjugated h.
    familial unconjugated h.
    idiopathic unconjugated h.
    neonatal conjugated h.
    unconjugated h.
hypercalcemia
hypercalcemic nephropathy
hypercalciuria
hypercaloric diet
hypercarbia
hypercatabolic
hypercatharsis
hypercathartic
hypercellularity
    interstitial h.
    mesangial h.
hyperchloremia
hyperchloremic
    h. metabolic acidosis
hyperchlorhydria

hypercholecystokininemia
hypercholesterolemia
    familial h.
    familial h. with hyperlipemia
hypercholesterolemic cadaveric renal
    transplant
hyperchromatic nucleus
hyperchylia
hyperchylomicronemia
    familial h.
    familial h. with
        hyperprebetalipoproteinemia
hypercoagulability
hypercoagulable state
hypercontractile external sphincter
    response
hyperdense
hyperdiploidy
hyper-dopaminemia
hyperdynamic
    h. circulation
    h. precordium
hyperechoic
    h. shadowing
    h. spot
hyperemesis
    h. gravidarum
hyperemetic
hyperemia
    gastric h.
    splanchnic h.
hyperemic
    h. border zone
    h. mucosa
hyperesthesia
    cutaneous h.
hyperfibrinogenemia
hyperfiltration
    capillary h.
    glomerular h.
    h. injury
    renal h.
hyperfunction
    antral gastrin cell h.
    gastrin cell h.
hyperganglionosis

NOTES

H

hypergastrinemia
  clinical h.
  h. with acid hypersecretion
hyperglobulinemic hepatitis
hyperglycemia
hypergonadotropic hypogonadism
HyperHep
hyperhidrosis
hyperhomocysteinemia
hyperhydrochloria
hyperinfection
hyperinsulinemia
  euglycemic h.
hyperinsulinism
  alimentary h.
hyperkalemia
hyperkeratosis
  esophageal h.
  h. palmaris et plantaris
hyperkinesia
  esophageal h.
hyperkinesis
  paroxysmal anal h.
hyperlipidemia
  carbohydrate-induced h.
  combined fat- and
    carbohydrate-induced h.
  familial fat-induced h.
  idiopathic h.
  mixed h.
hyperlipoproteinemia
  acquired h.
  familial h.
  type I familial h.
  type II familial h.
  type III familial h.
  type IV familial h.
  type V familial h.
hypermagnesemia
hypermetabolic state
hypermobility
  urethral h.
hypernatremia
hypernephroid
hypernephroma
hypernephronia
hyperorchidism
hyperosmolar
  h. liquid
  h. perfusate
hyperosmolarity
  extracellular h.
hyperosmotic feeding

hyperoxaluria
  absorptive h.
  acquired h.
  enteric h.
  idiopathic h.
  primary h.
hyperoxaluric stone
hyperpancreatism
hyperparathyroidism (HPT)
hyperpepsia
hyperpepsinia
hyperpepsinogenemia
hyperperfusion
hyperperistalsis
hyperphagia
  weight loss with h.
hyperphosphatemia
hyperplasia
  adenomatous h. (AH)
  adrenal h.
  antral G-cell h.
  atypical adenomatous h. (AAH)
  benign prostatic h. (BPH)
  bilobar h.
  Brunner gland h.
  colonic nodular lymphoid h.
  congenital adrenal h. (CAH)
  crypt h.
  diffuse nodular h. (DNH)
  ductal epithelial h.
  ECL cell h.
  fibromuscular h.
  focal nodular h. (FNH)
  follicular lymphoid h.
  foveolar h.
  G-cell h.
  goblet cell h.
  incomplete basal cell h.
  intimal h.
  islet cell h.
  lymphoid h.
  lymphoid nodular h.
  median lobe h.
  mesonephric h.
  mesothelial h. (MH)
  neointimal h.
  nodular h.
  nodular lymphoid h. (NLH)
  nodular h. of prostate
  nodular regenerative h. (NRH)
  papillary h.
  parathyroid h.
  polypoid lymphoid h.

post-atrophic h.
prostatic h.
Rokitansky-Aschoff sinus h.
trilobar h.
hyperplasiogenic polyp
hyperplasmic obesity
hyperplastic
  h. adenomatous polyp
  h. epithelial gastric polyp
  h. foveolar epithelium
  h. gastric polyp
  h. nodule
  h. obesity
  h. polyp (HP)
  h. polyposis
hyperplasticity
hyperprebetalipoproteinemia
  familial h.
hyperprochoresis
hyperprolactinemia
hyperproliferation
hyperprotidic diet
hyperpyrexia
hyperreflexia
  detrusor h.
hyperreflexic bladder
hyperresonance
hyperresonant abdomen
hyperresponsiveness
hyperrugosity
hypersalivation
hypersecreting tumor
hypersecretion
  acid h.
  gastric h.
  hypergastrinemia with acid h.
  h. obstruction hypothesis
  salivary h.
hypersensitivity
  cholestatic h.
  para-aminosalicylate h.
  phenindione h.
  h. reaction
hypersplenism
hyperstimulation
hypertension
  accelerated h.

allograft-mediated h.
ductal h.
extrahepatic portal venous h.
glomerular capillary h.
Goldblatt h.
idiopathic portal h. (IPH)
intraglomerular h.
intrahepatic portal h.
lithotripsy-induced h.
noncirrhotic portal h.
pancreatic ductal h.
portal h.
presinusoidal intrahepatic
  portal h.
renal h.
renin-mediated renovascular h.
renovascular h.
salt-sensitive h.
splenoportal h.
systemic h.
hypertensive
  h. autosomal dominant
    polycystic kidney disease
  h. end-organ damage
  h. LES
  h. lower esophageal sphincter
  h. lower esophageal sphincter
    syndrome
  h. nephrosclerosis (HN)
  h. renal injury
hyperthermia
  microwave h.
  transrectal prostatic h. (TPH)
hyperthyroidism
hypertonic
  h. bladder
  h. saline
  h. saline-epinephrine
  h. saline-epinephrine solution
    (HSE)
hypertonicity
hypertriglyceridemia
  familial h.
hypertrophic
  h. cirrhosis
  h. gastritis
  h. gastropathy

NOTES

hypertrophic *(continued)*
   h. lymphocytic gastritis (HLG)
   h. obesity
   h. osteoarthropathy
   h. pyloric stenosis
   h. pylorus
hypertrophy
   benign prostatic h. (BPH)
   bilobar h.
   h. of column of Bertin
   compensatory testicular h.
   glomerular h.
   muscle h.
   prostatic h.
   renal h.
   renovascular h.
   rugal h.
   trilobar h.
hyperuricemia
hyperuricosuria
hypervariable region 1 (HVR1)
hypervolemia
hyphema
hyphemia
   intertropical h., tropical h.
hypoacidity
   luminal h.
hypoactive bowel sounds
hypoalbuminemia
hypobetalipoproteinemia
hypocalcemia
hypocapnia
hypochloremic hypokalemic
   metabolic alkalosis
hypochlorhydria
hypochlorhydric cirrhotic
hypocholia
hypochondria (*pl. of*
   hypochondrium)
hypochondriacal patient
hypochondriac fossa
hypochondriasis
hypochondrium, pl. **hypochondria**
hypochylia
hypocitraturia
hypocomplementemia
hypocystotomy
hypodiploidy
hypoechoic
   h. cancer
   h. lesion
   h. periphery
   h. ringed layer

hypoestrogenic urethritis
hypoestrogenism
hypofibrinogenemia
hypogammaglobulinemia
hypogammaglobulinemic
hypoganglionosis
   h. of colon
hypogastric
   h. artery
   h. region
hypogastrium
hypogastrocele
hypogeusia
hypoglycemia
   postprandial h.
hypogonadal
   h. state
hypogonadism
   hypergonadotropic h.
   hypogonadotropic h.
hypogonadotropic hypogonadism
hypohepatia
hypohydrochloria
hypokalemia
hypokalemic
   h. metabolic alkalosis
   h. nephropathy
   h. renal tubular acidosis
hypolactasia
   adult h.
hypomagnesemia
hypometabolism
hypomethylation
   DNA h.
hyponatremia
   dilutional h.
   thiazide-induced h.
hypopancreatism
hypopancreorrhea
hypoparathyroidism
hypopepsia
hypoperfusion
   renal h.
hypopharyngeal
   h. cancer
   h. diverticulum
hypopharynx
hypophosphatemia
hypophosphatemic rickets
hypophysectomy
hypoplasia
   bile duct h.
   congenital h.

germ cell h.
intrahepatic biliary duct h.
thymic h.
unilateral renal h.
hypoplastic
    h. blind-ending spermatic
      vessels
    h. kidney
hypoproteinemia
hypoproteinosis
hypoprothrombinemia
hypopyon
hyporesponsiveness
    cardiac beta-adrenoreceptor h.
hypospadiac
hypospadias
    balanic h.
    coronal h.
    glandular h.
    penile h.
    penoscrotal h.
    perineal h.
    pseudovaginal perineoscrotal h.
    subcoronal h.
hyposplenism
hyposthenuria
    renal h.
hypotension
    dialysis-associated h.
    systemic h.
hypotestosteronism
hypothalamic-pituitary-adrenal
    (HPA)
hypothalamic-pituitary axis (HPA)
hypothalamic-pituitary-testicular-
    penile axis
hypothalamus
hypothenar eminence
hypothermia
    gastric h.
    renal h.
hypothermic
    h. effect

h. pulsatile perfusion
h. storage
hypothesis
    affinity-avidity h.
    hypersecretion obstruction h.
hypothyroidism
hypotonia
    rectal h.
hypotonic
    h. bladder
    h. duodenography
hypouricemia
hypoventilation
    benzodiazepine-induced h.
    sedation-induced h.
hypovolemia
hypovolemic
    h. anemia
    h. shock
hypoxanthine
hypoxemia
hypoxia
    pericentral h.
hypoxia-induced rhabdomyolysis
Hyrtl sphincter
hysterectomy
hysterical
    h. vomiting
hystericus
    globus h.
hysterocele
hysterocystopexy
hysterosacropexy
    Ivalon sponge h.
    polyvinyl alcohol sponge h.
hysterosalpingectomy
    laparoscopic h.
hysteroscopy
Hytrin
    H. Dosepak

NOTES

H

IA
> intra-arterial

IAS
> internal anal sphincter
> intra-abdominal sepsis

iatrogenic
> i. chymobilia
> i. coagulopathy
> i. colitis
> i. immunodeficiency syndrome
> i. malabsorption
> i. pancreatic trauma
> i. pneumothorax
> i. trauma

IBD
> inflammatory bowel disease

IBS
> inflammatory bowel syndrome
> irritable bowel syndrome

ibuprofen

IBW
> ideal body weight

IC
> intracisternal

ice
> i. cooling
> i. slush
> i. water test

ice-cold buffered picroformaldehyde fixative

iced
> i. lactated Ringer solution
> i. saline lavage

ice-water swallow

ICG
> indocyanine green dye
> ICG test

IC-GN
> immune complex glomerulonephritis

ICL
> intracorporeal laser lithotripsy

ICP
> intrahepatic cholestasis of pregnancy

ICSI
> intracytoplasmic sperm injection

ICT
> isolated cortical tubule

ictal

icteric
> i. sclera
> i. skin

icterogenic

icterohepatitis

icteroid

icterus
> benign familial i.
> conjunctival i.
> i. gravidarum
> i. gravis
> i. melas
> i. neonatorum
> i. praecox
> scleral i.

ictus

ID
> inner diameter

I&D
> incision and drainage

IDA
> iminodiacetic acid

IDD
> intraluminal duodenal diverticulum

IDDM
> insulin-dependent diabetes mellitus

ideal body weight (IBW)

identification
> colonic lesion i.
> lesion i.

idiopathic
> i. achalasia
> i. ascites
> i. autoimmune cholangitis
> i. autoimmune chronic hepatitis
> i. chronic erosion
> i. chronic erosive gastritis
> i. colitis
> i. constipation
> i. crescentic glomerulonephritis
> i. diffuse ulcerative nongranulomatous enteritis
> i. edema
> i. enteropathy
> i. esophageal ulcer (IEU)
> i. fibrosing pancreatitis
> i. fibrous retroperitonitis
> i. gastric acid secretion
> i. gastritis
> i. gastroparesis

idiopathic *(continued)*
- i. gastropathy
- i. hematuria
- i. hemochromatosis
- i. hypereosinophilic syndrome (IHES)
- i. hyperlipidemia
- i. hyperoxaluria
- i. hypertrophic gastropathy
- i. inflammatory bowel disease
- i. intestinal pseudo-obstruction
- i. megacolon
- i. membranous glomerulonephritis
- i. nephrotic syndrome
- i. obstruction
- i. pancreatitis
- i. portal hypertension (IPH)
- i. proctitis
- i. proctocolitis
- i. rapidly progressive glomerulonephritis (IRPGN)
- i. recurrent pancreatitis (IRP)
- i. retroperitoneal fibrosis
- i. steatorrhea
- i. thrombocytopenic purpura
- i. unconjugated hyperbilirubinemia
- i. varices
- i. volvulus

idiotype-anti-idiotype interaction
idioventricular
IDL
  intermediate-density lipoprotein
IDPN
  intradialytic parenteral nutrition
IDST
  intraductal secretin test
IDUS
  intraductal ultrasonography
  intraductal ultrasound
IEBD
  intraesophageal balloon distention
IEL
  intestinal epithelial cell
  intraepithelial leukocyte
  intraepithelial lymphocyte
    IEL T cell
IEM
  ineffective esophageal motility
IEU
  idiopathic esophageal ulcer

IF
  intrinsic factor
IFN-a
  interferon-alfa
IFN-gamma
  interferon-gamma
IFOBT
  immunological fecal occult blood test
ifosfamide
IFP
  inflammatory fibroid polyp
IG
  image guide
    IG bundle
Ig
  immunoglobulin
IgA
  immunoglobulin A
    IgA deficiency
    dimeric IgA
    endomysial IgA
    gliadin IgA
    IgA glomerulonephritis
    IgA immunological study
    jejunal IgA
    IgA neuropathy
    IgA polymerization
    secretory IgA (sIgA)
IgA1
IgA2
IgA-producing cell
IgD
  immunoglobulin D
IgE
  immunoglobulin E
IGF
  insulin-like growth factor
IGF-1
  insulin-like growth factor-1
    exogenous IGF-1
IGF-2
  insulin-like growth factor-2
IGF-binding protein-1 mRNA
IGFBP-1
  insulin-like growth factor-binding protein-1
IGF-1R
  I. mRNA
  I. RNA
IgG
  immunoglobulin G
    IgG anti-HAV-positive

IgG α-gliadin antibody
horseradish peroxidase-
    conjugated anti-rabbit IgG
IgG immunological study
polyclonal IgG
IgG reticulin antibody
IgG1
    immunoglobulin G1
IgG2a
    immunoglobulin G2a
    IgG2a antibody
IgG-producing cell
Iglesias
    I. fiberoptic resectoscope
    I. resectoscope
IgM
    immunoglobulin M
    IgM antibody
    IgM anti-HAV
    IgM anti-HAV antibody
    IgM anti-HBc antibody
    anti-*Helicobacter pylori* IgM
    IgM immunological study
    monoclonal IgM
    IgM nephropathy
IgM-HA antibody
IgM-HEV antibody titer
IHA
    indirect hemagglutination
    intrahepatic atresia
    IHA determination
IHb
    hemoglobin content indices
IHES
    idiopathic hypereosinophilic
    syndrome
Iα-hydroxyvitamin D3
II
    Cytocare Prolase II
    ELISA-II
        enzyme-linked
            immunosorbent assay II
    enzyme-linked immunosorbent
        assay II (ELISA-II)
    Gastrin RIA kit II
    GE RT 3200 Advantage II
    HCV EIA II

membranoproliferative
    glomerulonephritis type II
    (MPGN type II)
MPGN type II
    membranoproliferative
        glomerulonephritis type II
phenol II
UROLAB Janus II
[¹²³I]IMP
    iodoamphetamine
IL
    interleukin
IL-1
    interleukin-1
IL-6
    interleukin-6
    IL-6 receptor
IL-2 receptor
IL-3 receptor
IL-4 receptor
IL-8 receptor
ILA surgical stapler
ileal
    i. biopsy
    i. bladder
    i. blood vessel
    i. conduit
    i. conduit urinary diversion
    i. crypt
    i. duplication cyst
    i. inflow tract
    i. interposition
    i. J-pouch
    i. loop
    i. loopography
    i. neobladder
    i. neobladder urinary pouch
    i. nipple valve
    i. orthotopic bladder substitute
    i. outflow tract
    i. patch ureteroplasty
    i. pouch
    i. pouch-anal anastomosis
        (IPAA)
    i. pouch distal rectal
        anastomosis
    i. pull-through

NOTES

ileal *(continued)*
  i. resection
  i. reservoir
  i. reservoir construction
  i. sleeve
  i. S-pouch
  i. spout
  i. stasis
  i. varix
  i. W-pouch
ileectomy
ileitis
  backwash i.
  Crohn i.
  distal i.
  granulomatous i.
  Meckel i.
  obstructive dysfunctional i.
  pouch i.
  prestomal i.
  regional i.
  terminal i.
ileoanal
  i. anastomosis
  i. endorectal pull-through
  i. pouch
  i. pull-through
  i. pull-through procedure
  i. reservoir
ileoascending colostomy
ileocecal
  i. bladder
  i. continent urinary reservoir
  i. fat pad
  i. intussusception
  i. junction
  i. pouch
  i. region
  i. reservoir
  i. segment
  i. sphincter
  i. syndrome
  i. tuberculosis
  i. ureterosigmoidostomy
  i. valve
ileocecocystoplasty
  i. bladder augmentation
ileocecostomy
ileococcygeus muscle
ileocolectomy
ileocolic
  i. disease
  i. fold

  i. intussusception
  i. plexus
  i. resection
  i. urinary diversion
  i. vessel
ileocolitis
  Crohn i.
  transmural i.
ileocolonic
  i. bladder
  i. Crohn disease
  i. neobladder
  i. pouch
  i. pouch urinary diversion
ileocolonoscopy
ileocolostomy
  end-loop i.
  LeDuc-Camey i.
ileoconduit
ileocystoplasty
  Camey i.
  clam i.
  LeDuc-Camey i.
ileocystostomy
  cutaneous i.
ileoentectropy
ileogastric reflex
ileogastrostomy
ileogram
ileography
  endoscopic retrograde i.
ileoileal intussusception
ileoileostomy
ileojejunitis
ileopexy
ileoproctostomy
ileorectal
  i. anastomosis (IRA)
ileorectostomy
ileorrhaphy
ileoscopy
ileosigmoid
  i. colostomy
  i. fistula
  i. knot
ileosigmoidostomy
ileostogram
ileostomate
ileostomist
ileostomy
  i. bag
  blow-hole i.
  Brooke i.

i. closure
continent i.
Dennis-Brooke i.
i. diarrhea
diversionary i.
diverting loop i.
double-barrel i.
i. effluent
end i.
end-loop i.
Goligher extraperitoneal i.
incontinent i.
J-loop i.
Kock i.
Kock continent i.
Kock reservoir i.
loop i. (LI)
permanent loop i.
pouched i.
i. rod
split i.
i. stoma
temporary loop i.
terminal i.
Turnbull end-loop i.
ileotomy
ileotransverse
  i. colon anastomosis
  i. colostomy
ileotransversostomy
ileoureteric stenosis
ileovesical
  i. anastomosis
  i. fistula
ileo-vesicostomy
  incontinent i.-v.
ileum
  antimesenteric border of
    distal i.
  hose-pipe appearance of
    terminal i.
  neoterminal i.
  i. nipple
  terminal i.
ileus
  adhesive i.
  adynamic i.

colonic i.
dynamic i.
focal i.
gallbladder i.
gallstone i.
gastric i.
mechanical i.
meconium i.
occlusive i.
paralytic i.
postoperative i.
spastic i.
i. subparta
terminal i.
verminous i.
ilia (*pl. of* ilium)
iliac
  i. artery
  i. colon
  i. roll
  i. vein
iliocolotomy
iliohypogastric nerve
ilioinguinal
  i. nerve
  i. ring
iliopectineal line
iliopsoas
  i. ring
  i. sign
  i. test
iliorenal bypass
ilium, pl. **ilia**
illumination system
Ilopan
Ilosone
Ilozyme
ILS
  intraluminal stapler
IMA
  inferior mesenteric artery
image
  i. analysis
  axial i.
  B-mode ultrasound i.
  i. cytometry

NOTES

image *(continued)*
    i. guide (IG)
    i. guide bundle
    longitudinal i.
    point-counting i.
    i. processing
    sagittal i.
    transverse i.
image-processing unit
imager
    Tesla Signa MR i.
imaging
    B-mode i.
    endorectal coil magnetic
      resonance i.
    endoscopic ultrasonographic i.
    gray scale i.
    LaparoScan laparoscopic
      ultrasonic i.
    magnetic resonance i. (MRI)
    nuclear hepatobiliary i.
    planar i.
    radiolabeled i.
    radionuclide renal i.
    sonoelasticity i.
    transcutaneous ultrasound i.
    uni-planar i.
imbalance
    acid base i.
imbibe
imbricate
IMCD
    inner medullary collecting duct
imidazolecarboxamide
imidoacetic acid radioactive agent
imiglucerase
iminodiacetic acid (IDA)
imipenem
imipenem-cilastatin
imipramine
immersion
    i. cooling
    water i.
immitis
    Candida i.
immortalization
Immu-4
immune
    i. complex glomerulonephritis
      (IC-GN)
    i. deficiency
    i. electron microscopy
    i. serum globulin
    i. suppression
    i. system
immune-mediated reaction
immunity
    cell-mediated i.
    cellular i.
    humoral i.
immunization
    parenteral i.
immunoadsorption
immunoassay
    Abbott TDx monoclonal
      fluorescence polarization i.
    enzyme i. (EIA)
    enzyme-linked i. (ELISA)
    hepatitis C virus enzyme i.
      (HCV EIA 20 test)
    Magic Lite
      chemiluminometric i.
    microparticle enzyme i.
      (MEIA)
    second-generation enzyme i.
      (EIA-2)
    TDX fluorescent polarization i.
immunobead-reacting antigen
immunobiology
immunocompetency
immunocompetent
    i. host
immunocompromised
    i. host
immunocytochemical stain
immunocytochemistry
    vacuolar type protein pump i.
immunodeficiency
    acquired i.
    common variable i. (CVI)
    i. disease
    severe combined i. (SCID)
immunodepression
immunodiffusion
    radial i.
immunodominant T cell epitope
immunoelectrophoresis
immunoenhancing
immunofixation electrophoresis
immunofluorescence
    indirect i.
    i. microscopy
    negative i.
immunogen
    enteric i.

I

immunogenic gene
immunoglobulin (Ig)
 i. A (IgA)
 i. A nephropathy
 i. D (IgD)
 i. E (IgE)
 i. G (IgG)
 i. G1 (IgG1)
 i. G2a (IgG2a)
 i. G2a antibody (IgG2a
  antibody)
 i. G clearance
 hepatitis B i. (HBIG)
 i. M (IgM)
 i. neuropathy
 secretory i. A
immunohistochemical
 i. detection
 i. method
 i. stain
 i. staining
immunohistochemistry
 p53 i.
immunohistology
immunologic abnormality
immunological
 A28 i. study
 i. fecal occult blood test
  (IFOBT)
 i. study
immunology
 intestinal i.
immunomodulatory
 i. action
 i. therapy
immunonephelometry
immunoneutralization
immunoperoxidase
 light and electron i.
 i. stain
 i. staining
 i. staining technique
immunopositivity
immunoprecipitation
**immunoproliferative small intestinal
disease (IPSID)**
immunoradiometric assay

**immunoreactive methionine-
enkephalin (IRME)**
immunoreactivity
 cholecystokinin-like i. (CCK-LI)
 PYY-like i.
 vasoactive intestinal
  polypeptide i. (VIP-IR)
immunoscintigraphy
 ^{111}In-CYT-103 i.
immunosorbent
immunostain
immunostaining
 in situ i.
immunosuppressed patient
immunosuppression
 posttransplant i.
immunosuppressive
 i. regimen
 i. therapy
immunotactoid
 i. glomerulonephritis
 i. glomerulopathy (ITGP)
immunotherapy
immunotyping
Imodium
Imodium A-D
Imotec needle hydrophone
Impact
 I. lithotriptor system
impacted
 i. ampullary stone
 i. calculus
 i. cystic duct
 i. feces
 i. stone
 i. stool
impaction
 endoscope i.
 fecal i.
 food bolus i.
 meat i.
 rectal i.
 stone i.
 stone and basket i.
impactor
 electromechanical i. (EMI)
 stone i.

NOTES

impaired
- i. cell differentiation
- i. colonic motor function
- i. gastric absorption
- i. lecithin synthesis
- i. regeneration syndrome (IRS)

impairment
- ethanol-specific i.
- memory i.

impassable ureter

impedance
- i. planimetry
- i. plethysmography (IPG)

imperforate
- i. anus

implant
- Deflux system i.
- Dynaflex penile i.
- i. erosion
- Flexi-Flate penile i.
- gold seed i.
- Hydroflex penile i.
- iridium-192 wire i.
- Jonas i.
- Lifecath peritoneal i.
- malleable i.
- palladium-103 seeds i.
- penile i.
- retropubic i.
- Surgitek Flexi-Flate II penile i.
- testicular i.
- transperineal seed i.
- Zoladex i.

implantable penile venous compression device

implantation
- gastric balloon i.
- intracavitary i.
- i. metastasis
- metastatic i.
- radioactive seed i.
- real-time 3-D biplanar transperineal prostate i.
- ureter i.

impotence
- arteriogenic i.
- diabetic i.
- ejaculatory i.
- psychogenic i.
- vasculogenic i.
- venogenic i.
- venous leak i.

Impra graft

impression
- cardiac i. on the liver
- colic i.
- colon i.
- digastric i.
- duodenal i.
- esophageal i.
- gastric i.
- liver i.
- renal i.
- suprarenal i.

Imuran

IMV
- inferior mesenteric vein

IMX
- I. Hg assay

IMx PSA system

in
- i. situ
- i. situ immunostaining
- i. vitro
- i. vitro fertilization
- i. vitro incubation
- i. vitro synergism
- i. vivo
- i. vivo veritas

Inactin

inadequate
- i. bowel prep
- i. dilation

inadvertent enterotomy

in-and-out catheterization

inanition
- i. fever

Inapsine

inborn error of metabolism

incarcerated
- i. bowel
- i. hernia
- i. omentum
- i. snare

incarceration
- colon i.
- colonoscopy-related i.
- hernia i.
- penile i.

incentive spirometry

incidence
- angle of i.
- gallstone i.

incidental
- i. adenoma

i. appendectomy
i. splenectomy
incipient nephropathy
incision
  Amussat i.
  anterolateral thoracotomy i.
  apron skin i.
  Battle i.
  Bevan abdominal i.
  bilateral i.
  bilateral subcostal i.
  bilateral transabdominal i.
  bucket-handle i.
  buttonhole i.
  celiotomy i.
  Cherney i.
  Chernez i.
  chevron i.
  choledochotomy i.
  circum-umbilical i.
  Connell i.
  cruciate i.
  darting i.
  Deaver i.
  dorsal lumbotomy i.
  i. and drainage (I&D)
  eleventh rib flank i.
  eleventh rib transperitoneal i.
  elliptical i.
  endoscopic i.
  endourological cold-knife i.
  epigastric i.
  extended left subcostal i.
  fish-mouth i.
  flank i.
  Gibson i.
  Gibson-type i.
  gridiron i.
  groin i.
  Heineke-Mikulicz i.
  hockey-stick i.
  infraumbilical i.
  inguinal i.
  inverted-U abdominal i.
  Kammerer-Battle i.
  Kehr i.
  Kocher i.

  LaRoque herniorrhaphy i.
  i. line
  lower abdominal transverse i.
  low transverse i.
  Mallard i.
  McBurney i.
  median i.
  midabdominal transverse i.
  midline i.
  midline lower abdominal i.
  midline upper abdominal i.
  modified Gibson i.
  muscle-splitting i.
  oblique i.
  omega-shaped i.
  paramedian i.
  pararectus i.
  perineal i.
  Pfannenstiel i.
  plaque i.
  posterior transthoracic i.
  precut i.
  relaxing i.
  Rockey-Davis i.
  Schuchardt relaxing i.
  smiling i.
  stab i.
  stepladder i. technique
  steri-stripped i.
  subcostal i.
  subcostal flank i.
  subcostal transperitoneal i.
  surgical i.
  thoracoabdominal i.
  transpubic i.
  transverse i.
  transverse semilunar skin i.
  unilateral subcostal i.
  vertical midline i.
  xiphoid-to-pubis midline
    abdominal i.
  xiphoid-to-umbilicus i.
  Y-shaped i.
incisional
  i. biopsy
  i. corporoplasty
  i. hernia

NOTES

incisor
incisura
  i. angularis
  i. vesicae felleae hepatis
inclusion
  i. body
  concentric hyaline i.
  i. cyst
  glomerular endothelial
    myxovirus-like microtubular i.
  intracytoplasmic tuboreticular i.
    (TRI)
  tubuloreticular i. (TRI)
incompetence
  gastroesophageal i.
  neurogenic sphincteric i.
incompetent
  i. ileocecal valve
  i. sphincter
  i. valve
incomplete
  i. basal cell hyperplasia
  i. cirrhosis
  i. duplication
  i. hernia
  i. passage
  i. polypectomy
  i. relaxation
  i. voiding
incontinence
  anatomic stress i.
  anterior fecal i.
  bladder i.
  bowel i.
  diurnal i.
  double i.
  fecal i.
  genuine stress urinary i.
    (GSUI)
  ischemic fecal i.
  mixed i.
  overflow i.
  overflow fecal i.
  paradoxical i.
  passive i.
  post-prostatectomy i.
  rectal i.
  reflex i.
  Resident Assessment Protocol
    for i.
  secondary i.
  stool i.
  stress i.

  stress urinary i. (SUI)
  type III i.
  type 0 stress urinary i.
  urge i., urgency i.
  urinary i.
  urinary exertional i.
  urinary stress i.
incontinent
  i. epispadias
  i. ileostomy
  i. ileo-vesicostomy
incoordination
  pharyngeal-UES i.
incrustation
  stent i.
incrusted cystitis
incubation
  in vitro i.
Incystene
¹¹¹In-CYT-103 immunoscintigraphy
indapamide
indentation
  haustral i.
independent-t test
Inderal
index, pl. **indices**
  American Urological
    Association symptom i.
  AUA symptom i.
  biliary saturation i.
  body mass i. (BMI)
  Bouchard i.
  Broder i.
  cardiac output/cardiac i.
    (CO/CI)
  CD activity i.
  i. of cell proliferation
  cholesterol saturation i. (CSI)
  creatinine height i. (CHI)
  Crohn disease activity i.
    (CDAI)
  detrusor activity i.
  frequency-duration i. (FDI)
  Gingival i. (GI)
  hepatic iron i. (HII)
  hepatic perfusion i. (HPI)
  histological activity i. (HAI)
  Johnson-DeMeester i.
  Karnofsky i.
  Kruger i.
  Maine Medical Assessment
    Program i. (MMAP index)
  i. of malnutrition

mean shunt i.
mitosis-karyorrhexis i. (MKI)
mitotic i.
MMAP i.
    Maine Medical Assessment
    Program index
nutritional i.
obesity i.
obstruction i.
parietal cell i.
PCNA-labeling i. (PCNA-LI)
penile-brachial i.
portal shunt i. (PSI)
post-thaw sperm motility i.
p_2 penile brachial i.
prognostic nutritional i. (PNI)
PSA i.
pulsatility i.
renal vascular resistance i.
    (RVRI)
saturation i. (SI)
spleen i.
symptom i.
symptom sensitivity i.
symptom severity i. (SSI)
systemic vascular resistance i.
    (SVRI)
thymidine-labeling i.
uroflow i.
Van Hees i.
India
    I. ink
    I. ink tattoo
Indiana
    I. continent reservoir
    I. urinary pouch
Indiana continent reservoir urinary
    diversion
Indian sickness
indication
    primary i.
indicator
    prognostic i.
indices (*pl. of* index)
    hemoglobin content i. (IHb)
    oxygen saturation i. (ISO2)
indifferent electrode

indigenous amebiasis
indigestion
    acid i.
    fat i.
    gastric i.
    nervous i.
indigo
    i. calculus
    i. carmine
    i. carmine dye
    i. carmine stain
indigo-carmine-stained normal saline
indirect
    i. bilirubin
    i. hemagglutination (IHA)
    i. hemagglutination
        determination
    i. hernial sac
    i. immunofluorescence
    i. immunofluorescence assay
    i. inguinal hernia
indium
    i.-III pentetreotide
    i. 64-labeled white blood cell
        scan
    i. leukocyte scan
indium-111 DTPA
[111]indium-labeled autologous
    leukocyte test
Indocin
indocyanine
    i. green
    i. green dye (ICG)
indolalkylamine alkaloid
indole
indolent radiation-induced rectal
    ulcer
indomethacin
indomethacin-induced mucosal
    damage
induced
inducer
    interferon i.
indurated
    i. appendix
induration
industrial toxin

NOTES

indwelling
   i. catheter
   i. stomal device
ineffective
   i. erythropoiesis
   i. esophageal motility (IEM)
inertia
   colonic i.
infant
   i. esophagoscope
   i. reflex
infantile
   i. colic
   i. diarrhea
   i. gastroenteritis
   i. hypertrophic pyloric stenosis
   i. leishmaniasis
   i. nephrotic syndrome
   i. pellagra
   i. polycystic disease (IPCD)
infarct
   Brewer i.'s
   small-bowel i.
   uric acid i.
   Zahn i.
infarcted bowel
infarction
   acute nonocclusive bowel i.
   intestinal i.
   mesenteric i.
   myocardial i.
   nonocclusive i.
   nonocclusive intestinal i.
   occlusive i.
   omental i.
   segmental testicular i.
   small intestinal i.
   total i.
infected
   i. bile duct
   i. necrosis
   i. pseudocyst
   i. tract
infection
   active systemic bacterial i.
   adenovirus i.
   antifungal esophageal i.
   antifungal-resistant
     opportunistic i.
   Aspergillus i.
   bacterial i.
   blood stream i. (BSI)
   i. calculus

candidal i.
catheter tunnel i.
Chlamydia trachomatis i.
CMV i.
   cytomegalovirus infection
coliform urinary i.
Coxsackievirus i.
Coxsackievirus A i.
Coxsackievirus B i.
cryptosporidial i.
cytomegalovirus i. (CMV
   infection)
deep-seated fungal i.
dengue hemorrhagic fever i.
disseminated CMV i.
echovirus i.
enteric i.
Epstein-Barr viral i.
esophageal i.
esophageal fungal i.
exit site i.
extrapulmonary *Pneumocystis
   carinii* i.
fungal i.
gas-forming pyogenic liver i.
helminth i.
hematogenous spread of i.
hepatic candidal i.
hepatitis A i.
hepatitis B i.
hepatitis C i.
hepatitis D i.
hepatitis E i.
herpes i.
herpes simplex i.
HIV i.
intestinal i.
intra-abdominal i.
liver cyst i.
metasynchronous bacterial
   urinary tract i.
monilial i.
multiple hepatitis virus i.
Mycobacterium i.
necrotizing i.
nematode i.
nosocomial i.
nosocomial fungal i.
opportunistic i.
parasitic i.
perianal i.
perineal i.
peristomal i.

peritoneal fungal i.
pneumococcal i.
polymicrobial i.
postsplenectomy i.
renal cyst i.
retrovirus i.
rotavirus i.
synchronous urinary tract i.
torulopsis i.
tunnel i.
urinary tract i. (UTI)
varicella-zoster i.
Vibrio i.
Vibrio fetus i.
viral i.
whipworm i.
wound i.
infectious
  i. colitis
  i. complication
  i. diarrhea
  i. esophagitis
  i. gastroenteritis
  i. hepatitis
  i. jaundice
  i. mononucleosis heterophil
   antibody
  i. splenomegaly
infective splenomegaly
INFeD
Infergen
inferior
  i. mesenteric artery (IMA)
  i. mesenteric vein (IMV)
  i. rectal nerve
  i. rectal vein
  i. vena cava (IVC)
  i. vena cava thrombosis
inferomedial
infertility
  tubal i.
infestation
  Ascaris i.
  biliary i.
  Fasciola hepatica i.
  parasitic i.

infiltrate
  lobular mononuclear cell i.
  MN i.
  mononuclear histiocytic
   portal i.
  PMN i.
  polymorphonuclear
   inflammatory i.
infiltrating adenocarcinoma
infiltration
  bacterial mucosal i.
  cellular i.
  colonic i.
  focal fatty i.
  gastric epithelial cell i.
  glomerular macrophage i.
  glomerular neutrophil i.
  massive malignant i.
  neutrophilic i.
  panmucosal inflammatory
   cell i.
  plasma cell portal i.
  tumor i.
infiltrative
  i. disease
  i. lymphoma
inflamed
  i. appendix
  i. gallbladder
  i. mucosa
inflammation
  cervical i.
  Hara classification of
   gallbladder i.
  interstitial i.
  intralobular i.
  i. marker
  microbiliary i.
  portal eosinophilic i.
  portal tract i.
  traumatic i.
  vaginal i.
inflammatory
  i. bowel disease (IBD)
  i. bowel syndrome (IBS)
  i. colitis
  i. diarrhea

NOTES

inflammatory *(continued)*
   i. fibroid polyp (IFP)
   i. glomerulopathy
   i. polyp
   i. pseudotumor
   i. renal mass
inflammatory bowel syndrome (IBS)
inflatable penile prosthesis (IPP)
inflator
   LeVeen i.
influenza
   i. virus
influenzae
   Haemophilus i.
influx
   Rb i.
infold
infolding
   complex papillary i.
infracolic compartment
infradiaphragmatic
infragastric
   i. pancreoscopy
infrahepatic
   i. vena cava
inframammary region
infraorbital
infrapatellar bursa
infrared
   i. coagulation
   i. coagulator
   i. photocoagulation (IRC)
   i. spectroscopy
   i. transillumination gastroscopy
infrarenal
   i. template procedure
infraumbilical
   i. incision
   i. mound
infravesical
   i. prostatic obstruction
infrequent defecation
infundibular
infundibulopelvic stenosis
infundibulum
   i. of bile duct
   caliceal i.
   i. of gallbladder
Infusaid
   I. chemotherapy implantable pump
   I. hepatic pump

infusion
   circadian-shaped i.
   insulin/glucagon i.
   intra-arterial vasopressin i.
   intravariceal i.
   intravenous urea i.
   intravenous vasopressin i.
   lipid i.
   mono-octanoin i.
   pentagastrin i.
   i. pump
   solvent i.
   vasopressin i.
ingested
   i. foreign body
   i. foreign object
ingestion
   acid i.
   alkali i.
   battery i.
   button battery i.
   caustic i.
   cocaine package i.
   fish bone i.
   foreign body i.
   lye i.
   mercuric oxide battery i.
   razor blade i.
   safety pin i.
ingrowth
   mesodermal i.
inguinal
   i. adenopathy
   i. bulge
   i. canal
   i. crease
   i. floor
   i. fold
   i. hernia
   i. incision
   i. ligament
   i. lymphadenopathy
   i. reservoir inserter
   i. ring
   i. sphincter
   i. triangle
inguinale
   granuloma i.
   hernia uteri i.
inguinalis
   hernia uteri i.
inguinofemoral hernia
inguinoperitoneal

inguinoscrotal
  i. hernia
inguinosuperficial hernia
inhalation
  i. aerosol
inhaler
  Allis i.
  Vanceril i.
inheritance
  kallikrein i.
inhibin
inhibition
  antisense DNA i.
  i. assay
  bladder i.
  cyclooxygenase i.
  glycolytic i.
  laminin receptor i.
inhibitor
  ACE i.
  alpha-glucosidase i.
  5-alpha-reductase i.
  angiotensin-converting
    enzyme i. (ACEI)
  azasteroid i.
  carbonic anhydrase i. (CAI)
  C-1 esterase i.
  chain-terminating i.
  collagen synthesis i.
  cyclooxygenase i.
  cytolysis i.
  gastric acid pump i.
  hepatocyte proliferation i.
    (HPI)
  H+,K+-ATPase acid pump i.
  monoamine oxidase i.
  nitric oxide synthase i.
  plasminogen activator i. (PAI)
  protease i.
  proton pump i. (PPI)
  rectoanal i.
  serum alpha₁-protease i.
  trypsin i.
  type-1 plasminogen activator i.
    (PAI-1)

  type-2 plasminogen activator i.
    (PAI-2)
  urinary trypsin i.
inhibitor-1
  plasminogen activator i.
inhibitory
  i. postsynaptic potential (IPSP)
  i. syndrome
INH isoniazid
initial hematuria
InjecAid system
injectable
  Macroplastique i.
injection
  collagen i.
  cyanocobalamin i.
  depot i.
  diazepam emulsified i.
  endoscopic i.
  endoscopic India ink i.
  ethanol i.
  intracytoplasmic sperm i.
    (ICSI)
  intralesional i.
  intralesional steroid i.
  intraperitoneal i.
  intravariceal i.
  lipiodol i.
  local depot i.
  moxisylyte i.
  papaverine i.
  paravariceal i.
  percutaneous ethanol i. (PEI)
  PGE1 i.
  polidocanol i.
  polytetrafluorethylene paste i.
  sclerosant i.
  i. sclerosis
  i. sclerotherapy
  sham i.
  i. site
  sodium morrhuate i.
  sodium tetradecyl i.
  somatropin i.
  submucosal Teflon i.

I

NOTES

injection *(continued)*
  tangential colonic
    submucosal i.
  i. therapy
injector
  Olympus i.
  Teflon i.
  Virag i.
injury
  acid i.
  Ajmalin liver i.
  alkaline i.
  antecedent pancreatic i.
  blast i.
  cell-mediated hepatic i.
  closed i.
  drug-induced acute hepatic i.
  duodenal i.
  gastric mucosal i.
  gastroduodenal mucosal i.
  glomerular i.
  Helicobacter-induced gastric i.
  hemorrhagic radiation i.
  hepatic vein i.
  H2O2-induced i.
  hyperfiltration i.
  hypertensive renal i.
  intestinal radiation i.
  ischemia-reperfusion i.
  juxtahepatic venous i.
  liver transplantation
    preservation i.
  medication-induced i.
  mucosal i.
  obstetric i.
  open i.
  oxidant i.
  oxidative cell i.
  pancreatic i.
  paraquat-induced upper
    gastrointestinal i.
  pill-induced esophageal i.
  pinch i.
  rectal i.
  renal vascular i.
  reperfusion i.
  spinal cord i. (SCI)
  splenic i.
  stress-related mucosal i.
  tubular epithelial cell i.
  tubular morphologic i.
  tubulointerstitial i.

  ureteral i.
  vascular i.
ink
  autoclaved India i.
  Higgins India i.
  India i.
  Koh-I-Noor Universal India i.
  osmolarity of the i.
  Pelikan brand India i.
  solution-diluted India i.
inlay
  Turner-Warwick i.
inlet
  esophageal i.
  i. patch mucosa
  i. port
  thoracic i.
in-line blood gas monitor
Inmed whistle tip urethral catheter
inner
  i. crossbar
  i. diameter (ID)
  i. medullary collecting duct
    (IMCD)
innervation
  cholinergic i.
  intrinsic excitatory i.
  striated muscle i.
innocent gallstone
innocuous
innominate
Innova home incontinence therapy
  system
inoculated medium
inoculum size
inorganic iodine
iNOS
  nitric oxide synthase
inositol
  i. ring
  i. triphosphate
  i. 1,4,5-triphosphate (IP3)
insemination
  intrauterine i. (IUI)
  subzonal i. (SUZI)
insert
  Hollister Convex i.
  Nu-Hope Convex i.
  Reliance urinary control i.
  United Surgical Convex i.
inserter
  Furlow cylinder i.
  inguinal reservoir i.

insertion
 biliary endoprosthesis i.
 flatus tube i.
 jejunal tube i.
 J-tube i.
 PEG i.
 Sengstaken-Blakemore tube i.
 i. tube
insipidus
 congenital nephrogenic
  diabetes i. (CNDI)
 diabetes i.
in-situ end labelling (ISEL)
inspiration
inspiratory
inspissated
 i. bile
 i. bile syndrome
 i. feces
 i. sump syndrome
instability
 detrusor i. (DI)
instant
 i. camera
 i. photography
instillation therapy
institutional colon
instrument
 Bard Biopty i.
 Bard BladderScan bladder
  volume i.
 biopsy i.
 BIP biopsy i.
 i. count
 CRIT-LINE i.
 DaVinci handle i.
 Dilamezinsert i.
 Duette double lumen ERCP i.
 endosonography i.
 GIA i.
 guide-eye i.
 mechanical radial-scanning i.
 oblique-forward-viewing i.
 ProLine endoscopic i.
 Quinton suction biopsy i.
 Roboprep G i.
 Sharpoint cutting i.

 slotted i.
 small-diameter
  endosonographic i.
 spring loaded type biopsy i.
 TA i.
 XQ video i.
instrumentation
 biliary i.
 Karl Storz i.
 Microvasive i.
instrument-tract seeding
insufficiency
 exocrine i.
 exocrine pancreatic i. (EPI)
 hepatic i.
 progressive renal i.
 pyloric i.
 renal i.
 vascular i.
insufflation
 air i.
 helium i.
 i. of stomach
insufflator
 carbon dioxide i.
 nitrous oxide i.
 nitrous oxide/carbon dioxide i.
insular structure
insulated
 i. curved scissors
 i. straight scissors
insulin
 human i.
 Lente i.
 NPH i.
 protamine zinc i.
 i. reaction
 i. resistance
 Semilente i.
 Ultralente i.
insulin-dependent
 i.-d. diabetes
 i.-d. diabetes mellitus (IDDM)
insulin/glucagon
 i. infusion
 putative hepatotrophic factors i.

NOTES

insulin-like
> i.-l. growth factor (IGF)
> i.-l. growth factor-1 (IGF-1)
> i.-l. growth factor-2 (IGF-2)
> i.-l. growth factor-binding
>   protein-1 (IGFBP-1)

insulinoma
insulin-transferrin-sodium selenite
insulin-treated diabetic
insult
> ischemic i.

intact
> i. hormone assay
> i. proprioception
> i. PTH

intake
> caloric i.
> clandestine i.
> daily protein i. (DPI)
> dietary energy i.
> i. and output (I&O)

Intal
integrated automatic stone-tissue detection system
integrating spherical power meter
integrin
> membrane-spanning i.

integrins
> α3β1 i.
> α5β1 i.
> B1 i.
> B2 i.
> beta-1 chain i.

intensified radiographic imaging system (IRIS)
intensity
> fluorescent light i. (FLI)

intention
> delayed primary i.
> healing by primary i.
> healing by secondary i.

interaction
> cell-cell i.
> crystal-phospholipid i.
> idiotype-anti-idiotype i.
> vasoactive peptide-cytokine i.

intercalated cell
intercellular space
interceptive conditioning
Interceptor M3 triple-channel, solid state monitor
inter-colonoscopy
interconversion

intercostal
> i. scan
> i. space

intercourse
> receptal anal i.

interdialytic
interdigestive
> i. antroduodenal motility
> i. migrating motor complex
> i. myoelectric complex

interdigitating teeth
inter-endoscopist
interesophageal variceal pressure (IOVP)
interface
> fluid-air i.

interference barrier filter
interferon
> i. alfa-2a
> i. alfa-2b
> i. alfa-2b, recombinant
> i. alfa-n1
> i. alfa-n3
> i. alpha
> alpha i.
> beta i.
> i. beta
> i. beta-2
> i. beta-1a
> i. beta-1b
> consensus i.
> gamma i.
> i. gamma
> i. gamma-1a
> i. gamma-1b
> i. inducer
> recombinant human alpha i.
> i. therapy
> i. treatment

interferon-α
> lymphoblastoid i.-α

α$_{2a}$-interferon
interferon-β
interferon-alfa (IFN-a)
> i.-a. 2β
> recombinant i.-a. (rIFN-a)

interferon-gamma (IFN-gamma)
> basal i.-g.
> HLA class II-restricted i.-g.
> nucleocapsid antigen-stimulated i.-g.
> i.-g. stimulation

interferon type I

Intergroup Rhabdomyosarcoma
Study (IRS)
interhaustral
   i. fold
   i. septum
interleukin (IL)
interleukin-1 (IL-1)
   i. receptor antagonist
interleukin-2
   serum i.
interleukin-6 (IL-6)
   serum i.
interleukin-8
interleukin-2 receptor-blocking
  agent
inter-liver competition
interlobar artery
interlobular bile duct
interlocking ligature
interloop abscess
intermediate
   i. biomarker
   i. junction
   i. mesenteric lymph node
   thiol i.
intermediate-density lipoprotein
  (IDL)
intermesenteric abscess
intermittent
   i. catheterization
   i. click
   i. diarrhea
   i. drip feeding
   i. obstruction
   i. pain
   i. positive pressure breathing
   (IPPB)
   i. pulse
   i. self-obturation
   i. suctioning
interna
   elastica i.
   lamina rara i. (LRI)
internal
   i. abdominal ring
   i. anal sphincter (IAS)
   i. biliary lavage

   i. fiberoptic cable
   i. hemorrhage
   i. hemorrhoid
   i. iliac artery
   i. inguinal ring
   i. oblique
   i. oblique fascia
   i. procidentia
   i. pudendal artery
   i. pudendal vein
   i. rectal sphincter
   i. ribosome entry site (IRES)
   i. rotation
   i. sphincter
   i. sphincterotomy
   i. urethrotomy
international
   I. Association for Enterostomal
   Therapy
   I. Biomedical Mode 745-100
   microcapillary infusion system
   I. Prognostic Index score
   I. Prostate Symptom Score
   (IPSS)
   i. units per liter (IU/L)
internuclear ophthalmoplegia
interosseous
interpersonal sensitivity
interphase PBMC
interposition
   colonic i.
   i. Dacron graft
   ileal i.
interrupted suture
intersex
   i. condition
   i. gonad
intersphincteric
   i. anal fistula
   i. anorectal space
   i. perirectal abscess
   i. space
interstitial
   i. brachytherapy
   i. cell
   i. cells of Cajal
   i. cell tumor of testis

NOTES

interstitial *(continued)*
 i. cystitis
 i. diffusion
 i. fibroblast
 i. fibrosis
 i. gastritis
 i. hernia
 i. hypercellularity
 i. inflammation
 i. irradiation
 i. mononuclear cell
 i. nephritis
 i. pancreatitis
 i. photodynamic therapy
 i. rejection
interstitium
 medullary i.
 renal i.
inter-symphyseal
 i.-s. bar
 i.-s. stitch
intertriginous
 i. region
intertrigo
intertropical hyphemia
interureteric ridge
interval appendectomy
intervention
 angiographic i.
interventricular defect
intestinal
 i. anastomosis
 i. angina
 i. anthrax
 i. atony
 i. atresia
 i. bacterium
 i. bag
 i. calculus
 i. capillariasis
 i. clamp
 i. colic
 i. contents
 i. decompression
 i. diverticulum
 i. endoscopy
 i. epithelial cell (IEL)
 i. fistula
 i. fixation
 i. flora
 i. hemorrhage
 i. histoplasmosis
 i. immunology

 i. infarction
 i. infection
 i. intoxication
 i. intussusception
 i. ischemia
 i. juice
 i. lamina propria
 i. lipodystrophy
 i. loop
 i. lumen
 i. lymphangiectasia
 i. metaplasia
 i. motility disorder
 i. mucosa
 i. myiasis
 i. necrosis
 i. obstruction
 i. parasite
 i. peptide
 i. perforation
 i. perfusion
 i. permeability
 i. permeability measurement
 i. polyposis
 i. prolapse
 i. pseudo-obstruction
 i. radiation injury
 i. schistosomiasis
 i. sling
 i. sling placement
 i. spirochete
 i. stasis
 i. steatorrhea
 i. stricture
 i. surgery
 i. tract
 i. tuberculosis
 i. ureteral replacement
 i. ureter replacement
 i. viability
 i. villous architecture
 i. villus
 i. volvulus
 i. web
intestinalis
 Giardia i.
 pneumatosis i.
 pneumatosis cystoides i. (PCI)
 Septata i.
intestine
 bacterial metabolism in i.'s
 Crohn small i.
 kink in i.

malrotation of i.
milking of i.
small i.
intestinofugal neuron
intimal
i. fibroplasia
i. hyperplasia
intolerance
fatty food i.
fructose i.
glucose i.
hereditary fructose i.
lactose i.
intoxication
intestinal i.
quinidine i.
systemic mercury i.
intra-abdominal
i.-a. abscess
i.-a. adhesion
i.-a. bile leakage
i.-a. desmoid tumor
i.-a. hemorrhage
i.-a. ileal reservoir
i.-a. infection
i.-a. mass
i.-a. pressure
i.-a. pressure gauge
i.-a. sepsis (IAS)
i.-a. transverse testicular
ectopia
i.-a. viscus
intra-anal
i.-a. electromyography
i.-a. pressure
i.-a. wart
intra-arterial (IA)
i.-a. chemotherapy catheter
i.-a. digital subtraction
angiography
i.-a. vasopressin infusion
intra-assay precision
intracapillary thrombosis
intracapsular dissection
intracavernosal injection treatment

intracavernous
i. injection therapy
i. therapy
intracavitary
i. implantation
i. radiation boost therapy
intracellular
i. acidity
i. acification
i. flush effect
i. pH
intracellulare
Mycobacterium i.
intracholedochal
i. manometric catheter
i. pressure
i. stent
intracisternal (IC)
intracolonic Kaposi sarcoma
intracorporeal
i. injection therapy
i. laser lithotripsy (ICL)
i. needle breakage
i. shock wave lithotripsy
intracranial pressure monitoring
intractable
i. constipation
i. diarrhea
i. ulcer
i. ulcerative colitis
i. vomiting
intracuticular suture
intracystic epithelial proliferation
intracytoplasmic
i. calcium
i. CMV inclusion body
i. mucin
i. sperm injection (ICSI)
i. tuboreticular inclusion (TRI)
intradermal
i. suture
i. tattooing technique
intradialytic
i. parenteral nutrition (IDPN)
i. symptom
Intradop intraoperative Doppler

NOTES

Intraducer
  I. peritoneal cannula
  I. peritoneal catheter
intraductal
  i. cholangioscopy
  i. imaging catheter
  i. lithiasis
  i. mucin-producing tumor
  i. pressure
  i. secretin test (IDST)
  i. ultrasonography (IDUS)
  i. ultrasound (IDUS)
  i. ultrasound probe
intraduodenal
intraepiploic hernia
intraepithelial
  i. body
  i. cancer
  i. leukocyte (IEL)
  i. lymphocyte (IEL)
  i. lymphocytosis
intraesophageal
  i. acid test
  i. balloon distention (IEBD)
  i. peristaltic pressure
  i. pH monitoring (EpHM)
  i. pH test
  i. stent
intrafamilial clustering of
  Helicobacter pylori
intragastric
  i. acidity
  i. balloon
  i. bubble
  i. continuous pH-meter meter
  i. EGF
  i. gallstone
  i. hydrolysis
  i. pH
  i. pH mapping
  i. pH monitor record
  i. pressure
intraglandular fluid
intraglomerular
  i. hemodynamics
  i. hypertension
  i. pressure
intragraft
intrahaustral contraction ring
intrahepatic
  i. abscess
  i. antigen-dependent
    lymphocyte-hepatocyte

  i. artery-systemic shunt
  i. ascariasis
  i. atresia (IHA)
  i. AV fistula
  i. bile duct
  i. biliary cystic dilation
  i. biliary duct
  i. biliary duct hypoplasia
  i. biliary stricture
  i. cholelithiasis
  i. cholestasis
  i. cholestasis of pregnancy
    (ICP)
  i. duct
  i. ductal dilation
  i. hematoma
  i. hepatitis
  i. invasion
  i. lymphocyte
  i. portal hypertension
  i. portal obstruction
  i. radicle
  i. sclerosing cholangitis
  i. shunt
  i. spontaneous arterioportal
    fistula
  i. stone
intrailiac hernia
intralesional
  i. injection
  i. steroid injection
  i. treatment
intralipid fat emulsion
intralobar
intralobular
  i. fibrosis
  i. inflammation
intraluminal
  i. clot
  i. cyst
  i. duodenal diverticulum (IDD)
  i. esophageal pressure
  i. filling defect
  i. pH-pressure relationship
  i. pouch
  i. pressure
  i. probe
  i. proliferation
  i. radiotherapy
  i. reference electrode
  i. Silastic esophageal stent
  i. stapler (ILS)

i. stone
i. urethral pressure
intramesenteric abscess
intramucosal
    i. cancer
    i. carcinoma
    i. metastasis
intramural
    i. air dissection
    i. atheromatous disease
    i. colonic air
    i. diverticulum
    i. fistulous tract
    i. ganglia
    i. hematoma
    i. intestinal hemorrhage
    i. lesion
    i. secretory reflex
    i. ureter
intramuscular
intranuclear CMV inclusion body
intraoperative
    i. autologous transfusion
    i. biliary endoscopy
    i. cavernous nerve stimulation
    i. cholangiogram
    i. electron beam radiotherapy
    i. endoscopy
    i. enteroscopy
    i. mortality
    i. penile erection
    i. phlebography
    i. transfusion
    i. ultrasonography and
      angiography
intrapancreatic
    i. bile duct
    i. nerve
intrapapillary terminus
intraparavariceal procedure
intraparenchymal tumor
intrapelvic filling defect
intraperitoneal (IP)
    i. abscess
    i. adhesion
    i. air
    i. cavity

i. chemotherapy
i. hemorrhage
i. hyperthermic perfusion
    (IPHP)
i. injection
i. perforation
i. viscus
i. viscus rupture
i. volume
intraportally
intraprostatic
    i. spiral
    i. stent
intrapulmonary shunting
intrarectal ultrasonography
intrarenal
    i. chemolysis
    i. collecting system
    i. hemodynamics
    i. matrix-degrading enzyme
      cascade
    i. reflux
IntraSonix TULIP laser device
intrathecal chemotherapy
intrathoracic
    i. esophagogastroscopy
    i. esophagogastrostomy
    i. Nissen fundoplication
    i. stomach
intratubular germ cell neoplasia
(ITGCN)
intratumoral
    i. heterogeneity
intraurethral
    i. coil
    i. pressure
    i. swab specimen
intrauterine insemination (IUI)
intravaginal
    i. electrical stimulation
    i. torsion
intravariceal
    i. ethanolamine oleate
    i. infusion
    i. injection
    i. pressure
    i. sclerotherapy

NOTES

intravasation
intravascular
    i. lipolysis
    i. thrombosis
    i. volume expansion
intravenous (IV)
    i. albumin
    i. cholangiogram (IVC)
    i. cholangiography (IVC)
    i. drip
    i. drug abuse
    i. feeding
    i. heme-albumin
    i. hydration
    i. hyperalimentation
    i. immune globulin (IVIg)
    i. lipid emulsion
    i. nitroglycerin
    i. pyelogram (IVP)
    i. secretin test
    i. urea infusion
    i. urogram (IVU)
    i. urography
    i. vasopressin infusion
intravesical
    i. alum irrigation
    i. anastomosis
    i. chemotherapy
    i. migration
    i. pressure
    i. ureterolysis
intrinsic
    i. enzymatic activity
    i. excitatory innervation
    i. factor (IF)
    i. factor secretion
    finger i.
    i. reflex
    i. sphincter deficiency (ISD)
    i. sphincter dysfunction (ISD)
    i. striated muscle of the
      urethra
    i. striated sphincter
introducer
    Atkinson i.
    Dumon-Gilliard prosthesis i.
    entrapment sack i.
    Hickman percutaneous i.
    Key-Med Nottingham i.
    Nottingham semirigid i.
    pull-apart i.
    semirigid Nottingham i.
    i. set

    split sheath i.
    Wilson-Cook prosthesis i.
introitus
    i. oesophagi
INTROL bladder neck support
   prosthesis
intromission
Intron-A
Intropin
intruducer gun
intubate
intubated ureterotomy
intubation
    catheter-guided endoscopic i.
      (CAGEIN)
    endotracheal i.
    esophageal i.
    esophagogastric i.
    i. failure
    nasal i.
    nasogastric i.
    nasotracheal i.
    oral i.
    orotracheal i.
    pyloric i.
    terminal ileum i. (TII)
intussuscepted ileal triple nipple
intussusception
    appendiceal i.
    bowel i.
    cecocolic i.
    colocolic i.
    ileocecal i.
    ileocolic i.
    ileoileal i.
    intestinal i.
    jejunogastric i.
    jejuno-jejuno-colic i.
    retrograde i.
    triple i.
intussuscipiens
inulin
    i. clearance
    plasma i.
    i. solution
Inutest test
invaginated membrane
invaginating ampulla of Vater
invagination
    i. of the ampulla
    stomal i.
    stump i.
    i. technique

invasion
>   capillary-lymphatic i.
>   dermatolymphatic i.
>   intrahepatic i.
>   neural i.
>   periportal i.
>   vascular i.
>   venous i.

invasive
>   i. adenocarcinoma
>   i. carcinoma
>   i. colorectal polyp
>   i. diagnostic test
>   i. enteric pathogen

invermination
Inversine
inversion appendectomy
inversus
>   abdominal situs i.
>   situs i.

inverted
>   i. papilloma
>   i. sigmoid diverticulum
>   i. testis
>   i.-U pouch
>   i.-V peritoneotomy
>   i.-V sign

inverted-U abdominal incision
inverting suture
investigation
>   Lapides cystometric i.

involuntary
>   i. guarding
>   i. reflex rigidity

involvement
>   tubercular i.

I&O
>   intake and output

iocetamic
>   i. acid
>   i. acid contrast medium

iodide
>   isopropamide i.
>   Lugol i.
>   propidium i.

iodinated contrast agent

iodine
>   i. dye
>   i. hippurate scanning
>   inorganic i.
>   i. scan

iodine-123 iodoamphetamine
iodine-125
iodine-131
>   radioactive i.

iodipamide
>   i. meglumine
>   i. meglumine contrast medium
>   sodium i.

iodism
iodoamphetamine ([^{123}I]IMP)
>   iodine-123 i.
>   [^{123}I]i. radionuclide

iodochlorhydroxyquin
iodoform gauze
Iodohippurate
iodophor
Iodopyracet
iodoquinol
Iodothalamate
>   Tc DTPA, I125 I.

iohexol
ion
>   i. beam-assisted deposition
>   i. chromatography
>   hydrogen i.
>   i. laser

Ionamin
ionizing radiation
ionomycin
ionophore
ion-sensitive field effect transistor
ion-specific electrode
iontophoresis
iopamidol
iopanoic
>   i. acid
>   i. acid contrast medium

iopdate
iopromide
IOT29, clone K20 monoclonal antibody

NOTES

iothalamate
  i. clearance
  ^{125}I i. clearance
  i. level
  sodium i.
125-iothalamate
iotroxate
  meglumine i.
IOVP
  interesophageal variceal pressure
IP
  intraperitoneal
IP3
  inositol 1,4,5-triphosphate
IPAA
  ileal pouch-anal anastomosis
IPCD
  infantile polycystic disease
ipecac
  i. abuse
  i. syrup
ipecac-induced
  i.-i. cardiotoxicity
  i.-i. myopathy
  i.-i. vomiting
IPG
  impedance plethysmography
IPH
  idiopathic portal hypertension
IPHP
  intraperitoneal hyperthermic
  perfusion
ipodate contrast medium
IPP
  inflatable penile prosthesis
IPPB
  intermittent positive pressure
  breathing
ipratropium
iproniazid-induced jaundice
IPSID
  immunoproliferative small intestinal
  disease
ipsilateral adrenalectomy
IPSP
  inhibitory postsynaptic potential
IPSS
  International Prostate Symptom
  Score
IRA
  ileorectal anastomosis
IRC
  infrared photocoagulation

IRES
  internal ribosome entry site
iridectomy
  i. scar
iridium
  i.-192-loaded stent
  i.-192 wire implant
  i. prosthesis
  i. ribbon
  i. seed
IRIS
  intensified radiographic imaging
  system
iritis
IRME
  immunoreactive methionine-
  enkephalin
iron
  i. deficiency
  i. deficiency anemia
  i. dextran
  oral i.
  i. overload disorder
  i. poisoning
  i. storage disease
iron-dependent oxidant
IRP
  idiopathic recurrent pancreatitis
IRPGN
  idiopathic rapidly progressive
  glomerulonephritis
irradiate
irradiated
  i. patient
  i. tumor vaccine
irradiation
  i. effect
  external-beam i.
  i. failure
  half-body i.
  interstitial i.
  Nd:YAG laser i.
  total body i. (TBI)
  ultraviolet i.
irreducible hernia
irregular
  i. amputated mucosal pattern
  i. pupil
  i. rhythm
irregularity
  cervical i.
irretrievable object

irrigating
    i. fluid
    i. patient
irrigation
    acetohydroxamic acid i.
    i. of colostomy
    continuous bladder i. (CBI)
    copious i.
    hemiacidrin i.
    H-600 normothermic i.
    intravesical alum i.
    pulsed i.
    rectal pulsed i.
    rectum i.
    Renacidin i.
    whole-gut i.
irrigation-suction
    postoperative i.-s.
irrigator/aspirator
    Nezhat-Dorsey i.
irritable
    i. bladder
    i. bowel syndrome (IBS)
    i. colon
    i. colon syndrome
    i. gut syndrome
    i. stricture
    i. testis
irritative
    i. diarrhea
    i. symptom
IRS
    impaired regeneration syndrome
    Intergroup Rhabdomyosarcoma
      Study
^{192}Ir wire
ischemia
    AVF-induced renal i.
    colonic i.
    intestinal i.
    mesenteric i.
    mucosal i.
    myocardial i.
    i. necrosis
    tubular i.
    visceral i.
ischemia-reperfusion injury

ischemic
    i. bowel
    i. bowel disease
    i. colitis
    i. fecal incontinence
    i. hepatitis
    i. insult
    i. tubular cell death
    i. tubular damage
ischial tuberosity
ischiorectal
    i. anorectal space
    i. fossa plane
    i. perirectal abscess
    i. space
ischochymia
ISD
    intrinsic sphincter deficiency
    intrinsic sphincter dysfunction
ISEL
    in-situ end labelling
isethionate
    pentamidine i.
island
    i. flap procedure
    lipid i.
    mucosal i.
    i. pedicle flap
islet
    i. amyloid polypeptide
    i. cell
    i. cell adenoma
    i. cell antibody
    i. cell carcinoma
    i. cell hyperplasia
    i. cell of Langerhans
    i. cell tumor
Ismelin
Is-5-Mn
    isosorbide-5-mononitrate
ISO2
    oxygen saturation indices
isoamyl alcohol
Isocal
    I. HCN
    I. HCN liquid feeding
isocarboxazid

isodose contour
isoechoic
isoenzyme
    Regan i.
isoflurane
isoform
    growth factor i.
isoiodide
isolate
isolated
    i. cortical tubule (ICT)
    i. generator
    i. granulomatous gastritis
    i. hepatocyte perfusion
    i. renal mucormycosis
    i. retained antrum syndrome
isoleucine
    peptide histidine i. (PHI)
isomannide
isomerase
    glucose-6-phosphate i.
isometric
    i. force
    i. tubular vacuolization
Isomil
    I. SF
    I. SF formula
isomotic lavage
isoniazid
    INH i.
isoniazid-induced hepatitis
iso-osmolar liquid
isopentane
isoperistaltic
    i. ileal reservoir
isoprenaline
isoprenologue
isopropamide
    i. iodide
isoproterenol
Isoptin
Isordil
isosorbide
    i. dinitrate
isosorbide-5-mononitrate (Is-5-Mn)
Isospora belli
isosporan parasite
isosporiasis
Isotein HN
Isotein HN feeding
isoterm
    Langmuir adsorption i.

isothiocyanate
    fluorescein i. (FITC)
isotonic
    i. contraction
    i. feeding
    i. saline
isotope
    i. meal
    i. renal scan
    i. renography
    i. study
    ^{99m}Tc-MAG-3 i.
    technetium-99m
      mercaptoacetythiglycine i.
isotopic scan
isotropic
    i. probe 2818
    i. scan
isovaleric
    i. acid
    i. acidemia
Isovue
isoxsuprine
I-Soyalac formula
ispaghula husk
isradipine
Israel retractor
Isuprel
ITGCN
    intratubular germ cell neoplasia
ITGP
    immunotactoid glomerulopathy
Itis
    bundle of I.
Ito
    I. cell
    I. cell sarcoma
itraconazole
^{125}I-Tyr1-somatostatin
IUI
    intrauterine insemination
IU/L
    international units per liter
IV
    intravenous
    IV fluids
    IV fluid therapy
    Pepcid I.V.
Ivac Needleless IV System
Ivalon
    I. sponge
    I. sponge hysterosacropexy

I. sponge rectopexy
I. sponge-wrap operation
IVC
    inferior vena cava
    intravenous cholangiogram
    intravenous cholangiography
Ivemark syndrome
IVIg
    intravenous immune globulin

Ivor
    I. Lewis esophagogastrectomy
    I. Lewis two-stage subtotal
        esophagectomy
IVP
    intravenous pyelogram
IVU
    intravenous urogram

NOTES

J

J chain
J versus S versus W pelvic
ileal pouch
J wire
Jaboulay
J. gastroduodenostomy
J. pyloroplasty
Jaboulay-Doyen-Winkleman
J.-D.-W. operation
J.-D.-W. technique
jackknife position
Jackson
J. esophageal bougie
J. esophagoscope
J. membrane
J. staging system
J. veil
Jackson-Pratt
J.-P. catheter
J.-P. drain
Jacobson needle holder
Jacobs-Palmer laparoscope
Jacoby test
Jadassohn syndrome
Jaffe picrate reaction
Jamaican
J. vomiting sickness
J. vomiting syndrome
Jamshidi
J. liver biopsy needle
J. needle
Janeway gastroscope
Jansen retractor
Janus System III
Japanese
J. cancer classification
J. classification of cancer
J. dysentery
J. schistosomiasis
Jarit rotator
Jarvis
J. hemorrhoid clamp
J. hemorrhoid forceps
J. pile clamp
Jasbee esophagoscope
Jatrox *Helicobacter pylori* **test**
jaundice
acholuric j.
benign postoperative j.

black j.
Budd j.
catarrhal j.
cholestatic j.
chronic idiopathic j.
cloxacillin-induced cholestatic j.
familial chronic idiopathic j.
familial nonhemolytic j.
hemolytic j.
hepatocellular j.
hepatogenous j.
homologous serum j.
infectious j.
iproniazid-induced j.
leptospiral j.
malignant j.
malignant obstructive j.
mechanical j.
neonatal j.
newborn j.
nonhemolytic j.
nonobstructive j.
obstructive j.
painless j.
parenchymal j.
physiologic j.
regurgitation j.
retention j.
shrapnel-induced obstructive j.
ticrynafen-induced j.
jaundiced
j. skin
Javorski test
Jaworski body
jaw wiring
J/cm
joules per centimeter
Jeffrey introducer set
jejunal
j. bypass
j. crest
j. feeding tube
j. IgA
j. interposition of Henle loop
j. limb
j. loop
j. pouch
j. syndrome
j. tube insertion

jejunal *(continued)*
  j. ulcer
  j. villus
jejunectomy
jejuni
  Campylobacter j.
jejunitis
  nongranulomatous j.
jejunocolic fistula
jejunocolostomy
jejunogastric intussusception
jejunoileal
  j. atresia
  j. bypass (JIB)
  j. bypass surgery
  j. shunt
jejunoileitis
  nongranulomatous ulcerative j.
jejunoileostomy
  Roux-en-Y distal j.
jejuno-jejuno-colic intussusception
jejunojejunostomy
jejunoplasty
jejunostomy
  j. elemental diet feeding
  endoscopic j.
  loop j.
  needle-catheter j.
  percutaneous endoscopic j.
  (PEJ)
  j. tract choledochoscopy
  j. tube
  j. tube feeding
  Witzel j.
jejunotomy
jejunum
  Roux-en-Y loop of j.
Jelco catheter
jelly
  electrode j.
  lidocaine hydrochloride j.
  LubraSeptic j.
  Snap-It lubricating j.
  spermicidal j.
  Xylocaine j.
JEM-100B and 100S electron microscope
Jenamicin
Jenckel cholecystoduodenostomy
Jenning-Streifeneder gastroscope
JEOL
  J. 100 CX electron microscope

J. JSM 35 CF scanning
  electron microscope
jerk
  absent ankle j.
  ankle j.
Jesberg esophagoscope
jet
  j. nebulizer
  j. stream phenomenon
Jetco-spray
jet-like bleeding
Jevity isotonic liquid nutrition
jeweler's forceps
Jewett sound
Jewett-Whitmore Cancer Staging System
JFB III endoscope
J-hooking
J-hook tip laparoscopic electrode
JIB
  jejunoileal bypass
J-loop ileostomy
J-Maxx stent
Jobert de Lamballe suture
Job syndrome
Joe hoe
Johne disease
Johns
  J. Hopkins gallbladder forceps
  J. Hopkins gallbladder retractor
  J. Hopkins prostate cancer
    grading system
Johnson
  J. esophagogastroscopy
  J. esophagogastrostomy
Johnson-DeMeester index
Johnston
  J. buttonhole procedure
  J. procedure
joint erythema
Jolles test
Jonas
  J. implant
  J. penile prosthesis
Jones
  J. and Boadi-Boatang method
  J. stain
Jones-Politano technique
Joseph hook
Joubert syndrome
joule
joules per centimeter (J/cm)

Joyce-Loebl Magiscan image
　analysis system
J-pexy
　　omental J.-p.
J-pouch
　　colonic J.-p.
J-scope esophagoscope
J-shaped
　　J.-s. endoscope
　　J.-s. ileal pouch
　　J.-s. ileal pouch-anal
　　　anastomosis
　　J.-s. reservoir
J-tube
　　J.-t. insertion
　　wire-guided J.-t.
J turn of the scope
J-type maneuver
Judd-Allis intestinal forceps
Judd cystoscope
Judd-DeMartel gallbladder forceps
jugular
juice
　　acid-peptic j.
　　duodenal j.
　　gastric j.
　　intestinal j.
　　pancreatic j.
　　pure pancreatic j. (PPJ)
Julian
　　J. cystoresectoscope
　　J. splenorenal forceps
jumbo
　　j. biopsy
　　j. biopsy forceps
junction
　　anorectal j.
　　cardioesophageal j. (CE)
　　cardioesophageal mucosal j.
　　choledochopancreatic ductal j.
　　cystic-choledochal j.
　　cysticohepatic j.
　　desmosomal j.
　　duodenojejunal j.
　　esophagogastric j.
　　fundic-antral j.

gap j.
gastroesophageal j.
hepatico-cystic j.
hyperactive rectosigmoid j.
ileocecal j.
intermediate j.
mucosal j.
NS3/NS4 j.
NS4/NS5 j.
pancreaticobiliary j.
pancreaticobiliary ductal j.
pancreaticocholedochoductal j.
patulous gastroesophageal j.
penopubic j.
penoscrotal j.
pharyngoesophageal j.
prostatovesical j.
pyloroduodenal j.
rectosigmoid j.
saphenofemoral j.
squamocolumnar mucosal j.
tracheoesophageal j.
ureteropelvic j. (UPJ)
junctional cyst
juvenile
　　j. cirrhosis
　　j. polyp
　　j. polyposis
　　j. polyposis coli
　　j. retention polyp
juxta-anal colostomy
juxtacapillary process
juxtaglomerular
　　j. apparatus
　　j. apparatus tumor
juxtahepatic venous injury
juxtamedullary arteriole
juxtapapillary duodenal diverticulum
juxtaposed mesenteric lymph node
juxtapyloric ulcer
J-Vac
　　J.-V. closed wound drainage
　　J.-V. drain
　　J.-V. suction reservoir
J-wave phenomenon
J-wire guide

J

NOTES

321

K2
   vitamin K.
K-141
   Dianeal K.
K+
   Ca2+-activated K.
K562 erythroid line
kabure
Kader gastrostomy
kala azar
Kaleorid
Kalk esophagoscope
kallidin
kallikrein
   k. inheritance
   k.-like gene
   plasma k.
   tissue k.
Kallmann syndrome
Kammerer-Battle incision
Kanagawa phenomenon
Kangaroo
   K. 324 feeding pump
   K. gastrostomy tube
Kantor sign
Kanulase
kanyemba
Kaodene
kaolin
Kaopectate
Kaplan-Meier
   K.-M. analysis
   K.-M. curves
   K.-M. method
Kaposi sarcoma (KS)
kappa light chain
Kapsinow test
Karaya
   K. gum
   K. 5 paste
   K. powder
   K. ring ileostomy appliance
   K. 5 seal
Karl
   K. Storz endoscope
   K. Storz instrumentation
   K. Storz-Lutzeyer lithotriptor
Karmen unit
Karnofsky
   K. index

   K. performance status
   K. performance status scale
   K. score
karyometry
Kasai
   K. operation
   K. portoenterostomy
   K. procedure
Kasai-type hepatoportoenterostomy
Kashiwado test
Kaslow intestinal tube
Kasof
Kasugai
   chronic pancreatitis K.
   K. classification
Katayama
   K. disease
   K. syndrome
Kato test
Kawasaki syndrome
Kayexalate
   K. enema
Kayser-Fleischer ring
KBR
   ketone body ratio
KCl
   potassium chloride
127 Kda protein
Kearns-Sayre syndrome (KSS)
Keeler
   K. Magnalite headlamp
   K. panoramic loupe
Keen Edge disposable biopsy
   forceps
Keflex
Keftab
Kefzol
Kegel pelvic muscle exercise
Kehr
   K. incision
   K. sign
Keith needle
Kelami classification
Keller hydrodynamic hypothesis of
   sieving
Kelling
   K. gastroscope
   K. test
Kelling-Madlener procedure

K

Kelly
- K. abdominal retractor
- K. clamp
- K. cystoscope
- K. fistula scissors
- K. forceps
- K. hemostat
- K. operation
- K. plication
- K. rectal speculum
- K. retractor

Kelly-Kennedy modification

Kelman
- K. air cystotome
- K. cystotome
- K. double-bladed cystotome
- K. knife-cannula cystotome
- K. knife cystotome

keloid
Kelsey pile clamp
Kemadrin
Keofeed feeding tube
keratin
- antibody to k.

keratinization
- single cell k.

keratinocyte
keratosis, pl. **keratoses**
- k. follicularis
- lace-like k.

Kerckring
- K. fold
- valves of K.

kerion formation
Kerlix
- K. wrap

kernicterus
Kernig sign
Kessler-Kleinert suture
keto
- k. acid
- k. acid-amino acid supplement

ketoacidosis
- diabetic k.

ketoconazole
ketogenesis
ketoglutaramate (KGM)
ketoglutarate (KG)
- k. dehydrogenase (KGDH)

ketone
- k. body
- k. body ratio (KBR)

ketoprofen
- k. analgesic therapy

ketorolac tromethamine
ketosteroid
ketotifen
keyhole
- k. deformity
- k. limpet hemocyanin (KLH)

Key-Med
- K.-M. advanced dilator
- K.-M. Atkinson endoprosthesis
- K.-M. Nottingham introducer

KeyMed
- K. automatic reprocessor
- K. disposable variceal injection needle
- K. heater probe thermocoagulation
- K. unit

Keystone technique
KG
- ketoglutarate
- α-KG

KGDH
- ketoglutarate dehydrogenase
- α-KGDH

KGM
- ketoglutaramate
- α-KGM

Khafagy modified ileocecal cystoplasty urinary diversion
KHB
- Krebs-Henseleit bicarbonate buffer

Kidd cystoscope
kidney
- k. allograft
- artificial k.
- Ask-Upmark k.
- cadaver k.
- k. carbuncle
- k. clearance
- k. cortice
- decapsulation of k.
- k. disease
- Dow Hollow Fiber k. (DHFK)
- dysplastic k.
- ectopic k.
- k. failure
- k. function
- horseshoe k.
- hypoplastic k.
- living donor k.
- medullary sponge k.

multicystic k. (MCK)
multicystic dysplastic k.
multilobar k.
murine k.
k. pedicle clamp
solitary k.
k. sparing operation
k. stone
thoracic k.
k. transplant
k. transplantation
k. weight (KW)
k. worm
kidney, ureter, bladder radiography (KUB radiography)
Kiernan space
killer
natural k. (NK)
k. T cell
Killian
K. dehiscence
K. rectal speculum
K. suction tube
kinase
myosin light-chain k.
pyruvate k.
tyrosine protein k.
3-kinase
PI -k.
Kinberg test
Kinesed
kinetic
bromodeoxyuridine cell k.'s
capacity-limited k.'s
first-order k.'s
k. gallbladder study
gastric cell k.'s
Gompertzian tumor k.'s
Michaelis-Menten k.'s
k. parameter
urea k.'s
Kinevac
King
5-15 K. Armstrong unit
K. technique
kinins

kink
k. in bowel
k. in intestine
Kinkiang fever
kinking
Kinnier Wilson disease
Ki-ras gene
Kirchner diverticulum
Kirschner abdominal retractor
Kirsten-ras
K.-r. oncogene
K.-r. oncogen mutation
"kissing" prostatic lobes
kissing ulcer
kit
Abbott HCV EIA 2nd
generation k.
Abbott HCV 2.0 test k.
Bard-Stiegmann-Goff variceal
ligation k.
BIO101MERmaid k.
Boehringer k.
Carey-Coons biliary
endoprosthesis k.
DNA labeling k.
EIA k.
Flexiflo k.
Flexiflo Inverta-PEG
gastrostomy k.
Flexiflo Lap-J laparoscopic
jejunostomy k.
Flexiflo over-the-guidewire
gastrostomy k.
Gene Clean II k.
Hashizume endoscopic
ligator k.
Histofine SAB k.
Hybritech Tandem-R assay k.
Mallinckrodt ultra tag
labeling k.
MERmaid k.
Moss G-tube PEG k.
Moss PEG k.
Nichols IRMA k.
OctreoScan k.
Ott/Mayo Channel Sampling k.
Percufix catheter cuff k.

K

NOTES

kit *(continued)*
  Predicta TGF-β1 k.
  propHiler urinary pH testing k.
  Pros-Check k.
  Pulse-Pak infusion k.
  Pyloritek test k.
  Random Primed DNA
    Labeling k.
  Russell gastrostomy k.
  Sacks-Vine gastrostomy k.
  Serodia (β HIV, β HTLV-1)
    commercial k.
  Steigmann-Goff endoscopic
    ligator k.
  StoneRisk diagnostic
    monitoring k.
  Tandem-R assay k.
  Uri-Kit culture k.
  Uri-Three culture k.
  Versa-PEG gastrostomy k.
  Vesica percutaneous bladder
    neck suspension k.
  Wilson-Cook feeding tube k.
Kitano knot
Kiton red dye
Klatskin
  K. biopsy needle
  K. liver biopsy needle
  K. tumor
Klebanoff
  K. common duct sound
  K. gallstone scoop
Klebsiella
  K. oxytoca
  K. pneumoniae
Kleinert
  K. pants
  K. Safe and Dry panty and
    pad system
Kleinschmidt appendectomy clamp
Klemm sign
Klemperer disease
Kleppinger forceps
KLH
  keyhole limpet hemocyanin
Klinefelter syndrome
Kling dressing
Klonopin
Km
  Michaelis constant
knee-chest position

knee-elbow position
knife, pl. **knives**
  Bard-Parker k.
  k. blade
  cautery k.
  cold k.
  Collin k.
  Collings electrosurgery k.
  Desmarres paracentesis k.
  electrocautery k.
  k. electrode
  electrosurgical cutting k.
  endarterectomy k.
  hernia k.
  hook k.
  Hulbert electrosurgical k.
  Lempert paracentesis k.
  Mori k.
  needle k.
  optical laser k.
  optical urethrotome k.
  Orandi k.
  skin k.
  urethrotome k.
knife-like pain
knob
  lateral deflection control k.
knobby process
knock
  pericardial k.
Knodell score
Knok ileal reservoir
knot
  curved-needle surgeon's k.
  externally releasable k.
  friction k.
  granny k.
  half-hitch k.
  ileosigmoid k.
  Kitano k.
  laparoscopic k.
  one-handed k.
  Roeder loop k.
  self-tightening slip k.
  surgeon's k.
  Tim k.
knot pusher
  Clarke-Reich k. p.
  Gazayerli k. p.
knotting
  stochastic k.
knuckle of colon

Kocher
  K. anastomosis
  K. clamp
  K. forceps
  K. gallbladder retractor
  K. hemostat
  K. incision
  K. maneuver
  K. procedure
  K. pylorectomy
  K. ulcer
  K. ureterosigmoidostomy
    procedure
Koch pouch
Kock
  K. continent ileostomy
  K. ileostomy
  K. nipple
  K. pouch cutaneous urinary
    diversion
  K. reservoir ileostomy
  K. technique
  K. urinary pouch
Kockogram
Kodak Ektachem 700 machine
Kodsi scale
Koenig, König
  K. syndrome
Koerte gallstone forceps
KOH
  potassium hydroxide
  KOH smear
Koh-I-Noor Universal India ink
Köhlmeier-Degos disease
koilocytosis
Kolantyl
Kollmann dilator
König (*var. of* Koenig)
Konigsberg
  K. catheter
  K. 5-channel solid-state
    catheter assembly
  K. microtransducer
Konsyl-D
Koplik spot
Korean hemorrhagic fever
Koro syndrome

Korsakoff syndrome
Kossa stain
K-Phos
  K.-P. Neutral
K-ras
  K.-r. gene
  K.-r. oncogene
Kraske
  K. operation
  K. parasacral approach
  K. position
Krause arm rest
Krazy Glue sclerosant
krebiozen false cancer cure
Krebs
  K. cycle
  K. solution
Krebs-Henseleit bicarbonate buffer
  (KHB)
Krebs-Ringer
  K.-R. bicarbonate buffer
  K.-R. solution
Kreha
  polysaccharide K. (PSK)
Krentz gastroscope
Kretz
  K. Combison 330 ultrasound
    scanner
  K. 311 ultrasound scanner
  K. ultrasound system
Kringle domain
Krokiewicz test
Kron
  K. bile duct dilator
  K. gall duct dilator
Krönlein hernia
Kropp
  K. cystourethroplasty
  K. operation
  K. procedure
Kruger index
Krukenberg tumor
krusei
  Candida k.
Kruskal-Wallis test
krypton laser

K

NOTES

KS
Kaposi sarcoma
KSS
Kearns-Sayre syndrome
KTP
K. 532 laser
K. laser probe
KTP 532
Laserscope K.
Kt/V urea
KUB radiography
Kulchitsky cell
Kumpe catheter
Kunkel syndrome

Kupffer
K. cell
K. cell sarcoma
Kussmaul endoscope
Ku-Zyme HP
KW
kidney weight
kwashiorkor
Kwell
Kyasanur Forest disease
kymography
balloon k.
kyphoscoliosis
kyphosis

LA
  lupus anticoagulant
LAAL
  lower anterior axillary line
Labbe triangle
labelling
  in-situ end l. (ISEL)
labetalol
labia
  l. major muscle
  l. minor muscle
labialis
  herpes l.
labial ulceration
lace-like keratosis
laceration
  concurrent hepatic l.
  longitudinal l.
  lower pole l.
  rectal l.
  vascular l.
lacrimal duct probe
Lactaid
β-lactam antibiotic
lactase
  l. deficiency
  l. enzyme
lactate
  l. dehydrogenase (LDH)
  Ringer l.
lactated Ringer solution
lacteal vessel
lactic
  l. acid
  l. acid dehydrogenase (LDH)
  l. acidosis
lactilol
Lactinex
lactobacilli preparation
Lactobacillus
  L. acidophilus
  L. bifidus
  L. bulgaricus
  L. casei
lactobezoar
lactobionate
  erythromycin l.
lactoferrin
lacto-N-fucopentaose
  sialylated l.-N.-f.

lactose
  l. breath hydrogen test
  l. hydrogen breath testing
    (LHBT)
  l. intolerance
  l. malabsorption (LMA)
  l. maldigestors
  l. tolerance test
lactose-associated diarrhea
lactose-free
  l.-f. diet
  l.-f. feeding
Lactrase
lactulose
  l. enema
  l. hydrogen breath test
lactulose-mannitol ratio
lacuna magna
Ladd
  L. band
  L. operation
  L. procedure
  L. syndrome
laddering
  DNA l.
Laënnec cirrhosis
Lafora body
lag phase
Lahey
  L. gall duct forceps
  L. liver transplant bag
Laidley double-catheterizing
  cystoscope
Laird-McMahon anorectoplasty
LAK cell
  lymphokine-activated killer cell
lake
  bile l.
Lalonde hook forceps
LAMA
  laser-assisted microanastomosis
L-AmB
  liposomal-amphotericin B
lamblia
  Giardia l.
lambliasis
lamina
  l. densa
  l. muscularis mucosa
  l. propria

L

lamina *(continued)*
l. propria lymphoid cell
l. rara externa (LRE)
l. rara interna (LRI)
laminectomy
laminin
l. receptor
l. receptor inhibition
lamp
Desmoreaux l.
slit l.
Wood l.
xenon l.
lanceolatus
lancet-shaped biopsy forceps
lancinating pain
Landau
L. reflex
L. trocar
landmarks
bony l.
Lane
L. band
L. disease
L. intestinal clamp
L. intestinal forceps
L. operation
Langerhans
L. cell
islet cell of L.
L. lineage
Lange skin-fold calipers
Langhans
L. cell
L. line
Langmuir adsorption isoterm
Lanoxin
lansoprazole
Lanza scale
Lanz point
LAP
leucine aminopeptidase
LAP test
lap
laparotomy
laparator
Weck high flow l.
laparectomy
laparocele
Laparofan
laparogastroscopy
Laparolift system
LaparoLith

laparorrhaphy
LaparoSAC
LaparoScan laparoscopic ultrasonic
imaging
laparoscope
50-degree Foroblique optic l.
0-degree forward optic l.
10-degree operating l.
diagnostic l.
EL2-LS2 flexible video l.
flexible video l. (FVL)
Jacobs-Palmer l.
operative l.
laparoscopic
l. Allis clamp
l. biopsy
l. cannula
l. cholecystectomy (LC)
l. clip application
l. colectomy
l. colposuspension technique
l. dismembered pyeloplasty
l. grasper
l. hysterosalpingectomy
l. knot
l. lymphocelectomy
l. needle colposuspension
l. needle driver
l. nephrectomy
l. orchiopexy
l. pelvic lymphadenectomy
l. pelvic lymph node
dissection (LPLND)
l. photography
l. retraction system
l. retropubic colposuspension
l. seromyotomy
l. tie clip
l. trocar sleeve
l. ultrasound (LUS)
l. ureteral reanastomosis
l. ureterolithotomy
l. uterolysis
l. vagotomy
l. varicocelectomy
l. varicocele repair
l. varix ligation
laparoscopically guided transcystic
exploration
laparoscopic-assisted hemicolectomy
laparoscopist
laparoscopy
double-puncture l.

flexible l.
gasless l.
gynecologic l.
single-puncture l.
therapeutic l.
laparoscopy-guided subhepatic cholecystostomy
laparotomy (lap)
emergency l.
exploratory l.
negative l.
l. pack
l. pad
l. pad cover
second-look l.
l. sponge
l. tape
Lapides
L. cystometric investigation
L. test
Lapides-Ball urethropexy
Laplace
L. forceps
L. law
LapSac
Lapwall laparotomy sponge
large
l. bowel
l. bowel carcinoma
l.-channel therapeutic duodenoscope
l. common duct stone
l. needle size
l. volume paracentesis (LVP)
large-bore
l.-b. biliary endoprosthesis
l.-b. cannula
l.-b. catheter
l.-b. gastric lavage tube
l.-b. rigid esophagoscope
l.-b. Tygon tubing
large-bowel obstruction
large-diameter bougie
large-droplet fatty liver
large-particle biopsy
L-arginine

lari
Campylobacter l.
Larodopa
LaRoque herniorrhaphy incision
Larry rectal probe
larva migrans
visceral l. m.
laryngeal
l. carcinoma
l. edema
l. vestibule
laryngopharyngectomy
laryngoscope
Olympus ENF-P-series l.
laryngoscopy
direct l.
laryngospasm
larynx
LAS
lymphadenopathy syndrome
laser
l. ablation
ADD'Stat l.
alexandrite l.
argon ion l.
argon-pumped dye l.
Candela Model MDL 2000 l.
Candela 405-nm pulsed dye l.
carbon dioxide l.
L. CHRP rigid fiber scope system
CO_2 l.
Coherent Model 90-K l.
coumarin dye l.
coumarin-flash-lamp pumped pulsed dye l.
l. disk
l. Doppler flowmeter
dye l.
endoscopic l.
endoscopic pulsed dye l.
helium-neon l.
l. hemorrhoidectomy
l. hemorrhoid excision
holmium:YAG l.
ion l.
krypton l.

NOTES

L

331

laser *(continued)*
KTP 532 l.
l. laparoscopic vagotomy
Lateralase l.
Lithognost flash-lamp pulsed
  dye l.
l. lithotripsy
l. lithotriptor
l. lithotriptor basket
LX-20 l.
medical l.
Medilas fiberTome l.
l. microscope
Myriadlase Side-Fire l.
Nd:YAG l.
  neodymium:yttrium garnet
    laser
neodymium:yttrium garnet l.
  (Nd:YAG laser)
l. partial nephrectomy
l. photoablation
l. photocoagulation
l. photodestruction
l. plume
Prolase II lateral firing
  Nd:YAG l.
pulsed dye neodymium:YAG l.
Pulsolith l.
pumped-dye l.
Q-switched alexandrite l.
Q-switched Nd:YAG l.
rhodamine l.
l. sclerosis
Side-Fire l.
SLT contact MTRL l.
l. surgery
l. temperature
l. therapy
l. thermocoagulation
l. tissue weld
l. tissue welding
l. tissue welding solder
tunable pulsed dye l.
Ultraline l.
ultrasound-guided l.
Urolase l.
l. vaporization
VersaPulse Select l.
visual endoscopically
  controlled l.
l. welding
l. welding technique

l. writer
YAG l.
**laser-assisted microanastomosis
  (LAMA)**
laser-Doppler Periflux PF-3 probe
laser-induced
  l.-i. fragmentation
  l.-i. intracorporeal shock wave
    lithotripsy (LISL)
LaserMed laser pointer
Laserscope
  L. KTP 532
  L. YAG 1064
Lasersonic ACMI Ultraline
lasertripsy
Lasertripter
  Candela MDA-200 L.
Lasix
L-asparaginase
Lassa hemorrhagic fever
lasso snare
last-generation serologic ELISA test
lata
  Diphyllobothrium l.
lata (*pl. of* latum)
Latarjet
  nerve of L.
late
  l. dumping
  l. dumping syndrome
  l. graft dysfunction
latency
  pudendal nerve terminal
    motor l.
late-onset
  l.-o. ataxia
  l.-o. hepatic failure
lateral
  l. bending technique
  l. decubitus
  l. decubitus position
  l. deflection control knob
  l. gutter
  l. internal pelvic reservoir
  l. lithotomy
  l. oblique fascia
  l. pancreaticojejunostomy
  l. reflection of colon
  l. ventral hernia
  l. window technique
Lateralase laser
lateralizing sensory deficit
lateral-lateral pouch

latex
  l. allergy
  l. fixation test
  l. hood
  l. sclerosant
latum, pl. lata
  condyloma l.
Latzko partial colpocleisis
Laubry-Soulle syndrome
Laugier hernia
Laurence-Moon-Bardet-Biedl
  syndrome
Laurence-Moon-Biedl syndrome
Lauren gastric carcinoma
  classification
lavage
  abdominal l.
  l. bowel preparation
  colonic l.
  l. cytology
  Easi-Lav l.
  external biliary l.
  gastric l.
  gastrointestinal l.
  HeatProbe l.
  iced saline l.
  internal biliary l.
  isomotic l.
  nasogastric l.
  norepinephrine l.
  oral l.
  PEG l.
  peritoneal l.
  polyethylene glycol-based l.
  rapid colonic l.
  l. solution
  stomach l.
  l. and suction
lavage-induced
  l.-i. cardiac asystole
  l.-i. pill malabsorption
law
  Courvoisier l.
  Laplace l.
  Poiseuille l.
  Poiseuille-Hagen l.

  Tait l.
  Weigert-Meyer l.
Laws
  L. gastroplasty
  L. gastroplasty with Silastic
    collar-reinforced stoma
laxative
  l. abuse
  anthracene-type l.
  bulk l.
  emollient l.
  Fleet Phospho-Soda buffered
    saline l.
  osmotic l.
  sodium phosphate-based l.
    (NaP)
  stimulant l.
LaxCaps
  Phillips L.
laxity
  ligamentous l.
layer
  echo-poor l.
  fascial l.
  glycosaminoglycans l.
  hypoechoic ringed l.
  seromuscular l.
  subcutaneous l.
  submucosal vaginal smooth
    musculofascial l.
  subserosal l.
laying-open fistulotomy
Lazarus-Nelson technique
LB 9501 luminometer
LBM
  lean body mass
LC
  laparoscopic cholecystectomy
  liver cirrhosis
LCA
  lithocholic acid
  liver cell adenoma
LCA-DCA ratio
L cell
LCG
  liquid chemical germicide

L

NOTES

LCHAD
    long-chain 3-hydroxyacyl coenzyme
    A dehydrogenase
L-citrulline
lck protein
LCT
    long-chain triglyceride
LDH
    lactate dehydrogenase
    lactic acid dehydrogenase
    LDH enzyme
    LDH isoenzyme 5
    LDH level of ascitic fluid
    LDH test
LDL
    low-density lipoprotein
LDL-C
    low-density lipoprotein cholesterol
LDS stapler
LE
    L. cell
Le
    L. Bag
    L. Bag ileocolonic pouch
    L. Bag pouch reservoir
    L. Bag urinary diversion
    L. Bag urinary pouch
    L. Fort sound
Lea
    disialosyl L.
    monosialosyl L.
Leach technique
lead
    l. citrate
    l. citrate stain
    l. colic
    l. poisoning
Leadbetter
    L. cystourethroplasty
    L. modification technique
    L. procedure
    L. tunneling technique
Leadbetter-Politano reimplantation
lead-pipe colon
leaf-like villus
leak
    l. point pressure (LPP)
    l. pressure
leakage
    anastomotic l.
    biliary l.
    l. bypass cable
    cavernovenous l.

    crural venous l.
    cystic duct l.
    intra-abdominal bile l.
    postmicturition continuous l.
    postoperative biliary l.
    tube l.
lean body mass (LBM)
leather-bottle stomach
leaves
    l. of diaphragm
    l. of mesentery
Leber amaurosis
lecimibide
lecithin
    polyunsaturated l.
lecithin-cholesterol acyltransferase
lectin
    hepatic l.
    l. reactivity
    l. staining
lecturescope
LeDuc-Camey
    L.-C. ileocolostomy
    L.-C. ileocystoplasty
LeDuc technique
leech
    mechanical l.
left
    l. colon
    l. colonic flexure
    l. decubitus position
    l. gutter
    l. hepatic duct
    l. hepatic vein (LHV)
    l. lateral decubitus position
    l. lobe
    l. lower quadrant (LLQ)
    l. upper quadrant (LUQ)
left-sided
    l.-s. clonus
    l.-s. colitis
left-to-right subtotal pancreatectomy
Legionella pneumophila
Leigh disease
Leiner disease
leiomyoblastoma
leiomyoma, pl. leiomyomata
    duodenal l.
    epithelioid l.
    esophageal l.
    gastric l.
leiomyosarcoma
    gastric l.

hepatic l.
    small intestine l.
leiomyosarcomatoid differentiation
Leishmania
    L. donovani
    L. esophagitis
leishmanial enteritis
leishmaniasis, leishmaniosis
    infantile l.
    visceral l.
Lell esophagoscope
Lembert
    L. inverting seromuscular
    suture
    L. suture
Lempert paracentesis knife
Lendrum stain
length
    functional profile l.
    peripheral capillary filtration
    slit l.
    total slit pore l.
Lennhoff sign
lens
    120-degree l.
    30-degree l.
    70-degree l.
    Foroblique l.
    Hopkins II rod l.
    narrow l.
    objective l.
    right-angle l.
Lente insulin
lentum
    Eubacterium l.
Leo test
Lepley-Ernst tube
leprae
    Mycobacterium l.
leptospiral jaundice
leptospirosis
LES
    lower esophageal sphincter
    hypertensive LES
    LES pressure
Lesch-Nyhan syndrome
Lescol

Leser-Trelal
    sign of L.-T.
Leser-Trelat sign
Lesgaft
    L. hernia
    L. space
    L. triangle
lesion
    acetowhite l.
    acute gastric mucosal l.
    anal l.
    angiodysplastic l.
    aphthous-type l.
    apple-core l.
    bilobed polypoid l.
    bleeding l.
    bull's eye l.
    cauda equina l.
    colonic l.
    colonic vascular l.
    cutaneous l.
    Dieulafoy l.
    Dieulafoy-like l.
    duodenal l.
    dye sham intrarenal l.
    ectatic vascular l.
    extramural l.
    fingertip l.
    flat depressed l.
    flat elevated l.
    florid duct l.
    Forest (I, II) l.
    gastric l.
    gastrointestinal l.
    glomerular tip l. (GTL)
    gunpowder l.
    hamartomatous l.
    hepatic mass l.
    high neurological l.
    hypoechoic l.
    l. identification
    intramural l.
    localized l.
    lower motor neuron l.
    lumbar spinal cord l.
    macroscopic l.
    Mallory-Weiss l.

L

NOTES

lesion *(continued)*
  mesenteric vascular l.
  metastatic l.
  minute l.
  minute polypoid l.
  mucosal l.
  mulberry l.
  napkin-ring annular l.
  neoplastic l.
  nodular l.
  nonerosive gastric mucosal l.
  non-neoplastic l.
  ocular l.
  pancreatic l.
  papillary l.
  penile l.
  perianal l.
  photon-deficient l.
  plaque-like l.
  polypoid l.
  precancerous l.
  preoperative l.
  primary glomerular l.
  right-sided l.
  ruptured peliotic l.
  satellite l.
  scirrhous l.
  semipedunculated l.
  sessile l.
  short-segment l.
  skip l.
  space-occupying l.
  stenotic l.
  stress l.
  subglottic l.
  submucosal l.
  submucosal upper
    gastrointestinal tract l.
  synchronous l.
  target l.
  traumatic l.
  tubulovillar l.
  uremic gastrointestinal l.
  vascular l.
  vasculitic l.
  vegetative l.
LESP
  lower esophageal sphincter pressure
lesser
  l. curvature of stomach
  l. curvature ulcer
  l. omentum

  l. pancreas
  l. peritoneal sac
**Lester Martin modification of
  Duhamel operation**
lethargic
leucine
  l. aminopeptidase (LAP)
  l. aminopeptidase test
  l. amniopeptidase
  l. metabolism
  radiolabeled l.
  l. zipper
  l. zipper sequence
leucine-enkephalin (1-ENK)
leucovorin
leu-enkephalin
leukemia
  acute myelomonocytic l.
  chylous l.
  l. patient
Leukeran
leukobilin
leukocyte
  chemotaxis of
    polymorphonuclear l.'s
  l. common antigen
  l. esterase
  fecal l.
  ^{111}In-l. technique
  intraepithelial l. (IEL)
  peritoneal l.
  polymorphonuclear l.
  tether circulating l.
  WBC l.'s
leukocytosis
leukopenia
  acute l.
leukoplakia
  hairy l.
  oral l.
leukotriene
  l. C4
  cysteinyl l.
leu-peptide
leupeptin
leuprolide acetate
Leutrol
levamfetamine
Levarterenol
Levatol
levator
  l. ani
  l. ani muscle

l. ani syndrome
l. span
l. syndrome
Levbid
LeVeen
L. ascites shunt
L. catheter
L. inflation syringe
L. inflator
L. inflator with pressure gauge
L. peritoneal shunt
L. peritoneovenous shunt
L. syringe
L. valve
level
air/fluid l.
ammonia l.
AMP l.
anti-M2 antimitochondrial
antibody l.
α_1-antitrypsin l.
blood alcohol l. (BAL)
blood urea l.
breath ethane l.
complement l.
des-γ-carboxy prothrombin l.
fasting serum gastrin l.
α-fetoprotein l.
gastrin mRNA l.
γ-glutamyl transferase l.
HSP-70 messenger
ribonucleoprotein acid l.
25-hydroxyvitamin D l.
iothalamate l.
lipoprotein l.
lipoprotein X l.
motilin plasma l.
pentane excretion l.
pepsinogen l.
pepsinogen A l.
pepsinogen C l.
polyamine l.
protein C l.
protein S l.
serum gastrin l.
somatostatin MRNA l.
stairstep air/fluid l.'s

theophylline l.
thyroid-stimulating hormone l.
uric acid l.
urinary cGMP l.
whole-blood trough l.
Levin tube
levodopa
l. dopaminergic medication
levorphanol
levothyroxine
Levsinex
L. Timecaps
Levsin/SL
levulose test
Lewis
L. A blood group antigen
L. acids
L. B antigen
L. blood group
L. X antigen
L. Y antigen
L. Y carbohydrate epitope
Lewy syringe
Leyden disease
Leydig
L. cell
L. cell adenoma
L. cell secretion
L. cell secretory function
L. cell tumor
LFT
liver function test
LG
light guide
lymphocytic gastritis
LG bundle
LGD
low-grade dysplasia
L-glutamine
LGV
lymphogranuloma venereum
LH
loop of Henle
luteinizing hormone
LHBT
lactose hydrogen breath testing
LH-FSH releasing hormone

L

NOTES

LHRH
    luteinizing hormone-releasing
    hormone
LHV
    left hepatic vein
LI
    loop ileostomy
libera
    tenia l.
libido
Librax
Lich
    L. extravesical technique
    L. procedure
    L. technique
lichen
    l. planus
    l. sclerosus
    l. sclerosus et atrophicus
Lich-Gregoire
    L.-G. anastomosis
    L.-G. repair
    L.-G. technique
    L.-G. ureterolysis
Lichtenstein
    L. hernial repair
    L. herniorrhaphy
    L. repair
lidamidine
Lidex
lidocaine
    l. hydrochloride jelly
    l. topical anesthetic
    viscous l.
lidocaine-prilocaine cream
lidofenin
    ^{99m}Tc l.
Lidox
Lieberkühn
    L. crypts
    L. glands
Liebermeister groove
lienophrenic ligament
lienorenal ligament
lienteric
    l. diarrhea
    l. stool
lientery
life
    l. cycle of *Echinococcus*
    quality of l. (QOL)
Lifecath peritoneal implant
lifelong obesity

Lifemed catheter
Life-Tech flowmeter
lift
    gallbladder l.
lift-and-cut biopsy
Ligaclip
ligament
    cholecystoduodenal l.
    Cooper l.
    coronary l.
    external l.
    falciform l.
    femoral l.
    gastrocolic l.
    gastrohepatic l.
    gastrolienal l.
    gastropancreatic l.
    gastrophrenic l.
    gastrosplenic l.
    hepatic l.
    hepatocolic l.
    hepatocystocolic l.
    hepatoduodenal l.
    hepatogastric l.
    hepatogastroduodenal l.
    hepatophrenic l.
    hepatorenal l.
    hepatoumbilical l.
    Hesselbach l.
    Huschke l.
    inguinal l.
    lienophrenic l.
    lienorenal l.
    l. of Mackenrodt
    medial umbilical l.
    median arcuate l.
    mucosal suspensory l.
    phrenicocolic l.
    phrenicoesophageal l.
    Poupart l.
    pubocervical l.
    pubourethral l.'s
    l. reflecting edge
    reflecting edge of l.
    round l.
    sacrotuberous l.
    shelving edge of Poupart l.
    splenocolic l.
    splenopancreatic l.
    splenorenal l.
    l. of Treitz
    triangular l.

umbilical l.
urethropelvic l.
ligamentous laxity
ligamentum
  l. teres
  l. venosum
ligand
  l. for ELAM-1
  reciprocal l.
ligand-dependent receptor
  homodimerization
ligand-gated channel
ligandin
ligated
  doubly l.
  suture l.
ligation
  band l.
  Barron l.
  bidirectional l.
  bile duct l. (BDL)
  l. device
  elastic band l.
  endoscopic band l.
  endoscopic esophagogastric
   variceal l.
  endoscopic variceal l. (EVL)
  esophageal band l.
  l. of hemorrhoids
  hepatic artery l.
  high l.
  laparoscopic varix l.
  open retroperitoneal high l.
  postureteral l.
  rubber band l.
  spermatic vein l.
  stump l.
  transesophageal l.
  transgastric l.
  tubal l.
  variceal band l.
  varix l.
ligator
  Barron rubber band l.
  DDV l.
  NAMI DDV l.

rubber band l. (RBL)
Rudd-Clinic hemorrhoidal l.
Stiegmann-Goff Clearvue
  endoscopic l.
Stiegmann-Goff variceal l.
variceal l.
Ligat test
ligature
  elastic l.
  interlocking l.
  pursestring l.
  retroperitoneoscopic vein l.
  silk l.
  Surgiwip suture l.
  suture l.
light
  l. cable
  l. chain deposition disease
  l. electrocautery
  l. and electron
   immunoperoxidase
  l. and electron
   immunoperoxidase observation
  l. emitter
  l. flow
  l. guide (LG)
  l. guide bundle
  l. micrographic study
  l. microscopy
  l. monitoring probe
  l. reflex
γ light chain
Likert scale
Lillie intestinal forceps
limb
  afferent l.
  ascending l.
  blind l.
  l. deformity
  efferent l.
  jejunal l.
  Roux l.
  Roux-en-Y jejunal l.
  thick ascending l. (TAL)
limerence
limit dextrinosis

L

NOTES

339

limited
l. obturator node dissection
l. range of motion
limiting
l. plate
l. plate erosion
limosum
Eubacterium l.
limy bile
lindane
line
anterior axillary l. (AAL)
arterial l.
B cell l.
Brodel l.
CaSki cell l.
cell l.
central venous pressure l.
colonic mucosal l.
dentate l.
Dul45 cell l.
gas density l.
Hampton l.
iliopectineal l.
incision l.
K562 erythroid l.
Langhans l.
lower anterior axillary l.
(LAAL)
lower midclavicular l. (LMCL)
lymphoblastoid cell l.
midaxillary l.
midclavicular l. (MCL)
mucosal l.
murine mesangial cell l.
myelomonocytic cell l.
neuronal cell l.
pararectal l.
pectinate l.
Poupart l.
pubic hair l.
pubococcygeal l.
Rex-Cantli-Serege l.
Richter-Monroe l.
SERAFLO blood l.
skin l.'s
suture l.
T-cell l.
l. of Toldt
transverse umbilical l.
upper midclavicular l. (UMCL)
white l.
Z l.

linea
l. alba
l. nigra
lineage
hematopoietic l.
Langerhans l.
linear
l. array transducer
l. convex array scanner
l. erosion
l. fluorescein
l. 35-Mhz transducer
l. regression
l. stapler
l. stapling device
l. streaks en face
l. ulcer
linear-type echoendoscope
Lingeman
L. 3 in 1 procedure drape
L. TUR drape
lingua
lingula
linitis
l. plastica
l. plastica carcinoma
link
cytoskeletal l.
Linnartz intestinal clamp
linsidomine
l. chlorohydrate
Linton
L. shunt
L. tourniquet clamp
Linton-Nachlas tube
liparocele
lipase
Cherry-Crandall method for
testing serum l.
l. enzyme
hepatic l. (HL)
hepatic triglyceride l. (HTGL)
lipoprotein l. (LPL)
pancreatic l.
serum l.
l. test
lipid
biliary l.
l. emulsion
l. hydroperoxide
l. infusion
l. island
membrane-based l.

l. metabolism
l. peroxidation
lipid-laden
l.-l. clear cell
l.-l. hepatocyte
lipid-lowering drug
lipidosis
Schwann cell l.
lipid-to-protein ratio
lipiodol
l. injection
l. transarterial embolization treatment
lipoblastic sarcoma
lipocele
lipodystrophy, lipodystrophia
intestinal l.
mesenteric l.
lipofection reagent
lipofuscin
lipogranuloma
mesenteric l.
lipogranulomatosis
lipoidal
lipoid nephrosis
lipolysis
heparin-induced l.
intravascular l.
LPL-mediated l.
lipolytic enzyme
lipoma
colonic l.
l. of cord
gastric l.
submucosal ileal l.
lipoma-like tissue
lipomatous
l. ileocecal valve
l. tissue
lipomeningocele
lipomyelocystocele
lipomyelomeningocele
lipophagia
l. granulomatosis
lipophagic intestinal granulomatosis
lipopolysaccharide (LPS)

lipoprotein
apolipoprotein B-containing l.
high-density l. (HDL)
intermediate-density l. (IDL)
l. level
l. lipase (LPL)
liver-specific membrane l. (LSP)
low-density l. (LDL)
very-low-density l. (VLDL)
l. X level
liposarcoma
liposclerotic mesenteritis
liposomal-amphotericin B (L-AmB)
Liposyn II fat emulsion solution
lipothymia
lipoxygenase pathway
liquefaciens
Aeromonas l.
Enterobacter l.
Serratia l.
liquefaction
liquefactive necrosis
liquid
l. antacid
l. chemical germicide (LCG)
l. chromatographic assay
l. diarrhea
l. diet
l. emptying
l. food dysphagia
hyperosmolar l.
iso-osmolar l.
L. Pred
l. scintillation spectrometer
l. stool
Liqui-E
lisinopril
LISL
laser-induced intracorporeal shock wave lithotripsy
Listeria monocytogenes
liter
international units per l. (IU/L)
lithagogue
lithectomy

L

NOTES

lithiasis
    cystine l.
    intraductal l.
    renal l.
    uric acid l.
lithium
    l. clearance (CLi)
    fractional excretion of l.
    (FELI)
lithocholate
lithocholic
    l. acid (LCA)
    l. acid-deoxycholic acid ratio
    (LCA-DCA ratio)
lithoclast
    L. lithotriptor
    Swiss L.
lithocystotomy
lithodialysis
lithogenesis
    urinary l.
lithogenic bile
**Lithognost flash-lamp pulsed dye
laser**
litholabe
litholapaxy
litholysis
    chemical l.
litholyte
lithometer
lithomyl
lithonephritis
lithophone
lithoscope
Lithostar
    L. nonimmersion lithotriptor
    L. Plus
    Siemens L.
Lithostat
lithostathine
    l. molecule
lithotome
lithotomist
lithotomy
    bilateral l.
    dorsal l.
    high l.
    lateral l.
    marian l.
    median l.
    perineal l.
    l. position
    prerectal l.

    suprapubic l.
    vaginal l.
    vesical l.
lithotresis
    ultrasonic l.
lithotripsy
    biliary l.
    blind l.
    coumarin green tunable dye
    laser l.
    cystoscopic electrohydraulic l.
    Dornier extracorporeal shock
    wave l.
    Dornier MPL 9000 gallstone l.
    electrohydraulic l. (EHL)
    electrohydraulic shock wave l.
    (ESWL)
    endoscopic-controlled l.
    endoscopic electrohydraulic l.
    endoscopic pulsed dye laser l.
    external shock wave l.
    extracorporeal piezoelectric l.
    (EPL)
    extracorporeal piezoelectric
    shockwave l.
    extracorporeal shock wave l.
    (ESWL)
    intracorporeal laser l. (ICL)
    intracorporeal shock wave l.
    laser l.
    laser-induced intracorporeal
    shock wave l. (LISL)
    mechanical l.
    Medstone extracorporeal shock
    wave l.
    piezoelectric l.
    pressure regulated
    electrohydraulic l.
    l. retreatment
    shock wave l., shock-wave l.
    l. table
    tunable dye laser l.
    ultrasonic l.
lithotripsy-induced hypertension
lithotripter
lithotriptic
lithotriptor, lithotripter
    American endoscopy
    mechanical l.
    Breakstone l.
    Calcutript electrohydraulic l.
    Circon-ACMI l.
    Diasonic Therasonic l.

Direx Tripter X-1 l.
Dornier compact l.
Dornier gallstone l.
Dornier HM4 l.
Dornier HM3 waterbath l.
EDAP LT.01 l.
electrohydraulic l.
electromagnetic l.
extracorporeal shock wave l.
HM4 l.
Karl Storz-Lutzeyer l.
laser l.
Lithoclast l.
Lithostar nonimmersion l.
manual l.
Medispec Econolith spark
  plug l.
Medstone STS l.
MFL 5000 l.
Modulith SL 20 l.
MonoLith single-piece
  mechanical l.
Northgate SD-3 dual-purpose l.
Olympus l.
percutaneous ultrasonic l.
piezoelectric shock wave l.
Piezolith (2300 and 2500
  model) l.
second generation l.
shock wave l.
Siemens l.
Siemens Lithostar Plus System
  C l.
Sonotrode l.
Storz Monolith l.
Technomed Sonolith 3000 l.
Therasonics l.
third generation l.
tubeless l.
ultrasonic l.
water cushion l.
Wilson-Cook mechanical l.
Wolf Piezolith 2300 l.
Wolf Sonolith l.
lithotriptoscope
lithotriptoscopy

lithotrite
  Marmite l.
  Wolf l.
lithotrity
lithuresis
lithureteria
litmus milk test
littoral cell
Littré
  L. gland
  L. hernia
live
  l. attenuated virus
  l. donor nephrectomy
liver
  l. abscess
  acute fatty l.
  l. Ah receptor
  alcoholic fatty l.
  ballotable l.
  l. bed
  l. biopsy
  l. cancer
  l. capsule
  cardiac impression on the l.
  caudate lobe of l.
  l. cell adenoma (LCA)
  l. cell plate
  centrilobular region of l.
  l. cirrhosis (LC)
  cirrhotic l.
  colic impression on the l.
  cut surface of l.
  l. cyst infection
  diaphragmatic surface of l.
  l. diet
  l. disease
  l. distribution
  dome of l.
  l. dullness
  duodenal impression on l.
  l. eater
  echogenic l.
  l. edge
  l. engorgement
  l. enzyme
  l. failure

L

NOTES

liver *(continued)*
fatty l.
fatty infiltration of l.
finely fatty foamy l.
l. flap
l. flap sign
l. fluke
foamy l.
focal fatty infiltration of l.
focal nonfatty infiltration of l.
l. function profile
l. function test (LFT)
gastric impression on l.
l. hilus
hobnail l.
l. impression
l. iron store
large-droplet fatty l.
lobular architecture of l.
l. lymphoma
macrovesicular fatty l.
l. meal
l. membrane antigen
nodular l.
l. nodule
noncirrhotic l.
non-parasitic cyst of l.
nutmeg l.
l. parenchyma
phlegmonous alcoholic fatty l.
polycystic l.
polycystic disease of l. (PDL)
polylobar l.
potato l.
l. protein store
pyogenic l.
quadrate lobe of l.
renal impression on l.
l. resection
segmentectomy of l.
shock l.
shrunken l.
l. sinusoid
small-droplet fatty l.
l. span
stasis l.
tender l.
l. transplant
l. transplantation
l. transplantation preservation
injury
l. trauma
undersurface of l.

undifferentiated embryonal
sarcoma of l.
l. volume
wandering l.
yellow atrophy of the l.
liver-deprived epithelial clonic cell
liver-directed autoreactivity
liver-kidney microsomal antibody
liver, kidneys, spleen (LKS)
liver-specific
l.-s. antigen
l.-s. membrane lipoprotein
(LSP)
l.-s. protein
liver-spleen scan
living
l. donor kidney
l. donor transplant
l. unrelated donor (LURD)
living-related donor
Livingston triangle
livor mortis
LKB
L. Optiphase 2 scintillation
fluid
LKB-Wallac scintillation counter
LKS
liver, kidneys, spleen
LLC-PK1-FBPase+ cell
LLCPK renal tubular cell
Lletz-Leep active loop electrode
Lloyd-Davis
L.-D. knee and leg holder
L.-D. sigmoidoscope
LLQ
left lower quadrant
LMA
lactose malabsorption
LMCL
lower midclavicular line
LMP gene
LMWH
low-molecular weight heparin
LNa
low sodium
LNaCl
low salt
L-NAME
NG-nitro-L-arginine methyl ester
L-N-monomethyl-arginine
loading
water l.

lobar
l. atrophy
l. nephronia
lobe
caudate l.
left l.
quadrate l.
Riedel l.
right l.
lobectomy
hepatic l.
lobes
"kissing" prostatic l.
lobular
l. architecture
l. architecture of liver
l. hepatitis
l. mononuclear cell infiltrate
lobulated
l. filling defect
l. mass
local
l. alcohol instillation effect
l. anesthesia
l. depot injection
l. scarring
localization
bleeding site l.
pancreatic tumor l.
target l.
localized
l. amyloidosis
l. lesion
l. pain
localizing tenderness
location
tumor l.
locker room syndrome
locking suture
lock-stitch suture
Lockwood-Allis intestinal forceps
LOCM
low-osmolar contrast medium
locomote
locomotor
Lofenalac formula
logarithmic rate

logistic regression analysis
log-rank test
loin pain
lollipop tree sign
lomefloxacin
l. HCl
l. hydrochloride
l. TMP/SMX
Lomotil
Lomustine (CCNU)
Lonalac
L. feeding
L. formula
long
l. incubation hepatitis
l. intestinal tube
long-chain
l.-c. acyl-CoA dehydrogenase deficiency
l.-c. 3-hydroxyacyl coenzyme A dehydrogenase (LCHAD)
l.-c. triglyceride (LCT)
longitudinal
l. choledochotomy
l. enterotomy
l. esophageal stricture
l. image
l. laceration
l. myotomy
l. nephrotomy of Boyce
l. pancreaticojejunostomy
l. subepithelial venous plexus
l. view
longitudinalis
plica l.
long-jaw disposable forceps
Longmire operation
long-nosed sphincterotome
long-nose retriever snare
loop
afferent l.
air-filled l.
alpha l.
alpha sigmoid l.
Biebl l.
blind l.
bowel l.

L

NOTES

loop *(continued)*
    Bradley l.
    brain stem-sacral l.
    cerebral-sacral l.
    l. choledochojejunostomy
    closed afferent l.
    closed efferent l.
    colonic l.
    contiguous l.
    Cordonnier ureteroileal l.
    Davis l.
    diathermic l.
    l. diuretic
    double reverse alpha-sigmoid l.
    duodenal l.
    efferent l.
    l. esophagojejunostomy
    l. forearm graft
    gamma transverse colon l.
    l. gastrojejunostomy
    Heiss l.
    Henle l.
    l. of Henle (LH)
    ileal l.
    l. ileostomy (LI)
    intestinal l.
    jejunal l.
    jejunal interposition of
      Henle l.
    l. jejunostomy
    N l.
    N-shaped sigmoid l.
    ostomy l.
    l. ostomy bridge
    puborectalis l.
    resectoscope l.
    reverse alpha sigmoid l.
    Roeder l.
    Roux-en-Y l.
    Roux-Y l.
    sentinel l.
    sigmoid l.
    l. stoma
    Surgitite ligating l.
    l. suture
    transverse l.
    l. transverse colostomy
    vesical-sacral-sphincter l.
looped cautery
loopogram
loopography
    ileal l.
loops of redundant colon

loop-tipped electrode
loop-type
    l.-t. snare forceps
    l.-t. stone-crushing forceps
loose stool
loperamide
Lopez enteral valve
Lopid
Lopressor
LoPresti
    L. endoscope
    L. fiberoptic esophagoscope
Lopurin
Lorabid
Lorad StereoGuide prone breast
  biopsy system
lorazepam
Lord
    L. dilation of hemorrhoids
    L. hemorrhoidectomy
lordosis
losartan
Losec
loss
    electrolyte l.
    estimated blood l. (EBL)
    fluid l.
    ganglion cell l.
    negligible blood l.
    nephron l.
    obligatory dialysate protein l.
    psoas l.
    sensory l.
    l. of sigmoid curve
    weight l.
Lotrel
Lotrimin
Lotrisone
loupe
    Keeler panoramic l.
    surgical l.
    wide-angled l.
lovastatin
Lovelace forceps
low
    l. calorie diet
    l. fat diet
    l. fiber diet
    l. flow priapism
    l. intermittent suction
    l. pressure bladder substitute
    l. residue diet
    l. roughage diet

l. salt (LNaCl)
l. small-bowel obstruction
l. sodium (LNa)
l. sodium diet
l. transverse incision
low-affinity, high-capacity system
low-affinity transporter
low-calcium dialysate
low-compliance
　l.-c. balloon
　l.-c. bladder
　l.-c. perfusion system
low-density
　l.-d. lipoprotein (LDL)
　l.-d. lipoprotein cholesterol
　　(LDL-C)
low-dose HpD
lower
　l. abdominal transverse incision
　l. anterior axillary line
　　(LAAL)
　l. esophageal B ring
　l. esophageal mucosal ring
　l. esophageal ring
　l. esophageal sphincter (LES)
　l. esophageal sphincter circular
　　muscle
　l. esophageal sphincter pressure
　　(LESP)
　l. esophageal sphincter tone
　L. gall duct forceps
　l. gastrointestinal hemorrhage
　l. GI bleeding
　l. GI tract foreign body
　l. midclavicular line (LMCL)
　l. motor neuron bladder
　　disorder
　l. motor neuron lesion
　l. panendoscopy
　l. pole laceration
Lowery method
low-flux,
　l.-f. cellulose-based membrane
　l.-f. cuprophane membrane
low-flux dialysis membrane

low-grade
　l.-g. dysplasia (LGD)
　l.-g. fever
low-loop cutaneous ureterostomy
low-magnification electron
　micrograph
low-molecular
　l.-m. weight heparin (LMWH)
　l.-m. weight protein
　l.-m. weight protein
　　ribonuclease
Lown criteria
low-osmolar contrast medium
　(LOCM)
low-pitched bowel sounds
low-power photomicrograph
low-pressure
　l.-p. cardiopulmonary
　　baroreceptor
　l.-p. venous system
low-pulsatility arterial waveform
low-residue feeding
Lowsley
　L. retractor
　L. tractor
Lowsley-Peterson cystoscope
low-volume sclerotherapy
loxiglumide
Lozol
L-PAM
LPL
　lipoprotein lipase
LPL-mediated lipolysis
LPLND
　laparoscopic pelvic lymph node
　　dissection
LPP
　leak point pressure
LPS
　lipopolysaccharide
LRE
　lamina rara externa
L-rhamnose
LRI
　lamina rara interna
LSC 7000 curved array transducer
L-selectins

L

NOTES

347

LSMB
   lumbar spine bone mineral density
LSP
   liver-specific membrane lipoprotein
LubraSeptic jelly
lubricant
   Surgilube l.
Lubri-flex ureteral stent
Lubriglide-coated guidewire
lucent cyst
Lucey-Driscoll syndrome
luer
   L. hemorrhoid forceps
   positioner l.
Luer-Lok
   L.-L. connector
   L.-L. syringe
lues
Lugol
   L. iodide
   L. iodine solution
   L. solution stain
Lukes-Collins classification
lumbar
   l. appendicitis
   l. nephrectomy
   l. spinal cord lesion
   l. spine bone mineral density
   (LSMB)
lumbocolostomy
lumbocolotomy
lumbocostoabdominal triangle
lumbosacral
   l. fascia
   l. trunk
lumbricoides
   Ascaris l.
lumen, pl. lumina
   bile duct l.
   bowel l.
   8-l. catheter assembly
   cystic duct l.
   duct l.
   duodenal l.
   esophageal l.
   gastroduodenal l.
   intestinal l.
   scalloped bowel l.
   single l.
Lumenator injectable guidewire
lumen-seeking catheter
lumen-to-bath sodium flux
lumina (*pl. of* lumen)

Lumina guidewire
luminal
   l. acid
   l. amoxicillin
   l. EGF
   l. glucose
   l. hypoacidity
   l. narrowing
   l. secretagogue
luminol-enhanced chemiluminescence
luminometer
   LB 9501 l.
Lumi-Phos 530
lumpectomy
   endoscopic aspiration l. (EAL)
Lunar DPX total-body scanner
lunatus
   penis l.
Lunderquist guidewire
Lunderquist-Ring torque guide
Lundh
   L. meal
   L. test
lung cancer
lupoid hepatitis
Lupron Depot
lupus
   l. anticoagulant (LA)
   l. erythematosus
   l. nephritis
LUQ
   left upper quadrant
LURD
   living unrelated donor
LUS
   laparoscopic ultrasound
Luschka
   accessory duct of L.
   L. duct
lusoria
   arteria l.
   dysphagia l.
luteinizing
   l. hormone (LH)
   l. hormone-releasing hormone
   (LHRH)
Lütkens sphincter
Lüttke test
Lutz automatic reprocessor
LVP
   large volume paracentesis
LX-20 laser

lye
l. ingestion
Lyell syndrome
lymph
l. channel
l. node
l. node adenopathy
l. node dissection
l. node metastasis
l. scrotum
lymphadenectomy
endocavitary pelvic l. (ECPL)
extended pelvic l.
laparoscopic pelvic l.
mediastinal l.
para-aortic l.
pelvic l.
prophylactic l.
retroperitoneal l.
thoracoabdominal
retroperitoneal l.
lymphadenitis
lymphadenopathy
cervical l.
inguinal l.
mediastinal l.
l. syndrome (LAS)
lymphangiectasia, lymphangiectasis
intestinal l.
pancreatic l.
peritoneal l.'s
primary intestinal l. (PIL)
lymphangiogram
lymphangiography
lymphangioma
lymphangitic streak
lymphatic
l. microcyst
l. obstruction
l. package
l. transport
l. vessel
lymphedema
filarial l.
lymphoblastoid
l. cell line
l. interferon-α

lymphocele
l. drainage
lymphocelectomy
laparoscopic l.
pelvic l.
lymphocyst
lymphocyte, pl. lymphocytes
B l.
CD8 l.
CD45RO l.
CD8+ T l.
cytolytic T l. (CTL)
l. cytotoxicity
cytotoxic T l. (CTL)
intraepithelial l. (IEL)
intrahepatic l.
l. migration
naive l.
peripheral blood l. (PBL)
sinusoidal l.
T l.
thymus-derived l.
total l. (TTL)
tumor infiltrating lymphocytes
(TIL)
virgin l.
WBC lymphocytes
lymphocyte-hepatocyte
intrahepatic antigen-
dependent l.-h.
lymphocyte-target cell
lymphocytic
l. colitis
l. gastritis (LG)
lymphocytosis
intraepithelial l.
lymphocytotoxic antibody
lymphogranuloma venereum (LGV)
lymphography
lymphoid
l. aggregate
l. aggregates at mucosal site
l. cholangitis
l. component
l. follicle
l. hyperplasia
l. interstitial pneumonia

L

NOTES

lymphoid *(continued)*
   l. nodular hyperplasia
   l. nodule
   l. polyp
   l. tumor
lymphokine
   l. production
lymphokine-activated killer cell (LAK cell)
lymphoma
   Burkitt l.
   colorectal l.
   duodenal l.
   gastric l.
   histiocytic l.
   infiltrative l.
   liver l.
   MALT l.
     mucosa-associated lymphoid
      tissue lymphoma
     mucosa-associated lymphoid
      tissue l. (MALT lymphoma)
   nodular l.
   non-Hodgkin l. (NHL)
   polypoid l.
   primary B-cell l.
   primary hepatosplenic l. (PHSL)
   small noncleaved-cell l.
   T-cell l.
   testicular l.
   ulcerative l.
lymphomatosis
lymphomatous nodule
lymphomononuclear cell
lymphoplasmacytosis

lymphoproliferative
   l. disorder
   l. syndrome
lymphosarcoma
lymphs
   lymphocytes
Lynch
   L. syndrome
   L. syndrome I
   L. syndrome II
lyn protein
LYOfoam dressing
Lyon
   L. ring
   L. ring-constrictive band
lyophilized
Lyphocin
lyse
lysine
lysis
   l. of adhesions
   colon tumor cell l.
   CTL-mediated l.
   mesangial l.
   tumor cell l.
lysolecithin
lysosomal
   l. enzyme
   l. membrane
   l. swelling
lysosome
   hepatocyte l.
lysozyme
lysyl-bradykinin
lytic cocktail
Lytren electrolyte solution

M
    M antibody
    M cell
M1
    antibody to Leu M.
M30
    Zeiss morphomate M.
MAA
    macroaggregated albumin
    ^{99m}Tc MAA
Maalox
    M. Plus
    M. Therapeutic Concentrate
    M. Whip
MAB
    maximal androgen blockade
    monoclonal antibody
mAb
    monoclonal antibody
    anti-class II mAb
    mAb IOT2-recognizing
      monomorphic DR determinant
MABP
    mean arterial blood pressure
Macaluso stent remover
MacConkey agar
Macdonald test
Macewen
    M. hernia operation
    M. herniorrhaphy
Machado-Guerreiro test
Machida choledochoscope
machine
    A2008 ABGII hemodialysis m.
    Accuson-128 color flow
      Doppler m.
    Belzer m.
    endoscopic sewing m.
    Endotek m.
    Gambro AK10 m.
    gastric hypothermia m.
    heart-lung m.
    Kodak Ektachem 700 m.
    MOX TM-100 portable renal
      preservation m.
    Narco esophageal motility m.
    Nova II m.
    perfusion m.
    portable renal preservation m.
    Primus Prostate M.

Mackenrodt
    ligament of M.
Mackenzie point
MacLean test
Maclet magnetic ring
macroaggregated albumin (MAA)
macroamylasemia
macroangiodynamic
macroangiopathic hemolytic anemia
Macrobid
macrocephaly
macrocrystal
macrocyst
    adrenocortical m.
Macrodantin
macroglobulinemia
    Waldenström m.
macrolide
    m. antimicrobial
macromolecular
    m. secretion
    m. uronate (MMUA)
macromolecule
    radiolabeled m.
macronidia
macronodular cirrhosis
macropenis
macrophage
    bile-laden m.
    ceroid-laden m.
    hemosiderin-laden m.
    parasitizing m.
    peritoneal m.
**macrophage-rich inflammatory
  response**
macrophage-TGF-β axis
macrophallus
Macroplastique injectable
macroregenerative nodule
macroscopic
    m. hematuria
    m. lesion
    m. liver cyst
macrothrombocyte
macrovascular disease
macrovesicular
    m. fat
    m. fatty liver
macula densa
macular degeneration

M

macule
maculopapular
Madden
    M. incisional herniorrhaphy
    M. repair
    M. repair of incisional hernia
Maddrey discriminant function
Mad Hatter syndrome
Madsen-Iversen
    M.-I. scale
    M.-I. scoring system
Maffucci syndrome
MAG
    multifocal atrophic gastritis
MAG-3
    mercaptotriglycylglycine
    Technescan MAG-3
magaldrate
Magic Lite chemiluminometric
  immunoassay
magna
    lacuna m.
Magnacal liquid feeding
MagnaScanner
    Picker Vista M.
Magnatril
magnesia
    citrate of m.
    milk of m. (MOM)
    Phillips Milk of M.
magnesium
    m. ammonium phosphate
    m. citrate
    m. hydroxide
    m. oxide
magnetic
    m. bore
    m. internal ureteral stent
    m. resonance angiography
    m. resonance imaging (MRI)
    m. resonance spectroscopy
    m. susceptibility test
magnetization prepared-rapid
  gradient-echo (MP-RAGE)
magnification
magnifying
    m. colonoscope
    m. endoscope
    m. enteroscope
Mag-Ox 400
MAGP
    microfil-associated glycoprotein
    MAGP microfibrillar protein

MAGPI
    meatal advancement and glansplasty
    MAGPI operation
mahogany-colored stool
Mahurkar catheter
MAI
    Mycobacterium avium
maina propria
Maine Medical Assessment Program
  index (MMAP index)
main pancreatic duct (MBD, MPD)
maintenance treatment
Mainz
    M. pouch augmentation
    M. pouch cutaneous urinary
      diversion
    M. pouch II
    M. pouch operation
    M. urinary pouch
major
    m. histocompatibility complex
      (MHC)
    m. papilla
majus
    omentum m.
Makler
    M. cannula
    M. counting chamber
    M. insemination device
    M. sperm counting device
malabsorption
    bile acid m. (BAM)
    m. disease
    D-xylose m.
    folate m.
    glucose-galactose m.
    iatrogenic m.
    lactose m. (LMA)
    lavage-induced pill m.
    m. syndrome
    vitamin B_{12} m.
malabsorptive diarrhea
malacoplakia, malakoplakia
malacotomy
Malakit *Helicobacter pylori* Biolab
malakoplakia (*var. of* malacoplakia)
malaria
    algid m.
    bilious remittent m.
    dysenteric algid m.
    falciparum m.
    gastric m.

malignant tertian m.
pernicious m.
malarial
    m. hepatitis
malate
maldescent
maldigestion
maldigestion/absorption syndrome
maldigestive diarrhea
maldigestors
    lactose m.
male
    m. catheter
    m. escutcheon
maleate
    methysergide m.
    perhexiline m.
Malecot
    M. gastrostomy tube
    M. nephrostomy tube
    M. reentry catheter
malemission
malformation
    anorectal m.
    arteriovenous m. (AVM)
    bronchopulmonary foregut m.
    Chiari m.
    cloacal m.
    Dieulafoy vascular m.
    dysraphic m.
    gastric arteriovenous m.
    mermaid m.
    pulmonary arteriovenous m.
    "sink-trap" m.
    vascular m.
malignancy
    m. associated cellular marker
    de novo m.
    esophageal m.
    esophagocardial m.
    hepatic m.
    hepatobiliary m.
    humoral hypercalcemia of m.
    (HHM)
    pancreaticobiliary m.
    paratesticular m.

periampullary m.
peritoneal m.
malignant
    m. ascites
    m. B-cell syndrome
    m. biliary obstruction
    m. biliary obstructive disease
    m. cachexia
    m. carcinoid syndrome
    m. dysentery
    m. dysplasia
    m. histiocytosis
    m. jaundice
    m. malnutrition
    m. melanoma
    m. meniscus sign
    m. mesenchymal tumor
    m. nephrosclerosis
    m. nuclear structure
    m. obstructive jaundice
    m. pheochromocytoma
    m. polyp
    m. potential
    m. renal mass
    m. seeding
    m. stenosis
    m. stricture
    m. tertian malaria
    m. ulcer
Mallard incision
malleable
    m. blade
    m. implant
    m. prosthesis
    m. retractor
    m. scoop
Mallinckrodt
    M. catheter
    M. ultra tag labeling kit
Mallory
    M. hyalin
    M. hyaline body
Mallory-Azan stain
Mallory-Weiss
    M.-W. lesion
    M.-W. mucosal rupture
    M.-W. mucosal syndrome

M

NOTES

Mallory-Weiss *(continued)*
    M.-W. syndrome
    M.-W. tear
malnourished
malnutrition
    index of m.
    malignant m.
    protein-calorie m. (PCM)
    protein-energy m.
malnutrition-related diabetes
  mellitus (MRDM)
malodorous
    m. fluid
    m. stool
Malone antegrade continence enema
Maloney
    M. bougie
    M. mercury-filled esophageal
      dilator
    M. tapered-tip dilator
Maloney-type bougie
malpighian body
malpighii
    stratum m.
malrotation
    m. of intestine
    midgut volvulus with m.
MALT
    mucosa-associated lymphoid tissue
    MALT lymphoma
maltase
Maltese cross
maltose tetrapalmitate
Maltsupex
malutinization
Maly test
mammalgia
mammalian cell membrane
mAMSA
    amsacrine
management
    m. algorithm
    endoscopic m.
    foreign body m.
    mechanical endoscopic m.
    seton m.
Manchurian hemorrhagic fever
Mancke flex-rigid gastroscope
Mandelamine
mandible
mandril set
maneuver
    alpha-loop m.

    avoidance m.
    bunching m.
    Crede m.
    Duecollement m.
    Fowler-Stephens m.
    Heimlich m.
    Hoguet m.
    Hueter m.
    J-type m.
    Kocher m.
    Mattox m.
    Müller m.
    peroral m.
    Prentiss m.
    Pringle m.
    straightening m.
    U-turn m.
    Valsalva m.
manifestation
    hepatobiliary m.
    otolaryngologic m.
Manifold II slot-blot apparatus
manipulation
    direct m.
    pancreatic duct m.
    postureteroscopic m.
Mann-Bollman fistula
mannitol
Mann-Whitney
    M.-W. rank sum test
    M.-W. test
    M.-W. U-test
Mann-Williamson
    M.-W. operation
    M.-W. ulcer
manometer
manometric
    m. catheter
    m. criterion
    m. evaluation
    m. feature
    m. finding
    m. pattern
    m. sensor
    m. study
manometry
    anal m.
    aneroid m.
    anorectal m.
    balloon reflex m.
    biliary m.
    dry swallow on esophageal m.
    endoscopic m.

endoscopic sphincter of
  Oddi m.
ERCP m.
esophageal m.
perendoscopic m.
PIP on esophageal m.
point of respiratory reversal on
  esophageal m.
rectosigmoid m.
sphincter of Oddi m. (SOM)
transileostomy m.
mansonelliasis
mansoni
  Schistosoma m.
Manson schistosomiasis
Mansson
  M. operation
  M. urinary pouch
Mantel-Haenszel test
manual lithotriptor
MAP
  mean arterial pressure
  MAP kinase signaling cascade
  systemic MAP
mapping
  anal m.
  bladder m.
  intragastric pH m.
Maquet endoscopy table
marantic endocarditis
marasmus
Marazide
Marblen
Marburg virus
Marcaine
marcescens
  Serratia m.
Marcillin
Mardis soft stent
Mardi test
Marechal-Rosen test
Marezine
Marfan syndrome
margin
  cell-positive m.
  costal m.
  dentate m.

disk m.
dissection m.
subcostal m.
marginal ulcer
margo, pl. **margines**
marian lithotomy
Marie-Strumpell disease
Marinol
Marion disease
marked tube
marker
  anthropometric m.
  antigen m.
  biochemical m.
  biological m.
  B5 tumor m.
  D4S231 m.
  D4S414 m.
  D16S283 m.
  D16S291 m.
  D16S84 m.
  DUPAN 2 tumor m.
  fecal m.
  fluid phase m.
  genetic m.
  hepatitis serologic m.'s
  HMB-45 monoclonal
   antibody m.
  inflammation m.
  malignancy associated
   cellular m.
  molecular m.
  OA-519 prognostic prostate
   carcinoma m.
  p-ANC genetic m.
  pancreatic cancer m.
  plasma membrane m.
  polycationic m.
  radiopaque m.
  serologic m.
  serum m.
  m. stitch
  surrogate m.
  m. transit study
  tumor m.
  viral hepatitis m.

M

NOTES

marking
    haustral m.
marks
    crosshatch m.
Marlen
    M. double-faced adhesive disk
    M. Gas Relief drainage pouch
    M. Neoprene All-Flexible
      faceplate
    M. Odor-Ban ileostomy pouch
    M. Solo ileostomy pouch
    M. Zip Klosed pouch
Marlex
    M. band
    M. graft
    M. hernial repair
    M. mesh
    M. mesh abdominal rectopexy
    M. plug technique
Marmite lithotrite
maroon-colored stool
marrow transplant recipient
Marseille
    M. classification
    M. pancreatitis classification
Marshall-Bonney test
Marshall-Marchetti-Krantz
    M.-M.-K. operation
    M.-M.-K. procedure
    M.-M.-K. urethropexy
Marshall-Marchetti test
Marshall test
marshmallow
    barium-impregnated m.
    m. bolus
marsupialization
    renal cyst m.
Martel clamp
Martin anoplasty
Martin-Davis rectal speculum
Martius
    M. fat pad
    M. flap
    M. scarlet blue stain
Martorell hypertensive ulcer
MAS
    mean allograft survival
masculinizing genitoplasty
MASE
    microsurgical extraction of sperm
    from epididymis
mask phenomenon

Mason
    M. operation
    M. vertical banded gastroplasty
mass
    abdominal m.
    abdominal wall m.
    adnexal m.
    appendiceal m.
    asymptomatic m.
    body cell m. (BCM)
    colonic m.
    congenital renal m.
    cul-de-sac m.
    cystic m.
    discrete m.
    duodenal m.
    dysplasia-associated lesion
      or m. (DALM)
    esophageal m.
    exophytic m.
    expansile abdominal m.
    extramucosal m.
    extrarenal m.
    extrinsic m.
    flank m.
    fluctuant m.
    gastric m.
    hilar m.
    inflammatory renal m.
    intra-abdominal m.
    lean body m. (LBM)
    lobulated m.
    malignant renal m.
    mediastinal m.
    mushroom-shaped m.
    neoplastic renal m.
    palpable m.
    parovarian m.
    periampullary m.
    perirectal m.
    phlegmonous m.
    pleural m.
    polypoid m.
    pulsatile m.
    rectal m.
    renal m.
    salivary m.
    scrotal m.
    soft tissue m.
    submucosal m.
    testicular m.
    transformary m.
    traumatic renal m.

tubular excretory m.
vaginal m.
vascular renal m.
massage
prostatic m.
masseter strength
Masset test
massive
m. bowel resection syndrome
m. hepatic necrosis
m. malignant infiltration
Masson
M. trichrome
M. trichrome stain
M. trichrome staining
technique
mast
m. cell
m. cell degranulation
master
m. duodenoscope
m. IG bundle
m. image guide
MasterFlex pump
Masters intestinal clamp
Masters-Schwartz liver clamp
Mastisol
mastocytosis
systemic m.
urticaria pigmentosa with
systemic m.
masturbation
traumatic m.
matching
HLA-DR m.
material
anastomotic m.
coffee-grounds m. (CGM)
congophilic m.
Conray (60, 70) contrast m.
extravasated iodinated
contrast m.
fecal m.
microcrystalline m.
proteinaceous cast m.
purulent m.
suture m.

Mathews rectal speculum
Mathieu
M. island onlay flap
M. procedure
M. technique
Mathieu-Horton-Devine flip-flap
Matrigel
matrix
m. calculus
m. deposition
extracellular m. (ECM)
glomerular extracellular m.
m. metalloproteinase (MMP)
matted node
Mattox maneuver
mattress suture
maturation
collagen m.
mucosal barrier m.
osteoclast m.
stone m.
maturing the stoma
**Mauch double-sheathed plastic wash
pipe**
Maunsell-Weir operation
Mavigraph color video printer
Maxaquin
MaxBloc
Max-EPA capsules
MaxForce
M. TTS balloon
M. TTS biliary balloon
dilatation catheter
M. TTS high performance
balloon dilatation catheter
maximal androgen blockade (MAB)
maximum
m. bladder capacity
m. cystometric capacity
m. diameter
maximus
gluteus m.
Maxisorb test plate
Maxum
M. reusable forceps
Maxzide

M

NOTES

Maydl
- M. hernia
- M. procedure
- M. ureterosigmoidostomy

Mayer acid alum hematoxylin stain
Mayer-hematoxylin solution
Mayer-Rokitansky syndrome
May-Grünwald-Giemsa stain
Mayo
- M. abdominal clamp
- M. abdominal retractor
- M. common duct probe
- M. common duct scoop
- M. common duct spoon
- M. gallstone scoop
- M. grading system
- M. needle
- M. operation
- M. scissors
- M. stand
- M. trocar-point needle

Mayo-Adams appendectomy retractor
Mayo-Blake gallstone forceps
Mayo-Hegar needle holder
Mayo-Ochsner suction trocar cannula
Mayo-Pean forceps
Mayo-Robson
- M.-R. clamp
- M.-R. intestinal clamp
- M.-R. intestinal forceps
- M.-R. position

Mazicon
mazindol
Mazzariello-Caprini forceps
MBD
  main pancreatic duct
MBS
  modified barium swallow
MC
  mesangial cell
MCA
  middle colic artery
MCAD
  medium-chain acyl-CoA dehydrogenase
McBurney
- M. incision
- M. point
- M. retractor
- M. sign

MCC
  mutated colorectal carcinoma
McCall culdoplasty
McCarthy-Campbell miniature cystoscope
McCarthy Foroblique panendoscope cystoscope
McCleery-Miller intestinal clamp
McCormack gastric mucosal sign
McCort sign
McCrea
- M. cystoscope
- M. sound

McDonald cerclage
MCF-7 tumor
MCFA
  medium-chain fatty acids
McGaw
- M. plastic bottle
- M. volumetric pump

McGill
- M. forceps
- M. pain questionnaire

McGivney hemorrhoid forceps
M-CH
  mitomycin adsorbed onto activated charcoal
MCH
  mean corpuscular hemoglobin
  microfibrillar collagen hemostat
  Endo-Avitene MCH
  MCH gene
MCHA
  microsome antibody
MCHC
  mean corpuscular hemoglobin concentration
McIndoe procedure
McIntyre reverse cystotome
MCK
  multicystic kidney
MCL
  midclavicular line
  MCL port
McLean pile clamp
McNealey-Glassman-Mixter forceps
McNeer classification
McNemar
- M. ascites test
- M. test for ascites

MCP
  membrane cofactor protein
  monocyte chemoattract protein

MCP-1
MCT
mean colonic transit
medium-chain triglyceride
medullary carcinoma of thyroid
MCT oil
MCTD
mixed connective tissue disease
MCV
mean corpuscular volume
molluscum contagiosum virus
McVay
M. herniorrhaphy
M. inguinal hernial repair
MD-60 contrast medium
MDCA
mean distal contraction amplitude
MDCK epithelial cell
MDP
^{99m}Tc M.
MDS
membrane-spanning domain
MDT renogram
Meadox Surgimed Doppler probe
MEA-I
multiple endocrine adenomatosis
type I
MeAIB
methylaminoisobutyric acid
MEA-II
multiple endocrine adenomatosis
type II
meal
barium m.
Boyden m.
butter m.
double contrast barium m.
Ewald test m.
fatty m.
isotope m.
liver m.
Lundh m.
motor test m.
normal saline m.
opaque m.
pH standardized m.
retention m.

small-bowel m.
solid egg white m.
standard fatty m.
test m.
meal-stimulated
m.-s. acid output (MSAO)
m.-s. pancreatic secretion
m.-s. secretion
mean
m. allograft survival (MAS)
m. arterial blood pressure
(MABP)
m. arterial pressure (MAP)
m. colonic transit (MCT)
m. corpuscular hemoglobin
(MCH)
m. corpuscular hemoglobin
concentration (MCHC)
m. corpuscular volume (MCV)
m. distal contraction amplitude
(MDCA)
m. input time (MIT)
m. renal volume
m. resistance time (MRT)
m. shunt index
m. TIMP-1/GAPDH rates
m. TIMP-3-GAPDH ratio
m. transit time
m. venous outflow (MVO)
Meares-Stamey technique
measles
measure
antiendotoxin m.
cGy radiation m.
measurement
anorectal m.
anthropometric m.
bulbocavernous reflex
latency m.
Doppler ultrasound intestinal
blood flow m.
intestinal permeability m.
microfluorometric m.
planimetric m.
plasma bile acid m.
pressure m.
RigiScan m.

M

NOTES

measurement *(continued)*
  serum bile acid m.
  m. test
  urethral pressure m.
  velocity m.
measurements
  voiding urethral pressure m.
  (VUPP)
meatal
  m. advancement
  m. advancement and
    glansplasty (MAGPI)
  m. spreader
  m. stenosis
meat impaction
meatoplasty
  V-flap m.
meatorrhaphy
meatoscope
meatoscopy
meatotome
meatotomy
  m. scissors
  ureteral m.
meatus
  retrusive m.
mebendazole
mebrofenin
mecamylamine
mechanical
  m. assist system
  m. biliary obstruction
  m. diarrhea
  m. duct obstruction
  m. endoscopic management
  m. extrahepatic obstruction
  m. ileus
  m. intestinal obstruction
  m. jaundice
  m. leech
  m. lithotripsy
  m. product
  m. radial-scanning instrument
  m. rotating probe
  m. small-bowel obstruction
  m. stress wave
  m. ureteral dilation
  m. variceal compression
  m. ventilation
mechanism
  Albarran m.
  antireflux flap-valve m.
  cell-mediated m.

countercurrent m.
cyclooxygenase-dependent m.
deglutition m.
deranged hemostatic m.
flap-valve m.
Mitrofanoff m.
neuroparacrine m.
peptidergic m.
pinchcock m.
renal autoregulatory m.
sphincteric m.
swallowing m.
T-cell-dependent m.
Tubuloglomerular Feedback M.
urethral closure m.
mechanoreceptor
Mecholyl
mecillinam
Meckel
  M. diverticulitis
  M. diverticulum
  M. ileitis
  M. rod
  M. scan
Meckel-Gruber syndrome
meclizine
meclofenamate
  sodium m.
meconium
  m. ileus
  m. ileus equivalent (MIE)
  m. peritonitis
  m. plug
  m. plug syndrome
Medena tube
media (*pl. of* medium)
medial
  m. fibroplasia
  m. umbilical ligament
median
  m. arcuate ligament
  m. bar formation
  m. furrow of the prostate
  m. incision
  m. lithotomy
  m. lobe hyperplasia
mediastinal
  m. crunch
  m. histoplasmosis
  m. lymphadenectomy
  m. lymphadenopathy
  m. lymph node sampling
  m. mass

m. shift
m. thickening
m. tube
m. tumor
m. widening
mediastinitis
mediastinum testis
mediated
plasmid m.
medical
m. dilation
m. evaluation
m. laser
m. therapy
m. vagotomy
medically-induced achlorhydria
medicamentosus
pseudopolyposis m.
medication
m. allergy
anticholinergic m.
m. bezoar
bromocriptine dopaminergic m.
carbidopa dopaminergic m.
dopaminergic m.
levodopa dopaminergic m.
pergolide dopaminergic m.
psychopharmacologic m.
psychotropic m.
m. teratogenesis
medication-associated suppression of
gastric secretion
medication-induced injury
medicine
nuclear m. (NM)
teratogenic m.
medicolith
Medicone
Medicon-Jackson rectal forceps
medicus
furor m.
Medicut catheter
Mediflex-Gazayerli retractor
Mediflex MD-7 endoscopic video
system
Medihistory
Medilas fiberTome laser

Medina
M. ileostomy catheter
M. tube
medionodular cirrhosis
medisect
Medispec Econolith spark plug
lithotriptor
Medi-Tech
M.-T. bipolar catheter
M.-T. bipolar probe
Mediterranean fever
Meditron EL-100 Endolav
medium, pl. media
Balch 1 broth m.
Baricon contrast m.
Baroflave contrast m.
Barosperse contrast m.
Biligrafin contrast m.
Biliscopin contrast m.
Bilivist contrast m.
Bilopaque contrast m.
Biloptin contrast m.
Campy-BAP culture m.
chocolate agar m.
Cholebrine contrast m.
Cholografin contrast m.
Conray 280 contrast m.
contrast m.
culture m.
dissociated m.
Dulbecco modified Eagle m.
Eagle minimal essential m.
Earle m.
extravasation of contrast m.
Gastrografin contrast m.
Gastrovist contrast m.
Ham F12 m.
Hypaque contrast m.
inoculated m.
iocetamic acid contrast m.
iodipamide meglumine
contrast m.
iopanoic acid contrast m.
ipodate contrast m.
low-osmolar contrast m.
(LOCM)
MD-60 contrast m.

M

NOTES

medium *(continued)*
    meglumine diatrizoate
      contrast m.
    meglumine iotroxate
      contrast m.
    Niopam contrast m.
    OCT m.
    Oragrafin contrast m.
    Reno-M contrast m.
    RPMI 1640 culture m.
    Skirrow m.
    sodium iodipamide contrast m.
    Solu-Biloptin contrast m.
    Telepaque contrast m.
    Thorotrast contrast m.
    tyropanoate contrast m.
    Urografin 290 contrast m.
    water-soluble contrast m.
medium-chain
    m.-c. acyl-CoA dehydrogenase
      (MCAD)
    m.-c. acyl-CoA dehydrogenase
      deficiency
    m.-c. fatty acids (MCFA)
    m.-c. triglyceride (MCT)
medium-power photomicrograph
medium-term result
Medivator automatic reprocessor
Medoc-Celestin
    M.-C. endoprosthesis
    M.-C. pulsion tube
Medrol
medronate
    ^{99m}Tc m.
medroxyprogesterone
    m. acetate
MEDS
    microsurgical extraction of ductal
    sperm
Medstone
    M. extracorporeal shock wave
      lithotripsy
    M. IRIS system
    M. STS lithotripsy system
    M. STS lithotriptor
Medtrax
    M. urology database
    M. urology software
medulla
medullaris
    conus m.

medullary
    m. carcinoma of thyroid
      (MCT)
    m. collecting duct
    m. interstitial osmolality
    m. interstitium
    m. oxygenation
    m. pyramid
    m. sponge kidney
    m. thyroid carcinoma
medulloblastoma
medusae
    caput m.
Medusa head
Meeker gallbladder clamp
Mefoxin
Mefoxin-saline solution
megabladder
megacalycosis
Megace
megacolon
    acquired m.
    congenital m.
    idiopathic m.
    toxic m.
megacystic
    m. mucinous neoplasm
    m. syndrome
megacystis
megacystis-megaureter
    m.-m. association
    m.-m. syndrome
megacystis-microcolon-intestinal
    hypoperistalsis syndrome
megaduodenum
megaesophagus
    Chagasic m.
20-megahertz endoscopic ultrasound
    probe
megakaryocyte
megalin
megaloblastic anemia
megalopenis
megalophallus
megaloureter
megalourethra
megamitochondria
megarectum
megasigmoid
    m. syndrome
megaureter
    primary m.

primary obstructive m.
secondary m.
megaurethra
megestrol acetate
meglumine
diatrizoate m.
m. diatrizoate
m. diatrizoate contrast medium
iodipamide m.
m. iotroxate
m. iotroxate contrast medium
Urovist M.
MEGX
monoethylglycinexylidide
MEIA
microparticle enzyme immunoassay
Meigs syndrome
Meissner plexus
melanogaster
Drosophila m.
melanoma
malignant m.
metastatic m.
melanorrhagia
melanorrhea
melanosis
m. coli
melanotic
melanotic neuroectodermal tumor of infancy
melas
icterus m.
melena
m. vera
melenemesis
melenic
m. stool
melitensis
Brucella m.
Melkersson-Rosenthal syndrome
mellitus
diabetes m.
insulin-dependent diabetes m. (IDDM)
malnutrition-related diabetes m. (MRDM)

non-insulin-dependent diabetes m. (NIDDM)
posttransplant diabetes m. (PTDM)
streptozotocin-induced diabetes m.
type II diabetes m.
melphalan
Meltzer-Lyon test
membrane
antiglomerular basement m.
antitubular basement m.
antral m.
basement m.
basolateral m. (BLM)
brush-border m. (BBM)
m. catheter technique
cell m.
cellulose-based m.
cloacal m.
m. cofactor protein (MCP)
congenital pyloric m.
m. current
dialyzer m.
dry mucous m.
elastic silicone m.
filtration-slit m.
glomerular basement m. (GBM)
HEMOPHAN m.
Hibond N+ nylon m.
high-flux dialysis m.
invaginated m.
Jackson m.
low-flux, cellulose-based m.
low-flux, cuprophane m.
low-flux dialysis m.
lysosomal m.
mammalian cell m.
microvillous m.
moist mucous m.
MSI nylon m.
mucous m.
NaK-ATPase m.
m. oxygenator
m. permeability
phrenoesophageal m.

M

NOTES

membrane *(continued)*
    porous filter m.
    posttransplant antiglomerular
      basement m.
    Preclude peritoneal m.
    serous m.
    small intestinal m.
    thin basement m. (TBM)
    m. trafficking
    m. transport protein
    tubular basement m.
    urea-impermeable m.
    urothelial basement m. (UBM)
    XM-50 Dialow m.
membrane-attack complex
membrane-based lipid
membrane-spanning
    m.-s. domain (MDS)
    m.-s. integrin
Membranfilter
    NY 13N M.
membranoproliferative
    m. glomerulonephritis (MPGN)
    m. glomerulonephritis type II
      (MPGN type II)
membranoproliferative
  glomerulonephritis type I (MPGN
  type I)
membranous
    m. glomerulonephritis (MGN)
    m. nephropathy
    m. neuropathy
    m. urethra
Memokath catheter
memory
    m. impairment
    m. T cell
    m. wire
Memotherm stent
MEN
    multiple endocrine neoplasia
    MEN 2A
      multiple endocrine neoplasia
      2A
    MEN 2B
      multiple endocrine neoplasia
      2B
    MEN I syndrome
    MEN syndrome
menaquinone (MK)
Mendelian pattern
Mendez ultrasonic cystotome
Ménétrier disease

Menghini
    M. biopsy needle
    M. liver biopsy needle
    M. needle
    M. technique
    M. technique for percutaneous
      liver biopsy
Ménière disease
meningismus
meningitis
    pyogenic m.
meningomyelocele
meningosepticum
    Flavobacterium m.
meniscus sign
Menoquinon
    sodium diatrizoate with M.
menouria
MENS
    multiple endocrine neoplasia
    syndrome
Mentor
    M. Alpha 1 inflatable penile
      prosthesis
    M. GFS penile prosthesis
    M. gun
    M. inflatable penile prosthesis
    M. IPP penile prosthesis
    M. malleable penile prosthesis
    M. Mark II penile prosthesis
    M. Response VCD
    M. straight catheter
Mentor-Piston VCD
Mentor-Touch VCD
Menuel cavernosometry
Menuet
    M. Compact primary
      urodynamic analyzer
    M. Compact urodynamics
      system
    M. Compact urodynamic
      testing device
    M. urodynamics system
mepenzolate
    m. bromide
meperidine
    m. conscious sedation
    m. HCl
    m. hydrochloride
mephentermine
mepiperphenidol
mercaptan

mercaptoethane sulfonate
6-mercaptopurine (6-MP)
mercaptotriglycylglycine (MAG-3)
Mercier bar
mercurialism
mercuric
    m. chloride-induced ARF
    m. chloride-induced nephritis
    m. chloride nephrotoxicity
    m. oxide
    m. oxide battery ingestion
mercury
    m. bougienage treatment
    m. chloride (HgCl2)
    millimeters of m. (mmHg, mm Hg)
    m. poisoning
mercury-containing balloon
mercury-filled dilator
mercury-weighted
    m.-w. dilator
    m.-w. rubber bougie
    m.-w. tube
Merindino operation
Meritene liquid feeding
MERmaid
    M. kit
mermaid malformation
meropenem
Merrem
Mersilene
    M. mesh
    M. strut
    M. suture
    M. tape
merthiolate fresh stool examination
merycism
MESA
    microsurgical epididymal sperm aspiration
mesalamine
    m. enema
    m. sodium
mesalzine
mesangial
    m. angle
    m. cell (MC)

    m. deposit
    m. hypercellularity
    m. lysis
    m. matrix expansion
    m. proliferation
    m. proliferative glomerulonephritis
    m. volume fraction
mesangiocapillary glomerulonephritis
mesangiolysis
mesangioproliferative glomerulonephritis
mesangium
    glomerular m.
mesenchymal
    m. change
    m. hamartoma
mesenchyme
mesenchymoma
mesenteric
    m. adenitis
    m. apoplexy
    m. arterial embolism
    m. arterial thrombosis
    m. arteriography
    m. arteriovenous fistula
    m. artery
    m. artery constriction
    m. attachment
    m. attachments of colon
    m. circulation
    m. cyst
    m. fibromatosis
    m. fistula
    m. hematoma
    m. hernia
    m. infarction
    m. inflammatory disease
    m. ischemia
    m. lipodystrophy
    m. lipogranuloma
    m. lymph node (MLN)
    m. panniculitis (MP)
    m. rupture
    m. sensory receptor
    m. stranding
    m. tear

M

NOTES

mesenteric *(continued)*
   m. triangle
   m. tumefaction
   m. varix
   m. vascular disease
   m. vascular lesion
   m. vascular occlusion
   m. venous thrombosis
   m. window
mesenteriopexy
mesenteriorrhaphy
mesenteriplication
mesenteritis
   liposclerotic m.
   retractile m.
mesenteroaxial gastric volvulus
mesenterorenal bypass
mesentery
   leaves of m.
   small intestine m. (SIM)
mesh
   Dacron m.
   Dexon polyglycolic acid m.
   Marlex m.
   Mersilene m.
   polypropylene m.
   m. stent
   m. stent prosthesis
   synthetic m.
mesher
   Collin m.
mesilate
   gabexate m.
mesoappendicitis
mesoappendix
mesoblastic nephroma
mesocaval
   m. anastomosis
   m. H-graft shunt
   m. interposition shunt
   m. shunt
mesocolic
   m. band
   m. hernia
   m. shelf
mesocolica
   taenia m.
mesocolon
mesocolonic vessel
mesocolopexy
mesocoloplication
mesodermal ingrowth
mesoileum

mesometrium
mesonephric
   m. duct
   m. hyperplasia
   m. remnant
mesopexy
mesophilic bacterium
Mesor
mesorectum
mesoridazine
mesorrhaphy
mesosigmoid colon
mesosigmoidopexy
mesothelial
   m. hyperplasia (MH)
   m. metaplasia
mesothelioma
   benign cystic m.
   benign m. of genital tract
   diffuse malignant m. (DMM)
   giant fibrous m.
   peritoneal m.
   well-differentiated papillary m.
      (WDPM)
mesotrypsin
message-2
   testosterone repressed
      prostate m. (TRPM-2)
messenger
   m. ribonucleoprotein acid
      (mRNA)
   m. RNA (mRNA)
   m. RNA molecule
   T-cell second m.'s
Messerklinger endoscope
Mestinon
mesylate
   doxazosin m.
meta-analysis
metabolic
   m. alkalosis
   m. balance
   m. bone survey
   m. calculus
   m. complication
   m. derangement from vomiting
   m. disorder
   m. effect
   m. evaluation
   m. liver disease
   m. range
   m. rate

m. stone
m. stone disease
metabolism
albumin m.
drug m.
first-pass m.
glomerular m.
glutathione m.
hepatic m.
inborn error of m.
leucine m.
lipid m.
protein m.
sulfur amino acid m.
tryptophan m.
metabolite
arachidonic acid m.
reactive oxygen m.
toxic m.
metachromatic dye
metachronous
m. adenoma
m. tumor
metadysentery
MetaFluor system
Metahydrin
metaicteric
metaiodobenzylguanidine (MIBG)
metal
m. ball-tip catheter
m. bar retractor
m. clip
m. olive
m. stent
M. Z stent
metallic
m. biliary stent
m. biliary stent migration
m. embolus
m. staple
metallic-tip catheter
metalloproteinase
matrix m. (MMP)
tissue m. (TIMP (-1, -2, -3))
metallothionein
metal-tipped stent pusher
metal-weighted Silastic feeding tube

metamass
metamorphosis
fatty m.
Metamucil
metanephrine
metaplasia
Barrett m.
columnar m.
gastric m.
goblet cell m.
intestinal m.
mesothelial m.
myeloid m.
osseous m.
**metaplasia-dysplasia-carcinoma
sequence**
metaplastic
m. epithelium
m. ossification
m. polyp
metaproterenol
metaraminol
metastasis, pl. metastases
brain m.
colonic m.
cutaneous m.
diffuse m.
duodenal m.
extrahepatic m. (EHM)
extralymphatic m.
implantation m.
intramucosal m.
lymph node m.
neoplasm m.
periesophagogastric lymph
node m.
metastatic
m. adenocarcinoma
m. cancer
m. carcinoid syndrome
m. carcinoma
m. cascade
m. cholangiocarcinoma
m. disease
m. dissemination
m. implantation
m. lesion

M

NOTES

metastatic *(continued)*
  m. melanoma
  m. prostatic carcinoma
  m. renal cell carcinoma
    (MRCC)
Metastron
metasulfobenzoate
  prednisolone m.
**metasynchronous bacterial urinary
  tract infection**
Metatensin
metaxalone
met-enkephalin
  methionine-enkephalin
  met-enkephalin peptide
  plasma met-enkephalin
meteorism
meter
  Aleo m.
  Fisher Accumet pH m.
  integrating spherical power m.
  intragastric continuous pH-
    meter m.
  Synectics 6000 digital pH-
    meter m.
methacholine
methadone
methamphetamine
methane (CH4) excretor
methanethiol
Methanobrevibacter smithii
methanogen
methanogenesis
methanogenic archaea
methantheline
  m. bromide
methapyrilene
methdilazine
Methedrine
methemalbumin
methenamine
methicillin
methicillin-resistant *Staphylococcus
  aureus* **(MRSA)**
Methiodal
methionine
**methionine-enkephalin (met-
  enkephalin)**
  immunoreactive m.-e. (IRME)
methixene
method
  acid guanidine thiocyanate-
    phenol-chloroform m.

  anthrone m.
  avidin-biotin-peroxidase
    complex m.
  barostat m.
  Beck m.
  Benedict-Talbot body surface
    area m.
  Biogenex antigen retrieval m.
  Brown and Wickham pressure
    profile m.
  cholesterol-cholesteroloxidase-
    phenol 4-aminophenazone m.
  cinefluoroscopic m.
  Cockroft m.
  dye scattering m.
  ellipsoid m.
  m. of Gates
  immunohistochemical m.
  Jones and Boadi-Boatang m.
  Kaplan-Meier m.
  Lowery m.
  Metzer-Boyce m.
  microwave-assisted streptavidin-
    biotin peroxidase m.
  Morison m.
  Okamoto m.
  Papanicolaou m.
  Parker-Kerr closed m.
  pause-squeeze m.
  percutaneous sampling m.
  phosphotungstic acid-magnesium
    chloride precipitation m.
  Reddick-Saye m.
  Rehfuss m.
  Schwartz m.
  Sengstaken-Blakemore m.
  standard radioenzymatic m.
  thermally active m.
  thiourea-resorcinol m.
  trapezoid m.
  triangulation stapling m.
  Waterston m.
  Woolf m.
methotrexate (MTX)
**methotrexate, vinblastine,
  Adriamycin, and cisplatin
  (MVAC)**
methotrimeprazine
methoxamine
methoxsalen
methoxyphenamine
methscopolamine
  m. bromide

methyclothiazide
methyl
   m. CCNU
   m. red test
   m. salicylate
   m. tert-butyl ether (MTBE)
   m. tertbutyl ether stone
    dissolution
   m. tertiary butyl ether
methylaminoisobutyric acid (MeAIB)
methylatropine nitrate
methylbromide
   anisotropine m.
   homatropine m.
methylcellulose
methyldopa
   parenteral m.
methyldopate
methylene
   m. blue
   m. blue dye
   m. blue enema
   m. blue stain
3-methylhistidine
   urinary -m.
methylnitrate
   atropine m.
methylphenidate
1-methyl-4-phenyl-1,2,3,6-
   tetrahydropyridine (MTPT)
methylprednisolone
   m. acetate
6-methylprednisolone
methyl-tert-butyl ether therapy
   (MTBE therapy)
methyltestosterone
methyltestosterone-induced cholestasis
methysergide
   m. maleate
Meticorten
metoclopramide
   m. premedication
metolazone
metoprolol
   m. tartrate
Metricide disinfectant
metrifonate

metrizamide
metrizoate
MetroGel
metronidazole
metronidazole-resistant strain
Metryl 500
mets
   metastases
metyrapone
   m. stimulation test
Metzenbaum scissors
Metzer-Boyce method
Meulengracht diet
Mevacor
Mewissen infusion catheter
Meyenburg complex
mezlocillin
MFL 5000 lithotriptor
Mg++-free
MGN
   membranous glomerulonephritis
MH
   mesothelial hyperplasia
MHC
   major histocompatibility complex
   MHC class I antigen
   MHC class II antigen
MHV
   middle hepatic vein
Miami pouch
MIB-1
   monoclonal antibody M.
   M. staining
MIBG
   metaiodobenzylguanidine
MIC
   minimal inhibitory concentration
   MIC gastrostomy tube
micelle
   m. formation
Michaelis constant (Km)
Michaelis-Gutmann body
Michaelis-Menten kinetics
Michal
   M. II procedure
   M. II technique
   M. I procedure

M

NOTES

Michigan Kidney Registry
Mick
    M. prostate template
    M. TP-200 applicator
miconazole
Micro-6 ureteroscope
microabscess
micro-acini
microadenoma
microaerophilic organism
microalbuminuria
microanastomosis
    laser-assisted m. (LAMA)
microaneurysm
microangiodynamic
microangiopathy
    diabetic m.
    thrombotic m.
microballoon probe
microbiliary inflammation
microbiology
microcalcification
Microcell chamber
microcephaly
microchimerism
    donor-type m.
microchromoendoscopy
microclimate
    acid m.
microcolitis
microcolon
microcrystalline material
microcrystals
microcyst
    lymphatic m.
microcystic disease of renal
  medulla
microdensitometer
    Vickers M85a m.
microdroplet fat deposition
Microelectrode
    M. MI-506 small-caliber pH
      electrode
    M. MI-506 small-caliber probe
micro-endoprobe
    Toshiba m.-e.
microenvironment
    gastric m.
microerosion
microfibril
microfibrillar
    m. collagen hemostat (MCH)
    m. protein (MP)

microfilament bundle
microfil-associated glycoprotein
  (MAGP)
microfilter
    Minnpure m.
microflora
    colonic m.
microfluorometric measurement
microgastria
Microglass pH electrode
microgram
micrograph
    low-magnification electron m.
Microgyn II urinary incontinence
  device
microhamartoma,
    pl. microhamartomata
    biliary m.
microhematuria
microimplant
microlens cystourethroscope
microlith
microlithiasis
microlithiasis-induced pancreatitis
MicroLyzer (model SC, model 12i)
micromanipulation
    gamete m.
    oocyte m.
micromedionodular cirrhosis
micromelena
micrometastases
micrometastasis
    hematogenous m.
Micronase
microneedle holder
micronidia
micronodular cirrhosis
microparticle enzyme immunoassay
  (MEIA)
micropenis
microperforation
microphallus
micropipette
micros
    Peptostreptococcus m.
microscope
    ELMISKOP 101 electron m.
    JEM-100B and 100S
      electron m.
    JEOL 100 CX electron m.
    JEOL JSM 35 CF scanning
      electron m.
    laser m.

Olympus BH2-
epifluorescence m.
Olympus BH2-RFCA
reflecting m.
Olympus BHT-2 m.
Olympus CBK fluorescence m.
Phillips CM 12 electron m.
real-time confocal scanning
laser m.
scanning electron m.
Zeiss IDO3 phase-contrast m.
Zeiss S9 electron m.

microscopic
m. colitis
m. colitis syndrome
m. epididymal sperm aspiration
m. hematuria
m. urine examination

microscopy
electron m.
immune electron m.
immunofluorescence m.
light m.
paraffin-section light m.
polarization m.
rotary shadowing electron m.
scanning electron m.
scanning force m. (SFM)
transmission electron m.
(TEM)

microsomal damage
microsome antibody (MCHA)
microsphere
biodegradable m.
Super-Bright m.
^{99m}Tc albumin m.

Microspike
M. approximator clamp
Microsporidia
microsporidia
microsporidian
microsporidiosis
Microsporium species
microsurgery
transanal endoscopic m. (TEM)

microsurgical
m. epididymal sperm aspiration
(MESA)
m. epididymal sperm aspiration
procedure
m. extraction of ductal sperm
(MEDS)
m. extraction of sperm from
epididymis (MASE)
m. inguinal varicocelectomy

microsuture
Sharpoint m.

microtelangiectasia
microtendon
micro-tip sensor catheter
microtitration plate reader
**microtrabecular hepatocellular
carcinoma**
microtransducer
Konigsberg m.
m. technique

microtubule (MT)
micro-tubulotomy technique
microvascular
m. clamp
m. needle holder

Microvasive
M. Altertome
M. ASAP 18
M. balloon catheter
M. 5F mini-snare
M. Geenen Endotorque
guidewire
M. Glidewire
M. Glidewire guidewire
M. instrumentation
M. papillotome
M. retrieval balloon
M. Rigiflex balloon dilator
M. Rigiflex through-the-scope
balloon
M. sclerotherapy needle
M. stent
M. Ultraflex esophageal stent
system

M

NOTES

microvesicular
   m. fat
   m. steatosis
microvillous membrane
microvillus, pl. microvilli
microvolt (Uv)
microwave
   m. coagulation
   endoscopic m.
   m. hyperthermia
   m. thermotherapy
microwave-assisted streptavidin-biotin
   peroxidase method
microwell plate
micturating cystogram
micturition
   m. cystourethrogram
   m. phase
midabdominal
   m. abscess
   m. transverse incision
   m. wall
midaxillary line
midazolam
   m. conscious sedation
   m. HCl
midclavicular line (MCL)
midcolon
middle
   m. colic artery (MCA)
   m. extrahepatic bile duct
   m. hepatic vein (MHV)
   m. rectal vein
   m. rectal venous plexus
midepigastric area
midepigastrium
midesophageal diverticulum
midesophagus
midgastric electrode
midgut
   m. volvulus with malrotation
midline
   m. abdominal crease
   m. incision
   m. lower abdominal incision
   m. upper abdominal incision
midrectal area
midregion PTH
midsigmoid colon
midstomach
midureteral calculus
MIE
   meconium ileus equivalent

Miescher cheilitis granulomatosa
migraine
   abdominal m.
migrating motor complex (MMC)
migration
   calculus m.
   gallstone m.
   gastrostomy tube m.
   intravesical m.
   lymphocyte m.
   metallic biliary stent m.
   tube m.
Mik
   Mikulicz
   Mik clamp
   Mik gastrostomy tube
   Mik retractor
Mikulicz (Mik)
   M. clamp
   M. colostomy
   M. drain
   M. gastroscope
   M. operation
   M. pad
   M. peritoneal forceps
   M. pyloroplasty
   M. retractor
mil
   delta per m.
mild distress
Miles
   M. abdominoperineal resection
   M. operation
   M. resection
   M. V.I.P. 300 vacuum
     infiltration processor
milia (pl. of milium)
miliaria rubra
miliary tuberculosis
milium, pl. milia
milk
   acidophilus m.
   m. diet
   m. of magnesia (MOM)
   m. protein antibody
   m. sickness
milk-alkali syndrome
milking
   m. of intestine
milk-sensitive colitis
milky
   m. ascites
   m. fluid

Millar catheter
Millard mouth gag
Miller
    M. cystoscope
    M. rectal forceps
    M. rectal scissors
Miller-Abbott
    M.-A. intestinal tube
    M.-A. tube
Miller-Senn retractor
Millex-GS 0.22 mm pore-size filter
Millex-GV 0.22-mm filter
"Millie" female urinal
millijoules (mJ)
milliliter (mL)
millimeters of mercury (mmHg,
    mm Hg)
millimolar concentration
millimoles per liter (mmol/L)
Millin
    M. bladder retractor
    M. forceps
milliosmole/kilogram (mosm/kg)
Millipore
    M. filter
milliwatts (mW)
Mill-Rose
    M.-R. flexible endoscopic
      overtube
    M.-R. RiteBite biopsy forceps
Milroy disease
mind-bladder syndrome
mineral
    divalent m.
mineralocorticoid
Ming gastric carcinoma
    classification
miniature
    m. probe
    m. ultrasound suction device
MiniBard catheter
minilaparoscope
    m. cholecystectomy
    Storz m.
minilaparotomy
minimal
    m. access surgery

    m. inhibitory concentration
      (MIC)
    m. transurethral resection of
      prostate (M-TURP)
minimal-change
    m.-c. disease
    m.-c. nephrotic syndrome
minimal-lesion nephrotic syndrome
minimicrosphere
minipapillotome
Minipress
minipump
    Alzer Model 2001 osmotic m.
Miniscope
    Candela M.
mini-snare
    Microvasive 5F m.-s.
mini-VAB
    vinblastine, actinomycin D, and
     bleomycin
mink cell bioassay
Minnesota
    M. antilymphocyte globulin
    M. tube
Minnpure microfilter
Minocin
minocycline
minor papilla
minoxidil
Mintezol
minus
    omentum m.
minute
    m. bleeding mucosal ulcer
    counts per m. (cpm, CPM)
    m. lesion
    m. polypoid lesion
mirabilis
    Proteus m.
Mirizzi syndrome
mirror-image artifact
misakiensis
    Streptomyces m.
mismatch
    HLA m.
    V/Q m.

M

NOTES

misoprostol
   m. protection
misperfusion
   gastroduodenal m.
misplaced gland
Mission VED VCD
Missouri catheter
**Misstique female external urinary
   collector**
MIT
   mean input time
Mitek bone anchor
mitochondria
   giant m.
mitochondrial
   m. antibody
   m. complex
   m. ethanol oxidase system
   m. fatty acid β-oxidation
   m. glutamate dehydrogenase
      pathway
   m. immunological study
   m. phosphate-dependent
      glutaminase
mitogen
mitogenic
   m. stimulation
   m. stimulus
mitomycin, mitomycin C
   m. adsorbed onto activated
      charcoal (M-CH)
   m. transarterial embolization
      treatment
mitosis count
mitosis-karyorrhexis index (MKI)
mitotic
   m. activity
   m. index
mitoxantrone
Mitrofanoff
   M. appendicovesicostomy
   M. catheterizable channel
   M. conduit
   M. continent urinary diversion
      technique
   M. mechanism
   M. neourethra
   M. principle
   M. procedure
   M. stoma
   M. technique
   M. valve
mitrogenic effect

Mitrolan
Mitscherlich test
mittelschmerz
Mivacron
mivacurium chloride
mixed
   m. cirrhosis
   m. connective tissue disease
      (MCTD)
   m. connective tissue disorder
   m. essential cryoglobulinemia
   m. germ cell-sex cord stromal
      tumor
   m. growth on culture
   m. hemorrhoids
   m. hyperlipidemia
   m. hyperplastic/adenomatous
      gastric polyp
   m. incontinence
   m. intralobular fibrosis
   m. structure
mixed-cholesterol gallstone
Mixter
   M. clamp
   M. dilating probe
   M. dissector
   M. forceps
   M. gallstone forceps
   M. hemostat
mixture
   amino acid-glucose m.
   citric acid bladder m.
   eutectic m.
   sodium citrate and potassium
      citrate m.
mizoribine
mJ
   millijoules
MK
   menaquinone
MKI
   mitosis-karyorrhexis index
MKII automated scanner
MKIII
   Digitrapper M.
mL
   milliliter
MLN
   mesenteric lymph node
MLP
   multiple lymphomatous polyposis
MMAP index

MMC
migrating motor complex
murine mesangial cell
mmHg, mm Hg
millimeters of mercury
mmol/L
millimoles per liter
MMP
matrix metalloproteinase
MMUA
macromolecular uronate
MN
mononuclear
MN cell
MN infiltrate
M-O
Haley M-O
MoAb
monoclonal antibody
Moban
mobile
m. gallbladder
mobility
electrophoretic m.
mobilization
Mobin-Uddin umbrella
Moctanin
modality
dialysis m.
Modane
M. Soft
M. Versabran
model
M. 500F electromagnetic
flowmeter
M. IL 750, AA
spectrophotometer
M. 3-60 mass spectroscopy
m. 440 M1.5, M4 electrode
M. 5500 vapor pressure
osmometer
moderate distress
moderately differentiated adenoma
Moderil
modification
Al-Ghorab m.
Kelly-Kennedy m.

Muzsnai m.
Raz m.
modified
m. barium swallow (MBS)
m. Cantwell technique
m. caulking gun
m. Essed-Schroeder
corporoplasty
m. Gibson incision
m. Hassan open technique
m. liver diet
m. method of Pugh
m. Minnesota tube
m. Norfolk procedure
m. polyethylene dilator
m. Sacks-Vine push-pull
technique
m. sham feeding
m. Whitehead
hemorrhoidectomy
m. Young urethroplasty
modulation
obstruction-induced m.
pressure amplitude m.
Modulith
M. SL20 device for ESWL
M. SL 20 lithotriptor
Moduretic
modus
Moersch esophagoscope
MOF
multiple organ failure
mofetil
mycophenolate m.
Mogen clamp
Moh microsurgery technique
Mohr test
moiety
steroid m.
moist
m. laparotomy pack
m. mucous membrane
Moi-Stir
molar
m. pregnancy
mold

M

NOTES

375

mole
    hydatidiform m.
molecular
    m. cloning
    m. cloning and sequencing
    m. genetic alteration
    m. marker
    m. study
    m. weight (mol wt)
molecule
    adhesion m.
    CD4 m.
    CD8 m.
    Class II MHC m.
    Class I MHC m.
    HLA-DQ2 m.
    lithostathine m.
    messenger RNA m.
    monocyte adhesion m.
molecule-1
    endothelial leukocyte
      adhesion m. (ELAM-1)
molindone
**molluscum contagiosum virus
(MCV)**
Molnar disk
mol wt
MOM
    milk of magnesia
Monfort operation
mongolian spot
monilial
    m. esophagitis
    m. infection
moniliasis
Monistat
monitor
    Contimed II pelvic floor
      muscle m.
    Dinamap Plus m.
    Dobbhoff biofeedback m.
    gastric pH m.
    Gould pressure m.
    24-hour ambulatory gastric
      pH m.
    in-line blood gas m.
    Interceptor M3 triple-channel,
      solid state m.
    return electrode m. (REM)
    RigiScan penile tumescence
      and rigidity m.
    television m.
    video m.

monitoring
    ambulatory m.
    ambulatory pH m.
    ambulatory urodynamic m.
    clinical m.
    esophageal pH m.
    fluoroscopic m.
    heart rate m.
    24-hour ambulatory esophageal
      pH m.
    intracranial pressure m.
    intraesophageal pH m. (EpHM)
    nocturnal penile tumescence m.
    NPT m.
    pH m.
monitor/recorder
    Gastroreflex ambulatory pH m.
Monitur
mono
    monocyte
monoamine oxidase inhibitor
monoclonal
    m. antibody (MAB, mAb,
      MoAb)
    m. antibody BR96
    m. antibody ED1
    m. antibody MIB-1
    m. antibody scintigraphic scan
    m. antibody therapy
    m. antigen
    m. anti-Hbc
    4B4 m. antibody
    m. IgM
    4KB5 m. antibody
    m. light chain
monoclonality by genetic analysis
Monocryl suture
monocyte (mono)
    m. adhesion molecule
    m. chemoattract protein (MCP)
    WBC m.'s
monocytes/macrophages
monocytogenes
    Listeria m.
Monodox
Monodral
monoethylglycinexylidide (MEGX)
**monoethyl glycine xylidide liver
function test**
monofilament
    m. nylon suture
    m. suture

monohydrate
  cefadroxil m.
  doxycycline m.
monohydroxy bile salt
monokine
monolayer
  cobblestone-like m.
MonoLith single-piece mechanical lithotriptor
monomicrobial bacterascites
mononuclear (MN)
  m. cell recruitment
  m. dyspepsia
  m. histiocytic portal infiltrate
mononucleotide
  flavin m.
mono-octanoin
  m.-o. infusion
monophosphate
  5'-m.
  adenosine m. (AMP)
  cyclic adenosine m. (cAMP)
  5'-cyclic adenosine m. (cAMP)
  cyclic guanosine m. (cGMP)
  5'-cyclic guanosine m. (cGMP)
  guanosine m.
  guanosine 5'-m. (GMP)
monopolar
  BICAP m.
  m. coagulation
  m. electrocautery
  m. electrocoagulation
  m. probe
monosaccharide
monosialoganglioside
monosialosyl Lea
monospot
monosymptomatic enuresis
monotherapy
  androgen ablative m.
mons
  m. plasty
  m. veneris
Montezuma revenge
Montgomery
  M. abdominal straps
  M. salivary bypass tube

  M. strap dressing
  M. tape
moon
  m. facies
  M. rectal retractor
Moore gallstone scoop
MOP-Videoplan morphometric system
Moraxella
morbidity
  febrile m.
  operative m.
  treatment m.
morbid obesity
morbus
  cholera m.
morcellation technique
morcellator
  Cook tissue m.
  electric tissue m.
  high-speed electrical tissue m.
  tissue m.
Morgagni
  M. appendix
  column of M.
  M. crypt
  M. hernia
Morganella morganii
morganii
  Morganella m.
  Proteus m.
Morganstern
  M. aspiration/injection system
  M. cystoscope
moribund
Mori knife
Morison
  M. method
  M. pouch
morning diarrhea
Moro-Heisler diet
Moro reflex
morphine
  m. narcotic analgesic therapy
morphine-neostigmine test
morphogenesis
morphologic stage

NOTES

M

morphology
Dogiel type (I, II) m.
Gram-stain m.
morphometric criteria
morphometry
nuclear m.
morrhuate
m. sclerosant
sodium m.
mortality
intraoperative m.
mortis
livor m.
rigor m.
mosaic duodenal mucosal pattern
mosaicism
XX male m.
Moschcowitz procedure
Moscontin
Mosher esophagoscope
mosm/kg
milliosmole/kilogram
**900 mOsmolar amino acid-glucose
solution (P-900)**
mosquito
m. forceps
m. hemostat
m. hemostatic clamp
Moss
M. gastrostomy tube
M. G-tube
M. G-tube PEG kit
M. Mark IV tube
M. PEG kit
M. T-anchor introducer gun
M. tube
Mosse syndrome
Mostofi grade prostate cancer
mother cyst
mother/daughter endoscope
mother-infant dyad
**mother-to-infant transmission of
hepatitis C virus**
motif
coiled coil m.
motilide
motilin
m. plasma level
motility
altered sperm m.
colon m.
colonic m.
m. disorder

esophageal m.
gastrointestinal m.
ineffective esophageal m.
(IEM)
interdigestive antroduodenal m.
prefreeze m.
reduced m.
sequential m.
Motilium
Motilyn
motion
full range of m.
limited range of m.
paradoxic m.
passive range of m.
m. picture camera
range of m.
m. sickness
motogenesis
motogenic
motoneuron
enteric excitatory m.
enteric inhibitory m.
motor
m. activity
m. meal barium GI series
m. oil peritoneal fluid
m. quiescence
m. syringe
m. test meal
m. urgency
motorneuron, motoneuron
Motrin
mottled testis
moulage sign
mound
infraumbilical m.
Moure esophagoscope
mouse
peritoneal m.
Mousseau-Barbin prosthetic tube
mouth
m. breathing
m. gag
m. guard
mouthguard
Oxyguard oxygenating m.
movable testis
movement
bowel m. (BM)
dys-coordinate hyoid m.
pelvic floor m.
periodic leg m. (PLM)

segmentation m.
symmetric face m.
tongue m.
vermicular m.
moxisylyte injection
MOX TM-100 portable renal
preservation machine
Moynihan
    M. bile duct probe
    M. clamp
    M. gall duct forceps
    M. gallstone probe
    M. gallstone scoop
    M. test
MP
  mesenteric panniculitis
  microfibrillar protein
6-MP
  6-mercaptopurine
MPD
  main pancreatic duct
MPGN
  membranoproliferative
    glomerulonephritis
    MPGN type II
MPGN type I
  membranoproliferative
    glomerulonephritis type I
M-phase
MP-RAGE
  magnetization prepared-rapid
    gradient-echo
MRCC
  metastatic renal cell carcinoma
MRDM
  malnutrition-related diabetes mellitus
MRI
  magnetic resonance imaging
    endorectal surface coil MRI
    rectal coil MRI
    MRI scan
mRNA
  messenger ribonucleoprotein acid
  messenger RNA
    β-actin mRNA
    AR mRNA
    clusterin mRNA

    cotransporter mRNA
    gastrin mRNA
    glomerular fibronectin mRNA
    HSP-70 mRNA
    IGF-binding protein-1 mRNA
    IGF-1R mRNA
    preproEt-1 mRNA
    taurine cotransporter mRNA
    TCT mRNA
MRSA
  methicillin-resistant *Staphylococcus*
    aureus
MRT
  mean resistance time
MS-1 hepatitis
MS-2 hepatitis
MSAO
  meal-stimulated acid output
MS Classique balloon dilatation
catheter
MSI nylon membrane
MSOF
  multiple system organ failure
MT
  microtubule
MTBE
  methyl tert-butyl ether
    MTBE gallstone dissolution
    MTBE therapy
MT12, MT20, MT24
  Ultrase M.
MTPT
  1-methyl-4-phenyl-1,2,3,6-
    tetrahydropyridine
M-TURP
  minimal transurethral resection of
    prostate
MTX
  methotrexate
MUC
  mucosal ulcerative colitis
mucin
  intracytoplasmic m.
mucin-hypersecreting tumor
mucinous
    m. adenocarcinoma
    m. adenoma

M

NOTES

mucinous *(continued)*
   m. carcinoma
   m. cystadenoma
   m. cystic neoplasm
   m. cystic tumor
   m. ductal ectasia
   m. pancreatic tumor
mucin-producing
   m.-p. adenocarcinoma
   m.-p. cancer
   m.-p. tumor
mucin-type glycolipid
mucocele
   m. of gallbladder
mucociliary clearance
mucocolitis
mucocutaneous
   m. hemorrhoids
   m. pigmentation of Peutz-
     Jeghers syndrome
mucoenteritis
mucoepidermoid carcinoma
mucoid
   m. secretion
   m. stool
mucolipidosis, pl. mucolipidoses
mucolytic
   m. agent
mucolytic-antifoam solution
mucomembranous enteritis
Mucomyst
mucoprotein
   Tamm-Horsfall m. (THM)
mucopurulent
   m. cervicitis
Mucor
   M. corymbifera
Mucorales
Mucoreae
mucormycosis
   m. esophagitis
   gastric m.
   isolated renal m.
   pulmonary m.
mucosa
   antral m.
   antrofundal m.
   biopsy of gastric m.
   blanching of m.
   buccal m.
   burned-out m.
   cardiac stomach m.
   cardiac-type m.

   cobblestone m.
   cobblestoning of m.
   colorectal m.
   congested m.
   corpus gastric m.
   denuded m.
   duodenal m.
   ectopic gastric m.
   edematous hyperemic m.
   esophageal m.
   foveolar gastric m.
   foveolosulciolar gastric m.
   friable m.
   fundic m.
   gastric m.
   gastric muscularis m.
   gastroduodenal m.
   heterotopic gastric m.
   hyperemic m.
   inflamed m.
   inlet patch m.
   intestinal m.
   lamina muscularis m.
   multifocal ectopic gastric m.
   muscularis m.
   normal-appearing m.
   oxyntic m.
   pyloric m.
   rectal m.
   rose thorn ulcer of m.
   sloughing of m.
   sulciolar gastric m.
   tethering of m.
   thumbprinting of m.
   vaginal m.
mucosa-associated
   m.-a. lymphoid tissue (MALT)
   m.-a. lymphoid tissue
     lymphoma (MALT lymphoma)
mucosal
   m. abnormality
   m. adenocarcinoma
   m. aneuploidy
   m. angiography
   m. atrophy
   m. background
   m. barrier maturation
   m. biopsy
   m. blood hemoglobin
   m. border
   m. bridge
   m. bridging
   m. cell proliferation

m. disease
m. diverticulum
m. dysplasia
m. esophageal ring
m. fatty acid
m. fold
m. gastric ulcer
m. graft
m. guideline pattern
m. hexosamine content
m. homogenate
m. ileal diaphragm
m. injury
m. ischemia
m. island
m. junction
m. lesion
m. line
m. lymphoid follicle
m. nodularity
m. pallor
m. pattern
m. pit
m. PMN grade
m. polyp
m. proctectomy
m. prostaglandin synthesis
m. ring
m. stripping
m. suspensory ligament
m. tear
m. tongue
m. ulcerative colitis (MUC)
m. urease
m. vaccine
m. vascular dilation
m. vascular permeability
m. washout
m. web
mucosa-to-mucosa anastomosis
mucosectomy
endoanal m.
rectal m.
mucositis
mucous
m. colitis
m. depletion

m. diarrhea
m. enteritis
m. fistula
m. gel thickness
m. lake of the stomach
m. membrane
m. membrane pemphigoid
m. neck cell
m. patch
m. stool
mucoviscidosis
mucus
excess m.
gastric m.
mucus-secreting
m.-s. cell
m.-s. gland
mud
biliary m.
Mueller-Hinton-supplemented agar plate
Muir hemorrhoid forceps
Muir-Torre syndrome
Mui Scientific pressurized capillary infusion system
mulberry
m. calculus
m. gallstone
m. lesion
m. stone
Mulholland sphincterotomy
muliebris
hydrocele m.
mulleri
Streptococcus m.
müllerian
m. duct
m. duct cyst
m. duct derivation syndrome
m. inhibiting factor
m. remnants
Müller maneuver
multiacinar regenerative nodule
multicentricity
multichannel cystometry
multicystic
m. dysplastic kidney

M

NOTES

multicystic *(continued)*
  m. kidney (MCK)
  m. renal dysplasia
multidrug regimen
multifiber catheter
multifire clip applicator
Multi-Flex stent
multifocal
  m. atrophic gastritis (MAG)
  m. ectopic gastric mucosa
multiforme
  erythema m. (EM)
multiloaded clip applier
multiload occlusive clip applicator
multilobar kidney
multilocular
  m. cyst
  m. cystic nephroma
multilocularis
  Echinococcus m.
multilumen
  m. manometric catheter
  m. probe
multimodal protocol
multiorgan
  m. hernia
  m. system failure
multiple
  m. biopsy
  m. concentric ring sign
  m. endocrine adenomatosis
    type I (MEA-I)
  m. endocrine adenomatosis
    type II (MEA-II)
  m. endocrine neoplasia (MEN)
  m. endocrine neoplasia 2A
    (MEN 2A)
  m. endocrine neoplasia 2B
    (MEN 2B)
  m. endocrine neoplasia I
  m. endocrine neoplasia
    syndrome (MENS)
  m. familial polyposis
  m. hamartoma syndrome
  m. hepatitis virus infection
  m. lymphomatous polyposis
    (MLP)
  m. myeloma
  m. nodule
  m. organ failure (MOF)
  m. polyp
  m. recurrent renal colic
  m. sclerosis

  m. stone
  m. system atrophy
  m. system organ failure
    (MSOF)
multipolar
  m. coagulation
  m. electrocoagulation
  m. neuron
multiseptate gallbladder
multishot speedbander
multisynaptic pathway
multivariate
  m. analysis
multocida
  Pasteurella m.
mumps
  m. epididymitis
Munich inclusion criteria
Munro point
mural thrombus
murine
  m. B16 cell
  m. graft
  m. hepatitis
  m. kidney
  m. lymphoid cell
  m. mesangial cell (MMC)
  m. mesangial cell line
  m. proximal tubule cell
  m. spleen
  3T3 m. fibroblast
muris
  Cryptosporidium m.
murmur
  continuous m.
  diastolic m.
  systolic m.
muromonab-CD3
Murphy
  M. button
  M. common duct dilator
  M. drip
  M. gallbladder retractor
  M. sign
muscarinic
  m. activity
  m. blockade
  m. cholinergic agonist
  m. receptor
muscle
  adductor brevis m.
  adductor longus m.
  m. atrophy

cremaster m.
cricopharyngeus m.
dartos m.
external anal sphincter m.
gastrointestinal smooth m.
gracilis m.
m. guarding
m. hypertrophy
ileococcygeus m.
labia major m.
labia minor m.
m. layer disease
levator ani m.
lower esophageal sphincter
  circular m.
obturator internus m.
paraspinous m.
pectoralis m.
periurethral striated m.
psoas m.
pubococcygeus m.
rectourethral m.
rectus abdominis m.
rhabdosphincter m.
m. sensory receptor
smooth m.
m. spasm
submucosal vaginal m.
superficial trigonal m.
urogenital sphincter m.
vascular smooth m.
m. wasting
muscle-splitting
  m.-s. incision
  m.-s. technique
muscular
  m. dystrophy
  m. esophageal ring
muscularis
  m. mucosa
  m. propria
  tunica m.
  m. tunnel closure
musculature
  electrophysiology of the
    gastric m.
musculocutaneous

mushroom
  Amanita m.
  m. catheter
  m. poisoning
mushroom-shaped mass
mushy stool
musical bowel sounds
mustard seed
mutagenic
  m. effect
Mutamycin
**mutated colorectal carcinoma
  (MCC)**
mutation
  endogenous m.
  germline m.
  Kirsten-ras oncogen m.
  p53 m.
  splice-cite m.
MutL
  gene M.
MutS gene
Muzsnai modification
MVAC
  methotrexate, vinblastine,
    Adriamycin, and cisplatin
MVO
  mean venous outflow
mW
  milliwatts
myasthenia
  m. gravis
mycelial
  m. antibody
  m. phase
mycetism, mycetismus
  m. gastrointestinalis
mycobacteria
  Runyon group III m.
mycobacterial
  m. antibody
  m. disease
  m. spheroplast
mycobacteriology
Mycobacterium
  M. avium (MAI)
  M. avium complex

M

NOTES

Mycobacterium (continued)
  M. avium-intracellulare
  M. bovis
  M. bovis BCG
  M. infection
  M. intracellulare
  M. leprae
  M. tuberculosis
mycogastritis
Mycolog-II
mycology
mycophenolate mofetil
Mycoplasma
  M. hominis
mycoplasma
  m. urethritis
mycosis, pl. mycoses
  endemic deep m.
  gastric m.
  m. intestinalis
Mycostatin
mycotic aneurysm
Mycotrim triphasic culture system
MycroMesh
myectomy
  anorectal m.
myelocele
myelocystocele
myelodysplasia
myelography
myeloid metaplasia
myelolipoma
  adrenal m.
myeloma
  multiple m.
  plasmablastic m.
  m. protein
myelomeningocele
myelomonocytic cell line
myelopathy
  HTLV-I-associated m.
myeloperoxidase
myeloperoxidase-H2O2-halide system
myelophthisic splenomegaly
myeloproliferative
  m. disease
  m. disorder
myelosuppression
myenteric
  m. ganglion cell
  m. plexus
myentericus
  plexus m.

Myers-Fine test
myiasis
  intestinal m.
Mylanta
Mylanta-II
Mylicon
Mylius test
myoblastic myoma
myoblastoma
  granular cell m.
myocardial
  m. infarction
  m. ischemia
  m. revascularization
myocelialgia
myoclonus
myoclonus-opsoclonus syndrome
myocutaneous flap
myoelectric activity
myoelectrical
myofibroblast
myofibroma
myogenic tumor
myoglobinuria
Myojector
myolysis
myoma
  ball m.
  myoblastic m.
  red degeneration of uterine m.
myopathy
  familial visceral m.
  hereditary internal anal
    sphincter m.
  ipecac-induced m.
  sporadic visceral m.
myorrhaphy
myosin
  m. light-chain kinase
myotomy
  circular m.
  cricoid m.
  cricopharyngeal m.
  esophageal m.
  Heller m.
  longitudinal m.
Myotonachol
myotonic
  m. dystrophy
  m. muscular dystrophy
MyoTrac EMG
Myriadlase Side-Fire laser
myringotomy tube

Mytelase
myxedema
    m. ascites
myxofibroma

myxomembranous colitis
myxorrhea
    m. gastrica

NOTES

NABS
    normoactive bowel sounds
N-acetyl-5-ASA (Ac-5-ASA)
N-**acetylecysteine**
N-acetyl-β-D-glucosaminidase
N-acetyl-β-glucosaminidase (NAG)
N-acetyl-p-benzoquinoneimine
    (NAPQI)
Nachlas-Linton esophagogastric
    balloon tamponade device
nadolol
NADPH
    nicotinamide adenine dinucleotide
    phosphate
      NADPH diaphorase stain
      NADPH oxidase
naeslundii
    Actinomyces n.
NaF
    sodium fluorescein
nafcillin
nafoxidine
NAG
    N-acetyl-β-glucosaminidase
    nonagglutinable
      NAG lysosomal marker
        enzyme
nagging pain
NA+-glucose cotransporter
Na+/H+ antiporter
    Na+/H+ a. activity
    amiloride-sensitive,
      electroneutral Na+/H+ a.
nail
    n. bed
    thickened n.
naive lymphocyte
Na/K-ATPase
    N.-A. activity
NaK-ATPase membrane
Nakayama test
nalbuphine
Naldecon
naldrolone decanoate
nalidixic acid
NA+-linked cotransport system
nalmefene
naloxone
naloxone hydrochloride
NAMI DDV ligator

[13N]ammonia
nana
    Hymenolepis n.
NANB
    non-A, non-B
      NANB hepatitis
NANC
    nonadrenergic noncholinergic
      NANC inhibitory transmitter
NaP
    sodium phosphate-based laxative
naphazoline
naphthylamine
napkin-ring annular lesion
nappies
    electronic recording n.
NAPQI
    N-acetyl-p-benzoquinoneimine
Naprosyn
naproxen
    n. sodium
napthylurea
    polysulfonated n.
Naqua
Narcan
Narco
    N. Bio-Systems rectilinear
      recorder
    N. Bio-Systems MMS 200
      physiograph tracing
    N. esophageal motility machine
narcotic
    n. bowel syndrome
Nardil
Nardi test
naris, pl. nares
narrow
    n. albumin gradient ascites
    n. lens
narrow-caliber duct
narrowing
    bird-beak n.
    hourglass n.
    luminal n.
nasal
    Concentraid N.
    n. deformity
    n. discharge
    n. feeding
    n. intubation

nasal *(continued)*
  n. polyp
  n. trumpet
Nasalcrom
Nasalide
nasobiliary
  n. drain
  n. drainage
  n. drainage catheter
  n. tube
nasocystic
  n. catheter
  n. drain
  n. drainage tube
nasoduodenal feeding tube
nasoenteric
  n. feeding tube
  n. tube
nasogastric (NG)
  n. aspirate
  n. decompression
  n. drainage
  n. feeding tube
  n. intubation
  n. lavage
  n. suction
  n. tube (NGT)
nasoileal tube
nasojejunal (NJ)
  n. feeding
  n. feeding tube
  n. tube
nasopancreatic
  n. catheter
  n. drainage
nasopharyngeal
  n. angiofibroma
  n. reflux
nasotracheal intubation
nasovesicular
  n. catheter
  n. catheter technique
natelenis
National
  N. Association of Anorexia Nervosa and Associated Disorders
  N. general purpose cystoscope
  N. Prostatic Cancer Project
  The N. Cooperative Dialysis Study
native
  n. pancreatic secretin receptor

  n. renal biopsy
  n. valve bacterial endocarditis
NA+ transport system
natriuresis
  pressure n.
natural
  n. killer (NK)
  n. killer cell
Naturetin
nausea
  epidemic n.
  postprandial n.
  n. and vomiting (N&V)
nauseant
nauseate
nauseous
Navane
navicular abdomen
navicularis
  fossa n.
NBC
  nephroblastomatosis complex
NBD
  nucleotide-binding domain
N-benzoyl-L-tyrosyl-P-aminobenzoic
  N.-b.-L.-t.-P.-a. acid
  N.-b.-L.-t.-P.-a. acid excretion test
NBP
  nonbacterial prostatitis
NBT-PABA test
NBVV
  nonbleeding visible vessel
NC
  nephrocalcin
NCPF
  noncirrhotic portal fibrosis
N-deethylation
NDF
  new differentiation factor
Nd:YAG
  N. laser
  N. laser irradiation
  N. laser therapy
near-infrared electronic endoscope
nebulizer
  jet n.
NEC
  necrotizing enterocolitis
Necator americanus
necatoriasis
neck
  humeral n.

n. of pancreas
tonic n.
necropsy
necrosectomy
necrosis
acute sclerosing hyaline n.
(ASHN)
acute tubular n.
avascular n.
Balser fatty n.
biliary piecemeal n.
bowel n.
bridging n.
cell n.
central n.
centrilobular acidophilic n.
coagulation n.
colonic n.
distal renal tubular n.
electrocoagulation n.
ethanol-induced tumor n.
(ETN)
fatty n.
fibrosing piecemeal n.
hepatocellular n.
hepatocyte n.
infected n.
intestinal n.
ischemia n.
liquefactive n.
massive hepatic n.
papillary n.
patchy n.
perivenular confluent n.
piecemeal n.
postischemic tubular n.
pressure n.
puromycin aminonucleoside n.
renal papillary n. (RPN)
spinal cord n.
spontaneous penile ischemic n.
sterile pancreatic n.
strangulation n.
subacute n.
subacute hepatic n.
submassive n.
tissue n.

tubular n.
tumor n.
necrotic
n. cirrhosis
n. hemorrhagic colitis
n. hemorrhoids
n. tissue
n. ulceration
necroticans
enteritis n.
necrotizing
n. bowel vasculitis
n. enterocolitis (NEC)
n. fasciitis
n. infection
n. pancreatitis
n. vasculitis
n. vasculitis of bowel
needle
ASAP channel cut automated
biopsy n.
ASAP prostate biopsy n.
aspirating n.
B-D Safety-Gard n.
bi-curved n.
n. biopsy
n. biopsy diagnosis
Biopty cut n.
blunt n.
butterfly n.
CE-24 n.
Chiba n.
circle n.
Cobb-Ragbe n.
Colopinto transjugular n.
concentric n.
Corson n.
n. count
curved transjugular n.
cutting n.
cutting LR n.
diathermic precut n.
n. driver
Durrani n.
Durrani dorsal vein complex
ligation n.
n. electrode

NOTES

N

needle *(continued)*
n. electrode electromyography
electrosurgical n.
fine n.
flexible aspiration n.
French eye n.
gastrointestinal n.
GIP/Medi-Globe prototype n.
Greenwald n.
Grice suture n.
Hemoject n.
n. holder
n. hydrophone
Jamshidi n.
Jamshidi liver biopsy n.
Keith n.
KeyMed disposable variceal
injection n.
Klatskin biopsy n.
Klatskin liver biopsy n.
n. knife
Mayo n.
Mayo trocar-point n.
Menghini n.
Menghini biopsy n.
Menghini liver biopsy n.
Microvasive sclerotherapy n.
Olympus NM-K-series
sclerotherapy n.
Olympus NM-L-series n.
optical n.
n. papillotome
Pentax prototype n.
pneumoperitoneum n.
Promex biopsy n.
PS-2 n.
sclerotherapy n.
Seldinger n.
Silverman n.
Silverman-Boeker n.
skinny n.
skinny Chiba n.
smaller gauge n.
Spinelli biopsy n.
Stifcore transbronchial
aspiration n.
Sure-Cut biopsy n.
n. suspension procedure
suture-release n.
swaged n.
swaged-on n.
tapered n.
through-the-scope injection n.

n. tip catheter
n. tracheoesophageal puncture
n. tract
Tru-Cut n.
Tru-Cut biopsy n.
Tru Taper Ethalloy n.
TT-3 n.
Turner-Warwick n.
Variject n.
Veress n.
Vim-Silverman n.
Vim-Silverman biopsy n.
Williams n.
winged steel n.
Yang n.
needle-catheter
n.-c. jejunostomy
needle-knife
n.-k. fistulotome
n.-k. papillotome
n.-k. papillotomy
n.-k. sphincterotome
n.-k. sphincterotomy
n.-k. technique
needleless system
needlescope device
needle-tip laparoscopic electrode
needle-tipped sphincterotome
needle-tract seeding
negative
n. immunofluorescence
n. laparotomy
n. nitrogen balance
n. pressure-controlled tube
n. pressure overtube
n. pressure tube
NegGram
negligible blood loss
Negus rigid esophagoscope
Neisseria gonorrhoeae
Neisser syringe
Neivert polyp hook
Nélaton
N. catheter
N. fold
N. rubber tube drain
N. sphincter
**Nellcor Durasensor adult oxygen
transducer**
Nelson
N. forceps
N. scissors

nematode
    n. infection
Nembutal
NEMD
    nonspecific esophageal motility
    disorder
neoadjuvant
    n. antiandrogenic treatment
    n. hormonal deprivation
    n. total androgen ablation
neo-anal sphincter
neobladder
    Camey n.
    decompensated n.
    gastric n.
    ileal n.
    ileocolonic n.
    sigmoid n.
neocholangiole
Neocholex
neocystostomy
neodymium:YAG laser therapy
neodymium:yttrium-aluminum garnet
neodymium:yttrium garnet laser
    (Nd:YAG laser)
neoformans
    Candida n.
neointimal
    n. hyperplasia
Neoloid
neomeatus
Neomed electrocautery
neomycin
neonatal
    n. cholestasis
    n. conjugated
      hyperbilirubinemia
    n. hepatitis
    n. jaundice
neonatorum
    icterus n.
neopenis
neophallus
neoplasia
    cervical intraepithelial n. (CIN)
    colonic n.

    intratubular germ cell n.
      (ITGCN)
    multiple endocrine n. (MEN)
    multiple endocrine n. 2A
      (MEN 2A)
    multiple endocrine n. 2B
      (MEN 2B)
    multiple endocrine n. I
    penile intraepithelial n.
    prostatic intraepithelial n. (PIN)
    n. risk
neoplasm
    bladder n.
    colorectal n.
    genitourinary n.
    megacystic mucinous n.
    n. metastasis
    mucinous cystic n.
    non-ductectatic cystic n.
    periampullary n.
    prostatic n.
    retroperitoneal n.
    n. staging
    stomach n.
neoplastic
    n. cell proliferation
    n. disease
    n. lesion
    n. polyp
    n. potential
    n. renal mass
    n. tissue
    n. transformation
Neopterin
Neoral
neorectal emptying
neorectum
neoscrotum
neosphincter
    gracilis n.
    stimulated gracilis n.
Neosporin G.U.
neostigmine
neoterminal ileum
neotransformation
    papillomatous n.

N

NOTES

neourethra
  Mitrofanoff n.
Neo-Vadrin
neovagina
  gracilis myocutaneous n.
  skin graft n.
neovascular bundle
neovascularization
nephelometry
nephradenoma
nephralgia
nephralgic
nephrasthenia
nephratonia, nephratony
nephrectasis, nephrectasia
nephrectomy
  abdominal n.
  adjuvant n.
  anterior n.
  apical polar n.
  Balkan n.
  extracorporeal partial n.
  extraperitoneal laparoscopic n.
  laparoscopic n.
  laser partial n.
  live donor n.
  lumbar n.
  paraperitoneal n.
  partial n.
  perifascial n.
  posterior n.
  radical n.
  transperitoneal laparoscopic n.
    (TLN)
  transplant n.
  unilateral n.
nephredema
nephrelcosis
nephritic
  n. calculus
  n. sediment
  n. syndrome
nephritis, pl. nephritides
  acute n.
  acute focal bacterial n.
    (AFBN)
  acute interstitial n. (AIN)
  allergic interstitial n.
  antiglomerular basement
    membrane n.
  antiglomerular basement
    membrane-negative crescentric
    glomerular n.

  anti-Thy-1 n.
  autoimmune interstitial n.
  crescentic n.
  hemorrhagic n.
  hereditary n.
  interstitial n.
  lupus n.
  mercuric chloride-induced n.
  nephrotoxic antiglomerular
    basement membrane
    antibody n.
  nephrotoxic serum n.
  passive Heymann n. (PHN)
  salt-losing n.
  serum n.
  suppurative n.
  trench n.
  tubulointerstitial n. (TIN)
  tubulointestinal n.
nephritogenic epitope
nephroangiosclerosis
nephroblastoma
nephroblastomatosis
  n. complex (NBC)
nephrocalcin (NC)
nephrocalcinosis
nephrocapsectomy
nephrocele
nephrocelom
nephrogenetic, nephrogenic
nephrogenous
nephrogram
  delayed n.
  diffuse patchy n.
nephrography
nephrohydrosis
nephrolith
nephrolithiasis
  autosomally inherited forms
    of n.
  calcium oxalate n.
  X-linked recessive n. (XRN)
nephrolitholapaxy
  percutaneous n.
nephrolithotomy
  anatrophic n.
  percutaneous n. (PCNL, PNL)
  simultaneous bilateral
    percutaneous n. (SBPN)
nephrologist
nephrology
nephrolysin
nephrolysis

nephrolytic
nephroma
    cystic n.
    mesoblastic n.
    multilocular cystic n.
nephron
    n. loss
    n. plasma flow
    proximal n.
    n. transport
nephronia
    lobar n.
nephron-sparing surgery
nephropathia epidemica
nephropathy
    amyloid n.
    analgesic n.
    Balkan n.
    Berger n.
    cast n.
    cisplatin n. (CPN)
    C1q n.
    Danubian endemic familial n.
    diabetic n.
    epidemic n.
    HIV-associated n. (HIVAN)
    hypercalcemic n.
    hypokalemic n.
    IgM n.
    immunoglobulin A n.
    incipient n.
    membranous n.
    non-nephrotic immunoglobulin
      A n.
    obstructive n.
    overt n.
    puromycin aminonucleoside n.
      (PAN)
    reflux n.
    tubulointerstitial n.
    urate n.
    uric acid n.
nephropexy
nephrophthiasis
    familial juvenile n.
nephrophthisis
    familial juvenile n.

nephroptosis, nephroptosia
nephropyelitis
nephropyeloplasty
nephropyosis
nephrorrhaphy
nephrosclerosis
    arteriolar n.
    hypertensive n. (HN)
    malignant n.
nephroscope
    flexible n.
    rigid n.
    n. sheath
    Storz n.
    Wolf percutaneous universal n.
nephroscopy
    anatrophic n.
    flexible n.
nephrosis
    acute n.
    Adriamycin-induced n.
    amyloid n.
    familial n.
    lipoid n.
    steroid resistant idiopathic n.
    steroid sensitive/dependent
      idiopathic n.
nephrospasia, nephrospasis
nephrostogram
nephrostolithotomy
    percutaneous n. (PCNL)
nephrostomy
    n. catheter
    percutaneous n.
    n. tube
nephrotic
    n. edema
    n. syndrome
nephrotomic cavity
nephrotomogram
nephrotomography
nephrotomy
    anatrophic n.
    n. tube
nephrotoxic
    n. acute renal failure

N

NOTES

nephrotoxic *(continued)*
  n. antiglomerular basement
    membrane antibody nephritis
  n. antiserum
  n. serum nephritis
nephrotoxicity
  cadmium-induced n.
  cyclosporine n.
  mercuric chloride n.
nephrotoxin
nephrotrophic
nephrotropic
nephrotuberculosis
nephroureterectomy
  bilateral n.
  radical n.
  transperitoneal laparoscopic n.
nephroureterocystectomy
nephroureteroscopy
Nephrox
Neptune girdle
nerve
  afferent renal n.
  n. block
  dorsal n. of penis
  genitofemoral n.
  n. growth factor receptor
    (NGFR)
  n. hook
  iliohypogastric n.
  ilioinguinal n.
  inferior rectal n.
  intrapancreatic n.
  n. of Latarjet
  noncholinergic n.
  pelvic autonomic n.
  perineal n.
  postganglionic cholinergic n.
  pudendal n.
  renal sympathetic n.
  n. sparing dissection
  splanchnic n.
  transcutaneous n.
  vagus n.
nerve-sparing
  n.-s. radical retropubic
    prostatectomy
nervosa
  anorexia n.
  bulimia n.
  dysphagia n.
nervous
  n. bladder

  n. dyspepsia
  n. gut
  n. indigestion
  n. vomiting
Nesbit
  N. cystoscope
  N. operation
  N. plication
  N. procedure
  N. tuck procedure
nesidiectomy
nesidioblastoma
nest
  Brunn n.
NESTED procedure
net
  Roth polyp retrieval n.
  ureteric retrieval n.
network
  capillary n.
  Pentax EndoNet digital
    endoscopy n.
  trans-Golgi n.
  vascular collateral n.
Neukomm test
Neu-Laxova syndrome
neural
  n. control
  n. invasion
  n. pathway
neuraminidase
**neuraminidase-treated sheep
  erythrocyte**
neurasthenia
  gastric n.
neurinoma
neuroaminidase
neuroblastoma
  presacral n.
neuroblockage
neurocutaneous syndrome
neurodegenerative disorder
neuroendocrine
  n. cell
  n. tumor
neuroendocrinology
  gastrointestinal n.
neurofibroma
  duodenal n.
  gastrointestinal n.

plexiform n.
Recklinghausen gastric n.
neurofibromatosis (NF)
von Recklinghausen n.
neurofilament protein triplet
neurogenic
n. bladder
n. erectile dysfunction
n. intestinal obstruction
n. sphincteric incompetence
n. tumor
neurohumoral
n. disease
neurohumoral-immune axis
neurokinin A
neurologic
n. complication
n. deficit
n. disorder
neurolytic
n. celiac plexus block
n. drug
neuron
adrenergic n.
afferent n.
alpha motor n.
argyrophilic and
argyophobic n.
bipolar n.
cholinergic n.
enteric n.
final motor n.
gamma aminobutyric
acidergic n.
intestinofugal n.
multipolar n.
nonadrenergic n.
noncholinergic n.
peptidergic n.
S n.
sensory n.
serotoninergic n.
unipolar n.
neuronal cell line
neuronoma
VIP-secreting n.
neuron-specific enolase (NSE)

neuroparacrine mechanism
neuropathic
n. bladder
n. dysfunction
neuropathy
autonomic n.
diabetic n.
IgA n.
immunoglobulin n.
membranous n.
polyradicular n.
vasculitic n.
visceral n.
neuropeptide
n. Y (NPY)
neuropharmacology
neurophysiology
pelvic floor n.
neuroplasticity
neuropsychotropic drug
neurosis
bladder n.
neurotensin
neurotransmitter
noncholinergic n.
neurotrophin
neurotropic
neuroureterectomy
neurourological
Neutral
K-Phos N.
Neutra-Phos
Neutra-Phos-K
neutrocytic ascites
neutron
neutropenia
neutrophil
n. chemotactic peptide
n. dysfunction
n. elastase
polymorphonuclear n. (PMN)
WBC n.'s
neutrophilia
neutrophilic
n. gastroduodenitis
n. infiltration
neutropic virus

N

NOTES

Neville tracheal reconstruction prosthesis
nevus, pl. **nevi**
   n. flammeus
   pigmented n.
   spider n.
newborn
   n. hepatitis
   n. jaundice
new differentiation factor (NDF)
newport
   Salmonella n.
nexus
Nezhat-Dorsey irrigator/aspirator
NF
   neurofibromatosis
NG
   nasogastric
      NG aspirate
      NG suction
NGFR
   nerve growth factor receptor
15Nglutamine
NG-nitro-L-arginine methyl ester (L-NAME)
NGT
   nasogastric tube
NH2-terminal SH2 domain
NHL
   non-Hodgkin lymphoma
nialamide
Niblitt dissector
nicardipine
Nichols-Condon bowel preparation
Nichols IRMA kit
nick
niclosamide
Nicolet SM-300 stimulator
Nicorette
nicotinamide adenine dinucleotide phosphate (NADPH)
nicotinic
   n. agonist
   n. receptor
   n. receptor blocker
NIDDM
   non-insulin-dependent diabetes mellitus
Niemann-Pick disease
Niemeier gallbladder perforation
nifedipine
nifedipine extended release
Niferex-150

niflutamide
nifurtimox
nigericin
nightly intermittent peritoneal dialysis (NIPD)
nighttime polyuria
nigra
   linea n.
nigricans
   acanthosis n.
Nihon tocodynamometer
nil disease
Nilstat
nilutamide
nimodipine
Ninhydrin
Niopam
   N. contrast medium
NIPD
   nightly intermittent peritoneal dialysis
nipple
   n. discharge
   ileum n.
   intussuscepted ileal triple n.
   Kock n.
   pigmented n.
   ureteral split cuff n.
   n. valve
nippled stoma
Nipride
niridazole
N-isopropyl-p-iodoamphetamine
   biodistribution of N.-i.-p.-i.
Nissen
   N. antireflux operation
   N. 360-degree wrap fundoplication
   N. fundoplication
   N. fundoplication wrap
   N. gall duct forceps
   N. repair
nitecapone
nitinol
   n. stent
   n. wire
nitrate
   amyl n.
   methylatropine n.
   organic n.
nitrate-induced venodilation
nitric
   n. oxide (NO)

n. oxide blocked sphincter relaxation
n. oxide synthase (iNOS, NOS)
n. oxide synthase inhibitor
n. oxide synthetase
nitrite
amyl n.
4-nitrobiphenyl
nitrofurantoin
n. hepatotoxicity
nitrofurazone
nitrogen
n. balance
blood urea n. (BUN)
glutamine n.
high n. (HN)
high calorie and n. (HCN)
n. overload
n. partition test
total body n. (TBN)
urine urea n. (UUN)
nitroglycerin
intravenous n.
vasopressin with n.
nitroimidazole
2-nitropropane hepatotoxicity
nitroprusside
sodium n. (SNP)
nitrosamine
carcinogenic n.
nitrosourea
Nitrostat
nitrous
n. oxide
n. oxide/carbon dioxide insufflator
n. oxide insufflator
nizatidine
Nizoral
NJ
nasojejunal
NJ feeding tube
NK
natural killer
NK cell
NK1 tachykinin receptor

NK2 tachykinin receptor
NLH
nodular lymphoid hyperplasia
N-linked glycoprotein
N loop
NM
nuclear medicine
N-methyl-D-glucamide (NMG)
NMG
N-methyl-D-glucamide
NMR
nuclear magnetic resonance
N-myc oncogene
N-nitrosamine
NO
nitric oxide
Noble
N. bowel plication
N. surgical plication of bowel
nociceptive
n. stimulation
n. structure
nociceptor
nocte
ranitidine n.
nocturia
nocturnal
n. acid reflux
n. diarrhea
n. emission
n. enuresis
n. erection
n. gastric reflux
n. heartburn
n. pain
n. penile tumescence (NPT)
n. penile tumescence monitoring
n. regurgitation
n. tumescence
n. tumescence self-monitoring
node
celiac lymph n.
n. of Cloquet
n. dissection
n. distribution

N

NOTES

node *(continued)*
    intermediate mesenteric
      lymph n.
    juxtaposed mesenteric lymph n.
    lymph n.
    matted n.
    mesenteric lymph n. (MLN)
    pelvic lymph n.
    retrorectal lymph n.
    sentinel n.
    shotty lymph n.
    Sister Mary Joseph lymph n.
    subcarinal n.
    succulent mesenteric lymph n.
    Virchow sentinel n.
    Virchow-Troisier n.

nodosa
    polyarteritis n.

nodosum
    erythema n.

nodular
    n. hyperplasia
    n. hyperplasia of prostate
    n. lesion
    n. liver
    n. lymphoid hyperplasia (NLH)
    n. lymphoma
    n. pancreatitis
    n. regenerative hyperplasia
      (NRH)
    n. transformation

nodularity
    coarse n.
    mucosal n.
    surface n.

nodule
    cecal mucosal n.
    colonic lymphoid n.
    daughter n.
    hyperplastic n.
    liver n.
    lymphoid n.
    lymphomatous n.
    macroregenerative n.
    multiacinar regenerative n.
    multiple n.
    pentastomum denticulatum n.
    peritoneal n.
    prostatic n.
    regenerative cirrhotic n.
    Sister Mary Joseph n.
    surface n.

    thyroid n.
    yellow n.

nodule-in-nodule pattern
Nolvadex
nomogram
non-A,
    n.-A. non-B (NANB)
    n.-A. non-B hepatitis
    n.-A. non-B posttransfusion
      hepatitis

nonabsorbable suture
non-adherent clot
nonadhesive dressing
nonadrenergic
    n. neuron
    n. noncholinergic (NANC)
    n. noncholinergic inhibitory
      transmitter

nonadrenergic noncholinergic
    inhibitory transmitter
nonagglutinable (NAG)
non-alcoholic steatohepatitis
non-alpha, non-beta pancreatic islet
    cell
nonamyloid glomerulopathy
nonaneuploid tumor
non-anion-gap metabolic acidosis
non-A, non-B (NANB)
nonantibiotic colitis
non-antigen expressing target cell
nonapoptotic pathway
nonazotemic
    n. cirrhotic

non-B
    n.-B islet cell tumor
    non-A, n.-B (NANB)

nonbacterial
    n. gastroenteritis
    n. prostatitis (NBP)

nonbench surgery
nonbilious vomitus
nonbleeding
    n. visible vessel (NBVV)

nonbloody stool
nonbuckling erection
noncalcified stone
noncalculous disease
noncardiac chest pain
noncaseating tubercle-like granuloma
noncerebral vasculopathy
non-CH4 excretor
noncholecystokinin substance

noncholinergic
  n. nerve
  n. neuron
  n. neurotransmitter
  nonadrenergic n. (NANC)
nonchylous ascites
noncirrhotic
  n. liver
  n. portal fibrosis (NCPF)
  n. portal hypertension
noncleaved B cell
noncollagen protein
noncommunicating
  n. biliary cyst
  n. diverticulum
  n. hydrocele
nonconductive guidewire
nonconfluent
noncontributory
noncrushing bowel clamp
nondiabetic
  n. gastroparesis
  n. neurogenic erectile
    dysfunction
nondilating reflux
nondismembered anastomosis
nondistended abdomen
nondistensible
non-ductectatic cystic neoplasm
nonenzymatic glycosylation
nonenzymic reaction
nonepithelial cyst
nonerosive
  n. gastric mucosal lesion
  n. gastritis
  n. nonspecific gastritis
nonestrogen-supplemented
nonfamilial
  n. gastrointestinal polyposis
  n. intestinal pseudo-obstruction
nonfluctuant
nonfunction
  primary graft n.
nonfusion
non-gas-forming liver abscess
nongene carrier
non-germ cell carcinoma

nonglycated albumin
nongonococcal urethritis
nongranulomatous
  n. jejunitis
  n. ulcerative jejunoileitis
nonhealing ulcer
non-heart beating donor protocol
nonhemolytic
  n. jaundice
  n. strep
non-hemolyzed blood
non-Hodgkin lymphoma (NHL)
nonicteric
  n. sclera
  n. skin
non-insulin-dependent diabetes
  mellitus (NIDDM)
nonintussuscepted valve
noninvasive
  n. assessment of urinary flow
  n. diagnosis
  n. diagnostic test
  n. intra-anal electromyography
  n. tumor
nonionizing radiation
nonirrigating patient
nonischemic tubule
nonkeratinizing squamous epithelium
nonmalodorous fluid
nonmetallic
non-neoplastic
  n.-n. lesion
  n.-n. polyp
non-nephrotic immunoglobulin A
  nephropathy
nonnephrotoxic
non-nephrotoxic drug
nonneurogenic bladder
NONOate
  spermine N.
nonobstructive
  n. hepatic parenchymal disease
  n. jaundice
nonocclusive
  n. infarction
  n. intestinal infarction
  n. mesenteric thrombosis

N

NOTES

nonoliguric acute renal failure
nonorgan confined disease
nonorganic dyspepsia
nonoxynol-9
nonparametric
   n. Wilcoxon statistics
non-parasitic cyst of liver
nonparasitic splenic cyst
nonparticulate radiation
nonperforated
   n. appendicitis
   n. appendix
nonpitting
nonpliable
nonplicated appendicocystostomy
nonpolypoid adenoma
nonpolyposis colorectal cancer
nonpruritic
nonreactive pupil
nonreflux esophagitis
nonrosetted cell
nonsecretory sigmoid cystoplasty
nonseminomatous
   n. germ cell tumor
   n. testicular carcinoma
   n. tumor
nonspecific
   n. colitis
   n. erosive gastritis
   n. esophageal motility disorder
   (NEMD)
   n. esophagitis
   n. gas pattern
   n. gastritis
   n. motility disorder
   n. reactive hepatitis
   n. ulcerative proctitis
nonsteroidal
   n. anti-inflammatory drug
   (NSAID)
   n. anti-inflammatory drug-
   induced intestinal stricture
nonstruvite
   n. calculus
   n. stone
nonsulfated bile acid
nonsuppurative destructive
  cholangitis
non-T-cell fraction
non-transected pancreatic duct
nontropical sprue
nontumorous and tumorous
  epithelia

nontyphoidal
   n. Salmonella
   n. salmonellosis
non-ulcer
   n.-u. dyspepsia (NUD)
   n.-u. dysplasia
nonulcer
   n. dyspepsia (NUD)
   n. dysplasia
nonvariceal upper GI hemorrhage
nonviable tissue
nonvisualization of gallbladder
Noonan syndrome
noradrenaline
   serum n.
no rejection (NR)
norepinephrine
   n. lavage
norestriol
norethandrolone
Norflex
norfloxacin
Norfolk technique
normal
   n. appendix
   n. caliber duct
   n. carrier hepatitis
   n. detrusor contractility
   eversion n.
   n. flora
   palpably n.
   n. saline meal
   n. saline solution
   visibly n.
normal-appearing mucosa
normalized protein catabolic rate
  (NPCR)
normeperidine
normoacidity
normoactive
   n. bowel sounds (NABS)
normocephalic
normochlorhydria
normochromic
normocytic
Normodyne
normoproliferative
normospermatogenic sterility
normotensive
Normotest test
normothermia
normothermic effect
Noroxin

Norplant
Norpramin
Nor-tet
North American Medical
    Incorporated deep dorsal vein
Northern blot analysis
Northgate SD-3 dual-purpose
    lithotriptor
nortriptyline
Norvasc
Norwalk
    N. agent
    N. gastroenteritis
    N. virus
Norwood rectal snare
NOS
    nitric oxide synthase
no-scalpel vasectomy
nosocomial
    n. fungal infection
    n. infection
nostril blood
notch
    splenic n.
note
    percussion n.
Nottingham
    N. Key-Med introducing device
    N. One-Step tapered dilator
    N. semirigid introducer
    N. ureteral dilator
Nova II machine
Novamine amino acid
novo
    de n.
Novocain
NovoNorm
NPCR
    normalized protein catabolic rate
NPH insulin
NPT
    nocturnal penile tumescence
    NPT monitoring
NPY
    neuropeptide Y
NR
    no rejection

NRH
    nodular regenerative hyperplasia
NS2 protein
NS3/NS4 junction
NS3 protein
NS4/NS5 junction
NS4 protein
NS5 protein
NSAID
    nonsteroidal anti-inflammatory drug
NSE
    neuron-specific enolase
N-shaped sigmoid loop
NT
    nucleation time
N-terminal
    N.-t. fragment
    N.-t. propeptide of type III
        procollagen
N-trimethylsilylimidazole
NTZ Long-acting
nuchal rigidity
Nuck
    canal of N.
    diverticulum of N.
    N. hydrocele
nuclear
    n. bleeding scan
    n. enema
    n. fragment
    n. hepatobiliary imaging
    n. hyperchromasia and
        pleomorphism
    n. isotope scan
    n. magnetic resonance (NMR)
    n. matrix alteration
    n. medicine (NM)
    n. medicine scan
    n. morphometry
    n. protein cyclin proliferating
        cell nuclear antigen
    n. roundness factor
    n. sclerosis
    n. transcriptional activation
nuclear-tagged
    n.-t. cell

N

NOTES

401

nuclear-tagged *(continued)*
  n.-t. red blood cell bleeding study
nuclear-to-cytoplasmic size ratio
nucleation
  epitaxial n.
  n. time (NT)
nucleic acid hybridization
nucleocapsid
  n. antigen-specific
  n. antigen-stimulated interferon-gamma
nucleotide
  guanine n.
nucleotide-binding domain (NBD)
nucleus
  cigar-shaped hyperchromatic n.
  elongated, pseudostratified n.
  hyperchromatic n.
  Onuf n.
  pyknotic n.
  n. tractus solitarius
NUD
  non-ulcer dyspepsia
  nonulcer dyspepsia
Nu-Hope
  N.-H. Adhesive waterproof skin barrier
  N.-H. Convex insert
  N.-H. ileostomy pouch
  N.-H. Nu-Self drainable pouch
  N.-H. Protective Skin Barrier
Nullo deodorant tablets
NuLYTELY
NuLytely enema
number
  n. connection test
  shock n.
numbness
Nupercainal
  N. ointment
Nuport PEG tube
Nursoy formula
Nussbaum
  N. intestinal clamp
  N. intestinal forceps

nutcracker
  n. esophagus
Nu-Tip laparoscopic scissors
nutmeg liver
Nutramigen formula
nutrient
  n. enema
nutrition
  enteral n. (EN)
  home parenteral n. (HPN)
  intradialytic parenteral n. (IDPN)
  Jevity isotonic liquid n.
  Nutri-Vent liquid n.
  parenteral n.
  Peptamen liquid n.
  perioperative n.
  Replete liquid n.
  support parenteral n. (SPN)
  total enteral n. (TEN)
  total parenteral n. (TPN)
nutritional
  n. cirrhosis
  n. deficiency
  n. dropsy
  n. index
  n. pancreatitis
  n. status
  n. support
  n. therapy
nutritive
nutriture
Nutri-Vent liquid nutrition
Nutromat Pad S feeding pump
Nutropin
N&V
  nausea and vomiting
nycturia
Nyhus-Nelson gastric decompression and jejunal feeding tube
nylidrin
NY 13N Membranfilter
nystagmus
nystatin
  n. suspension
Nystex

O2
fMLP-stimulated O.
PMA-stimulated O.
OA-519 prognostic prostate carcinoma marker
OASIS
One Action, Stent Introduction System
oasthouse urine disease
oat
o. cell
o. cell carcinoma
oatmeal
colloidal o.
OB-10 Comfort bite block
OBA
oral bile acid
O'Beirne sphincter
obesity
adult-onset o.
alimentary o.
endogenous o.
exogenous o.
hyperplasmic o.
hyperplastic o.
hypertrophic o.
o. hypoventilation syndrome (OHS)
o. index
lifelong o.
morbid o.
object
foreign o.
ingested foreign o.
irretrievable o.
radiolucent o.
objective
o. lens
o. vertigo
obligate anaerobe
obligatory dialysate protein loss
oblique
aponeurosis of external o.
aponeurosis of internal o.
external o.
o. incision
internal o.
o. obturator
oblique-forward-viewing instrument
oblique-viewing endoscope

obliterans
appendicitis o.
balanitis xerotica o. (BXO)
endophlebitis hepatica o.
obliterated varices
obliteration
balloon-occluded retrograde transvenous o. (B-RTO)
endoscopic extirpation cicatricial o.
percutaneous transhepatic o.
o. of psoas shadow
observation
electron immunoperoxidase o.
light and electron immunoperoxidase o.
obsolescent glomeruli
obstetric injury
obstipation
obstipum
abdomen o.
obstructed
o. defecation
o. pelvis
o. testis
obstructing
o. carcinoma
obstruction
adynamic intestinal o.
airflow o.
airway o.
o. of bile flow
biliary tract o.
bladder outflow o.
bladder outlet o. (BOO)
bowel o.
cerumen o.
closed-loop intestinal o.
clot-induced urinary tract o.
colonic o.
common bile duct o.
complete bowel o.
duodenal o.
o. duodenum
ejaculatory duct o.
esophageal o.
extrahepatic o.
extrahepatic bile duct o.
extrahepatic biliary o.

O

obstruction (*continued*)
extrahepatic portal vein o.
(EHPVO)
false colonic o.
fecal o.
food bolus o.
functional cystic duct o.
gastric outlet o. (GOO)
hepatic venous outflow o.
(HVOO)
high-grade o.
high small-bowel o.
idiopathic o.
o. index
infravesical prostatic o.
intermittent o.
intestinal o.
intrahepatic portal o.
large-bowel o.
low small-bowel o.
lymphatic o.
malignant biliary o.
mechanical biliary o.
mechanical duct o.
mechanical extrahepatic o.
mechanical intestinal o.
mechanical small-bowel o.
neurogenic intestinal o.
outlet o.
paralytic colonic o.
paralytic intestinal o.
partial bile outflow o.
partial bowel o.
portal vein o.
pyloric o.
pyloric outlet o.
pyloroduodenal o.
shrapnel-induced biliary o.
simple mechanical o.
small-bowel o. (SBO)
splenic vein o. (SVO)
strangulated bowel o.
unilateral ureteral o. (UUO)
ureteral o.
ureteric o.
ureteropelvic junction o.
ureterovesical o.
urethral o.
urinary o.
urodynamic o.
obstruction-induced modulation
obstructive
o. appendicitis

o. biliary cirrhosis
o. dysfunctional ileitis
o. gastroduodenal Crohn
disease
o. jaundice
o. nephropathy
o. pancreatitis
o. uropathy
obtunded
obturation
obturator
blunt-tipped o.
Endopath Optiview
laparoscopic o.
o. internus muscle
o. lymphatic chain
oblique o.
Optiview o.
o. shelf cystourethropexy
o. sign
o. test
Timberlake o.
OCBF
outer cortical blood flow
occipital
occiput
occlusion
o. balloon
balloon ureteral o.
mesenteric vascular o.
portal triad o.
retinal artery o.
retinal vein o.
o. of TIPS
tourniquet o.
urethral o.
occlusive
o. azoospermia
o. clamp
o. collodion dressing
o. dressing
o. ileus
o. infarction
occult
o. bleeding
o. blood
o. GI bleeding
o. hepatitis
o. spinal dysraphism
occupational
o. toxin
o. toxin exposure

OCG
oral cholecystogram
Ochoa syndrome
Ochsner
O. flexible spiral gallstone probe
O. forceps
O. gallbladder probe
O. gallbladder trocar
O. hemostat
O. retractor
O. ring
Ockerblad-Boari flap
OCL bowel prep
OCLG
osteoclast-like giant cell
O'Connor drape
Octamide
octapeptide
cholecystokinin o. (CCK-8, CCK-OP)
OCT medium
OctreoScan
O. kit
O. scintigraphy
octreotide
o. acetate
o. effect
somatostatin analog o.
octreotide-induced hepatic toxicity
OCTT
orocecal transit time
ocular
o. abnormality
o. lesion
OD
outer diameter
overdose
ODC
ornithine decarboxylase
Oddi
sphincter of O. (SO)
O'Donoghue cystourethroscope
odor
breath o.
foul-smelling o.
fruity o.

odynophagia
OEIS
omphalocele, exstrophy of the bladder, imperforate anus and spinal abnormalities
OEIS complex
OES
Olympus endoscopy system
oesophagi
introitus o.
Oettingen abdominal retractor
offset lens ureteroscope
ofloxacin
Ogen
Ogilvie syndrome
O'Hanlon intestinal clamp
O'Hara forceps
25-OH-D3
25-hydroxyvitamin D
OHS
obesity hypoventilation syndrome
oil
arachis o.
castor o.
cottonseed o.
olive o.
peppermint o.
o. red O stain
o. retention enema
oily stool
ointment
Nupercainal o.
Tucks o.
OK432 streptococcal suspension
Okamoto method
OK cell
OKT3
O. anti-T-cell antibody
O. monoclonal antibody
OKT4
OKT8
Okuda transhepatic obliteration of varix
Olbert balloon dilator
Oldfield syndrome
O'Leary lesser curvature gastroplasty

O

NOTES

oleate
ethanolamine o.
intravariceal ethanolamine o.
olestra fat substitute
oligoasthenospermia
oligoasthenoteratospermia
oligoasthenoteratozoospermia
oligoazoospermia
oligocholia
oligochylia
oligochymia
oligocilia
oligohydramnios
o. complex
oligomerize
oligometric complex
oligonucleotide
o. probe
specific o.
oligopepsia
oligosaccharidase
oligospermia, oligospermatism
oligosymptomatic ADPKD
oligosynaptic pathway
oligozoospermatism, oligozoospermia
oliguresia, oliguresis
oliguria
oliguric renal failure
olive
Eder-Puestow o.
expandable o.
metal o.
o. oil
o. over guidewire
palpable pyloric o.
Savary-Gilliard metal o.
o. shaped
olive-tipped catheter
olsalazine
o. sodium
olsalazine-S
OLT
orthotopic liver transplant
orthotopic liver transplantation
Olympus
O. adapter
O. alligator-jaw endoscopic forceps
O. Aloka EU-MI ultrasound gastrointestinal fiberscope
O. Aloka GF-EU-series endoscope
O. automatic reprocessor

O. basket-type endoscopic forceps
O. BH2-epifluorescence microscope
O. BH2-RFCA reflecting microscope
O. BHT-2 microscope
O. CBK fluorescence microscope
O. CD-20Z heater probe
O. CD-Z-series heat probe thermocoagulator
O. CF-HM-series magnifying colonoscope
O. CF-L-series flexible sigmoidoscope
O. CF-MB-series colonoscope
O. CF-OSF-series flexible sigmoidoscope
O. CF-PL-series colonoscope
O. CF-TL-series forward-viewing video colonoscope
O. CF-T-series colonoscope
O. CF-TVL-series colonoscope
O. CF-UHM-series colonoscope
O. CF-UM-series colonoscope
O. CF-UM-series echoendoscope
O. CF-VL-series colonoscope
O. CG-P-series colonofiberscope
O. CHF-P-series choledochoscope
O. clip-fixing device
O. CLV-series fiberoptic system
O. continuous flow resectoscope
O. CV-series colonoscope
O. CV-series endoscope
O. CYF-series OES cystofiberscope
O. cytology brush
O. DES-series endoscope
O. EF-series esophagoscope
O. endoscopy system (OES)
O. Endo-Therapy disposable biopsy forceps
O. ENF-P-series laryngoscope
O. EU-M-series endosonography image processor

O. Europe ETD automated endoscope washer
O. EUS-series endoscope
O. EVIS color computer chip system
O. EVIS Q-series endoscope
O. EVIS video colonoscope
O. EW-series fiberoptic duodenoscope
O. FB-series forceps
O. FG-series forceps
O. fiberoptic cystoscope
O. FS-K-series endoscopic suture-cutting forceps
O. gastrostomy
O. GF-EU-series ultrasound gastrointestinal fiberscope
O. GF-UM-series echoendoscope
O. GF-UM-series endoscope
O. GIF-D-series panendoscope
O. GIF-EUM-series echoendoscope
O. GIF-HM-series endoscope
O. GIF-J-series endoscope
O. GIF-K-series gastroscope
O. GIF-Q-series endoscope
O. GIF-series double-channel therapeutic videoendoscope
O. GIF-series echoendoscope
O. GIF-series videoendoscope
O. GIF-SQ-series videoendoscope
O. GIF-T-series endoscope
O. GIF-T-series videoendoscope
O. GIF-XP-series endoscope
O. GIF-XQ-series panendoscope
O. GIF-XV-series endoscope
O. grasping rat-tooth forceps
O. GTF-A gastrocamera
O. heat probe
O. hot biopsy forceps
O. injector
O. JF-series video duodenoscope
O. JF-T-series endoscope
O. JF-TV-series endoscope

O. JF-UM-series echoendoscope
O. JF-V-series endoscope
O. JF-V-series video duodenoscope
O. JT-series video duodenoscope
O. lithotriptor
O. magnetic extractor forceps
O. mini-snare forceps
O. monopolar cannula
O. needle-knife papillotome
O. NM-K-series sclerotherapy needle
O. NM-L-series needle
O. OES fiberscope
O. OM-2 camera with SM-45 enlarging adapter
O. OM-series endoscopic camera
O. one-step button gastrostomy tube
O. OSP fluorescence measuring system
O. OTV-S-series miniature camera
O. PCF-series pediatric colonoscope
O. pelican-type endoscopic forceps
O. PJF-series pediatric duodenoscope
O. PJF-series pediatric endoscope
O. P-series endoscope
O. PW-1L wash catheter
O. rat-tooth endoscopic forceps
O. rubber-tip endoscopic forceps
O. SCA-series endoscopic camera
O. shark-tooth endoscopic forceps
O. SIF-M-series video enteroscope
O. SIF-series video enteroscope
O. SIF-SW-series video enteroscope

O

NOTES

Olympus *(continued)*
O. sphincterotome
O. SP-series image analyzer
O. SSIF-series video
   enteroscope
O. stone retrieval basket
O. TJF-series endoscope
O. tripod-type endoscopic
   forceps
O. UES-series snare cautery
   device
O. ultrasonic esophagoprobe
O. ultrathin balloon-fitted
   ultrasound probe
O. UM-R-series miniature
   ultrasonic probe
O. UM-series echoendoscope
O. UM-series endoscope
O. UM-W-series endoscopic
   probe
O. URF-P2
   choledochofiberscope
O. video endoscopy system
O. video urology procedure
   system
O. V-series endoscope
O. VU-M-series echoendoscope
O. W-shaped endoscopic
   forceps
O. XCF-XK-series endoscope
O. XIF-UM-series
   echoendoscope
O. XJF-UM20
   echoduodenoscope
O. XK-series oblique-viewing
   flexible fiberscope
O. XMP-U2 catheter echoprobe
O. XP-series endoscope
O. XQ-series endoscope
O. XSIF-series video
   enteroscope
Olympus P20
Ombredanne forceps
Ombrédanne operation
OME
   omeprazole
OmegaPort access port
omega-shaped incision
omenta (*pl. of* omentum)
omental
   o. adhesion
   o. band
   o. cyst

o. enterocleisis
o. infarction
o. J-pexy
o. patch
o. pedicle
o. pedicle flap graft
o. studding
o. vein
omentalis
   taenia o.
   tenia o.
omentectomy
omentofixation
omentopexy
omentoplasty
   pedicled o.
omentorrhaphy
omentovolvulus
omentum, pl. **omenta**
   bowel adherent to o.
   colic o.
   gastric o.
   gastrocolic o.
   gastrohepatic o.
   gastrosplenic o.
   greater o.
   incarcerated o.
   lesser o.
   o. majus
   o. majus flap procedure
   o. minus
   pancreaticosplenic o.
   splenogastric o.
omentumectomy
omeprazole (OME)
   o. therapy
omeprazole/amoxicillin
**omeprazole-clarithromycin-amoxicillin
   therapy**
Omnicide disinfectant
Omni-LapoTract support system
Omnipaque
Omnipen
Omnipen-N
Omniphase penile prosthesis
OMNI Prep
Omnitract retractor
omphalectomy
omphalocele
**omphalocele, exstrophy of the
   bladder, imperforate anus and
   spinal abnormalities (OEIS)**
omphalodiverticular band

oncoantigen 519
oncocytoma
oncogene
    c-met o.
    c-myc o.
    Her-2/neu o.
    Kirsten-ras o.
    K-ras o.
    N-myc o.
    polyoma middle T o.
    ras o.
oncogene-induced carcinogenesis
oncoprotein
OncoScint
    O. colorectal/ovarian carcinoma
    localization scintigraphy
    (OncoScint CR/OV)
    O. CR/OV
OncoSpect
ondansetron
One Action, Stent Introduction
  System (OASIS)
one-handed knot
one-hour office pad test
oneirogmus
one-minute endoscopy room test
one-piece
    o.-p. disposable plug
    o.-p. ostomy pouch
one-stage
    o.-s. hypospadias repair
    o.-s. procedure
One-Step
    O.-S. gastric button
    Surgitek O.-S. (SOS)
onlay
    o. island flap
    o. island flap urethroplasty
    o. technique
onlay-tube-onlay urethroplasty
  technique
onset of pain
Onuf nucleus
oocyst
    Cryptosporidium o.
oocyte
    o. micromanipulation

oolemma
oophorectomy
ooplasm
ooze
oozing
    o. blood
O&P
    ova and parasites
opacification
opacify
opaque meal
open
    o. biopsy
    o. drainage
    o. electrocautery snare
    o. end flo-thru radiopaque tip
    o. hemorrhoidectomy
    o. injury
    o. pyelolithotomy
    o. pyelotomy
    o. renal descent
    o. retroperitoneal high ligation
    o. sphincterotome
    o. ulcer
    o. wound
open-ended ureteral catheter
open-end ostomy pouch
opening
    appendiceal o.
operation (*See also* procedure, repair)
    Abbe o.
    Amussat o.
    antireflux o.
    Aylett o.
    bariatric o.
    Bassini o.
    Battle o.
    Belsey Mark IV antireflux o.
    Bloch-Paul-Mikulicz o.
    bottle o.
    Bozeman o.
    Bricker o.
    Brunschwig o.
    Camey I, II o.
    Collis antireflux o.
    Crespo o.
    Delorme rectal prolapse o.

NOTES

O

operation *(continued)*
Duhamel colon o.
eversion o.
Finney o.
Foley o.
Fredet-Ramstedt o.
Furlow-Fisher modification of
  Virag 1 o.
Gauderer-Ponsky PEG o.
Gil-Vernet o.
Hartmann o.
Heller o.
Hill antireflux o.
Hofmeister o.
Huggins o.
Ivalon sponge-wrap o.
Jaboulay-Doyen-Winkleman o.
Kasai o.
Kelly o.
kidney sparing o.
Kraske o.
Kropp o.
Ladd o.
Lane o.
Lester Martin modification of
  Duhamel o.
Longmire o.
Macewen hernia o.
MAGPI o.
Mainz pouch o.
Mann-Williamson o.
Mansson o.
Marshall-Marchetti-Krantz o.
Mason o.
Maunsell-Weir o.
Mayo o.
Merindino o.
Mikulicz o.
Miles o.
Monfort o.
Nesbit o.
Nissen antireflux o.
Ombrédanne o.
orthotopic hemi-Kock o.
Palomo o.
Payne o.
Pólya o.
pubovaginal o.
Puestow-Gillesby o.
Ramstedt o.
Ripstein rectal prolapse o.
Roux-en-Y o.
Rovsing o.

sacrofixation o.
Scott o.
scrotal pouch o.
second-look o.
Smith-Boyce o.
Soave o.
staging o.
Tanner o.
Thal fundic patch o.
Thiersch anal incontinence o.
Torek o.
transection and
  devascularization o.
Turnbull multiple ostomy o.
Virag o.
Wheelhouse o.
Whipple o.
Whitehead o.
Young-Dees o.
Young-Dees-Leadbetter o.
operative
  o. cholangiogram
  o. choledochoscopy
  o. decompression
  o. laparoscope
  o. morbidity
  o. staging
o-phenantrolin
ophthalmoplegia
  internuclear o.
opiate
  o. antagonist
opioid
  o. antidiarrheal
  antisecretory o.
  endogenous o.
  o. peptide
opioid-mediated pruritus
opisthorchiasis
opium
  deodorized tincture of o.
  (DTO)
opportunistic
  o. complication
  o. infection
opposure
OpSite dressing
opsonic activity
opsonization
opsonized zymosan
optical
  o. esophagoscope
  o. fiber

o. laser knife
o. multichannel analyzer system
o. needle
o. switch
o. system
o. ureterotome
o. urethrotome knife
optics
fiber o.
Wappler cystoscope with microlens o.
Optilume prostate balloon dilator
optimum cooling range
Optiview obturator
OPUS-1
Ausonics O.
Oracit
orad
o. propagation
Oragrafin
O. contrast medium
oral
o. barium suspension
o. bile acid (OBA)
o. cholecystogram (OCG)
o. disease
o. intubation
o. iron
o. iron preparation
o. lavage
o. leukoplakia
o. preparation
o. purge
o. suction catheter
o. thermometer
o. thrush
o. tolerance
o. transmission
o. ulcer
Orandi
O. knife
O. technique
orange-colored tonsil
Orasone
OraSure salivary collection device
OraVax vaccine

orbital
o. depression
o. exenteration gastroscopic access technique
Orcein stain
orchectomy
orchialgia
orchiatrophy
orchichorea
orchidalgia
orchidectomy
partial o.
radical o.
orchiditis
orchidometer
Prader o.
punched-out o.
Test-Size o.
orchidoptosis
orchidorraphy
orchiectomy
prophylactic o.
radical inguinal o.
orchiepididymitis
orchilytic
orchiocele
orchiodynia
orchioneuralgia
orchiopathy
orchiopexy
Bevan o.
Cabot-Nesbit o.
eversion o.
Fowler-Stephens o.
Fowler-Stephens o.
laparoscopic o.
scrotal pouch o.
staged o.
Torek o.
transseptal o.
two-step o.
orchioplasty
orchiorrhaphy
orchiotherapy
orchiotomy
orchitic

NOTES

orchitis
  o. parotidea
  Salmonella enteritidis o.
  traumatic o.
  o. variolosa
orchotomy
Oreopoulos Zellerman catheter
Oresus Potentest test
Oretic
Oreticyl
Orex
organ
  artificial o.
  o. donation
  O. Procurement Program
  o. transplantation
organelle
organic
  o. neurologic disease
  o. nitrate
organism
  Campylobacter-like o.
  enteropathic o.
  H. pylori-like o. (HPLO)
  microaerophilic o.
  urea-splitting o.
organized germinal center
organoaxial gastric volvulus
organogenesis
organomegaly
organoscopy
Oriental
  O. cholangiohepatitis
  O. schistosomiasis
β-orientation
orienting reflex
orifice
  appendiceal o.
  bell-shaped o.
  duodenal o.
  epispadiac o.
  fistulous o.
  sharp-edged o.
  ureteral o.
Origin trocar
O-rings
Orion model AE 940 ion analyzer
Ormond disease
ornithine
  o. carbamoyl transferase
    deficiency
  o. decarboxylase (ODC)
orocecal transit time (OCTT)

oroesophageal overtube
orogastric Ewald tube
oropharyngeal
  o. carcinoma
  o. damage
  o. dysphagia
  o. tube
oro-respiratory tract
orosomucoid
orotracheal intubation
orphenadrine
Orr
  O. automatic reprocessor
  O. gall duct forceps
Orr-Loygue transabdominal
  proctopexy
Ortho
  O. Diagnostic System
  O. HCV ELISA test system
    second generation
orthochromatic dye
Orthoclone OKT 3
Orthohepadnavirus
Orthopara-DDD
orthostatic change
orthostatism
orthotopic
  o. appendicocystostomy
  o. bladder
  o. colonic reservoir
  o. continent reservoir
  o. hemi-Kock operation
  o. liver transplant (OLT)
  o. liver transplantation (OLT)
  o. remodeled ileocolonic
    reservoir
  o. transplantation
  o. voiding
orthovoltage teletherapy
Orthoxine
Orudis
Osbon
  O. ErecAid VCD
  O. pressure-point tension ring
Os-Cal
oscheitis
oschelephantiasis
oscheohydrocele
oscheoplasty
oscillatory potential
oscilloscope
  Tektronix digital o.

Osler-Weber-Rendu
    O.-W.-R. disease
    O.-W.-R. syndrome
    O.-W.-R. telangiectasia
Osmette osmometer
osmium tetroxide
osmolality
    diurnal urine o.
    medullary interstitial o.
    plasma o.
    urine o.
osmolarity
    o. of the ink
    urine o. (Uosm)
Osmolite HN enteral feeding
osmometer
    Model 5500 vapor pressure o.
    Osmette o.
osmoreceptor
OSMO reverse osmosis unit
osmotic
    o. diarrhea
    o. diuretic
    o. laxative
osseous metaplasia
ossification
    metaplastic o.
osteitis
    o. pubis
osteoarthropathy
    hypertrophic o.
osteoblast-like proliferation
osteoclast-like giant cell (OCLG)
osteoclast maturation
osteodystrophy
    hepatic o.
    renal o.
osteogenic
    o. differentiation
    o. sarcoma
osteomalacia
osteopenia
osteophyte
    esophageal o.
osteopontin
osteoporosis
osteosarcoma

osteotomy
    anterior innominate o.
    pelvic o.
ostial atherosclerotic plaque
ostium
ostomate
ostomy
    o. appliance
    o. bag
    ConvaTec Durahesive Wafer o.
    o. loop
    o. skin
O'Sullivan-O'Connor abdominal
    retractor
O'Sullivan scoring system
12-O-tetradecanoylphorbol-13-acetate
    (TPA)
    phorbol ester -O.-t.-a. (phorbol
    ester TPA)
Otis urethrotome
otolaryngologic manifestation
Otrivin
Ott/Mayo Channel Sampling kit
ouabain
outcome and process assessment
outer
    o. cortical blood flow (OCBF)
    o. crossbar
    o. diameter (OD)
outflow
    hepatic venous o.
    mean venous o. (MVO)
    pulmonary o.
    o. tract
outlet
    bladder o.
    o. dysfunction
    gastric o.
    o. obstruction
    o. obstruction constipation
    pyloric o.
outline
    gastric o.
outpatient endoscopy
output
    basal acid o. (BAO)
    intake and o. (I&O)

O

NOTES

output *(continued)*
  meal-stimulated acid o.
  (MSAO)
  peak acid o. (PAO)
oval
  o. esophagoscope
  o. snare
oval-form colonic groove
oval-open esophagoscope
ova and parasites (O&P)
ovarian
  o. cancer
  o. carcinoma
  o. dermoid cyst
  o. disease
  o. endometrioma
  o. enlargement
  o. fibroma
  o. hyperstimulation syndrome
  o. overstimulation syndrome
  o. remnant syndrome
  o. vein syndrome
ovarii
  stroma o.
  struma o.
  tunica albuginea o.
ovary
  streak o.
ovatus
  Bacteroides o.
over-and-over suture
overdistension
overdose (OD)
  acetaminophen o.
overdosing
overexpression
  p53 o.
overflow
  o. fecal incontinence
  o. incontinence
  o. theory
overgrowth
  bacterial o.
  gastric bacterial o. (GBO)
  small intestinal bacterial o.
  (SIBO)
  tube o.
overlap syndrome
overload
  hepatic copper o.
  nitrogen o.
  volume o.
overlying clot

oversedation
over-the-wire
  o.-t.-w. balloon catheter
  o.-t.-w. set
  o.-t.-w. technique
overt nephropathy
overtube
  Christopher-Williams o.
  flexible endoscopic o.
  Mill-Rose flexible
  endoscopic o.
  negative pressure o.
  oroesophageal o.
  o. sheath
  split o.
  Steigmann-Goff endoscopic
  ligature o.
  Williams varices injection o.
oviductal fluid
oviduct epithelia
ovoid fungi
oxacillin
**oxacillin-associated anicteric
  hepatitis**
oxalate
  calcium o.
  o. calculus
  o. crystal
oxaloacetate
oxalosis
oxaluria
  calcium o.
  enteric o.
oxamniquine
oxandrolone
  o. treatment
oxazepam
oxidant
  o. injury
  iron-dependent o.
oxidase
  o. cytosolic factor
  NADPH o.
  xanthine o.
oxidation
  arachidonic acid o.
  xanthine o.
β-oxidation
  mitochondrial fatty acid β-o.
  β-o. pathway
oxidative
  o. cell injury

o. phosphorylation
slow-twitch o.
oxidative-glycolytic fiber
oxide
deuterium o.
donor of nitric o.
endothelium-derived nitric o.
(EDNO)
ethylene o.
magnesium o.
mercuric o.
nitric o. (NO)
nitrous o.
propylene o.
oxidoreductase activity
oxime
sugar o.
oximetry
pulse o.
oxybutynin
o. chloride
Oxycel
oxychlorosene sodium
oxycodone
oxygen
blood gas on o.

o. desaturation
fractional percentage of
inspired o. (FiO$_2$)
o. radical
o. saturation
o. saturation indices (ISO2)
oxygenation
medullary o.
oxygenator
membrane o.
oxygen-derived free radical
oxygen-free radical
Oxyguard oxygenating mouthguard
oxymorphone
oxyntic
o. cell
o. gland
o. mucosa
oxyphenbutazone
oxyphencyclimine
o. hydrochloride
oxyphenonium
oxytoca
Klebsiella o.

NOTES

O

415

P-900
    900 mOsmolar amino acid-glucose
    solution
p21
    ras p21
p53
    p53 allelotyping
    p53 antibody
    p53 expression
    p53 gene
    p53 immunohistochemistry
    p53 mutation
    p53 nuclear protein
    p53 nuclear staining
    p53 overexpression
    p53 protein
    p53 proto-oncogene
    p53 reactivity
    p53 tumor suppressor gene
    analysis
    p53 wild-type
P23b Statham pressure transducer
P24 antigen
P450 function
p47 cytosolic protein
p67 cytosolic protein
PA
    plasminogen activator
PAb
    protein antibody
    PAb 1801 monoclonal antibody
PABA
    para-aminobenzoic acid
    PABA test
PACAP
    pituitary adenylate cyclase activating
    polypeptide
paced rhythm
pacemaker cell
pachycholia
pachychymia
pacinian corpuscle
pack
    gauze p.
    laparotomy p.
    moist laparotomy p.
    petrolatum gauze p.
package
    lymphatic p.

Packard Auto-Gamma 5650
    analyzer
packed red blood cells
packing
    Adaptic p.
    p. forceps
    p. fraction
Pacquin ureterolysis
pad
    abdominal p.
    abdominal fat p.
    abdominal laparotomy p.
    Active Living incontinence p.
    antimesenteric fat p.
    bulbocavernosus fat p.
    p. cover
    dinner p.
    esophagogastric fat p.
    fat p.
    ileocecal fat p.
    laparotomy p.
    Martius fat p.
    Mikulicz p.
    Sani Pads medicated
    cleansing p.
padding
    Spenco p.
Padua bladder urinary pouch
Paecilomyces
PAF
    platelet activating factor
PAGE
    polyacrylamide gel electrophoresis
Pagenstecher circle
Paget
    P. disease
    P. disease of perianal area
    P. extramammary disease
    P. perianal disease
Pagitane
PAH
    para-aminohippurate
    PAH clearance
PAI
    plasminogen activator inhibitor
PAI-1
    type-1 plasminogen activator
    inhibitor

P

PAI-2
　　type-2 plasminogen activator
　　　inhibitor
pain
　　abdominal p.
　　biliary p.
　　boring p.
　　burning p.
　　chest p.
　　colicky abdominal p.
　　constricting p.
　　p. control
　　cramping p.
　　crampy abdominal p.
　　deep p.
　　diffuse p.
　　drug-induced p.
　　dull p.
　　epicritic p.
　　epigastric p.
　　exacerbation of p.
　　exquisite p.
　　functional p.
　　gnawing p.
　　hunger p.
　　intermittent p.
　　knife-like p.
　　lancinating p.
　　localized p.
　　loin p.
　　nagging p.
　　nocturnal p.
　　noncardiac chest p.
　　onset of p.
　　palliation of p.
　　parietal p.
　　perianal p.
　　perirectal p.
　　poorly localized p.
　　postprandial p.
　　posture-dependent p.
　　protopathic p.
　　radiating p.
　　rebound p.
　　recurrent p.
　　recurring p.
　　referred p.
　　remission of p.
　　retrosternal chest p.
　　scrotal p.
　　severe p.
　　somatic p.
　　steady p.

　　sudden onset of p.
　　tearing p.
　　terrifying p.
　　testicular p.
　　unrelenting p.
　　unrelieved p.
　　unremitting p.
　　visceral p.
painful
　　p. defecation
　　p. hematuria
painless
　　p. hematuria
　　p. jaundice
　　p. rectal bleeding
painter's colic
Pak
　　SCD MaleFactor P.
palate
　　cleft p.
　　smoker's p.
palatine pillar
palatinus
　　torus p.
palatopharyngeal fold
Palco enuretic alarm system
pale
　　p. cell
　　p. stool
palindromic rheumatism
palladium-103
　　p. seeds implant
palliation
　　p. of pain
palliative
　　p. exeresis
　　p. therapy
pallidum
　　Treponema p.
pallor
　　mucosal p.
palmar
　　p. erythema
　　p. grasp
palmatus
　　penis p.
Palmaz
　　P. balloon-expandable stent
　　P. stent
Palmer acid test for peptic ulcer
palmin test
palmitin test

Palomo
P. operation
P. procedure
P. technique
palp
palpable
p. adenopathy
p. cord
p. gallbladder
p. mass
p. pyloric olive
p. rib diastasis
p. stool
palpably
p. normal
palpating probe
palpation
p. tenderness
Pamelor
Pamine
p-aminohippurate
p-amino-hippuric acid
pamoate
pyrantel p.
pampinocele
PAN
puromycin aminonucleoside
nephropathy
panacinar
p. disease
p. emphysema
p-ANC
perinuclear antineutrophil
cytoplasmic
p-ANC antibody
p-ANC genetic marker
pancolectomy
pancolitis
steroid responsive p.
pancolonoscopy
pancreas
aberrant p.
accessory p.
anlage of p.
annular p.
Aselli p.

Christmas tree appearance
of p.
p. divisum (PD)
ectopic p.
endoscopic retrograde
parenchymography of p.
(ERPP)
head of p.
heterotopic p.
lesser p.
neck of p.
tail of p.
uncinate process of p.
Willis p.
Winslow p.
Pancrease (MT 10, 4, 16, 25)
pancreas-kidney
simultaneous p.-k. (SPK)
p.-k. transplant
pancreatalgia
pancreatectomy
distal p.
en bloc distal p.
left-to-right subtotal p.
partial p.
subtotal p.
total p.
Whipple p.
pancreatic
p. abscess
p. acinar cell
p. acinar cell carcinoma
p. acini
p. alpha-amylase
p. amylase
p. ascariasis
p. ascites
p. bladder
p. calcification
p. calculus
p. cancer (PC)
p. cancer marker
p. carcinoma (PCA)
p. cholera
p. cholera syndrome
p. colic
p. cutaneous fistula

NOTES

P

pancreatic *(continued)*
p. cyst
p. disease
p. diverticulum
p. duct
p. ductal hypertension
p. ductal morphological change
p. duct disruption
p. duct manipulation
p. duct sphincter
p. duct sphincterotomy
p. ducts pressure (PDP)
p. duct stent
p. duct stone
p. duct stricture
p. endoprosthesis
p. enzyme
p. enzyme replacement therapy
p. fibrosis
p. fistula
p. hamartoma
p. injury
p. intraluminal radiation
  therapy
p. islet cell
p. islet cell carcinoma
p. islet cell tumor
p. juice
p. lesion
p. lipase
p. lipase deficiency
p. lymphangiectasia
p. mucinous
  cystadenocarcinoma
p. oncofetal antigen (POA)
p. phlegmon
p. polypeptide (PP)
p. pseudocyst
p. pseudocyst abscess
p. pseudocystogastrostomy
p. rest
p. sarcoidosis
p. secretory flow rate (PSFR)
p. secretory test
p. sepsis
p. sphincteroplasty
p. steatorrhea
p. stent
p. stone
p. stone protein (PSP)
p. tail resection
p. transpapillary stenting
p. trauma

p. tumor diagnosis
p. tumor localization
pancreatica
achylia p.
ansa p.
diarrhea p.
pancreaticobiliary
p. common channel
p. disease
p. ductal junction
p. ductal system
p. endoscopy
p. junction
p. malignancy
p. septum
p. sphincter
p. tract
pancreaticocholedochoductal junction
pancreaticocystostomy
pancreaticoduodenal
p. transplantation
p. vein
pancreaticoduodenectomy
pylorus sparing p.
Whipple p.
pancreaticoduodenostomy
Child p.
Dennis-Varco p.
Waugh-Clagett p.
Whipple p.
pancreaticogastrostomy
pancreaticohepatic syndrome
pancreaticojejunostomy
caudal p.
Duval p.
lateral p.
longitudinal p.
Puestow p.
Roux-en-Y p.
p. stenosis
pancreaticopleural fistula
pancreaticosplenic omentum
pancreatin
pancreatis
caput p.
pancreatitis
acquired p.
acute p.
acute gallstone p.
acute hemorrhagic p.
acute recurrent p. (ARP)
acute relapsing p.
alcoholic p.

biliary p.
calcereous p.
calcific p.
calcifying p.
centrilobular p.
chronic p. (CP)
chronic alcoholic p.
chronic calcifying p. (CCP)
chronic relapsing p.
coagulopathy p.
diffuse p.
drug-induced p.
edematous p.
endoscopic sphincterotomy-
 induced p.
familial p.
focal p.
fulminating p.
gallstone p.
groove p.
hemoductal p.
hemorrhagic p.
hemorrhagic necrotizing p.
hereditary p. (HP)
idiopathic p.
idiopathic fibrosing p.
idiopathic recurrent p. (IRP)
interstitial p.
microlithiasis-induced p.
necrotizing p.
nodular p.
nutritional p.
obstructive p.
pentamidine-induced p.
perilobar p.
post-ERCP induced p.
post-procedure p.
purulent p.
recurrent p.
segmentary p.
tropical calcific p.
ventral chronic calcific p.
pancreatitis-related
 p.-r. bleeding
 p.-r. hemorrhage

pancreatobiliary
 p. canal
 p. region
pancreatocholangiography
 retrograde p.
pancreatocholecystostomy
pancreatoduodenal cancer
pancreatoduodenectomy
pancreatoduodenostomy
pancreatogastrostomy
pancreatogenic, pancreatogenous
pancreatogram
 endoscopic retrograde p. (ERP)
 rat-tail appearance on p.
pancreatography
 endoscopic p.
 endoscopic retrograde p. (ERP)
 retrograde p.
pancreatojejunostomy
 cystolateral p.
 retrocolic end-to-end p.
pancreatolith
pancreatolithectomy
pancreatolithiasis
pancreatolithotomy
pancreatolysis
pancreatolytic
pancreatomy
pancreatopathy
pancreatoscope
 ultrathin p.
pancreatoscopy
 peroral p.
pancreatotomy
pancreectomy
pancrelipase
pancreolith
pancreopathy
pancreoprivic
pancreoscopy
 infragastric p.
pancreostatin
pancreozymin
Pancrex
panel-reactive antibody (PRA)
panendoscope
 cap-fitted p.

NOTES

P

panendoscope *(continued)*
    flexible forward-viewing p.
    Olympus GIF-D-series p.
    Olympus GIF-XQ-series p.
    Storz p.
    Wolf rigid p.
panendoscopy
    fiberoptic p.
    lower p.
    primary p.
    upper gastrointestinal p.
Paneth cell
panlobular emphysema
panmucosal inflammatory cell infiltration
Panmycin
panniculectomy
panniculitis
    mesenteric p. (MP)
panniculus
    hanging p.
pannus
Panoview rod-lens ureteroscope
panproctocolectomy
pantaloon hernia
Pantopaque
pantothenic
    p. acid
    p. acid deficiency-induced colitis
pants
    Ashton p.
    Dignity incontinence p.
    Endo p.
    Holyoke p.
    Kleinert p.
    Suretys p.
    Ultrafem p.
pants-over-vest
    p.-o.-v. hernial repair
    p.-o.-v. herniorrhaphy
Panzer gallbladder scissors
PAO
    peak acid output
PAP
    prostatic acid phosphatase
    PAP test
Pap
    Papanicolaou
    Pap smear
    Pap test

papain
Papanicolaou (Pap)
    P. method
    P. stain
papaverine
    p. hydrochloride
    p. injection
PAP-HT25 cell
papilla, pl. **papillae**
    balloon dilation of the p.
    duodenal p.
    major p.
    minor p.
    sloughed p.
    Suda (type I, II, III) classification of p.
    p. of Vater
papillary
    p. adenocarcinoma
    p. adenoma
    p. gastric carcinoma
    p. hyperplasia
    p. lesion
    p. necrosis
    p. renal cell carcinoma
    p. stenosis
    p. tip
    p. transitional cell carcinoma
papilledema
papillitis
papilloma
    esophageal squamous p.
    hirsuitoid p.
    inverted p.
    squamous cell p. (SCP)
papilloma-carcinoma sequence
papillomatosis
    biliary p.
    p. coronae
    p. of intrahepatic bile duct
papillomatous neotransformation
papillomavirus
    human p. (HPV)
    human p. 16 (HPV 16)
papillotome
    30-30 p.
    Accuratome pre-curved p.
    BILISYSTEM wire-guided p.
    Classen-Demling p.
    Cremer-Ikeda p.
    double-lumen tapered-tip p.
    dual-lumen p.

Erlangen p.
Erlangen-type p.
Frimberger-Karpiel 12
  o'clock p.
Howell Rotatable BII p.
Huibregtse-Katon p.
Microvasive p.
needle p.
needle-knife p.
Olympus needle-knife p.
Piggyback needle-knife p.
precut p.
shark fin p.
Swenson p.
Wilson-Cook p.
Wiltek p.
papillotome/sphincterotome
Zimmon p.
papillotomy
endoscopic p. (EPT)
needle-knife p.
precut p.
Pap-Kaps
papule
Bowen p.
papulosis
bowenoid p.
papulous gastropathy
Paque
E-Z P.
Paquin technique
PAR
postanesthesia recovery
para-aminobenzoic acid (PABA)
para-aminohippurate (PAH)
^{131}I para-aminohippuric acid
para-aminosalicylate hypersensitivity
para-aortic
p.-a. lymphadenectomy
p.-a. region
parabola
paracancerous tissue
paracecal appendix
paracellular
p. pathway
p. route

paracentesis
abdominal p.
diagnostic p.
large volume p. (LVP)
paracervical tenderness
paracetamol absorption
parachute reflex
paracoccidiodomycosis
paracolic
p. abscess
p. gutter
paracollicular biopsy
paracrine
p. cell
p. factor
p. peptide
paradoxical
p. contraction
p. incontinence
p. puborectalis contraction
p. renal response
paradoxic motion
paradoxus
pulsus p.
paraductal adenopathy
paraduodenal pseudocyst
paraesophageal
p. diaphragmatic hernia
p. hiatal hernia
p. varices
p. varix
paraesophagogastric
devascularization
para-exstrophy skin flap
paraffin-embedded
p.-e. specimen
p.-e. tissue
paraffin-section light microscopy
paraformaldehyde
paragastric pseudocyst
parahaemolyticus
Vibrio p.
parahiatal hernia
paraileostomal hernia
para-isopropyliminodiacetic acid
(PIPIDA)
parakeratosis

NOTES

P

paralytic
  p. colonic obstruction
  p. ileus
  p. intestinal obstruction
paramedian
  p. incision
parameter
  anthropomorphic p.
  chronobiological p.
  clinical p.
  clotting p.
  DIC p.
  kinetic p.
paraneoplastic syndrome
paranephric abscess
para-nitroaniline release
paraparesis
  spastic p.
paraperitoneal nephrectomy
paraphasias
paraphimosis
paraplegia
paraprostatitis
paraproteinemia
parapubic hernia
paraquat
paraquat-induced upper gastrointestinal injury
pararectal
  p. abscess
  p. fistula
  p. line
pararectus incision
parasite
  intestinal p.
  isosporan p.
  protozoan p.
  stool for ova and p.'s
parasitic
  p. chylocele
  p. cyst
  p. disease
  p. infection
  p. infestation
  p. liver disease
  p. peritonitis
parasitizing macrophage
parasitology
paraspadia, paraspadias
paraspinous
  p. aspect
  p. muscle
parasternum

parastomal hernia
parasympathetic projection
parasympatholytic drugs
parasympathomimetic
  p. agent
  p. anticholinesterase
  p. drugs
paratesticular
  p. fat
  p. malignancy
  p. rhabdomyosarcoma
parathyroid
  p. disease
  p. hormone (PTH)
  p. hyperplasia
paraumbilical
  p. vein
  p. vein tumor (PUVT)
parauresis
paravariceal
  p. fibrosis
  p. injection
  p. sclerotherapy
paravesical pouch
paregoric
parenchyma
  allograft p.
  hepatic p.
  liver p.
  renal p.
parenchymal
  p. hematoma
  p. jaundice
  p. liver disease
  p. sparing surgery
  p. tissue
  p. tumor
parenchymatous acute renal failure
parenchymography
  endoscopic retrograde p. (ERP)
parenteral
  p. alimentation
  p. feeding
  p. guanethidine
  p. hyperalimentation
  p. immunization
  p. methyldopa
  p. nutrition
pargyline
parietal
  p. cell
  p. cell index
  p. cell vagotomy (PCV)

p. epithelium
p. fistula
p. hernia
p. pain
p. peritoneum
parietography
Paris renal adenocarcinoma
Parker-Kerr
  P.-K. closed method
  P.-K. enteroenterostomy
  P.-K. suture
Parker retractor
parkinsonian gait
Parks
  P. ileal reservoir
  P. ileoanal anastomosis
  P. ileoanal reservoir
  P. ileostomy pouch
  P. method of anal fistulotomy
  P. partial sphincterotomy
  P. retractor
  P. staged fistulotomy
Parnate
paromomycin
paromphalocele
paronychia
parorchidium
parotid
  p. gland enlargement
parotidea
  orchitis p.
parovarian
  p. cyst
  p. mass
paroxysmal
  p. anal hyperkinesis
  p. motor disease
  p. nocturnal hemoglobinemia
  p. nocturnal hemoglobinuria
    (PNH)
Parsidol
partial
  p. bile outflow obstruction
  p. bowel obstruction
  p. cystectomy
  p. enterocele
  p. gastrectomy

p. hepatectomy
p. ileal bypass
p. nephrectomy
p. orchidectomy
p. pancreatectomy
p. thromboplastin time (PTT)
p. water bath and water
  cushion
p. zonal dissection (PZD)
partial-occlusion clamp
particle
  Dane p.
  food p.
  virus-like p. (VLP)
particulate
  p. radiation
  p. silicone
Partipilo gastrostomy
partition
  gastric p.
partitioning
  abdominal p.
paruresis
parvum
  Corynebacterium p.
  Cryptosporidium p.
PAS
  periodic acid-Schiff
  PAS stain
  PAS test
PAS-AB
  periodic acid Schiff-Alcian blue
  combination stain
PAS-Alcian blue
passage
  biliary p.'s
  p. biliary dilatation catheter
  p. of flatus per vagina
  guidewire p.
  incomplete p.
  p. pressure
  spontaneous p.
  p. of stool
passive
  p. congestion
  p. Heymann nephritis (PHN)

NOTES

P

passive *(continued)*
    p. incontinence
    p. range of motion
Passport Balloon-on-a-Wire dilatation catheter
paste
    Anatrast barium sulfate p.
    Hollister Premium p.
    Karaya 5 p.
    sandy skin prepping p.
    Stomahesive P.
Pasteurella
    P. multocida
past pointing
PAT
    prophylactic antibiotic treatment
patch
    aortic p.
    Bowen p.
    Carrel aortic p.
    colic p.
    colonic p.
    estradiol transderm p.
    Gore-Tex soft tissue p.
    p. graft
    herald p.
    mucous p.
    omental p.
    Peyer p.
    p. technique
    vein p.
    white p.
patchy
    p. colonic ulceration
    p. necrosis
patella disease
patency
    biliary stent p.
    p. rate
    stent p.
patent
    p. airway
    p. urachus
Paterson-Brown-Kelly syndrome
Paterson-Kelly syndrome
pathergy phenomenon
Pathfinder exchange guidewire
Pathibamate-200
Pathilon
pathogen
    blood-borne p.
    invasive enteric p.
    protozoan p.

pathogenesis
pathogenetic
    p. factor
pathogenic bacterium
pathognomonic feature
pathologic
    p. reflux
    p. substaging
pathological hypersecretory condition
pathology
    renal p.
    thoracic aortic p.
pathophysiology
pathway
    antigen-dependent p.
    antigen-independent p.
    cyclooxygenase p.
    gluconeogenic p.
    glutamine aminotransferase p.
    guanosine monophosphate p.
    lipoxygenase p.
    mitochondrial glutamate dehydrogenase p.
    multisynaptic p.
    neural p.
    nonapoptotic p.
    oligosynaptic p.
    β-oxidation p.
    paracellular p.
    receptor-mediated endocytosis p.
    renal transduction p.
    signal-transduction p.
patient
    Child class A p.
    Child class B p.
    Child class C p.
    Child C-minus p.
    cholestasis p.
    cirrhotic p.
    diabetic p.
    endoscopically normal p.
    gastrectomized p.
    hypochondriacal p.
    immunosuppressed p.
    irradiated p.
    irrigating p.
    leukemia p.
    nonirrigating p.
    p. positioning
    posttransplant p.
    p. selection

shock p.
tube-fed p.

pattern

abdominal wall venous p.
anhaustral colonic gas p.
circadian testosterone p.
cobblestone p.
colonic mucosal p.
cytometric p.
DNA ploidy p.
echo p.
fine gastric mucosal p.
fine reticular p.
fold p.
gallstone p.
gas p.
haustral p.
hindgut p.
histochemical p.
irregular amputated mucosal p.
manometric p.
Mendelian p.
mosaic duodenal mucosal p.
mucosal p.
mucosal guideline p.
nodule-in-nodule p.
nonspecific gas p.
reticulonodular p.
rugal p.
snake-skin mucosal p.
sonographic p.
sonographic gallstone p.
trabecular/sinusoidal p.
vascular p.
venous p.

patulous

p. anus
p. cardia
p. gastroesophageal junction
p. hiatus
p. pylorus

Pauchet procedure
pauciimmune crescentic
   glomerulonephritis
paucity

bile duct p.

Paul-Mikulicz resection
Paul-Mixter tube
pause-squeeze method
Pavabid
Pavacap
Pavacen
Pavatest
Pavatine
Payne-DeWind jejunoileal bypass
Payne operation
Payr

P. pyloric clamp
P. pyloric forceps

Pazo
PBC

primary biliary cirrhosis

PBC-associated antibody
PBD

percutaneous biliary drainage

PBL

peripheral blood lymphocyte

PBMC

peripheral blood mononuclear cell
   interphase PBMC

PBS

phosphate-buffered saline

PC

pancreatic cancer
principal cell

PC10 monoclonal antibody
PCA

pancreatic carcinoma

PCa

prostate cancer

PCC

peripheral cholangiocarcinoma

P cell
PCI

pneumatosis cystoides intestinalis

PCIVOT

Prostate Cancer Intervention Versus
   Observation Trial

PCLD

polycystic liver disease

PCM

protein-calorie malnutrition

NOTES

P

PCNA
  proliferating cell nuclear antigen
PCNA-labeling index (PCNA-LI)
PCNA-LI
  PCNA-labeling index
PCNL
  percutaneous nephrolithotomy
  percutaneous nephrostolithotomy
PCPS
  peroral cholangiopancreatoscopy
PCR
  polymerase chain reaction
  protein catabolic rate
PCRC
  primary colorectal cancer
PCS
  peroral cholangioscopy
  postcholecystectomy syndrome
PCT
  porphyria cutanea tarda
  proximal convoluted tubule
PCV
  parietal cell vagotomy
PD
  pancreas divisum
  peritoneal dialysis
  potential difference
PDE
  peritoneal dialysis effluent
PDG
  phosphate-dependent glutaminase
PDGF
  platelet-derived growth factor
PDL
  polycystic disease of liver
PDP
  pancreatic ducts pressure
PDS
  PDS suture
  PDS Vicryl suture
PDT
  photodynamic therapy
peak
  p. acid output (PAO)
  p. flow rate
  p. pressure
  p. response
  p. secretory flow rate (PSFR)
  p. secretory flow rate test
  p. urinary flow study
  p. uroflow

Péan
  P. clamp
  P. forceps
peanut
  p. agglutinin (PNA)
  p. sponge
Pearson
  P. correlation
  P. marrow-pancreas syndrome
  P. $\chi 2$ test
pea soup stool
peau d'orange
pecten band
pectin
pectinate line
pectoralis muscle
pectoriloquy
  whispered p.
pectus excavatum
pedal
  p. control venography
  p. edema
  suction foot p.
Pedialyte RS electrolyte solution
Pediapred
pediatric
  p. carcinoma
  p. colonoscope
  p. colonoscopy
  p. endoscope
  p. endoscopy
  p. esophagogastroduodenoscopy
  p. feeding tube
  p. gastroscope
  p. nasogastric tube
  P. Peritoneal Dialysis Study
    consortium
  p. stirrups
Pediazole
pedicle
  p. clamp
  p. flap urethroplasty
  omental p.
  renal p.
  vascular p.
pedicled omentoplasty
pediculicide
pediculosis
Pedi PEG tube
pedunculated
  p. polyp
pedunculation
peel-away sheath

peeping testis
Pee Wee low profile gastrostomy tube
pefloxacin
PEG
 percutaneous endoscopic gastrostomy
 polyethylene glycol
  Bard PEG
  PEG bumper
  complete replacement PEG
  PEG insertion
  PEG lavage
  Ponsky-Gauderer type PEG
  PEG pull
  PEG push
  replacement PEG
  Sacks-Vine type PEG
  Sandoz Caluso 22F, 28F super PEG
  PEG tube
peg
 rete p.
PEG-400 tube
PEG-assisted decompression
PEG-ELS
 polyethylene glycol electrolyte lavage solution
PEI
 percutaneous ethanol injection
 polyethylenimine
  PEI therapy
PEJ
 percutaneous endoscopic jejunostomy
  PEJ tube
pelican biopsy forceps
Pelikan brand India ink
peliosis
 bacillary p.
 hepatic p.
 p. hepaticus
 p. hepatis
pellagra
 infantile p.
pellagroid
pellagrous

pellet
 radiopaque p.
 ^{99m}Tc-labeled Amberlite p.
pelleted stool
pellucida
 zona p. (ZP)
pelvic
 p. abscess
 p. adhesion
 p. appendicitis
 p. autonomic nerve
 p. brim
 p. colon
 p. colonic surgery
 p. diaphragm
 p. discontinuity
 p. exenteration
 p. floor
 p. floor disorder
 p. floor dysfunction
 p. floor dyssynergia
 p. floor electromyography
 p. floor exercise (PFE)
 p. floor movement
 p. floor neurophysiology
 p. floor syndrome
 p. ileal reservoir construction
 p. inflammatory disease (PID)
 p. lymphadenectomy
 p. lymph node
 p. lymphocelectomy
 p. muscle training
 p. osteotomy
 p. peritoneum
 p. phased-array coil (PPA)
 p. plexus
 p. pouch
 p. pouchoscopy
 p. pouch procedure
 p. prolapse
 p. sidewall
 p. stimulation
 p. stone
pelvicaliceal
 p. stasis
 p. system
pelviectasis

NOTES

P

pelvilithotomy, pelviolithotomy
pelvioplasty
pelviotomy, pelvitomy
pelvirectal achalasia
pelvis
    arcus tendineus fasciae p.
    obstructed p.
    renal p.
pelviscope
pelviscopic clip ligation technique
pelvitomy (*var. of* pelviotomy)
Pemberton sigmoid clamp
pemphigoid
    benign mucous membrane p.
    bullous p.
    mucous membrane p.
pemphigus
    p. vulgaris
PE-MV balloon dilatation catheter
penbutolol
pencil
    cautery p.
    electrocautery p.
pencil-like stool
pencil-tipped electrode
pendiomide
pendulous abdomen
penectomy
penes (*pl. of* penis)
Penetrak
penetrating
    p. abdominal trauma
    p. pancreatic trauma
    p. trauma
    p. ulcer
    p. wound
penetration
    capsular p.
    splenic p.
Penetrex
Pen-F half-frame camera
penicillamine
penicillin
    benzathine p.
    beta-lactamase-resistant p.
    procaine p.
penicillin-streptomycin
penile
    p. amputation
    p. biothesiometry
    p. carcinoma
    p. curvature
    p. deformity

    p. duplex ultrasonography
    p. epispadias
    p. erection
    p. extensibility
    p. fibromatosis
    p. hypospadias
    p. implant
    p. incarceration
    p. injection testing
    p. injection therapy
    p. intraepithelial neoplasia
    p. island flap
    p. lesion
    p. plethysmography
    p. raphe
    p. revascularization
    p. rupture
    p. schwannoma
    p. sensitivity
    p. synechiae
    p. torsion
    p. turgescence
    p. urethra
    p. vascular function assessment
    p. vein occlusion therapy
    p. venous ligation surgery
penile-brachial index
penis, pl. penes
    bifid p.
    bulbus p.
    buried p.
    clubbed p.
    concealed p.
    double p.
    p. lunatus
    p. palmatus
    retractile concealed p.
    webbed p.
penischisis
penitis
Penn
    P. pouch
    P. umbilical scissors
Pennington
    P. clamp
    P. forceps
    P. rectal speculum
penoid tissue
penoplasty
penopubic
    p. epispadias
    p. junction

penoscrotal
- p. hypospadias
- p. junction
- p. transposition
- p. transposition complex
- p. trapping
- p. webbing

penotomy

Penrose
- P. drain
- P. seton
- P. sump drain

pentagastrin
- p. gastric secretory test
- p. infusion
- p. infusion test
- p. provocative test
- p. stimulated analysis
- p. stimulated analysis test

pentamidine
- p. isethionate

pentamidine-induced pancreatitis

pentane excretion level

pentapiperium

Pentasa

pentastomiasis

pentastomum
- p. denticulatum
- p. denticulatum fibrosis
- p. denticulatum nodule

Pentax
- P. EC-series video endoscope
- P. EG-series video endoscope
- P. EndoNet
- P. EndoNet digital endoscopy network
- P. endoscopic camera
- P. FC-series colonoscope
- P. FD-series video endoscope
- P. FG-series video endoscope
- P. fiberscope
- P. FS-series flexible fiberoptic video sigmoidoscope
- P. gastroscope
- P. prototype needle
- P. VSB-P-series enteroscope

Pentax/Hitachi FG-32UA

pentazocine

pentetreotide
- indium-III p.

penthienate

pentolinium

pentosan
- p. polysulfate sodium
- p. sodium polysulfate

pentose phosphate shunt

pentoxifylline

Pento-X syndrome

Pen-Vee K

Pepcid
- P. AC
- P. I.V.

PEPCK
- phosphoenolpyruvate carboxykinase

peplomycin

peppermint oil

pepsic

pepsin
- p. secretion

pepsinogen
- p. A-C ratio
- p. A level
- p. C level
- p. I
- p. level

pepstatin

Peptamen
- P. liquid nutrition

Peptavlon
- P. stimulation test

peptic
- p. cell
- p. cell receptor
- p. esophageal stricture
- p. esophagitis
- p. reflux
- p. reflux disease
- p. stricture
- p. ulcer
- p. ulcer bleeding
- p. ulcer disease (PUD)

peptidase

peptide
- antral p.

NOTES

P

peptide *(continued)*
  atrial natriuretic p. (ANP)
  brain-gut p.
  calcitonin gene-related p.
    (CGRP)
  cellular p.
  chemotactic p.
  C-type atrial natriuretic p. (C-ANP)
  gastrin-releasing p. (GRP)
  gastrointestinal regularity p.
  p. HI
  p. histidine isoleucine (PHI)
  p. hormone
  intestinal p.
  met-enkephalin p.
  neutrophil chemotactic p.
  opioid p.
  paracrine p.
  plasma atrial natriuretic p.
  posttranslational processing of
    the p.
  regulatory p.
  somatostatin p.
  trefoil p.
  p. tyrosine
  vasoactive intestinal p. (VIP)
  p. YY (PYY)
peptide/bombesin
  gastrin-releasing p./b.
peptidergic
  p. mechanism
  p. neuron
Pepto-Bismol
peptone
Peptostreptococcus
  P. micros
percent transferrin saturation
Percival gastric balloon
Percodan
Percoll
  P. bead
  P. filter
Percufix catheter cuff kit
Percuflex
  P. Amsterdam stent
  P. biliary stent
  P. catheter
  P. endopyelotomy stent
  P. Plus ureteral stent
percussion
  dullness to p.

  p. note
  p. tenderness
percutaneous
  p. abscess drainage
  p. antegrade biliary drainage
  p. bacille Calmette-Guérin
    administration
  p. balloon aspiration
  p. balloon dilation
  p. biliary drainage (PBD)
  p. biopsy
  p. catheter cecostomy
  p. cholangiography
  p. cholecystolithotomy
  p. cholecystostomy
  p. CT-guided aspiration
  p. debulking
  p. drainage catheter
  p. embolization therapy
  p. endopyeloureterotomy
  p. endoscopic gastrostomy
    (PEG)
  p. endoscopic jejunostomy
    (PEJ)
  p. endoscopic removal
  p. epididymal sperm aspiration
  p. ethanol injection (PEI)
  p. ethanol injection therapy
    (PEI therapy)
  p. femoral vein catheter
  p. fetal cystoscopy
  p. fine-needle pancreatic biopsy
  p. liver biopsy
  p. native renal biopsy
  p. needle aspiration
  p. nephrolitholapaxy
  p. nephrolithotomy (PCNL,
    PNL)
  p. nephrostolithotomy (PCNL)
  p. nephrostomy
  p. nephrostomy Malecot
    catheter
  p. nephrostomy tube placement
  p. pancreas biopsy
  p. pressure ureteral perfusion
    test
  p. radical cryosurgical ablation
    of prostate
  p. sampling method
  p. stent
  p. stone removal
  p. transcatheter perfusion
  p. transhepatic approach

p. transhepatic biliary drainage (PTBD)
p. transhepatic biliary drainage catheter
p. transhepatic cholangiogram (PTHC)
p. transhepatic cholangiography (PTC)
p. transhepatic cholangioscopy
p. transhepatic cholecystoscopy
p. transhepatic choledochoscopic electrohydraulic
p. transhepatic decompression
p. transhepatic drainage (PTD)
p. transhepatic obliteration
p. transhepatic obliteration of esophageal varix
p. transhepatic pigtail catheter
p. transhepatic portography
p. transluminal renal angioplasty (PTRA)
p. ultrasonic lithotriptor
percutanoue endoscopic placement of jejunal tube
Percy intestinal forceps
Percy-Wolfson gallbladder retractor
Perdiem
perendoscopic manometry
Pereyra
P. bladder neck suspension
P. ligature carrier
P. procedure
Pereyra-Raz cystourethropexy
perforate
perforated
p. acid peptic ulcer
p. appendicitis
p. appendix
p. carcinoma
p. cholecystitis
p. diverticulum
p. nasal septum
p. peptic ulcer
p. ulcer disease
p. viscus

perforating
p. aneurysm
p. forceps
p. ulcer
perforation
appendiceal p.
barogenic p.
bladder p.
bowel p.
p. of colon
colonic p.
ductal system p.
duodenal p.
endoscopic sphincterotomy-induced duodenal p.
eosinophilic ileal p.
esophageal p.
p. of gallbladder
gastric p.
intestinal p.
intraperitoneal p.
Niemeier gallbladder p.
peritoneal p.
polyethylene p.
prepyloric p.
retroduodenal p.
retroperitoneal p.
Performa ultrasound system
perfringens
Clostridium p.
perfusate
p. bag
esophageal p.
hyperosmolar p.
p. solution
perfusion
allogenic liver p.
p. cannula
CCD p.
con A-anti-con A p.
continuous hypothermic pulsatile p.
p. cooling
extracorporeal liver p. (ECLP)
ex vivo p.
heterologous liver p.
p. hypothermia technique

NOTES

perfusion (*continued*)
  hypothermic pulsatile p.
  intestinal p.
  intraperitoneal hyperthermic p.
  (IPHP)
  isolated hepatocyte p.
  p. machine
  percutaneous transcatheter p.
  plasma p.
  transcatheter p.
  transvenous p.
  trickle p.
pergolide dopaminergic medication
perhexiline maleate
Periactin
periadvential tissue
periampullary
  p. carcinoma
  p. duodenal diverticulum
  p. duodenal tumor
  p. malignancy
  p. mass
  p. neoplasm
  p. pseudotumor
  p. tumor
perianal
  p. abscess
  p. anorectal space
  p. area
  p. condyloma
  p. disease
  p. edema
  p. fistula
  p. fistula abscess
  p. hematoma
  p. hygiene
  p. infection
  p. lesion
  p. pain
  p. region
  p. skin tag
  p. soak
  p. space
  p. wart
pericapillary diffusion
pericardial
  p. decompression
  p. knock
pericecal abscess
pericentral
  p. hypoxia
  p. pyridine nucleotide
    fluorescence

pericholangiolar
pericholangitis
pericholecystic
  p. abscess
  p. edema
  p. stranding
Peri-Colace
pericolic
  p. abscess
  p. membrane syndrome
  p. phlegmon
pericolitis
pericolonic
  p. abscess
  p. fat
pericolostomy area
pericostal suture
periductal
  p. fibrosis
  p. gland
periesophagogastric lymph node
  metastasis
perifascial nephrectomy
periglandular nonspecific
  inflammatory reaction
periglomerular
perihepatic adhesion
perihepatitis
  p. syndrome
peri-ileal
perikaryon
perilobar pancreatitis
perilobular
  p. duct
  p. fibrosis
perimedial fibroplasia
perimesangial GBM
perimylolysis
perinatal
  p. hemochromatosis
  p. torsion
  p. urology
perinea (*pl. of* perineum)
perineal
  p. abscess
  p. descent
  p. drain
  p. fistula
  p. hypospadias
  p. impact trauma
  p. incision
  p. infection
  p. lithotomy

p. nerve
p. nerve terminal motor
latency test
p. polyp
p. prostatectomy
p. section
p. sinus
p. sinus tract
p. skin tag
p. ulcer
p. urethrostomy
p. urethrotomy
p. urinary fistula
perineobulbar
p. detrusor facilitative reflex
p. detrusor inhibitory reflex
perineodetrusor inhibitory reflex
perineometer
perineostomy
perineotomy
perinephric
p. abscess
p. fluid collection
p. tissue
perineum, pl. **perinea**
watering-can p.
water pot p.
perinuclear antineutrophil
cytoplasmic (p-ANC)
period
dwell p.
periodic
p. acid-Schiff (PAS)
p. acid Schiff-Alcian blue
combination stain (PAS-AB)
p. acid-Schiff stain
p. acid-Schiff test
p. leg movement (PLM)
p. peritonitis
p. polyserositis
p. vomiting
periodicity
circadian p.
perioperative
p. antibiotic
p. nutrition
p. vomiting

peripancreatic
p. area
p. fibrosis
p. fluid
peripapillary diverticulum
peripartum endoscopy
peripelvic extravasation
peripheral
p. acinar vein
p. adrenergic agent
p. blood lymphocyte (PBL)
p. blood mononuclear cell
(PBMC)
p. capillary filtration slit
length
p. cholangiocarcinoma (PCC)
p. edema
p. extremity edema
p. hyperalimentation
p. intrahepatic
cholangiocarcinoma
p. intravenous alimentation
p. T cell
p. vascular
p. venous thrombosis
periphery
hypoechoic p.
periportal
p. area
p. fibrosis
p. hepatocyte
p. invasion
p. pyridine nucleotide
fluorescence
p. sinusoidal dilation
periprostatic
p. tissue
perirectal
p. abscess
p. mass
p. pain
perirenal
p. abscess
p. hematoma
perisigmoid colon
perisinusoidal
p. fibrin deposition

NOTES

P

435

perisinusoidal *(continued)*
  p. fibrosis
  p. space
perisplenitis
  fibropurulent p.
peristalsis
  absent p.
  decreased p.
  esophageal p.
  reversed p.
  visible p.
peristaltic
  p. contraction
  p. pump
  p. reflex
  p. rushes
  p. wave
peristomal
  p. area
  p. infection
  p. skin
  p. varix
peritoneal
  p. access
  p. adenocarcinoma
  p. adhesion
  p. anatomy
  p. aspiration
  p. attachment
  p. band
  p. biopsy
  p. blastomycosis
  p. button
  p. carcinomatosis
  p. catheter
  p. cavity
  p. cavity abscess
  p. dialysate
  p. dialysis (PD)
  p. dialysis catheter
  p. dialysis effluent (PDE)
  p. dropsy
  p. encapsulation
  p. equilibration test (PET)
  p. fluid
  p. friction rub
  p. fungal infection
  p. lavage
  p. leukocyte
  p. lymphangiectasis
  p. macrophage
  p. malignancy
  p. membrane permeability

  p. membrane solute transport capacity
  p. membrane transport
  p. mesothelioma
  p. mouse
  p. nodule
  p. perforation
  p. reflection
  p. sac
  p. seeding
  p. sign
  p. soilage
  p. solute transport
  p. space
  p. studding
  p. tap
  p. toilet
  p. transfusion
  p. tuberculosis
  p. vein
  p. window
peritoneal-atrial shunt
peritonealgia
peritonealize
peritonei
  carcinomatosis p.
  pseudomyxoma p.
peritoneocaval shunt
peritoneocentesis
peritoneoclysis
peritoneogram
peritoneojugular shunt
peritoneopathy
peritoneopexy
peritoneoplasty
peritoneoscope
peritoneoscopy
peritoneotomy
  inverted-V p.
peritoneovenous
  p. shunt (PVS)
  p. shunt patency scan
peritoneum
  abdominal p.
  parietal p.
  pelvic p.
  visceral p.
peritonism
peritonitis
  bacterial p.
  barium p.
  benign paroxysmal p.
  bile p.

Candida p.
chemical p.
coccidioidal p.
Coccidioides immitis p.
p. deformans
exudative p.
fecal p.
fungal p.
generalized p.
granulomatous p.
meconium p.
parasitic p.
periodic p.
postsclerotherapy bacterial p.
primary p.
sclerosing p.
secondary bacterial p.
spontaneous bacterial p. (SBP)
starch granulomatous p.
sterile p.
subacute nonspecific p.
tuberculous p.
peritonize
peritubular
p. capillary
p. fluid
periumbilical
p. port
p. region
periureteral
p. abscess
p. fibrosis
p. stone
periureteritis
p. plastica
periurethral
p. abscess
p. striated muscle
perivascular
p. fibroblast
p. sheath
peri-Vaterian therapeutic endoscopic procedure
perivenular
p. confluent necrosis
p. fibrosis
perivesical fat

Perkin-Elmer model 5000 atomic absorption spectrophotometer
Perls stain
Perma-hand silk suture
permanent
p. end colostomy
p. loop ileostomy
p. section
p. stoma
permanganate
potassium p.
PermCath
P. dual lumen catheter
permeability
capillary p.
colonic p.
intestinal p.
membrane p.
mucosal vascular p.
peritoneal membrane p.
transurothelial p.
urea p.
permeable
Permitil
permselectivity
pernasal cholangiogram
pernicious
p. anemia
p. malaria
p. vomiting
p. vomiting of pregnancy
peroral
p. approach
p. bougienage
p. cholangiopancreatoscopy (PCPS)
p. cholangioscopy (PCS)
p. endoprosthesis
p. endoscopy
p. esophageal dilation
p. gastroscope
p. maneuver
p. pancreatoscopy
peroxidase
endogenous p.
p. stain
peroxidase-conjugated streptavidin

NOTES

P

peroxidation
lipid p.
peroxide
hydrogen p.
Peroxynitrite-induced colitis
perphenazine
per-rectal portal scintigraphy
per rectum
Perry bag
Persantine
perseverating
persimmon bezoar
persistence
persistent
p. chronic hepatitis
p. müllerian duct syndrome
p. pylorospasm
p. viral hepatitis (PVH)
p. viral hepatitis, non-A, non-B (PVH-NANB)
p. viral hepatitis, type B (PVH-B)
p. vomiting
personality
histrionic p.
ulcer-prone p.
pertechnetate
^{99m}Tc sodium p.
technetium-99m p.
Pertofrane
pertussin toxin-sensitive G protein
pertussis
perversion
taste p.
pessary
Smith-Hodge p.
PET
peritoneal equilibration test
PET dialysate volume
petal-fugal flow
petechia, pl. petechiae
gastric p.
petechial
p. angioma
p. rash
Petersen bag
pethidine
p. premedication
Petit triangle
petrolatum gauze pack
Pettenkofer test
Petz clamp

Peutz-Jeghers
P.-J. gastrointestinal polyposis
P.-J. hamartoma
P.-J. polyp
P.-J. syndrome
Peyer patch
Peyronie
P. disease
P. plaque
Pezzer
P. catheter
P. drain
Pfannenstiel incision
PFE
pelvic floor exercise
PFGE
pulsed field gel electrophoresis
PG
prostaglandin
pyoderma gangrenosum
PGE2
prostaglandin E2
exogenous PGE2
ratio of PGF2-α PGE2
PGE1 injection
PGF2α
prostaglandin F2α
PGG
prostaglandin G
PGG2 endoperoxide
PGH
prostaglandin H
PGH2 endoperoxide
PGI
prostaglandin I
serum PGI
PGI2
prostaglandin I2
PGV
proximal gastric vagotomy
pH
pH electrode placement
gastric luminal pH
pH holding time
intracellular pH
intragastric pH
pH monitoring
pH probe
pH recording
pH standardized meal
pH threshold
Phadebas angiotensin-I test
phage type

phagocyte respiratory burst
phagocytes
bactericidal function of p.
phagocytic stellate cell
phagocytosis
phallalgia
phallectomy
phallitis
phalloarteriography
phallocampsis
phallocrypsis
phallodynia
phalloplasty
phalloplethysmography (PPG)
phallorrhagia
phallorrhea
phallotomy
phallus
phantom
P. 5 Plus ST balloon
dilatation catheter
p. ulcer
pharmacoangiography
pharmacoarteriography
pharmacocavernosogram
pharmacocavernosometry
pharmaco-duplex ultrasonography
pharmacodynamic
pharmacokinetic
famotidine p.'s
pharmacologically induced erection
pharmacomechanical coupling
pharyngeal
p. anesthesia
p. diverticulum
p. exudate
p. pouch
p. pouch syndrome
p. wall
pharyngeal-UES incoordination
pharyngis
globus p.
pharyngitis
herpes p.
pharyngoesophageal
p. diverticulectomy
p. diverticulum

p. function
p. junction
p. sphincter
p. tear
pharyngoesophagogastroduodenoscopy
pharynx
phase
complement-independent
autologous p.
p. III marrow transplant
recipient
p. II marrow transplant
recipient
lag p.
micturition p.
mycelial p.
predialysis p.
pre-S p.
prolonged expiratory p.
reservoir p.
phasic
p. contraction
p. fluctuation on squeeze
p. wave sequence
phasic-free tone variation
Phazyme
Phazyme-125
Phazyme-95
Phazyme-PB
pHCV31 antigen
pHCV34 antigen
phenacetin
phenazopyridine
p. hydrochloride
sulfamethoxazole and p.
sulfisoxazole and p.
phencyclidine abuse
phendimetrazine
phenelzine
Phenergan
phenindamine
phenindione hypersensitivity
phenmetrazine
phenobarbital
phenol
aqueous p.
p. II

NOTES

P

439

Phenolax
phenolphthalein
phenolsulfonphthalein
phenoltetrachlorophthalein test
phenomenon, pl. phenomena
    capillary-leak p.
    cloud p.
    common cavity p.
    disappearing p.
    dystonic p.
    Goldblatt kidney p.
    jet stream p.
    J-wave p.
    Kanagawa p.
    mask p.
    pathergy p.
    walking stick p.
    yo-yo weight fluctuation p.
phenothiazine
phenotype
    antigenic p.
    B-cellular p.
    CD4 p.
    CD8 p.
    HLA class II p.
    Potter p.
    replication error p.
    slow bilirubin
        glucuronidation p.
    ZZ p.
phenotypic
    p. sex
    p. study
Phenoxine
phenoxybenzamine
phenoxymethylpenicillin
phentermine
phentolamine
    p. test
phentosanpolysulfate
phenylacetate
phenylalanine
phenylbutazone hepatotoxicity
phenylephrine
phenyl ethyl alcohol agar
phenylethylamine N-methyl
    transferase (PNMT)
phenylhydrazine
phenyl-methane-sulfonyl fluoride
phenylpropanolamine
phenylpropylmethylamine
phenytoin

pheochromocytoma
    familial p.
    malignant p.
PHG
    portal hypertensive gastropathy
PHI
    peptide histidine isoleucine
Phillips
    P. catheter
    P. CM 12 electron microscope
    P. LaxCaps
    P. Milk of Magnesia
phimosis, pl. phimoses
    adult p.
phimotic
phisoHex scrub
PHIV
    portal hypertensive intestinal
        vasculopathy
phlebitis
phlebography
    intraoperative p.
phlebolith
phleborrheograph
    Cranley p.
phleborrheography
phlegmon
    pancreatic p.
    pericolic p.
phlegmonous
    p. abscess
    p. alcoholic fatty liver
    p. change
    p. enteritis
    p. gastritis
    p. mass
phlorizin
pH-metry
    esophagogastric p.-m.
    24-hour ambulatory p.-m.
    24-hour home p.-m.
PHN
    passive Heymann nephritis
pholedrine
phonoenterography
phonorenogram
phorbol
    p. ester 12-O-
        tetradecanoylphorbol-13-acetate
        (phorbol ester TPA)
    p. ester TPA
    p. myristate acetate (PMA)
PhosLo

Phosphaljel
phosphatase
    alkaline p. (ALP, AP)
    Bessey-Lowry unit for
        alkaline p.
    placental alkaline p. (PIAP)
    prostatic acid p. (PAP)
    protein-tyrosine p.
phosphate
    p. binder therapy
    p. buffered saline solution
    calcium hydrogen p.
    chloroquine p.
    p. crystal
    dexamethasone sodium p.
    elemental p.
    p. enema
    estramustine p.
    magnesium ammonium p.
    nicotinamide adenine
        dinucleotide p. (NADPH)
    phosphatidylinositol p. (PI4P)
    potassium p.
    pyridoxal p.
    sodium p.
phosphate-buffered saline (PBS)
phosphate-dependent glutaminase
    (PDG)
phosphatidyl
    p. choline
    p. inositol 4,5-biphosphate
        (PI4,5P2)
phosphatidylethanolamine
phosphatidylinositol (PI)
    p. phosphate (PI4P)
phosphatidyl-inositol 4,5-bisphosphate
phosphatidylserine
phosphodiester
phosphoenolpyruvate carboxykinase
    (PEPCK)
phosphofructokinase
phosphoglucomutase
phosphoinositide
phosphokinase
    creatine p. (CPK)
phospholipase

    p. A2 (PLA2)
    p. A2 catalytic activity
    p. C (PLC)
    p. D
phospholipid
    p. bilayer
    p. ratio
    serum p.
phospholipidase A
phospholipidosis
phosphonoformate
phosphoramidite chemistry
phosphorhylates
phosphorous-31 magnetic resonance
    spectroscopy
phosphorus
    p. poisoning
    tubular reabsorption of p.
phosphorylase
    glycogen p.
    uridine p.
phosphorylated growth factor
    receptor
phosphorylation
    oxidative p.
    src p.
    tyrosine p.
phosphotyrosyl protein profile
Phospho-Soda
    P.-S. enema
    Fleet P.-S.
phosphotungstic acid-magnesium
    chloride precipitation method
phosphotyrosine antibody
phosphotyrosine-SH2 binding
photoablation
    laser p.
photoaffinity
photochemotherapy
photocoagulation
    infrared p. (IRC)
    laser p.
    transendoscopic laser p.
    p. treatment
photodestruction
    laser p.
photodiode

NOTES

P

photodocumentation
photodynamic therapy (PDT)
Photofrin
    P. derivative
photogastroscope
photography
    endoscopic p.
    instant p.
    laparoscopic p.
    television p.
photoirradiation
photometer
    transurethral resection
    TUR-Cue photometer
    transurethral resection
photometry
    flame p.
photomicrograph
    high-power p.
    low-power p.
    medium-power p.
photomicrography
photomultiplier
    EMI 9813B p.
    p. tube
photon-deficient lesion
photophobia
photoradiation
    p. therapy
photosensitivity
photosensitizer
    porphyrin p.
photosensitizing hemoporphyrin
    derivative
phrenicocolic, phrenocolic
    p. ligament
phrenicoesophageal,
    phrenoesophageal
    p. ligament
phrenocolopexy
phrenogastric
phrygian
    p. cap
    p. cap deformity
pH-sensitive radiotelemetry capsule
PHSL
    primary hepatosplenic lymphoma
    B-cell PHSL
phthiriasis
Phthirus pubis
phycomycetes
phycomycosis
phylloquinone

phylogenetic tree
physic
Physick pouch
physicochemical basis of gallstone
    formation
physiograph
physiologic
    p. jaundice
    p. reflux test (PRT)
    p. role in acid secretion
    p. salt solution (PSS)
    p. testosterone-replacement
    therapy
physiological trophic effect
physiology
    anorectal p.
    p. testing
phytobezoar
phytohemagglutinin
phytonadione
phytosterolemia
phytyl group
PI
    phosphatidylinositol
    PI 3-kinase
    PI surgical stapler
PI90 double-headed stapler
PIAP
    placental alkaline phosphatase
pica
pick
    P. cell
    P. tubular adenoma
Picker Vista MagnaScanner
picket fence appearance
picosulfate
    sodium p.
PID
    pelvic inflammatory disease
piecemeal necrosis
piezoelectric
    p. lithotripsy
    p. shock wave lithotriptor
    p. transducer
Piezolith
    P. EPL
    P. (2300 and 2500 model)
    lithotriptor
pigbel
piggyback
    p. liver transplantation
piggybacking of I.V.
Piggyback needle-knife papillotome

pigment
    p. gallstone
    gastric p.
pigmentary cirrhosis
pigmentation
pigmented
    p. gallstone
    p. histiocyte
    p. nevus
    p. nipple
pigmentosa
    urticaria p.
pIgR
    polyimmunoglobulin receptor
pigtail
    p. biliary stent
    p. catheter
    p. endoprosthesis
    p. nephrostomy tube
    p. stent
PIL
    primary intestinal lymphangiectasia
pile, pl. **piles**
    sentinel p.
pili
    p. torti et canaliculi
pillar
    palatine p.
pill esophagitis
pill-induced esophageal injury
pillow
    Bedge p.
    Sand-Eze EGD p.
    p. sign
pilonidal
    p. cyst
    p. cystectomy
    p. disease
    p. perirectal abscess
    p. sinus
    p. sinus disease
pimelorrhea
PIN
    prostatic intraepithelial neoplasia
pinch
    p. biopsy
    diaphragmatic p.

    p. forceps
    p. injury
pinchcock
    diaphragmatic p.
    p. mechanism
pindolol
pineoblastoma
pinguecula
pinocytosis
    fluid-phase p.
    p. vacuole
pinpoint pupil
PIP
    pressure inversion point
    PIP on esophageal manometry
PI4P
    phosphatidylinositol phosphate
PI4,5P2
    phosphatidyl inositol
    4,5-bisphosphate
pipe
    endoscopic washing p.
    Mauch double-sheathed plastic
    wash p.
    p. stem cirrhosis
pipenzolate
piperacillin
piperazine citrate
piperidolate
piperoxan
pipestem stool
PIPIDA
    para-isopropyliminodiacetic acid
    PIPIDA scan
    ^{99m}Tc PIPIDA
Pipracil
Pipradol
PIR
    pressure increment rate
pirenzepine
piritramide
piroxicam
piston-type syringe
pit
    anal p.
    clathrin-coated p.
    colonic p.
    gastric p.

NOTES

P

pit *(continued)*
    mucosal p.
    postanal p.
Pitressin
pitting
    anal p.
    colonic p.
    p. edema
    gastric p.
pituitary
    p. adenylate cyclase activating
      polypeptide (PACAP)
    p. tumor
pituitary-gonadal axis
PIVKA
    protein in vitamin K absence
PIVKA-II antagonist
pixel
PiZZ alpha$_1$-antitrypsin deficiency
PKC
    protein kinase C
PKD1 gene
PLA2
    phospholipase A2
placebo
    p. effect
    p. therapy
placement
    band p.
    dilator p.
    electrode p.
    endoscopic biliary stent p.
    endotracheal tube p.
    feeding tube p.
    five-port "fan" p.
    four-port "diamond" p.
    graft p.
    intestinal sling p.
    percutaneous nephrostomy
      tube p.
    pH electrode p.
    radiologic biliary stent p.
    tube p.
    ultrasound-assisted PEG p.
    ureteral stent p.
    wire-guided p.
placental alkaline phosphatase
(PIAP)
Placer guidewire
plain
    p. catgut suture
    p. film
    p. film of abdomen

    p. gut
    p. gut suture
planar
    p. imaging
    p. xanthoma
plane
    Addison clinical p.'s
    cleavage p.
    p. of dissection
    ischiorectal fossa p.
planimeter
planimetric measurement
planimetry
    impedance p.
plantar
    p. grasp
plantaris
    hyperkeratosis palmaris et p.
    Tylosis palmaris et p.
planuria
planus
    lichen p.
plaque
    atherosclerotic p.
    augmentation p.
    Hollenhorst p.
    p. incision
    ostial atherosclerotic p.
    Peyronie p.
    Randall p.
plaque-like
    p.-l. lesion
    p.-l. linear defect
    p.-l. thickening
plasma
    p. albumin
    p. ammonia
    p. atrial natriuretic peptide
    p. bile acid measurement
    p. caffeine concentration
    p. cell
    p. cell balanitis
    p. cell granuloma
    p. cell hepatitis
    p. cell portal infiltration
    p. clearance
    p. cloud
    p. creatinine
    cryoprecipitated p.
    dialysis to p. (D-P)
    p. enzyme
    p. exchange
    p. fibronectin

p. flow
fresh frozen p. (FFP)
gastric p.
p. gastrin concentration
p. inulin
p. ionized calcium
p. kallikrein
p. membrane marker
p. met-enkephalin
p. norepinephrine concentration
p. oncotic pressure
p. osmolality
p. parathyroid hormone (PTH)
p. perfusion
p. protein
p. protein fraction
p. renin activity (PRA)
p. renin concentration
p. urea concentration
p. viscosity
p. volume depletion
plasma-activated complement 3 (C3a)
plasma-activated complement 4 (C4a)
plasma-activated complement 5 (C5a)
plasmablastic myeloma
plasmacellularis
balanitis circumscripta p.
plasmacytoma
extramedullary p.
gastric p.
radioresistant gastric p.
plasmacytosis
Plasmalyte
Plasmanate
plasmapheresis
plasmid
p. mediated
p. profile
p. profile role
plasminogen
p. activator (PA)
p. activator inhibitor (PAI)
p. activator inhibitor-1

plasmodium
encapsulated p.
Plastibell circumcision
plastic
p. cylinder Hostaform
p. endoprosthesis
plastica
linitis p.
periureteritis p.
plasty
Foley Y-V p.
mons p.
posterior bladder flap p.
V-Y p.
Y-V p.
plate
anal p.
blood agar p.
bowel p.
cloacal p.
exstrophic bladder p.
hilar p.
limiting p.
liver cell p.
Maxisorb test p.
microwell p.
Mueller-Hinton-supplemented
    agar p.
Skirrow agar p.
trigonal p.
urethral p.
plateau
dieting p.
p. response
platelet
p. abnormality
p. activating factor (PAF)
p. count
p. dysfunction
p. transfusion
platelet-derived growth factor (PDGF)
Platinol
platinum

NOTES

P

platinum-based consolidation
chemotherapy
platinum, Velban and bleomycin
(PVB)
platysma
plaunotol
PLC
  phospholipase C
PLD
  polycystic liver disease
pleating of small bowel
Plegine
pleiotropic
pleomorphic destructive cholangitis
pleomorphism
  nuclear hyperchromasia and p.
Plesiomonas shigelloides
plethora
plethoric
plethysmography
  impedance p. (IPG)
  penile p.
pleural
  p. mass
  p. rub
  p. tube
pleuritis
  bile p.
pleurobiliary fistula
pleuroperitoneal canal
plexiform neurofibroma
plexus
  Auerbach and Meissner p.
  Auerbach mesenteric p.
  biliary p.
  colonic myenteric p.
  cystic p.
  distal venous p.
  esophageal p.
  extrapancreatic nerve p.
  gastric p.
  gastroesophageal variceal p.
  gastrointestinal myenteric p.
  hemorrhoidal p.
  ileocolic p.
  longitudinal subepithelial
    venous p.
  Meissner p.
  middle rectal venous p.
  myenteric p.
  p. myentericus
  pelvic p.
  proximal venous p.

  rectal p.
  Santorini venous p.
  submucosal p.
  submucosal venous p.
  suburothelial nerve p.
  superior rectal venous p.
  thyreoideus impar p.
  vascular p.
plica
  p. longitudinalis
plicae circulares
plicated appendicocystostomy
plication
  Child-Phillips bowel p.
  fundal p.
  Graham p.
  Kelly p.
  Nesbit p.
  Noble bowel p.
  Rehne-Delorme p.
  p. suture
  suture p.
  transgastric p.
  transmesenteric p.
PLM
  periodic leg movement
ploidy
  p. analysis
plot
  Eadie-Hofstee p.
plug
  bile p.
  meconium p.
  one-piece disposable p.
  urethral p.
plumbism
plume
  laser p.
Plummer
  P. bag
  P. dilator
Plummer-Vinson syndrome
Plus
  Candela MiniScope P.
  Charcoal P.
  Ensure P.
  Lithostar P.
  Maalox P.
  Pyridium P.
  Riopan P.
  Titralac P.
PMA
  phorbol myristate acetate

PMA-stimulated O2
PMC
    pseudomembranous colitis
PMMA
    polymethyl methacrylate
        PMMA beads
PMN
    polymorphonuclear
    polymorphonuclear neutrophil
        PMN cell
        PMN infiltrate
        PMN leukocyte
        PMN oxidative burst capacity
        uremic PMN
PMN-elastase
    fecal P.-e.
PNA
    peanut agglutinin
PNET
    primitive neuroectodermal tumor
pneumatic
    p. bag
    p. bag dilation
    p. bag dilation of esophagus
    p. bag esophageal dilation
    p. balloon catheter dilation
    p. balloon dilator
    p. compression device
    p. leg pump
pneumatinuria
pneumatosis
    p. coli
    p. cystoides coli
    p. cystoides intestinalis (PCI)
    p. intestinalis
pneumaturia
pneumobilia
pneumocholecystitis
pneumococcal infection
pneumococcus
pneumocolon
Pneumocystis
    P. carinii
    P. carinii pneumonia
pneumocystosis
    gastric p.
pneumodissection

pneumogastrography
pneumography
    retroperitoneal p.
pneumohydraulic capillary infusion system
pneumohydroperitoneum
pneumomediastinum
pneumonectomy
pneumonia
    aspiration p.
    lymphoid interstitial p.
    Pneumocystis carinii p.
    Proteus p.
    Pseudomonas aeruginosa p.
    Pseudomonas pseudomallei p.
pneumoniae
    Klebsiella p.
pneumopenis
pneumopericardium
pneumoperitoneum
    benign p.
    p. needle
    stent-induced p.
    tension p.
pneumophila
    Legionella p.
pneumoretroperitoneum
pneumoscrotum
pneumostatic dilation
pneumothorax
    iatrogenic p.
    tension p.
PNH
    paroxysmal nocturnal hemoglobinuria
PNI
    prognostic nutritional index
PNL
    percutaneous nephrolithotomy
PNMT
    phenylethylamine N-methyl transferase
POA
    pancreatic oncofetal antigen
    POA test
Pockel cell
pocketed calculus

NOTES

P

447

podagra
podocalyxin
podocyte
  p. glycocalyx
podofilox
  p. solution
Podophyllin
podophyllotoxin
poikilocyte
  teardrop p.
point
  Addison p.
  APACHE-II p.
  bleeding p.
  Boas p.
  Chauffard p.
  Desjardins p.
  dorsal p.
  F2 focal p.
  Hartmann p.
  Lanz p.
  Mackenzie p.
  McBurney p.
  Munro p.
  pressure inversion p. (PIP)
  Ramond p.
  respiratory inversion p. (RIP)
  p. of respiratory reversal on
    esophageal manometry
  Robson p.
  Sudeck p.
  p. tenderness
point-counting image
pointer
  LaserMed laser p.
POINTER computer program
pointing
  past p.
Poiseuille-Hagen law
Poiseuille law
poison
poisoning
  ackee fruit p.
  bacterial food p.
  ferrous salts p.
  food p.
  iron p.
  lead p., acute lead p., chronic
    lead p.
  mercury p., acute mercury p.,
    chronic mercury p.
  mushroom p.
  phosphorus p.

  Salmonella food p.
  Staphylococcus food p.
  thallium p.
Poisson regression
Polachrome 35-mm slide system
polar
  p. body
  p. sheathed flagella
Polaris grasper
polarization microscopy
polarized
  p. glucose transporter
  p. reflex
  p. standing reflex
polarographic study
Polaroid
  P. camera
  P. endocamera EC-3
  P. SX-70 with ACMI adapter
Polhemus-Schafer-Ivemark syndrome
polidocanol
  p. injection
  p. injection therapy
  p. sclerosant
POLIP
  polyneuropathy, ophthalmoplegia,
    leukoencephalopathy, and
    intestinal pseudo-obstruction
  POLIP syndrome
Politano-Leadbetter
  P.-L. anastomosis
  P.-L. tunnel creation
  P.-L. ureterolysis
polka fever
pollakiuria
Pólya
  P. anastomosis
  P. gastrectomy
  P. gastroenterostomy
  P. operation
  P. technique
polyacrylamide
  p. gel
  p. gel electrophoresis (PAGE)
polyamine
  p. level
  p. spermine
polyanion
  GBM p.
polyantibiotic chemotherapy
polyarteritis nodosa
polyarthritis
  seronegative p.

polycationic
    p. histochemical probe
    p. marker
Polycillin-N
Polycitra
Polycitra-K
Polycitra-LC
polyclonal
    p. epidermal growth factor
      antibody
    p. IgG
Polycose glucose supplement
polycystic
    p. chronic esophagitis
    p. disease of liver (PDL)
    p. kidney disease
    p. liver
    p. liver disease (PCLD, PLD)
polycythemia vera
Polydek suture
polydimethylsiloxane
polydioxan
polydioxanone
    p. suture
polydipsia
polyester-reinforced Dacron tape
polyestradiol phosphate therapy
polyethylene
    p. balloon dilator
    p. cannula
    p. catheter
    p. glycol (PEG)
    p. glycol-based lavage
    p. glycol electrolyte lavage
      solution (PEG-ELS)
    p. glycol electrolyte solution
    p. perforation
    p. stent
    p. tube
polyethylene glycol 600
polyethylenimine (PEI)
polyglactin
    p. suture
polyglecaprone 25 suture
polyglutamate folate
polyglycolic
    p. acid

    p. acid collar
    p. acid suture
polyglyconate suture
polygonal hepatocyte
polyhydramnios
polyimmunoglobulin receptor (pIgR)
poly-L-lysine-coated glass slide
polylobar liver
polymerase
    p. chain reaction (PCR)
    p. chain reaction technology
    DNA p.
    HBV-associated DNA p.
    Taq p.
polymerization
    IgA p.
polymethyl methacrylate (PMMA)
polymicrobial
    p. bacterascites
    p. infection
polymorphic
    p. gene
    p. reticulosis
polymorphism
    DNA p.
    restriction fragment length p.
      (RLP)
polymorphonuclear (PMN)
    p. cell
    p. inflammatory infiltrate
    p. leukocyte
    p. neutrophil (PMN)
Polymox
polymyositis
polymyositis-dermatomyositis
polymyxin B
polyneuropathy
**polyneuropathy, ophthalmoplegia,
   leukoencephalopathy, and
   intestinal pseudo-obstruction
   (POLIP)**
polyoma middle T oncogene
polyorchism, polyorchidism
polyp
    adenomatous p. (AP)
    adenomatous colorectal p.
    adenomatous gastric p.

NOTES

P

polyp *(continued)*
antral p.
benign adenomatous p.
bleeding p.
broad-based p.
cervical p.
cholesterol p.
cloacogenic p.
colonic p.
colorectal p.
diminutive adenomatous p.
diminutive colonic p.
diminutive hyperplastic p.
duodenal p.
elusive p.
eroded p.
esophageal p.
fibroid p.
fibrovascular p.
filiform p.
fundic gland p.
gastric p.
gastric antral sessile p.
gastric hyperplastic p.
gastric inflammatory fibroid p.
hamartomatous p.
hamartomatous gastric p.
hyperplasiogenic p.
hyperplastic p. (HP)
hyperplastic adenomatous p.
hyperplastic epithelial gastric p.
hyperplastic gastric p.
inflammatory p.
inflammatory fibroid p. (IFP)
invasive colorectal p.
juvenile p.
juvenile retention p.
lymphoid p.
malignant p.
metaplastic p.
mixed hyperplastic/adenomatous
    gastric p.
mucosal p.
multiple p.
nasal p.
neoplastic p.
non-neoplastic p.
pedunculated p.
perineal p.
Peutz-Jeghers p.
polypoid p.
postinflammatory p.
prepyloric p.

rectal p.
p. relocation
retention p.
sentinel hyperplastic p.
sessile p.
p. stalk
synchronous p.
tuberculosis p.
tubular p.
tubulovillous p.
villoglandular p.
villous p.
polypectomized
polypectomy
colonoscopic p.
duodenal endoscopic p.
electrosurgical snare p.
endoscopic p.
endoscopic sessile p.
gastric p.
incomplete p.
p. snare
polypeptide
gastric inhibitory p. (GIP)
p. growth factor
islet amyloid p.
pancreatic p. (PP)
pituitary adenylate cyclase
    activating p. (PACAP)
vasoactive intestinal p. (VIP)
polyphagia
polyphosphate
^{99m}Tc p.
polyphosphoinositide
polypoid
p. cancer
p. carcinoma
p. dysplasia
p. exophytic non-ulcerating
    carcinosarcoma
p. lesion
p. lymphoid hyperplasia
p. lymphoma
p. mass
p. polyp
p. tumor
polyposa
enteritis p.
gastritis cystica p.
polyposis
adenomatous p.
cap p.
p. coli

colonic p.
diffuse mucosal p.
duodenal p.
familial adenomatous p. (FAP)
familial colorectal p.
familial gastrointestinal p.
familial hamartomatous p.
familial intestinal p.
familial juvenile p.
filiform p.
florid p.
gastric p.
gastrointestinal p.
hamartomatous p.
hyperplastic p.
intestinal p.
juvenile p.
multiple familial p.
multiple lymphomatous p.
(MLP)
nonfamilial gastrointestinal p.
Peutz-Jeghers gastrointestinal p.
p. syndrome
polypous gastritis
Polyprep centrifugation
polypropylene
p. mesh
p. suture
polyradicular neuropathy
polyribosome
polysaccharide
p. antigen
p. capsule
p. Kreha (PSK)
polysaccharide-iron complex
polyserositis
familial paroxysmal p., familial
recurrent p. (FPP)
periodic p.
polysome
endoplasmic reticulum-bound p.
polysomnography
polyspermy, polyspermia
polysplenia syndrome
polysulfate
pentosan sodium p.
polysulfonated napthylurea

760 **polysulfone dialyzer**
polysulphone
F60S p.
high-flux p.
polysynaptic reflex
Polytef
polytetrafluorethylene paste injection
polytetrafluoroethylene
p. sock
Polytrac Gomez retractor
polyunsaturated lecithin
polyurethane nasoenteric catheter
polyuria
nighttime p.
polyvinyl
p. alcohol
p. alcohol sponge
p. alcohol sponge
hysterosacropexy
p. bougie
p. dilator
p. tubing
Pompe disease
Pondimin
Ponka
P. herniorrhaphy
P. technique for local
anesthesia
Ponsky
P. pull
P. pull or guidewire insertion
technique
P. technique
Ponsky-Gauderer type PEG
pontine micturition center
pool
abdominal p.
bile acid p.
gastric p.
pooled saliva
Poole suction tube
pooling
pyriform p.
vallecular p.
venous p.
poorly
p. compliant bladder

NOTES

P

poorly *(continued)*
    p. differentiated adenoma
    p. localized pain
popliteal
    p. swelling
    p. tenderness
pop-off suture
population
    gluten-dependent p.
porcelain gallbladder
porcine carboxypeptidase B
pore
    shunt-like p.
Porges catheter
porin channel protein
pork tapeworm
porotomy
porous filter membrane
porphyria
    acute p.
    acute intermittent p. (AIP)
    p. cutanea tarda (PCT)
    erythropoietic p. (EPP)
    hepatic p.
porphyrin
    p. photosensitizer
port
    inlet p.
    MCL p.
    OmegaPort access p.
    periumbilical p.
    subcostal p.
    suprapubic p.
    umbilical p.
portable
    p. digital data recorder
    p. renal preservation machine
Port-A-Cath
portacaval shunt
Portagen
    P. diet
    P. feeding
    P. formula
Port-A-Germ anaerobic transport vial
porta hepatis
portal
    p. cannula
    p. catheter
    p. cirrhosis
    p. decompression
    p. eosinophilic inflammation
    p. fissure
    p. hypertension

    p. hypertensive gastropathy (PHG)
    p. hypertensive intestinal vasculopathy (PHIV)
    p. pressure
    p. pyemia
    p. shunt index (PSI)
    p. tract
    p. tract fibrosis
    p. tract inflammation
    p. triad
    p. triaditis
    p. triad occlusion
    p. trunk
    p. vascular bed
    p. vein (PV)
    p. vein obstruction
    p. vein thrombosis (PVT)
    p. venous pressure (PVP)
    p. venous system
    p. venule
    p. zone
    p. zone granuloma
portal-collateral circulation
portal-systemic, portosystemic
    p.-s. encephalopathy (PSE)
    p.-s. shunt
    p.-s. shunt surgery
portal-to-portal
    p.-t.-p. bridging
    p.-t.-p. fibrosis
portasystemic shunt
Porter duodenal forceps
portoenterostomy
    Kasai p.
portography
    arterial p.
    percutaneous transhepatic p.
    transhepatic p.
portopulmonary shunt
portosystemic *(var. of* portal-systemic)
    p. shunting (PSS)
PortSaver PercLoop device
position
    antero-oblique p.
    body p.
    Buie p.
    cervical p.
    curved flank p.
    decubitus p.
    dorsal p.
    dorsal lithotomy p.

dorsosacral p.
Elliot p.
final p.
flank p.
Fowler p.
greater curve p.
jackknife p.
knee-chest p.
knee-elbow p.
Kraske p.
lateral decubitus p.
left decubitus p.
left lateral decubitus p.
lithotomy p.
Mayo-Robson p.
prone p.
prone split leg p.
reverse Trendelenburg p.
right antero-oblique p.
Robson p.
Scultetus p.
semioblique p.
Sims p.
ski p.
supine p.
Trendelenburg p.
positional obstructive uropathy
positioner
gallbladder bag p.
p. luer
positioning
automated endoscopic system
for optimal p. (AESOP)
flank roll p.
patient p.
positive
p. bowel sounds
extradomain A p. (EDA+)
p. nitrogen balance
p. secretin stimulation study
Positrap
P. mini-retrieval basket
P. retriever
P. three prong non-retracting
grasping forceps
positron camera

post
status p. (S/P)
**postage stamp penile tumescence
test**
postanal
p. dimpling
p. pit
p. repair
postanesthesia recovery (PAR)
post-atrophic hyperplasia
post-autoclave contamination
postbiopsy
p. fistula
p. vascular complication
postbulbar duodenal ulcer
postcholecystectomy
p. flatulent dyspepsia
p. syndrome (PCS)
postcholecystitis adhesion
postcibal symptom
postcoital test
postcolonoscopy distention syndrome
postcricoid
p. area
p. web
postdialysis
post-dilation meglumine diatrizoate
postdystrophic scarring
postendoscopic cholangitis
postendoscopy
post-ERCP induced pancreatitis
posterior
p. abdominal wall
p. approach
p. bladder flap plasty
p. duodenal ulcer
p. flap vaginoplasty
p. lumbar approach
p. nephrectomy
p. pararenal compartment
p. pelvic exenteration
p. rectopexy
p. rectus sheath
p. renal fascia
p. transthoracic incision
p. urethra
p. urethral valve (PUV)

NOTES

P

posterolateral
postevacuation
  p. film
  p. view
postfundoplication syndrome
postganglionic cholinergic nerve
postgastrectomy
  p. bleed
  p. cancer
  p. dysfunction
  p. gastritis
  p. hemorrhage
  p. stasis
  p. syndrome
posthepatic, posthepatitic
  posthepatic cirrhosis,
    posthepatitic cirrhosis
posthepatitis aplastic anemia
posthetomy
posthioplasty
posthitis
posthoc test
postholith
postictal
postinflammatory
  p. contracture
  p. polyp
postischemic
  p. acute renal failure
  p. tubular necrosis
post-jejunoileal-bypass hepatic
  disease
postligation ulcer
postmenopausal
postmicturition
  p. continuous leakage
  p. dribble
postmyotomy reflux
postnasal drip
postnecrotic, post-necrotic
  p. cirrhosis
  p. scarring
post-obstructive diuresis
postoperative
  p. abscess
  p. adhesion
  p. anticoagulation therapy
  p. autologous transfusion
  p. biliary leakage
  p. choledochoscopy
  p. complication
  p. fistula

  p. gastritis
  p. hydrocele
  p. ileus
  p. irrigation-suction
  p. irrigation-suction drainage
  p. pleurobiliary fistula
  p. reflux
  p. stricture
  p. transfusion
  p. urinary retention
  p. vomiting
postpartum constipation
post-perfusion
postpolypectomy
  p. bleed
  p. coagulation syndrome
  p. hemorrhage
postprandial
  p. distention
  p. fullness
  p. hypoglycemia
  p. nausea
  p. pain
  p. vomiting
post-procedure pancreatitis
post-prostatectomy incontinence
post-pyloric feeding tube
postreceptor signaling of parietal
  cell
post-rubber band sepsis
postsclerotherapy bacterial
  peritonitis
postsecretory processing
postshunt encephalopathy
post-sphincterotomy
  p.-s. ductography
  p.-s. ERCP cannulation
postsplenectomy infection
poststreptococcal
  p. acute glomerulonephritis
  p. glomerulonephritis (PSGN)
postsurgical
  p. change
  p. endoscopy
  p. gastric stasis
  p. recurrent ulcer
post-thaw sperm motility index
post-thrombotic syndrome
post-TNM stage (I, II, III, IV)
posttransfusion hepatitis
posttranslational processing of the
  peptide

posttransplant
p. antiglomerular basement membrane
p. diabetes mellitus (PTDM)
p. immunosuppression
p. immunosuppression therapy
p. lymphoproliferative disorder (PTLD)
p. patient
p. renal dysfunction
posttraumatic
p. autotransplantation
p. pancreatic-cutaneous fistula
post-tussive vomiting
postural regurgitation
posture-dependent pain
postureteral ligation
postureteroscopic manipulation
posturing
decerebrate p.
decorticate p.
post-UUO time
Pos-T-Vac
P.-T.-V. vacuum erection device
P.-T.-V. VCD
postvagotomy
p. diarrhea
p. dysphagia
p. gastroparesis
p. syndrome
postvoid residual (PVR)
Potaba
potassium
aminobenzoate p.
p. balance
p. chloride (KCl)
p. citrate
p. cyanide
p. electrolyte
fractional excretion of p. (FEFEK)
p. hydroxide (KOH)
p. hydroxide smear
p. permanganate
p. phosphate
potassium-canrenoate antagonist

potato liver
potency
erectile p.
potential
p. difference (PD)
evoked p.
excitatory junction p. (EJP)
inhibitory postsynaptic p. (IPSP)
malignant p.
neoplastic p.
oscillatory p.
pudendal evoked p.
redox p.
resting membrane p.
spike p.
stromal tumors of unknown malignant p. (STUMP)
visual evoked p.
potentiation
alcohol p.
p. of drug hepatotoxicity
Potter
P. facies
P. phenotype
P. syndrome
Potts
P. forceps
P. scissors
Potts-Smith
P.-S. forceps
P.-S. scissors
pouch
anal p.
Bard Extra Ileo B p.
Bard Integrale p.
Benchekroun p.
p. biopsy
bladder replacement urinary p.
blind upper esophageal p.
Bricker p.
Camey urinary p.
closed-end ostomy p.
Coloplast Flange p.
Coloplast mini p.
coloplasty p.
continent ileal p.

NOTES

P

pouch *(continued)*
ConvaTec colostomy p.
ConvaTec Little One Sur-Fit p.
ConvaTec Sur-Fit two-piece p.
Cymed Micro Skin one-piece drainage p.
Dansac Karaya Seal one-piece drainage p.
Dansac Standard Ileo p.
Denis Browne p.
double loop p.
Douglas p.
drainable ostomy p.
Duke p.
endorectal ileal p.
Florida urinary p.
gastric p.
Graham closure with omental p.
Greer EZ Access drainage p.
Hartmann p.
haustral p.
hernia p.
Hollister First Choice p.
Hollister Holligard p.
Hollister Karaya 5 ostomy p.
Hollister Karaya Seal p.
Hollister Premium p.
Hunt-Lawrence p.
ileal p.
ileal J-p.
ileal neobladder urinary p.
ileal S-p.
ileal W-p.
p. ileitis
ileoanal p.
ileocecal p.
ileocolonic p.
Indiana urinary p.
intraluminal p.
inverted-U p.
jejunal p.
J-shaped ileal p.
J versus S versus W pelvic ileal p.
Koch p.
Kock urinary p.
lateral-lateral p.
Le Bag ileocolonic p.
Le Bag urinary p.
Mainz p. II
Mainz urinary p.

Mansson urinary p.
Marlen Gas Relief drainage p.
Marlen Odor-Ban ileostomy p.
Marlen Solo ileostomy p.
Marlen Zip Klosed p.
Miami p.
Morison p.
Nu-Hope ileostomy p.
Nu-Hope Nu-Self drainable p.
one-piece ostomy p.
open-end ostomy p.
Padua bladder urinary p.
paravesical p.
Parks ileostomy p.
pelvic p.
Penn p.
pharyngeal p.
Physick p.
rectal p.
rectouterine p.
rectovaginal p.
renal p.
sigma rectum p.
sigmoid rectum p.
S-shaped p.
superficial inguinal p.
Sur-Fit Mini p.
Tena p.
terminal ileal p.
three-loop ileal p.
triple loop p.
two-loop J-shaped ileal p.
two-piece ostomy p.
U p.
United Bongort Life-style p.
United Max-E drainable p.
United Surgical Bongort Life-style p.
United Surgical Featherlite ileostomy p.
United Surgical Shear Plus drainable p.
United Surgical Soft & Secure p.
VPI nonadhesive open-end p.
Willis p.
W-shaped p.
Zenker p.
pouched ileostomy
pouchitis
wastebasket p.
pouchogram

pouchography
  evacuation p.
pouchoscopy
  pelvic p.
Poupart
  P. ligament
  P. ligament shelving edge
  P. line
povidone-iodine
powder
  Karaya p.
  p. pyelogram
  Seidlitz p.
  Sween Micro Guard p.
power
  p. Doppler ultrasound
  p. grip
PP
  pancreatic polypeptide
PPA
  pelvic phased-array coil
PPAF
  progressive perivenular alcoholic
    fibrosis
PPC
  prostatic pressure coefficient
PPD immunological study
p$_2$ penile brachial index
PPG
  phalloplethysmography
PPI
  proton pump inhibitor
PP-immunoreactive cell
PPJ
  pure pancreatic juice
PPTT
  prepubertal testicular tumor
PRA
  panel-reactive antibody
  plasma renin activity
Prader orchidometer
Prader-Willi syndrome
praeacutus
  Bacteroides p.
praecox
  ejaculatio p.
  icterus p.

pralidoxime
pramoxine hydrochloride
Pratt
  P. bivalve retractor
  P. crypt hook
  P. rectal hook
  P. rectal probe
  P. rectal scissors
  P. rectal speculum
  P. scissors
  P. speculum
praziquantel
prazosin
PRCA
  pure red cell aplasia
preadventitial dissection
preampullary portion of bile duct
preauricular
precancerous lesion
precipitation
  glucagon p.
precirrhosis
precirrhotic hemochromatosis
Precision
  P. Isotein HN powdered
    feeding
  P. Isotonic powdered feeding
  P. LR powdered feeding
precision
  p. grip
  intra-assay p.
Precision-HN
Precision-LR
Precisor disposable biopsy forceps
Preclude peritoneal membrane
precordium
  hyperdynamic p.
**precore mutant strain of hepatitis
  B**
Precose
precursor
  benign neoplastic p.
precut, pre-cut
  p. incision
  p. papillotome
  p. papillotomy
  p. sphincterotome

NOTES

P

457

Pred
  prednisone
  Liquid Pred
predialysis
  p. phase
  p. plasma phosphate
    concentration
Predicta TGF-β1 kit
predictive value
predigested protein formula
predigestion
  diastase p.
predisposition
  genetic p.
prednisolone
  p. enema
  p. metasulfobenzoate
prednisone (Pred)
prednisone-colchicine combination
pre-eclamptic liver disease
pre-endoscopy
pre-esophageal · dysphagia
prefreeze
  p. motility
  p. semen analysis
Pregestimil formula
preglomerular
  p. arteriole
  p. vasculature
pregnancy
  abdominal ectopic p.
  acute fatty liver of p. (AFLP)
  ectopic p.
  ectopic sigmoid p.
  fatty liver of p.
  heartburn of p.
  intrahepatic cholestasis of p.
    (ICP)
  molar p.
  pernicious vomiting of p.
  subacute fatty liver of p.
  toxemia of p.
  tubal ectopic p.
  voluntary interruption of p.
    (VIP)
  p. wastage
pregnant uterus
Prehn sign
preileal appendix
prekallikrein
Prelone
Preludin
Premarin

premature
  p. ejaculation
  p. stop codon
premedication
  metoclopramide p.
  pethidine p.
  viscous lidocaine p.
premenarchal
premicturition pressure
Premium Barrier
Premix-Slip
Prempree modification staging
  system
prenatal
  p. diagnosis
  p. fetal hydronephrosis
Prentiss maneuver
preoperative
  p. antibiotic
  p. lesion
prep
  preparation
    Colonlite bowel prep
    Colyte bowel prep
    Dulcolax bowel prep
    Evac-Q-Kit bowel prep
    Evac-Q-Kwik bowel prep
    Fleet bowel prep
    GoLYTELY bowel prep
    OMNI Prep
    Sween Prep
    United Skin Prep
prepancreatic anlagen
prepapillary bile duct
preparation (prep)
  bowel p. (bowel prep)
  Brown dietary method for
    colon p.
  electrolyte p.
  galenic p.
  P. H
  lactobacilli p.
  lavage bowel p.
  Nichols-Condon bowel p.
  oral p.
  oral iron p.
  renal proximal tubule p.
  Touch p.
pre-perfusion
preperitoneal
  p. anesthesia
  p. approach
  p. fat
  p. space

preproenkephalin A
preproEt-1 mRNA
prepubertal testicular tumor (PPTT)
prepuce
    hooded p.
preputial
    p. calculus
    p. collar
    p. continent vesicostomy
    p. stenosis
prepyloric
    p. antrum
    p. atresia
    p. gastric ulcer
    p. perforation
    p. polyp
    p. sphincter
    p. ulcer
prerectal lithotomy
prerenal azotemia
presacral
    p. neuroblastoma
    p. rectopexy
    p. space
presbyesophagus
presentation
    rectocele p.
    trismus p.
preservation
    cadaver renal p.
    extracorporeal renal p.
    renal p.
    simple cold storage p.
    p. time
    p. times effect
presinusoidal intrahepatic portal
  hypertension
pre-S phase
pressure
    abdominal p.
    p. amplitude modulation
    anal p.
    anal sphincter squeeze p.
    basal p.
    basal anal canal p.
    basal anal sphincter p.
    bile duct p.

    biliary tract p.
    bladder p. (BP)
    blood p. (BP)
    central venous p. (CVP)
    cerebral perfusion p. (CPP)
    choledochal basal p.
    closing p.
    colloid osmotic p.
    detrusor p.
    p. dressing
    dynamic closure p.
    end-expiratory intragastric p.
    esophageal peristaltic p.
    free hepatic venous p. (FHVP)
    glomerular capillary p.
    hepatic vein wedge p.
    hepatic venous p.
    hepatic wedge p.
    high intraluminal p.
    hydrostatic p.
    p. increment rate (PIR)
    interesophageal variceal p.
      (IOVP)
    intra-abdominal p.
    intra-anal p.
    intracholedochal p.
    intraductal p.
    intraesophageal peristaltic p.
    intragastric p.
    intraglomerular p.
    intraluminal p.
    intraluminal esophageal p.
    intraluminal urethral p.
    intraurethral p.
    intravariceal p.
    intravesical p.
    p. inversion point (PIP)
    leak p.
    leak point p. (LPP)
    LES p.
    lower esophageal sphincter p.
      (LESP)
    mean arterial p. (MAP)
    mean arterial blood p.
      (MABP)
    p. measurement
    p. natriuresis

NOTES

P

pressure *(continued)*
p. necrosis
pancreatic ducts p. (PDP)
passage p.
peak p.
plasma oncotic p.
portal p.
portal venous p. (PVP)
premicturition p.
proximal p.
p. regulated electrohydraulic
  lithotripsy
resting anal sphincter p.
sinusoidal capillary p.
p. sore
sphincter of Oddi p. (SOP)
splanchnic capillary p.
squeeze p.
static closure p.
p. study
systemic arterial p.
p. transducer
transglomerular hydrostatic
  filtration p.
transmembrane hydraulic p.
p. transmission ratio (PTR)
ureteral p.
urethral p.
variceal p.
wedge p.
wedged hepatic venous p.
  (WHVP)
pressure-flow
p.-f. electromyography study
pressure-point tension ring
pressure-specific bladder capacity
prestomal ileitis
presurgical medical evaluation
preternatural anus
pretransplant evaluation
Prevacid
prevalence
cholelithiasis p.
prevention
acute pancreatitis p.
somatostatin p.
preventive intravesical therapy
Prevenzyme
prevertebral fascia
PRF
pulse repetition frequency
priapism
arterial p.

drug-induced p.
high flow p.
low flow p.
stuttering p.
priapitis
prifinium bromide
prilocaine
Prilosec
primary
p. anastomosis
p. antiphospholipid syndrome
p. B-cell lymphoma
p. biliary cirrhosis (PBC)
p. closure
p. colorectal cancer (PCRC)
p. contraction
p. diagnostic endoscopy
p. gastric lymphoma staging
p. glomerular disease
p. glomerular lesion
p. graft nonfunction
p. hepatosplenic lymphoma
  (PHSL)
p. hyperoxaluria
p. indication
p. intestinal lymphangiectasia
  (PIL)
p. megaureter
p. obstructive megaureter
p. panendoscopy
p. perineal hypospadias surgery
p. peristaltic wave
p. peritonitis
p. procedure
p. pseudo-obstruction syndrome
p. renal calculus
p. sclerosing cholangitis (PSC)
p. suture
p. syphilis
p. transitional cell carcinoma
p. urinary diversion
primed cell
priming
androgen p.
primitive neuroectodermal tumor
(PNET)
Primus
P. Prostate Machine
P. transrectal thermography
principal cell (PC)
Principen
principle
Boari-Ockerblad p.

Goodwin cup-patch p.
Heineke-Mikulicz p.
Mitrofanoff p.
Sarfeh p.
Pringle maneuver
printer
Mavigraph color video p.
Priscoline
privileges
bathroom p.
Proaqua
proband
Pro-Banthine
probe
β-actin cDNA p.
Aloka MP-PN ultrasound p.
ambulatory p.
antisense RNA p.
Barr fistula p.
Beckman 39042 pH p.
BICAP p.
BICAP bipolar hemostasis p.
BICAP electrocoagulation p.
BICAP electrode p.
BICAP endoscopic p.
biliary balloon p.
biotinylated DNA p.
biplane sector p.
bipolar p.
Bipolar Circumactive p.
(BICAP)
Bipolar EndoStasis p. (BESP)
bipolar hemostasis p.
blunt p.
Buie fistula p.
bullet p.
Cameron-Miller monopolar p.
cDNA p.
8-channel cross-sectional anal
sphincter p.
coagulation p.
CO_2 laser p.
continuously perfused p.
Corson needle
electrosurgical p.
C-Trak p.
cystic fibrosis gene p.

Desjardins gallbladder p.
Desjardins gallstone p.
p. dilator
Dobbhoff bipolar
coagulation p.
Doppler p.
dot-plotted p.
Earle rectal p.
EHL p.
electrode p.
electrohydraulic lithotripsy p.
electrohydraulic lithotriptor p.
electrosurgical monopolar
spatula p.
end-fire transrectal p.
endorectal p.
endoscopic BICAP p.
endoscopic Doppler p.
endoscopic heat p.
Fenger gallbladder p.
FIDUS p.
fistula p.
Fluhrer rectal p.
Fogarty biliary p.
gallstone p.
galvanic p.
genomic DNA p.
Gold p.
p. gorget
G3PDH CDNA p.
heat p.
heater p.
24-hour esophageal pH p.
human apo A-I DNA p.
human fibronectin cDNA p.
human gastrin p.
intraductal ultrasound p.
intraluminal p.
KTP laser p.
lacrimal duct p.
Larry rectal p.
laser-Doppler Periflux PF-3 p.
light monitoring p.
Mayo common duct p.
Meadox Surgimed Doppler p.
mechanical rotating p.
Medi-Tech bipolar p.

NOTES

P

probe *(continued)*
20-megahertz endoscopic ultrasound p.
microballoon p.
Microelectrode MI-506 small-caliber p.
miniature p.
Mixter dilating p.
monopolar p.
Moynihan bile duct p.
Moynihan gallstone p.
multilumen p.
Ochsner flexible spiral gallstone p.
Ochsner gallbladder p.
oligonucleotide p.
Olympus CD-20Z heater p.
Olympus heat p.
Olympus ultrathin balloon-fitted ultrasound p.
Olympus UM-R-series miniature ultrasonic p.
Olympus UM-W-series endoscopic p.
palpating p.
pH p.
polycationic histochemical p.
Pratt rectal p.
Radiometer GK2803C pH p.
rectal p.
reflectance spectrophotometric p.
RNA p.
Sandhill P32 pH antimony p.
silver p.
Sonocath ultrasound p.
stimulation p.
tactile p.
transrectal p.
tumor p.
ultrasonic lithotriptor p.
V33W high density endocavity p.
water p.
probenecid
probenecid-containing solution
probenecid-inhibited organic anion transport system
problem
benign pneumatic p.
bone marrow transplantation-related p.
probucol

procainamide
procainamide-induced systemic lupus erythematosus
procaine
p. hydrochloride
p. penicillin
Procaltrol
procarbazine
Procardia
P. XL
procedural amnesia
procedure *(See also* operation, repair)
abdominal p.
Al-Ghorab p.
antegrade continence enema p. (ACE)
anti-incontinence p.
antireflux . p.
bladder chimney p.
Boari bladder flap p.
bowel refashioning p.
Boyce-Vest p.
Camey p.
cecal imbrication p.
Cecil p.
Chester-Winter p.
Cleveland Clinic weighted scale of endoscopic p.'s
Cohen antireflux p.
colon p.
corporeal rotation p.
dartos pouch p.
Datta p.
DAWG p.
Devine-Devine p.
Duckett p.
Duval p.
Ebbehoj p.
endoscopic p.
endoscopy p.
flip-flap p.
Fowler-Stephens p.
Gilchrist p.
Gil-Vernet p.
Gittes p.
Gittes-Loughlin p.
Goulding p.
Gregoir-Lich p.
Halban p.
Hanley rectal bladder p.
Harewood suspension p.
Hartmann p.
hemi-Kock p.

Hinman p.
Hodgson technique of modified
  Lich p.
Hofmeister p.
ileoanal pull-through p.
infrarenal template p.
intraparavariceal p.
island flap p.
Johnston p.
Johnston buttonhole p.
Kasai p.
Kelling-Madlener p.
Kocher p.
Kocher ureterosigmoidostomy p.
Kropp p.
Ladd p.
Leadbetter p.
Lich p.
Marshall-Marchetti-Krantz p.
Mathieu p.
Maydl p.
McIndoe p.
Michal I p.
Michal II p.
microsurgical epididymal sperm
  aspiration p.
Mitrofanoff p.
modified Norfolk p.
Moschcowitz p.
needle suspension p.
Nesbit p.
Nesbit tuck p.
NESTED p.
omentum majus flap p.
one-stage p.
Palomo p.
Pauchet p.
pelvic pouch p.
Pereyra p.
peri-Vaterian therapeutic
  endoscopic p.
primary p.
Puestow p.
Puestow-Gillesby p.
pull-through p.
Ransley p.

Raz p.
repeat p.
Richardson p.
Righini p.
Ripstein p.
Roux-en-Y p.
Salle p.
Schoemaker p.
Snow p.
Spence p.
Stamey p.
Stamey-Martius p.
Studer pouch p.
suburethral rectus fascial
  sling p.
suburethral sling p.
Sugiura p.
takedown of pelvic sling p.
Thiersch p.
Thiersch-Duplay proximal
  tube p.
Thompson p.
TIPS p.
transhepatic antegrade biliary
  drainage p.
transvaginal Burch p.
untethering p.
ureteral patch p.
vaginal needle suspension p.
vaginal wall sling p.
Van de Kramer fecal fat p.
Whipple p.
Winter p.
Young-Dees p.

process
  finger-like epithelial p.
  foot p. (FP)
  juxtacapillary p.
  knobby p.
  signal transduction p.
  sodium-linked p.
  spinous p.
  transverse p.
  uncinate p.
processing
  image p.

NOTES

P

processing *(continued)*
   postsecretory p.
   swim-up p.
processor
   Miles V.I.P. 300 vacuum
     infiltration p.
   Olympus EU-M-series
     endosonography image p.
   video p.
processus vaginalis
prochlorperazine
ProCide disinfectant
procidentia
   anal p.
   internal p.
   rectal p.
   p. recti
procoagulant
procollagen
   C-terminal propeptide of type
     I p.
   N-terminal propeptide of type
     III p.
Procrit
proctalgia fugax
proctectomy
   mucosal p.
Procter-Livingstone
   P.-L. endoprosthesis
   P.-L. tube
proctitis
   acute p.
   allergic p.
   chronic ulcerative p.
   diversion p.
   epidemic gangrenous p.
   factitial p.
   glutaraldehyde-induced p.
   gonococcal p.
   gonorrheal p.
   idiopathic p.
   nonspecific ulcerative p.
   radiation p.
   traumatic p.
   ulcerative p.
proctoclysis
proctocolectomy
   restorative p. (RP)
   single-stage total p.
   totally stapled restorative p.
     (TSRPC)
proctocolitis
   aphthoid p.

   idiopathic p.
   radiation p.
   venereal p.
proctocolonoscopy
ProctoCream-HC
ProctoCream HC
proctocystocele
proctocystoplasty
proctocystotomy
Procto-Esthesia
ProctoFoam
Proctofoam-HC
proctogenous constipation
proctogram
   balloon p.
   defecating p.
proctography
   evacuation p.
   quantitative scintigraphic
     evacuation p.
proctopexy
   Orr-Loygue transabdominal p.
proctoscope
   Salvati p.
proctoscopy
   rigid p.
proctosigmoidectomy
proctosigmoiditis
proctosigmoidoscopy
   rigid p.
procyclidine
Prodium
prodromal symptom
prodrome
product
   fibrinogen degradation p.
   mechanical p.
   secretory p.
production
   ammonia p.
   autoantibody p.
   chylomicron p.
   lymphokine p.
   superoxide p.
   unilateral renin p.
products
   Amadori p.
prodynorphin gene
proenkephalin
   p. gene
profile
   ASTRA p.
   liver function p.

phosphotyrosyl protein p.
plasmid p.
resting urethral pressure p.
Sickness Impact p.
spicules in p.
StoneRisk diagnostic p.
stress urethral pressure p.
urethral closure pressure p.
urethral pressure p.
Profile pediatric polypectomy snare
profound acid reduction
profunda
gastritis cystic p.
profuse vomiting
progesteronal agent
progesterone
progesterone-associated colitis
prognostic
p. factor
p. indicator
p. nutritional index (PNI)
prograde
p. technique
Prograf
Program
Organ Procurement P.
program
CLIM computer p.
POINTER computer p.
Stat-View computer p.
Synectics computer p.
progression factor
progressive
p. diet
p. dysphagia
p. familial cirrhosis
p. perivenular alcoholic fibrosis
(PPAF)
p. renal insufficiency
p. suppurative cholangitis
p. systemic sclerosis (PSS)
p. toxicity
Project
National Prostatic Cancer P.
projectile vomiting
projection
afferent p.

parasympathetic p.
sympathetic p.
prokinetic
p. agent
p. drug
p. effect
prolactin
Prolamine
prolapse
anal p.
bladder p.
gastric mucosal p.
p. gastropathy
genitourinary p.
hemorrhoidal p.
intestinal p.
pelvic p.
rectal p.
stomal p.
urethral p.
valve p.
prolapsed
p. bowel
p. hemorrhoids
p. rectum
p. stoma
prolapsing internal hemorrhoids
Prolase II
Cytocare P. II
P. II lateral firing Nd:YAG
laser
Prolene suture
Proleukin
P. aldesleukin
proliferating
p. cell
p. cell nuclear antigen (PCNA)
p. tubular cell
proliferation
bile duct p.
cell p.
cellular p.
colonic epithelial p.
cystic epithelial p.
diffuse mesangial p.
DNA p.
extraglandular endocrine cell p.

NOTES

P

proliferation *(continued)*
   p. of the gastric epithelium
   glomerular cell p.
   index of cell p.
   intracystic epithelial p.
   intraluminal p.
   mesangial p.
   mucosal cell p.
   neoplastic cell p.
   osteoblast-like p.
   rectal cell p.
proliferative hypertrophic gastritis
Proline endoscopic instrument
Prolixin
prolonged expiratory phase
Proloprim
promazine
promethazine
Promex biopsy needle
promontory
   sacral p.
promulgated
Pronase
pronation
pronator drift
prone
   p. position
   p. split leg position
Pronestyl
pronuclei
proopiomelanocortin gene
propagation
   p. of contraction
   orad p.
propantheline
   p. bromide
propendens
   venter p.
properitoneal
   p. fat
   p. flank stripe
   p. hernia
propHiler urinary pH testing kit
prophylactic
   p. antibiotic
   p. antibiotic treatment (PAT)
   p. cephalosporin
   p. cholecystectomy
   p. gamma globulin
   p. lymphadenectomy
   p. orchiectomy
   p. sclerotherapy
   p. treatment

prophylaxis
   antibiotic p.
   antimicrobial p.
   continuous p.
   stress ulcer p.
   stricture p.
propidium iodide
Propionibacterium acnes
propofol
propoxyphene
   p. hydrochloride
propranolol
propria
   intestinal lamina p.
   lamina p.
   maina p.
   muscularis p.
   ratio of 1:1:1 of mucosa to
     submucosa to muscularis p.
   tunica p.
proprioception
   intact p.
Propulsid
propulsive waves
propylene oxide
propylhexedrine
propylthiouracil
prorenin
   serine protease-activated p.
Proscan
   P. ultrasound imaging
     system
   P. ultrasound unit
Proscar
Pros-Check
   P.-C. kit
   P.-C. PSA assay
Prosed/DS
ProSobee
   P. formula
   P. liquid formula
prospermia
Prostacoil
   P. stent
prostacyclin
prostaglandin (PG)
   p. analog
   colonic p.'s
   cytoprotective p.
   p. E
   p. E1
   p. E2 (PGE2)

p. E$_2$
p. F
p. F2α (PGF2α)
p. F2 alpha
p. G (PGG)
p. H (PGH)
p. I (PGI)
p. I2 (PGI2)
renal p.
renal vasodilator p.
p. supplementation
p. synthesis
Prostakath urethral stent
prostatalgia
prostate
p. balloon dilator
boggy p.
p. cancer (PCa)
P. Cancer Intervention Versus Observation Trial (PCIVOT)
carcinoma of p. (CAP)
coagulation and hemostatic resection of the p. (CHRP)
enlarged p.
median furrow of the p.
minimal transurethral resection of p. (M-TURP)
percutaneous radical cryosurgical ablation of p.
p. rhabdomyosarcoma
total transurethral resection of p. (T-TURP)
transurethral evaporation of p. (TUEP)
transurethral grooving of p.
transurethral incision of p. (TUIP)
transurethral laser incision of the p.
transurethral resection of p. (TURP)
transurethral vaporization of p. (TUVP)
visual laser ablation of p. (VLAP)
prostatectomy
anatomical radical retropubic p.

cavernous nerve-sparing p.
nerve-sparing radical retropubic p.
perineal p.
radical p.
radical perineal p.
radical retropubic p. (RRP)
radical transcoccygeal p.
salvage p.
Stanford radical retropubic p.
suprapubic p.
total perineal p.
transurethral p.
transurethral ablative p.
transurethral ultrasound-guided laser-induced p.
visual laser assisted p. (VLAP)
Walsh radical retropubic p.
prostate-specific
p.-s. antigen (PSA)
p.-s. antigen density (PSAD)
p.-s. antigen velocity (PSAV)
Prostathermer
Biodan P.
P. 99D
P. prostatic hyperthermia system
prostatic
p. acid phosphatase (PAP)
p. adenocarcinoma
p. adenoma
p. calculus
p. capsule
p. carcinoma
p. catheter
p. chips
p. fossa
p. hyperplasia
p. hypertrophy
p. intraepithelial neoplasia (PIN)
p. massage
p. mesonephric remnant
p. neoplasm
p. nodule
p. pressure coefficient (PPC)
p. stent

NOTES

P

prostatic *(continued)*
  p. thermal treatment
  p. urethra
  p. urethral transitional cell
    carcinoma
  p. utricle
  p. volume
prostatism
prostatitic
prostatitis
  chemical p.
  chronic p.
  granulomatous p.
  nonbacterial p. (NBP)
prostatocystitis
prostatocystotomy
prostatodynia
prostatolith
prostatolithotomy
prostatomegaly
prostatomy
prostatorrhea
prostatoseminal vesiculectomy
prostatotomy
prostatovesical junction
prostatovesiculectomy
prostatovesiculitis
Prostatron transurethral
  thermotherapy device
prosthesis
  Alpha I inflatable penile p.
  Ambicor penile p.
  AMS Hydroflex penile p.
  AMS 700 inflatable penile p.
  AMS 600 malleable penile p.
  AMS Ultrex penile p.
  Angelchik antireflux p.
  Angelchik ring p.
  antireflux p.
  Atkinson p.
  balloon tamponade p.
  biliary p.
  bilioduodenal p.
  Celestin p.
  double-pigtail p.
  Dura-II positionable penile p.
  Duraphase inflatable penile p.
  Dynaflex penile p.
  ERCP conventional p.
  esophageal p.
  Finney Flexirod penile p.
  Flexi-Flate (I, II) penile p.
  Flexirod penile p.

GFS Mark II inflatable
  penile p.
glass penile p.
Hydroflex penile p.
inflatable penile p. (IPP)
INTROL bladder neck
  support p.
iridium p.
Jonas penile p.
malleable p.
Mentor Alpha 1 inflatable
  penile p.
Mentor GFS penile p.
Mentor inflatable penile p.
Mentor IPP penile p.
Mentor malleable penile p.
Mentor Mark II penile p.
mesh stent p.
Neville tracheal
  reconstruction p.
Omniphase penile p.
Scott AMS inflatable penile p.
silicone donut p.
Small-Carrion penile p.
Subrini penile p.
testicular p.
Ultraflex esophageal p.
Ultrex Plus penile p.
Uni-Flate 1000 penile p.
Unitary inflatable penile p.
UroLume Endourethral
  Wallstent p.
UroLume urethral p.
valved voice p.
Wallstent esophageal p.
Wilson-Cook plastic p.
prosthetic
  p. arterial graft
  p. bladder
  p. valve click
prosthetics
prosthetist
Prosthex sponge
Prostigmin
Protalba-R
protamine
  p. sulfate
  p. zinc insulin
protease
  p. inhibitor
  serine p.
  V8 p.
proteasome

protection
> gastroduodenal mucosal p.
> misoprostol p.

protein
> A-4 p.
> adenovirus-12 viral p.
> p. antibody (PAb)
> antibody to c100 p.
> anti-Tamm-Horsfall p.
> ascitic fluid total p. (AFTP)
> P. A Sepharose
> B p.
> band 3 p.
> basement membrane p.
> Bence Jones p.
> p. C
> p. catabolic rate (PCR)
> CDC42 p.
> p. C deficiency
> cholesterol ester transfer p. (CETP)
> p. C level
> complement regulatory p.
> copper-binding p. (CBP)
> C-reactive p.
> CSF p.
> cytoplasmic p.
> p. depletion
> dipstick p.
> downstream signaling p.
> E1 p.
> E2 p.
> E1b p.
> enzymic p.
> fatty acid binding p. (FABP)
> fibronectin-binding p.
> fyn p.
> G p.
> GTPase activating p.
> GTP-dependent signaling p.
> GTP-regulatory p.
> HCV p.
> heat shock p. (HSP)
> hepatocellular p.
> heterodimeric p.
> 127 Kda p.
> 87kDa p.

> p. kinase A
> p. kinase C (PKC)
> lck p.
> liver-specific p.
> low-molecular weight p.
> lyn p.
> MAGP microfibrillar p.
> membrane cofactor p. (MCP)
> membrane transport p.
> p. metabolism
> microfibrillar p. (MP)
> monocyte chemoattract p. (MCP)
> myeloma p.
> noncollagen p.
> NS2 p.
> NS3 p.
> NS4 p.
> NS5 p.
> p53 p.
> pancreatic stone p. (PSP)
> p47 cytosolic p.
> p67 cytosolic p.
> pertussin toxin-sensitive G p.
> plasma p.
> p53 nuclear p.
> porin channel p.
> PTH-related p. (PTH-rP)
> R p.
> rac p.
> ras-related p.
> receptor-associated p. (RAP)
> p. restriction
> retinol-binding p. (RBP)
> rho p.
> p. S
> S-100 p.
> Scrapie p.
> p. S deficiency
> p. serine/threonine kinase activity
> serum p.
> p. S level
> stress p.
> p. supplement
> p. synthesis
> Tamm-Horsfall p.

NOTES

P

protein *(continued)*
    T cell-specific p.
    testicular androgen-binding p.
    tight-junction p.
    total p.
    transmembrane p.
    urinary marker p.
    uronic acid-rich p.
protein-1
    insulin-like growth factor-
        binding p. (IGFBP-1)
proteinaceous
    p. cast
    p. cast material
proteinase
    p. enzyme
protein-bound homocysteine
protein-calorie malnutrition (PCM)
protein-energy malnutrition
protein-glutathione-S-transferase
    receptor-associated p.-g.-S.-t.
protein-losing
    p.-l. enteropathy
    p.-l. gastroenteropathy
    p.-l. gastropathy
protein-mediated tubular toxicity
protein-overload proteinuria
protein-tyrosine phosphatase
proteinuria
    BSA-induced overload p.
    glomerular p.
    protein-overload p.
proteinuric state
protein in vitamin K absence (PIVKA)
proteoglycan
    p. biglycan
    p. decorin
    heparan sulfate p. (HSPG)
proteolysis
proteolytic
    p. degradation
    p. digestion
    p. enzyme
Proteus
    P. mirabilis
    P. morganii
    P. pneumonia
    P. rettgeri
    P. vulgaris
prothrombin
    des-γ-carboxy p. (DCP)
    p. time (pro-time, PT)

    p. time/partial thromboplastin
        time (PT/PTT)
prothrombin time/partial thromboplastin time (PT/PTT)
Protilase
protocol
    CISCA p.
    clinical p.
    multimodal p.
    non-heart beating donor p.
    surveillance p.
    treatment p.
Protokylol
proton
    p. flux
    p. pump
    p. pump blocker
    p. pump inhibition therapy
    p. pump inhibitor (PPI)
protonated
proto-oncogene
    c-fos p.-o.
    c-jun p.-o.
    c-myc p.-o.
    p53 p.-o.
    RET p.-o.
Protopam
protopathic pain
protoporphyria
    erythropoietic p.
Protostat
prototype cholangioscope
protozoa
protozoan
    p. parasite
    p. pathogen
protriptyline
protruding fat
protrusion
    anal p.
protuberant abdomen
Provera
Providencia
    P. alcalifaciens
    P. rettgeri
    P. stuartii
provocative
    P. sensitivity balloon
    p. test
provoked cystometry
proxetil
    cefpodoxime p.

proximal
- p. bile duct
- p. convoluted tubule (PCT)
- p. gastrectomy
- p. gastric vagotomy (PGV)
- p. human colonic flora
- p. muscle weakness
- p. nephron
- p. pressure
- p. splenorenal shunt
- p. straight tubule (PST)
- p. superior mesenteric artery
- p. tubule (PT)
- p. venous plexus

Proximate
- P. flexible linear stapler
- P. intraluminal stapler
- P. linear cutter

Prozac
PRT
physiologic reflux test
Prulet
prune-belly syndrome
prune juice peritoneal fluid
pruning
- p. abnormality
- p. sign

pruritic
pruritus
- p. ani
- opioid-mediated p.

PS-2 needle
PSA
prostate-specific antigen
PSA doubling time
PSA index
PSAD
prostate-specific antigen density
PSAV
prostate-specific antigen velocity
PSC
primary sclerosing cholangitis
PSE
portal-systemic encephalopathy
Pseudallescheria boydii
pseudoachalasia
pseudoalcoholic liver disease

pseudoallergy
pseudoaneurysm
- p. formation
- ruptured p.

pseudoaneurysmal roof
pseudocapsule
pseudocholangiocarcinoma sign
pseudochylous ascites
pseudocirrhosis
cholangiodysplastic p.
pseudocolitis
pseudocryptorchism
pseudocyst
- p. communication
- drainage-resistant p.
- endosonography-guided drainage of pancreatic p.
- extramural p.
- extrapancreatic p.
- heterogenous p.
- infected p.
- pancreatic p.
- paraduodenal p.
- paragastric p.
- retrogastric p.

pseudocystobiliary fistula
pseudocystogastrostomy
pancreatic p.
pseudodefecation
pseudodiverticula
pseudodiverticulosis
pseudodiverticulum
pseudoductular transformation of hepatocytes
pseudodysentery
pseudoephedrine
pseudoesophageal colic
pseudohermaphroditism
pseudohyphae
pseudoileus
pseudolipomatosis
pseudolithiasis
ceftriaxone p.
pseudolymphoma
gastric p.
pseudomelanosis

NOTES

P

pseudomembranous
p. colitis (PMC)
p. enteritis
p. enterocolitis
p. gastritis
pseudomigration
Pseudomonas
P. aeruginosa
P. aeruginosa pneumonia
P. exotoxin A
P. pseudomallei pneumonia
pseudomononucleosis
pseudomyxoma
p. peritonei
pseudoneurogenic bladder
pseudo-obstruction
bowel p.-o.
chronic idiopathic intestinal p.-o. (CIIP)
colonic p.-o.
familial intestinal p.-o.
idiopathic intestinal p.-o.
intestinal p.-o.
nonfamilial intestinal p.-o.
polyneuropathy, ophthalmoplegia, leukoencephalopathy, and intestinal p.-o. (POLIP)
p.-o. syndrome
pseudopancreatic cholera syndrome
pseudoparallel channel sign
pseudopelade
pseudoperoxidase
pseudophimosis
pseudopodia
tumorous p.
pseudopolyp
chili bean p.
pseudopolyposis
p. medicamentosus
pseudosac
pseudosacculation
pseudosarcoma
pseudostone
pseudostricture
pseudotubercle
pseudotuberculosis
Yersinia p.
pseudotumor
helminthic p.
inflammatory p.
periampullary p.
urethral p.

pseudovaginal perineoscrotal hypospadias
pseudoxanthoma elasticum
PSFR
pancreatic secretory flow rate
peak secretory flow rate
PSFR test
PSGN
poststreptococcal glomerulonephritis
PSI
portal shunt index
PSK
polysaccharide Kreha
psoas
p. abscess
p. hitch
p. loss
p. muscle
p. shadow
p. sign
psorenteritis
psoriasis
psoriatic arthropathy
PSP
pancreatic stone protein
PSS
physiologic salt solution
portosystemic shunting
progressive systemic sclerosis
PST
proximal straight tubule
psychogenic
p. constipation
p. erectile dysfunction
p. impotence
p. vomiting
psychological
p. disorder
p. factor
p. support
psychologic dysfunction
psychometric test
psychopharmacologic medication
psychosexual support
psychosis
psychosomatic disorder
psychotropic
p. drug
p. medication
psychrophore
psyllium

PT
>prothrombin time
>proximal tubule

PTBD
>percutaneous transhepatic biliary
>drainage
>>PTBD catheter

PTC
>percutaneous transhepatic
>cholangiography

PTD
>percutaneous transhepatic drainage

PTDM
>posttransplant diabetes mellitus

pteroylglutamic acid
pterygium
pterygoid depression
PTH
>parathyroid hormone
>plasma parathyroid hormone
>>carboxyterminal PTH
>>intact PTH
>>midregion PTH

PTHC
>percutaneous transhepatic
>cholangiogram

PTH-related protein (PTH-rP)
PTH-rP
>PTH-related protein
>>PTH-rP by immunoradiometric
>>assay

PTLD
>posttransplant lymphoproliferative
>disorder

PT/PTT
>prothrombin time/partial
>thromboplastin time

PTR
>pressure transmission ratio

PTRA
>percutaneous transluminal renal
>angioplasty

PTT
>partial thromboplastin time

ptyocrinous cell
P-type amylase

pubic
>p. arch
>p. diastasis
>p. fixation
>p. hair line
>p. rami
>p. ramus
>p. symphysis
>p. tubercle

pubis
>osteitis p.
>symphysis p.

pubis
>*Phthirus p.*

pubocervical ligament
pubococcygeal
>p. line
>p. muscle training

pubococcygeus muscle
puboprostatic sling
puborectalis
>p. dysfunction
>dyskinetic p.
>p. loop
>p. muscle function
>p. sling
>p. syndrome

pubourethral
>p. ligaments
>p. sling

pubovaginal
>p. operation
>p. sling

Pucci-Seed
>P.-S. hook
>P.-S. spatula

pucker
PUD
>peptic ulcer disease

pudding
>Ensure p.
>Sustacal p.

puddle sign
puddling on barium enema
pudendal
>p.-anal reflex
>p. evoked potential

NOTES

P

pudendal *(continued)*
    p. nerve
    p. nerve function
    p. nerve terminal motor
      latency
    p. nerve terminal motor
      latency test
puerperium
Puestow
    P. pancreaticojejunostomy
    P. procedure
Puestow-Gillesby
    P.-G. operation
    P.-G. procedure
Pugh
    P. classification
    P. modification of Child
      criteria
    modified method of P.
Pugh-Child scoring system
pull
    complete PEG p.
    PEG p.
    Ponsky p.
pull-apart introducer
pull-enteroscopy
pull-through
    Duhamel p.-t.
    endorectal p.-t.
    endorectal ileal p.-t.
    ileal p.-t.
    ileoanal p.-t.
    ileoanal endorectal p.-t.
    p.-t. procedure
    rapid p.-t. (RPT)
    sacroabdominoperineal p.-t.
    Soave endorectal p.-t.
    station p.-t. (SPT)
    Swenson abdominal p.-t.
    p.-t. technique
pulmonary
    p. arteriovenous malformation
    p. aspiration
    p. cavitation
    p. complication
    p. disorder
    p. edema
    p. embolism
    p. embolus
    p. methane excretion
    p. mucormycosis
    p. outflow

pulp
    splenic p.
pulpar cell
pulsatile
    p. hematoma
    p. mass
pulsatility index
pulse
    abdominal p.
    abrupt p.
    Altmann p.
    atrial liver p.
    Corrigan p.
    intermittent p.
    p. oximetry
    Quincke p.
    p. repetition frequency (PRF)
    p. spray catheter
    thready p.
    p. volume recording
pulsed
    p. Doppler
    p. Doppler ultrasound
    p. dye neodymium:YAG laser
    p. field gel electrophoresis
      (PFGE)
    p. irrigation
    p. Solu-Medrol
Pulse-Pak infusion kit
pulse-width analysis
Pulsolith laser
pulsus
    p. abdominalis
    p. paradoxus
pulverizer
    Thermovac tissue p.
Pulvules
    Cinobac P.
pump
    Abbott LifeCare p.
    AS 800 p.
    ASID Bonz PP infusion p.
    Bluemle p.
    calcium ATPase p.
    centrifugal p.
    Companion feeding p.
    Compat feeding p.
    Endolav lavage p.
    Enteroport feeding p.
    Flexiflo feeding p.
    Flocare 500 feeding p.
    Flo-Gard p.
    Frenta Mat feeding p.

Frenta System II feeding p.
Harvard p.
hepatic artery infusion p.
Infusaid chemotherapy
  implantable p.
Infusaid hepatic p.
infusion p.
Kangaroo 324 feeding p.
MasterFlex p.
McGaw volumetric p.
Nutromat Pad S feeding p.
peristaltic p.
pneumatic leg p.
proton p.
reverse osmosis p.
roller p.
Sarns Siok II blood p.
sodium p.
stomach p.
subcutaneous morphine p.
  (SQMP)
suction p.
Tonkaflo p.
pumped-dye laser
punch
aortic p.
biopsy p.
p. biopsy
punched-out
p.-o. orchidometer
p.-o. ulcer
punctata
Aeromonas p.
punctate
p. area
p. ulcer
puncture
calix p.
cystic p.
direct cautery p.
endoscopic fine needle p.
needle tracheoesophageal p.
pupil
asymmetric p.'s
blown p.
dilated p.
irregular p.

nonreactive p.
pinpoint p.
pure
p. pancreatic juice (PPJ)
p. red cell aplasia (PRCA)
purgation
purge
oral p.
purging
self-induced p.
purified
p. HBeAg
p. T cell
purine
dietary p.
puromycin
p. aminonucleoside
p. aminonucleoside necrosis
p. aminonucleoside nephropathy
  (PAN)
purpura
anaphylactoid p.
Henoch-Schönlein p.
idiopathic thrombocytopenic p.
thrombocytopenic p.
thrombotic thrombocytopenic p.
  (TTP)
pursestring
p. ligature
p. suture
pursestringed
Pursuer helical basket
purulent
p. debris
p. discharge
p. material
p. pancreatitis
pus
p. collection
frank p.
push
complete PEG p.
p. enteroscopy
PEG p.
p. technique
pusher
p. catheter

NOTES

pusher *(continued)*
    Endo-Assist reusable knot p.
    Gazayerli knot p.
    metal-tipped stent p.
    p. tube
push-pull T technique
push-type enteroscopy
pustule
putative
    p. hepatotrophic factors
      insulin/glucagon
    p. host restriction
putredinis
    Bacteroides p.
putrescine
PUV
    posterior urethral valve
PUVT
    paraumbilical vein tumor
PV
    portal vein
PVB
    platinum, Velban and bleomycin
PVH
    persistent viral hepatitis
PVH-B
    persistent viral hepatitis, type B
PVH-NANB
    persistent viral hepatitis, non-A,
      non-B
PVP
    portal venous pressure
PVR
    postvoid residual
PVS
    peritoneovenous shunt
PVT
    portal vein thrombosis
pyelectasis, pyelectasia
pyelitic
pyelitis
pyelocaliectasis
pyelocalycotomy
pyelocystitis
pyelofluoroscopy
pyelogram
    antegrade p.
    intravenous p. (IVP)
    powder p.
    retrograde p.
pyelolithotomy
    coagulum p.
    open p.

pyelolymphatic backflow
pyelonephritis
    acute p.
    ascending p.
    chronic p.
    emphysematous p.
    xanthogranulomatous p. (XGP)
pyelonephrosis
pyeloplasty
    Anderson-Hynes p.
    Anderson-Hynes
      dismembered p.
    capsular flap p.
    Culp p.
    Culp spiral flap p.
    disjoined p., dismembered p.
    Foley Y-plasty p.
    laparoscopic dismembered p.
    Scardino vertical flap p.
    Thompson capsule flap p.
pyeloplication
pyeloscopy
pyelostomy
pyelotomy
    extended p.
    open p.
pyelotubular reflux
pyeloureteral catheter
pyeloureterectasis
pyeloureterography
pyeloureterostomy
pyelovenous
    p. backflow
pyelovesicostomy
pyemesis
pyemia
    portal p.
pyknotic nucleus
pylephlebitis
pyloralgia
pylorectomy
    Kocher p.
pylori
    Campylobacter p.
    Helicobacter p. (HP)
    intrafamilial clustering of
      Helicobacter p.
pyloric
    p. autotransplantation
    p. cap
    p. channel
    p. channel ulcer
    p. dilation

p. fullness
p. gland
p. insufficiency
p. intubation
p. mucosa
p. obstruction
p. outlet
p. outlet obstruction
p. ring
p. sphincter
p. spreader
p. stenosis
p. stricture
p. string sign
PyloriScreen test
pyloristenosis
Pyloritek
P. reagent strip
P. test kit
pylorodiosis
pyloroduodenal
p. junction
p. obstruction
pylorogastrectomy
pyloromyotomy
Ramstedt-Fredet p.
pyloroplasty
double p.
Finney p.
Heineke-Mikulicz p.
Jaboulay p.
Mikulicz p.
Ramstedt p.
reconstructive p.
truncal vagotomy and p.
vagotomy and p.
Weinberg p.
Weinberg modification of p.
pyloroptosis, pyloroptosia
pylorospasm
persistent p.
pylorostenosis
pylorostomy
pylorotomy
pylorus
closed p.
double p.

hypertrophic p.
patulous p.
p. sparing
pancreaticoduodenectomy
PyNPase activity
pyochezia
pyocystis
pyocystitis
pyoderma gangrenosum (PG)
pyogenes
Streptococcus p.
pyogenic
p. abscess
p. bacterium
p. cholangitis
p. liver
p. meningitis
pyohydronephrotic
pyonephritis
pyonephrolithiasis
pyonephrosis
pyopneumocholecystitis
pyopneumohepatitis
pyopneumoperitoneum
pyopneumoperitonitis
pyopyelectasis
pyosemia
pyospermia
pyostomatitis vegetans
pyoureter
PYP
pyrophosphate
^{99m}Tc PYP
pyramid
medullary p.
renal p.
pyramidal trocar
Pyraminyl
pyrantel pamoate
pyrazinamide
pyrexia
pyrexial
Pyribenzamine
Pyridium
P. Plus
pyridostigmine

NOTES

P

pyridoxal
 p. phosphate
 p. 5'-phosphate deficiency
pyriform
 p. fossa
 p. pooling
 p. sinus
pyrilamine
pyrimethamine
pyrimidine
Pyrinyl
pyrogen
 endogenous p.
pyrophosphate (PYP)
 stannous p. (SPP)

pyrosis
pyruvate
 p. kinase
pyuria
pyxigraphic
 p. device
 p. sampling capsule
pyxigraphy
PYY
 beta-endorphin peptide YY
 peptide YY
PYY-like immunoreactivity
PZD
 partial zonal dissection

Q
Q cell
Q fever
QAD-1
Doppler Q.
Q. sonography unit
QHS
quantitative hepatobiliary
scintigraphy
QID
Quantum inflation device
Q-Maxx side-firing laser device
QOL
quality of life
Q-switched
Q.-s. alexandrite laser
Q.-s. Nd:YAG laser
Q-tip test
Quad-Lumen drain
quadrant
all four q.'s
left lower q. (LLQ)
left upper q. (LUQ)
right lower q. (RLQ)
right upper q. (RUQ)
q. sampling technique
quadrate
q. lobe
q. lobe of liver
quadriplegia
quadruple therapy
qualitative
q. fecal fat test
q. microculture assay
quality of life (QOL)
quantified protein excretion
Quantikine quantitative
immunoenzymatometric sandwich
technique
quantitative
q. fecal fat test
q. hepatobiliary scintigraphy
(QHS)
q. liquid hybridization
q. scintigraphic evacuation
proctography
q. stool collection
Quantum
Q. inflation device (QID)
Q. TTC balloon dilator

Quartey technique
quartz waveguide
Quarzan
quasispecies
quatro therapy
queasiness
queasy
Quervain abdominal retractor
query
questionnaire
McGill pain q.
Questran
Queyrat
erythroplasia of Q.
Quick test
Quidel-Quick-Vue H. pylori test
quiescence
motor q.
quiescent
q. hepatitis
q. human fibroblast
quiet bowel sounds
quill sheath
quilted suture
quinacrine
Quinaglute
Quincke pulse
quinidine
q. gluconate
q. intoxication
q. sulfate
quinine ureahydrochloride
Quinlan test
quinolone
Quinton
Q. catheter
Q. Mahurkar dual-lumen
peritoneal catheter
Q. single port scissor-valve
Q. suction biopsy instrument
Q. tube
Quintron
Q. AlveoSampler
Q. Microlyzer 12
chromatograph

R
   resistance
      R protein
      R wave coordination
R5
      Salmonella typhimurium R5
RAAS
   renin-angiotensin-aldosterone system
rabbit stool
Rabuteau test
racephedrine
RackBeta scintillation counter
Racobalamin-57 radioactive agent
rac protein
RAD
   reactive airway disease
radial
   r. groove
   r. immunodiffusion
   r. jaw biopsy forceps
   r. jaw bladder biopsy forceps
   r. jaw hot biopsy forceps
   r. jaw 3 single-use biopsy
     forceps
   r. sector scanning
     echoendoscope
   r. suture tracks
radiata
   coronal r.
radiating pain
radiation
   r. cystitis
   effective dose equivalent r.
   r. enteritis
   r. enterocolitis
   r. enteropathy
   r. esophagitis
   5-fluorouracil, mitomycin C r.
     (FUMIR)
   r. gastritis
   r. hepatopathy
   ionizing r.
   nonionizing r.
   nonparticulate r.
   particulate r.
   r. proctitis
   r. proctocolitis
   radiotracer half-life r.
   rectosigmoid r.
   r. stenosis

   r. telangiectasia
   r. therapy
radiation-induced
   r.-i. angiosarcoma
   r.-i. colitis
   r.-i. disease
   r.-i. ulceration
radical
   r. cystectomy
   r. en bloc removal
   ferryl-free r.
   free r.
   r. hemorrhoidectomy
   hydroxyl r.
   hydroxyl-free r.
   r. inguinal orchiectomy
   r. nephrectomy
   r. nephroureterectomy
   r. orchidectomy
   oxygen r.
   oxygen-derived free r.
   oxygen-free r.
   r. perineal prostatectomy
   r. prostatectomy
   r. retropubic prostatectomy
     (RRP)
   superoxide r.
   r. surgery
   r. transcoccygeal prostatectomy
radicle
   biliary r.
   intrahepatic r.
   right hepatic r.
   tertiary r.
radioactive
   r. cholesterol
   r. iodine-131
   r. seed implantation
radioallergosorbent test (RAST)
radioautography
   thaw-mount r.
radiobiology
radiochemotherapy
radiocolloid
radiocontrast-induced
   r.-i. acute renal failure
   r.-i. renal vasoconstriction
radiodensity
radioenzymatic assay
radiographic triad

R

radiography
  barium contrast r.
  double contrast r.
  kidney, ureter, bladder r.
  (KUB radiography)
  KUB r.
    kidney, ureter, bladder
    radiography
  single contrast r.
radioimmunoassay (RIA)
  Cyclotrac-SP r.
  homogenous r.
  solid-phase r.
  Yang PSA r.
radioimmunodetection
radioimmunoguided surgery (RIGS)
radioimmunoinhibition assay
radioimmunoprecipitation assay
radioimmunoscintimetry
radioiodination
radioisotope
  r. capsule
  r. renography
  r. scan
  r. scanning
  r. scintigraphy
radiolabeled
  r. imaging
  r. leucine
  r. macromolecule
radiologic
  r. biliary stent placement
  r. portacaval shunt
radiological study
radiolucent
  r. gallstone
  r. object
Radiometer GK2803C pH probe
radionecrosis
radionuclide
  r. esophageal emptying time
  [^{123}I]iodoamphetamine r.
  r. renal imaging
  r. scan
  r. scintigraphy
  r. transit study
radiopaque
  r. density
  r. dye
  r. ERCP catheter
  r. marker
  r. pellet
radioresistant gastric plasmacytoma

radioscintigraphy
radioscopically
radiotherapy
  intraluminal r.
  intraoperative electron beam r.
radiotracer half-life radiation
radium-226
radius of varix
ragged-red fibers
railroad track scars
rake
  r. retractor
  r. ulcer
ramification
ramipril
Ramirez Silastic cannula
Ramond point
ramosum
  Absidia r.
  Clostridium r.
ramotomy
  superior pubic r.
Ramstedt
  R. operation
  R. pyloroplasty
Ramstedt-Fredet pyloromyotomy
ramus
  pubic r., pl. pubic rami
Randall
  R. plaque
  R. stone forceps
random
  r. bladder biopsy
  R. Primed DNA Labeling kit
  r. stool sample
randomized
Ranfac catheter
range
  dilation r.
  haptotoxic r.
  metabolic r.
  r. of motion
  optimum cooling r.
ranitidine
  r. hydrochloride
  r. nocte
  r. therapy
rank
  Spearman r.
Rankin clamp
Ransley-Cantwell repair
Ransley procedure

Ranson

R. acute pancreatitis classification

R. criterion

R. grading system

RANTES

regulated upon activation, normal T cell expressed and secreted

RAP

receptor-associated protein

rapamycin

raphe

anococcygeal r.

penile r.

rapid

r. colonic lavage

r. emptying of dye

r. pull-through (RPT)

r. pull-through esophageal manometry technique

r. serum amylase test

r. urease test

Rapid-hyb buffer

rapidly progressive glomerulonephritis (RPGN)

Rapoport test

Rappaport classification

Rapunzel syndrome

RAS

renin-angiotensin-aldosterone system

renin-angiotensin system

ras

r. oncogene

r. p21

rash

genital r.

petechial r.

scarlatiniform r.

ras-related protein

RAST

radioallergosorbent test

rate

albumin excretion r. (AER)

allograft survival r.

amphotericin B-induced reduction glomerular

filtration r. (AmB-induced reduction GFR)

average flow r.

basal metabolic r. (BMR)

basal secretory flow r. (BSFR)

blood flow r. (BFR)

erythrocyte sedimentation r. (ESR)

flow r.

gallbladder ejection r. (GBER)

glomerular filtration r. (GFR)

logarithmic r.

metabolic r.

normalized protein catabolic r. (NPCR)

pancreatic secretory flow r. (PSFR)

patency r.

peak flow r.

peak secretory flow r. (PSFR)

pressure increment r. (PIR)

protein catabolic r. (PCR)

r. ratio (RR)

rebleeding r.

respiratory r.

seroconversion r.

seroprevalence r.

stone-free r.

survival r.

transcapillary escape r.

voiding flow r.

rates

mean TIMP-1/GAPDH r.

Rathke duct

ratio

adenoma-hyperplastic polyp r.

adenoma-nonadenoma r.

amylase/creatinine clearance r.

androstenedione-to-testosterone r.

apolipoprotein CII-CIII r.

AST-ALT r.

BCAA/AAA plasma r.

bile salt-phospholipid r.

BUN-to-creatinine r.

CD4+-CD8+ T-cell r.

CO_2-CO_2 abundance r.

dialysate-to-plasma r.

NOTES

ratio *(continued)*
dialysis-to-plasma urea r. (D-P urea ratio)
D-P urea r.
dialysis-to-plasma urea ratio
foveola-gland r.
free-to-total PSA r.
G:D-cell r.
ketone body r. (KBR)
lactulose-mannitol r.
LCA-DCA r.
lithocholic acid-deoxycholic acid ratio
lipid-to-protein r.
lithocholic acid-deoxycholic acid r. (LCA-DCA ratio)
mean TIMP-3-GAPDH r.
r. of 1:1:1 of mucosa to submucosa to muscularis propria
nuclear-to-cytoplasmic size r.
pepsinogen A-C r.
r. of PGF2-α PGE2
phospholipid r.
pressure transmission r. (PTR)
rate r. (RR)
renal vein renin r.
signal-to-cutoff r.
somatostatin mRNA-D-cell density r.
surface-to-volume r.
urea reduction r.
Valsalva r.
Xc/R r.
Ratliff-Blake gallstone forceps
Ratliff-Mayo forceps
rat-tail
r.-t. appearance on pancreatogram
r.-t. sign
rat-tooth forceps
Raudixin
Rautina
Rauval
Rauverat
rauwolfia
Rauzide
raw
r. milk-associated diarrhea
r. surface of liver bed
Rayer disease
Raz
R. bladder neck suspension

R. 4-corner vaginal wall sling
R. four-quadrant suspension
R. modification
R. needle suspension
R. procedure
R. urethral suspension
razor
r. blade
r. blade ingestion
RBC
red blood cell
technetium-99m pyrophosphate-tagged RBC
Rb influx
RBL
rubber band ligator
RBP
retinol-binding protein
RCC
renal cell carcinoma
RCF
Ross carbohydrate free
RCF formula
RCRC
recurrent colorectal cancer
RCS
red-color sign
RCS sign
RCT
rectal carcinoid tumor
RCU
recurrent calcium urolithiasis
RDA
recommended daily allowance
RDG
retrograde duodenogastroscopy
R&D System
RDW
red cell distribution width
RE
reflux esophagitis
reabsorption
fractional proximal r.
spontaneous cyst r.
reactance (Xc)
r. and resistance (Xc/R)
reaction
acrosome r.
anaphylactic r.
cholestatic r.
desmoplastic r.
drug r.
Feulgen r.

foreign body r.
hypersensitivity r.
immune-mediated r.
insulin r.
Jaffe picrate r.
nonenzymic r.
periglandular nonspecific
inflammatory r.
polymerase chain r. (PCR)
reverse transcriptase r.
reverse transcriptase-polymerase
chain r.
scar tissue r.
sphincter r.
T-lymphocyte-mediated
cytotoxic r.
urticarial r.
Weiss r.

reactive
r. airway disease (RAD)
r. arthritis
r. oxygen metabolite
r. oxygen species (ROS)

reactivity
Goodpasture r.
lectin r.
p53 r.

reader
microtitration plate r.

reagent
ABC r.
CHOD-PAP cholesterol r.
Ehrlich r.
Folin phenol r.
lipofection r.
SAB r.
streptavidin-biotin peroxidase
complex

real focus shock wave
real-time
r.-t. confocal scanning laser
microscope
r.-t. 3-D biplanar transperineal
prostate implantation
r.-t. endoscopic ultrasound-
guided fine-needle aspiration

r.-t. fine-needle aspiration
(RTFNA)
r.-t. gallbladder ultrasound
r.-t. sonographic unit
r.-t. spectral analysis
r.-t. ultrasonography
r.-t. ultrasound

reanastomosis
end-to-end branch r.
laparoscopic ureteral r.
Roux-en-Y r.

reapproximate
reassignment
gender r.

rebleed
rebleeding
r. rate

rebound
gastric r.
gastric acid r.
r. pain
r. sign
r. tenderness

recanalization
r. of clogged biliary stent
umbilical vein r.

receiver-operating characteristic
(ROC)
receptal anal intercourse
receptor
adhesive protein r.
adrenergic r.
alpha-adrenergic r.
$alpha_1$-adrenergic r.
androgen r.
ANP r.
antidiuretic arginine vasopressin
V2 r. (AVPR2)
asialoglycoprotein r.
beta-adrenergic r.
C3 r.
C5 r.
cardiac beta r.
C3b r.
C4b r.
cell surface r.
c-met r.

NOTES

receptor *(continued)*
  endothelin A r.
  epidermal growth factor r.
   (EGFR)
  EtA r.
  EtB r.
  fMLP chemoattractant r.
  formyl peptide r.
  gastric mucosal laminin r.
  gastric oxyntic cell r.
  gastrin r.
  gp330 r.
  H2 r.'s
  histaminergic type 2 r.
  5HTM3 r. antagonist
  human PDGF r.
  IL-2 r.
  IL-3 r.
  IL-4 r.
  IL-6 r.
  IL-8 r.
  laminin r.
  liver Ah r.
  mesenteric sensory r.
  muscarinic r.
  muscle sensory r.
  native pancreatic secretin r.
  nerve growth factor r. (NGFR)
  nicotinic r.
  NK1 tachykinin r.
  NK2 tachykinin r.
  peptic cell r.
  phosphorylated growth factor r.
  polyimmunoglobulin r. (pIgR)
  recombinant pancreatic
   secretin r.
  sensory r.
  serotonergic type 3 r.
  r. and signal transduction
  smooth muscle motilin r.
  somatostatin r. (SSR)
  stretch r.
  T-cell r. (TCR)
  tyrosine kinase growth
   factor r.
  uroepithelial glycoid r.
receptor-associated
  r.-a. protein (RAP)
  r.-a. protein-glutathione-S-
   transferase
receptor-blocker
  H2 r.-b.

**receptor-mediated endocytosis
 pathway**
recess
  splenorenal r.
recession
  clitoral r.
recessive polycystic kidney disease
recipient
  r. hepatectomy
  marrow transplant r.
  phase II marrow transplant r.
  phase III marrow transplant r.
  renal transplant r.
reciprocal ligand
Recklinghausen
  R. disease
  R. gastric neurofibroma
  R. tumor
recombinant
  r. erythropoietin
  r. HBcAg (rHBcAg)
  r. human alpha interferon
  r. human erythropoietin (rh-
   EPO)
  r. human gelsolin
  r. immunoblot assay (RIBA)
  r. interferon-alfa (rIFN-a)
  r. interferon alfa-2a
   interferon alfa-2b, r.
  r. pancreatic secretin receptor
Recombivax HB
**recommended daily allowance
 (RDA)**
reconstruction
  anal sphincter r.
  Billroth I r.
  Billroth II r.
  bladder outlet r.
  corporeal r.
  3-D computer r.
  dural patch r.
  genital r.
  Roux-en-Y r.
  Roux-Y r.
  sphincter r.
  synchronous bladder r.
  Tanagho bladder neck r.
  r. technique
  tubularized bladder neck r.
  Young-Dees bladder neck r.
  Young-Dees-Leadbetter bladder
   neck r.
reconstructive pyloroplasty

R

record
 intragastric pH monitor r.
recorder
 Narco Bio-Systems
  rectilinear r.
 portable digital data r.
 Rectigraph-8K r.
 rectilinear r.
 Sandhill-800 TDS chart r.
 Sekomic SS-100F r.
 Toshiba ERVF 1A video
  floppy r.
 video r.
recording
 pH r.
 pulse volume r.
Recormon
recovery
 postanesthesia r. (PAR)
recreational drug
recrudescence
recruitment
 mononuclear cell r.
recta
 vas r.
 vasa r.
rectal
 r. abscess
 r. alimentation
 r. ampulla
 r. amyloidosis
 r. balloon
 r. biopsy
 r. bleeding
 r. cancer
 r. carcinoid tumor (RCT)
 r. carcinoma
 r. cell proliferation
 r. coil MRI
 r. compliance
 r. cream
 r. dilation
 r. dilator
 r. disease
 r. distention
 r. emptying

 r. endoscopic ultrasonography
  (REUS)
 r. epithelial cell
 r. evacuation
 r. examination
 r. fascia
 r. fistula
 r. fold
 r. foreign body
 r. gluten challenge
 r. gonorrhea
 r. hypotonia
 r. impaction
 r. incontinence
 r. inhibitory reflex
 r. injury
 r. laceration
 r. mass
 r. mucosa
 r. mucosectomy
 r. muscle cuff
 r. plexus
 r. polyp
 r. pouch
 r. probe
 r. probe electroejaculation
 r. procidentia
 r. prolapse
 r. pulsed irrigation
 r. reflex
 r. sensation
 r. shelf
 r. snare
 r. sparing
 r. speculum
 r. sphincter
 r. stenosis
 r. stricture
 r. stump
 r. suppository
 r. tenderness
 r. tenesmus
 r. thermometer
 r. trauma
 r. tube
 r. ulcer
 r. valve

NOTES

rectal *(continued)*
  r. varix
  r. vault
  r. villous adenoma
rectal-anal inhibitory reflex
recti
  procidentia r.
Rectigraph-8K recorder
rectilinear recorder
rectoabdominal
rectoanal
  r. dyssynergia
  r. function
  r. inhibitor
rectocele
  r. presentation
rectoclysis
rectolabial fistula
rectopexy
  abdominal r.
  anterior r.
  Ivalon sponge r.
  Marlex mesh abdominal r.
  posterior r.
  presacral r.
  Ripstein anterior sling r.
  Teflon sling r.
  Wells posterior r.
rectorrhagia
rectosigmoid
  r. anastomosis
  r. colon
  r. function
  r. junction
  r. manometry
  r. radiation
  r. region
  r. varix
rectosigmoidoscopy
rectosphincteric reflex (RSR)
rectosphincteromanometric study,
  rectosphincter manometric study
rectourethral
  r. fistula
  r. muscle
rectourinary fistula
rectouterina
  excavatio r.
rectouterine pouch
rectovaginal
  r. fistula
  r. pouch

  r. surgery
  r. surgical treatment
rectovesical
  r. center
  r. fistula
rectovestibular fistula
rectovulvar fistula
rectum
  bleeding per r.
  bright red blood per r.
  (BRBPR)
  gastric mucosal ectopia in r.
  (GMER)
  Hartmann closure of r.
  r. irrigation
  per r.
  prolapsed r.
  watermelon r.
rectus
  r. abdominis
  r. abdominis muscle
  r. diastasis
  r. fascial sling
  r. fascial wrap
  r. sheath
  r. sheath hematoma
recurrence
  anastomotic r.
recurrent
  r. appendicitis
  r. bouts of vomiting
  r. calcium urolithiasis (RCU)
  r. colonic histoplasmosis
  r. colorectal cancer (RCRC)
  r. focal sclerosing
    glomerulonephritis
  r. pain
  r. pancreatitis
  r. pyogenic cholangiohepatitis
  (RPC)
  r. stricture
  r. ulcer
recurring pain
red
  r. blood cell (RBC)
  r. blood cell cast
  r. blood cell count
  r. blood cell extravasation
  r. cell distribution width
  (RDW)
  r. degeneration of uterine
  myoma
  r. ring sign

r. rubber catheter
r. rubber Robinson catheter
ruthenium r.
red-color sign (RCS)
Reddick-Saye method
Redfield infrared coagulator
Redivac suction drain
Rediwash skin cleanser
Redman approach
redness
diffuse r. (DR)
Redo intestinal clamp
Redon drain
redox potential
reduced motility
reduced-size graft
reducible hernia
reducing
r. diet
r. substances test
r. substance in stool
reductase
aldose r. (AR)
5-alpha-r. inhibitor
hepatic 3-methylglutaryl
coenzyme A r. (HMG-CoA)
reduction
air pressure enema r.
barium enema r.
dissimilatory sulfate r.
gastric acidity r.
hepatic venous pressure
gradient r.
profound acid r.
sigmoid loop r.
volvulus r.
redundant sac tissue
redux
testis r.
Redy hemodialysis system
REE
resting energy expenditure
reefing
stomach r.
reentry
reexploration

refeeding
casein r.
reference values
referred pain
refill
capillary r.
delayed capillary r.
refined carbohydrate complex
reflectance
endoscopic r.
r. spectrophotometer
r. spectrophotometric probe
r. spectrophotometry
r. TS-200 spectrum analyzer
reflecting edge of ligament
reflection
hepatoduodenal r.
hepatoduodenal-peritoneal r.
peritoneal r.
total internal r.
reflex
absent gag r.
anocutaneous r.
anorectal inhibitory r.
axon r.
Babinski r.
Barrington third r.
bladder cooling r.
blinking r.
r. bradycardia
bulbocavernosus r. (BCR)
celiac plexus r.
consensual r.
corneal r.
cremasteric r.
descending inhibitory r.
detrusodetrusor facilitative r.
r. detrusor contraction
detrusosphincteric inhibitory r.
detrusourethral inhibitory r.
diminished gag r.
r. dyspepsia
emetic r.
enteric neuronal r.
r. erection
esophagosalivary r.

NOTES

R

reflex *(continued)*
fencing r.
gag r.
Galant r.
gastrocolic r.
gastroileal r.
gastropancreatic r.
glabella r.
ileogastric r.
r. incontinence
infant r.
intramural secretory r.
intrinsic r.
Landau r.
light r.
Moro r.
r. neurogenic bladder
r. neuropathic bladder
orienting r.
parachute r.
perineobulbar detrusor
  facilitative r.
perineobulbar detrusor
  inhibitory r.
perineodetrusor inhibitory r.
peristaltic r.
polarized r.
polarized standing · r.
polysynaptic r.
pudendal-anal r.
rectal r.
rectal-anal inhibitory r.
rectal inhibitory r.
rectosphincteric r. (RSR)
renal r.
Roger r.
rooting r.
secretory r.
single lens r. (SLR)
skin-CNS-bladder r.
somatointestinal r.
spinobulbar-spinal micturition r.
r. splanchnic vasoconstriction
stepping r.
sympathetic sphincter
  constrictor r.
urethral sphincter recruitment r.
urethrodetrusor facilitative r.
urethrosphincteric guarding r.
urethrosphincteric inhibitory r.
vasovagal r.
vesicoanal r.
visceral traction r.

viscerosensory r.
r. voiding
reflexogenic erection
reflux
acid r.
bile r.
r. bile gastritis
cholangiovenous r.
contralateral r.
delayed vesicoureteral r.
r. disease
duodenal r.
duodenobiliary r.
duodenogastric r. (DGR)
duodenogastroesophageal r.
  (DGER)
duodenopancreatic r.
ejaculatory duct r.
esophageal r.
r. esophagitis (RE)
free r.
r. gastritis
gastroesophageal r. (GER)
gastrointestinal r.
hepatojugular r.
intrarenal r.
nasopharyngeal r.
r. nephropathy
nocturnal acid r.
nocturnal gastric r.
nondilating r.
pathologic r.
peptic r.
postmyotomy r.
postoperative r.
pyelotubular r.
Roux-gastric r.
scintigraphic r.
ureterorenal r.
vesicoileal r.
vesicoureteral r. (VUR)
vesicoureteric r.
refluxant
refluxate
reflux-related stricture
refraction
refractory
r. ascites
r. duodenal ulcer
r. esophagitis
r. variceal hemorrhage
Regan isoenzyme

regeneration
carbon tetrachloride-induced
liver r.
tubular r.
regenerative cirrhotic nodule
regimen
antireflux r.
dietetic r.
immunosuppressive r.
multidrug r.
sequential quadruple drug r.
three-drug r.
region
antro-pyloro-duodenal r.
capsid-encoding r.
choledochal r.
floor of inguinal r.
gastric pacemaker r.
hepatic hilar r.
hydrophobic binding r.
hypogastric r.
ileocecal r.
inframammary r.
intertriginous r.
pancreatobiliary r.
para-aortic r.
perianal r.
periumbilical r.
rectosigmoid r.
retroperitoneal r.
suprapubic r.
regional
r. enteritis
r. enterocolitis
r. ileitis
registration
transcutaneous r.
Registry
Michigan Kidney R.
Regitine
Reglan
regression
r. analysis
linear r.
Poisson r.
spontaneous r.
Regroton

regular diet
**regulated upon activation, normal
T cell expressed and secreted
(RANTES)**
regulation
autocrine r.
growth r.
regulator
cystic fibrosis transmembrane
conductance r. (CFTR)
regulatory peptide
regurgitation
acid r.
chronic r.
r. jaundice
nocturnal r.
postural r.
Regutol
rehabilitation
renal r.
sexual r.
Rehfuss
R. method
R. stomach tube
R. test
Rehne abdominal retractor
Rehne-Delorme plication
rehydrating solution (RS)
rehydration therapy
Reichel-Pólya stomach resection
Reichert
R. FLPS-series flexible
fiberoptic sigmoidoscope
R. MH-series flexible
fiberoptic sigmoidoscope
R. MS-series flexible fiberoptic
sigmoidoscope
R. SC-series flexible fiberoptic
sigmoidoscope
Reichmann
R. rod
R. syndrome
Reich-Nechtow forceps
reimplantation
aortorenal r.
Cohen cross-trigonal r.
end-to-side r.

R

NOTES

reimplantation *(continued)*
  Leadbetter-Politano r.
  ureteral r.
reinforcing suture
reinsertion
reintubation
Reitan trail making test
Reiter syndrome
Reitman-Frankel test
rejection
  accelerated transplant r.
  acute cellular r.
  acute vascular r.
  allograft r.
  chronic transplant r.
  delayed hyperacute transplant r.
  ductopenic r.
  hyperacute r.
  interstitial r.
  no r. (NR)
  renal allograft r.
  transplant r.
  vascular r.
relationship
  dyadic r.
  endoscope-body position r.
  intraluminal pH-pressure r.
Relaxadon
relaxant
  cGMP-mediated r.
  smooth muscle r.
relaxation
  adaptive r.
  cardioesophageal r.
  endothelial-dependent r.
  esophageal sphincter r.
  incomplete r.
  nitric oxide blocked
    sphincter r.
  r. suture
  r. technique
  upper esophageal sphincter r.
    (UESR)
relaxatory response
relaxing incision
Relay suture delivery system
release
  nifedipine extended r.
  para-nitroaniline r.
  renin r.
  stimulated r.
  tethered-cord r.
  twin pulse shock wave r.

Reliance urinary control insert
ReliaSeal Skin Barrier
Relia-Vac drain
relocation
  polyp r.
REM
  return electrode monitor
Remegel
remission
  r. of pain
remnant
  cloacal r.
  gastric r.
  mesonephric r.
  prostatic mesonephric r.
remnants
  müllerian r.
removal
  colonoscopic r.
  endoscopic r.
  forceps r.
  foreign body r.
  gastric coin r.
  percutaneous endoscopic r.
  percutaneous stone r.
  radical en bloc r.
  small polyp r.
  through-the-scope balloon r.
  tube r.
  ureteral stoma r.
remover
  Macaluso stent r.
Renacidin
  R. irrigation
Renaflo hollow fiber dialyzer
Renal
  R. System HF250 filter
  R. systems dialyzer
renal
  r. abscess
  r. acid excretion
  r. adenocarcinoma
  r. afferent arteriolar resistance
  r. agenesis
  r. allograft
  r. allograft rejection
  r. allograft rupture
  r. amyloidosis
  r. angiography
  r. arterial occlusive disease
  r. arteriography
  r. artery aneurysm
  r. artery graft

r. artery stenosis
r. autoregulation
r. autoregulatory ability
r. autoregulatory mechanism
r. autotransplantation
r. baroreceptor
r. biopsy
r. bone disease
r. calculus
r. capsulotomy
r. carbuncle
r. carcinosarcoma
r. cell carcinoma (RCC)
r. colic
r. collecting duct cell
r. complication
r. concentrating defect
r. cortex
r. cortical abscess
r. cortical adenoma
r. cortical malondialdehyde content
r. cortical tubule cell
r. corticoadrenal
r. cyst
r. cyst decortication
r. cyst hemorrhage
r. cystic disease
r. cyst infection
r. cyst marsupialization
r. dialysis
r. disease
r. duplication
r. duplication with segmental renal dysplasia
r. dysplasia
r. epistaxis
r. epithelial cell
r. failure
r. Fanconi-like syndrome
r. fascia
r. function
r. gallium 67 scintigraphy
r. hematoma
r. hematuria
r. hemodynamics
r. hemophilia

r. hemorrhage
r. histologic sections
r. histopathology
r. hydatid disease
r. hydatidosis
r. hyperfiltration
r. hypertension
r. hypertrophy
r. hypoperfusion
r. hyposthenuria
r. hypothermia
r. impression
r. impression on liver
r. injury repair
r. insufficiency
r. interstitium
r. kallikrein-kinin system
r. lithiasis
r. mass
r. medullary carcinoma
r. messenger ribonucleoprotein acid
r. morphometric analysis
r. osteodystrophy
r. papillary necrosis (RPN)
r. parenchyma
r. pathology
r. pedicle
r. pelvic transitional cell carcinoma
r. pelvis
r. plasma flow (RPF)
r. pouch
r. preservation
r. preservation perfusion system
r. prostaglandin
r. proximal tubular cell
r. proximal tubule preparation
r. pyramid
r. reflex
r. rehabilitation
r. replacement therapy
r. retention
r. revascularization
r. scan
r. sinus

NOTES

renal *(continued)*
r. sodium
r. sodium retention
r. sodium wasting
r. sonography
r. stone
r. sympathetic activity
r. sympathetic nerve
r. sympathetic nerve activity recording electrode
r. thromboendarterectomy
r. toxicity
r. transduction pathway
r. transplant
r. transplantation
r. transplant recipient
r. trauma
r. tuberculosis
r. tubular acidosis
r. tubular acidosis I (RTA-I)
r. tubular fluid
r. tubular sodium handling
r. tubule
r. vascular injury
r. vascular resistance (RVR)
r. vascular resistance index (RVRI)
r. vascular tone
r. vasculitis
r. vasodilation
r. vasodilator
r. vasodilator prostaglandin
r. vein
r. vein renin
r. vein renin ratio
r. vein thrombosis
r. volume
r. xanthine oxidase-xanthine dehydrogenase activity
Renalin dialyzer
Renalyzer
Renatron dialyzer
Rendu-Olser-Weber syndrome
Rendu-Osler-Weber disease
Renese
renewal
epithelial restitution and r.
tissue r.
renin
active r.
r. release
renal vein r.

r. secreting juxtaglomerular cell tumor
r. secretion
renin-aldosterone system
renin-angiotensin-aldosterone
r.-a.-a. axis
r.-a.-a. system (RAAS, RAS)
renin-angiotensin system (RAS)
renin-mediated renovascular hypertension
reninoma
renogastric fistula
Renografin
renogram
MDT r.
renography
captopril r.
diethylenetriamine pentaacetic acid r. (DTPA renography)
diuretic nuclear r.
DTPA r.
diethylenetriamine pentaacetic acid renography
isotope r.
radioisotope r.
Reno-M contrast medium
renomedullary interstitial cell
renomegaly
renopathy
renoprival
Renoquid
renorrhaphy
renovascular
r. hypertension
r. hypertrophy
Renovist
Renovue
Renu enteral feeding
reoperative ureteroneocystostomy
reovirus
reoxygenation
repair *(See also* operation, procedure)
Allison gastroesophageal reflux r.
anal sphincter r.
Bassini inguinal hernia r.
Belsey Mark IV r.
Belt-Fuqua hypospadias r.
Boari ureteral flap r.
Cantwell-Ransley epispadias r.
Collis r.
cross-trigonal r.
Devine hypospadias r.

extracorporeal r.
first-stage r.
Halsted-Bassini hernia r.
hernia r.
hernial r.
Hill r.
Hill hiatus hernia r.
Hill median arcuate r.
laparoscopic varicocele r.
Lich-Gregoire r.
Lichtenstein r.
Lichtenstein hernial r.
Madden r.
Marlex hernial r.
McVay inguinal hernial r.
Nissen r.
one-stage hypospadias r.
pants-over-vest hernial r.
postanal r.
Ransley-Cantwell r.
renal injury r.
reverse sigma penoscrotal
transposition r.
Rodney Smith biliary
stricture r.
slipped Nissen r.
sphincter r.
Thal esophageal stricture r.
Thiersch-Duplay r.
tight Nissen r.
transabdominal r.
two-stage r.
vascular laceration r.
vest-over-pants hernial r.
Young type epispadias r.
repeat procedure
reperfusion
r. injury
reperitonealization
replaced hepatic vessel
replacement
bladder r.
buccal mucosal urethral r.
intestinal ureter r.
intestinal ureteral r.
r. PEG
tube r.

tunica r.
volume r.
Replete liquid nutrition
replication
r. error phenotype
gastric epithelial cell r.
viral r.
replicator
Steers r.
Replogle tube
repopulation
clonogenic r.
reprep
repreparation
repreparation (reprep)
reprocessor
American Endoscopy
automatic r.
Bard automatic r.
Custom Ultrasonic automatic r.
ECI automatic r.
KeyMed automatic r.
Lutz automatic r.
Medivator automatic r.
Olympus automatic r.
Orr automatic r.
Steris automatic r.
reproduction
assisted r.
reproductive system
reptilase acid
requirement
analgesic r.
rescinnamine
rescue
r. therapy
uridine r.
resectable
resection
abdominoperineal r., abdominal-
perineal r. (APR)
anterior r.
bowel r.
cold-cup r.
colon r.
colosigmoid r.
curative r.

NOTES

resection *(continued)*
 diathermic r.
 electrocautery r.
 en bloc r.
 endoscopic mucosal r.
 endoscopic snare r.
 esophageal r.
 hepatic r.
 ileal r.
 ileocolic r.
 liver r.
 Miles r.
 Miles abdominoperineal r.
 pancreatic tail r.
 Paul-Mikulicz r.
 Reichel-Pólya stomach r.
 segmental colonic r.
 strip r.
 terminal ileal r.
 transanal endoscopic
  microsurgical r.
 transurethral r. (photometer,
  TUR, TUR-Cue photometer,
  TUR-Cue photometer)
 transurethral r. of prostate
  (TURP)
 transverse r.
 wedge r.
 Whipple r.
resective colostomy
resectoscope
 continuous-flow r.
 Foroblique r.
 Iglesias r.
 Iglesias fiberoptic r.
 r. loop
 Olympus continuous flow r.
 Richard Wolf video r.
 r. sheath
 Storz r.
 Wolf r.
resectoscopy
resedation
Resercen
reserpine
 hydrochlorothiazide and r.
reserpine-induced ulcer
reservoir
 continent ileal r.
 detubularized right colon r.
 double-barrel r.
 double J-shaped r.
 double-stapled ileal r.

 fecal r.
 ileal r.
 ileoanal r.
 ileocecal r.
 ileocecal continent urinary r.
 Indiana continent r.
 intra-abdominal ileal r.
 isoperistaltic ileal r.
 J-shaped r.
 J-Vac suction r.
 Knok ileal r.
 lateral internal pelvic r.
 Le Bag pouch r.
 r. mucosal absorption
 orthotopic colonic r.
 orthotopic continent r.
 orthotopic remodeled
  ileocolonic r.
 Parks ileal r.
 Parks ileoanal r.
 r. phase
 S-shaped r.
reservoirography
**Resident Assessment Protocol for
 incontinence**
residual
 r. barium
 r. fragment
 postvoid r. (PVR)
 r. stone
 r. stool
 r. urine
 r. urine volume (RUV)
residue
 fecal r.
 food r. ·
 sialic acid r.
 sialyl r.
resin
 anion exchange r.
 bile-salt binding r.
 Epon 812 r.
resistance (R)
 basal renal vascular r.
 drug r.
 insulin r.
 reactance and r. (Xc/R)
 renal afferent arteriolar r.
 renal vascular r. (RVR)
 systemic vascular r.
 tissue r.
 transhepatic vascular r.

urethral r.
vesical neck r.
resistant ascites
Resol electrolyte solution
resonance
  nuclear magnetic r. (NMR)
resonant abdomen
resorbable thread clip applicator
resorption
  tubular r.
Resource enteral feeding
respiratory
  r. acidosis
  r. alkalosis
  r. burst
  r. depression
  r. distress
  r. distress syndrome
  r. embarrassment
  r. excursion
  r. failure
  r. inversion point (RIP)
  r. rate
respiratory-esophageal fistula
response
  alloantigen r.
  ameliorated vasodilating r.
  antibody directed cytotoxic r.
  cell-mediated
    immunohistological r.
  cellular immune r.
  cytotoxic T-cell r.
  desmopressin r.
  fed r.
  gag r.
  hypercontractile external
    sphincter r.
  macrophage-rich
    inflammatory r.
  paradoxical renal r.
  peak r.
  plateau r.
  relaxatory r.
responsiveness
  vasculature r.
rest
  adrenal r.

R

bowel r.
ectopic adrenal r.
gut r.
Krause arm r.
pancreatic r.
testicular adrenal r.
total bowel r.
restaging of cancer
resting
  r. anal sphincter pressure
  r. energy expenditure (REE)
  r. membrane potential
  r. tremor
  r. urethral pressure profile
restless leg syndrome
restoration
  foreskin r.
  voice r.
restorative proctocolectomy (RP)
Restoril
restricted
  HLA class II r.
restriction
  dietary protein r.
  fluid r.
  r. fragment length
    polymorphism (RLP)
  protein r.
  putative host r.
  sodium r.
result
  medium-term r.
resuscitation
  fluid r.
retained
  r. antrum
  r. antrum syndrome
  r. barium
  r. feces
  r. gallstone
  r. testis
retardata
  ejaculatio r.
retch
retching
rete, pl. **retia**
  r. peg

NOTES

rete *(continued)*
  r. ridge
  r. testis
retention
  barium r.
  BSP r.
  r. cyst
  r. enema
  r. esophagitis
  gastric r.
  r. jaundice
  r. meal
  r. polyp
  postoperative urinary r.
  renal r.
  renal sodium r.
  sodium r.
  stool r.
  r. suture
  urinary r.
  r. vomiting
re-tethering
retia (*pl. of* rete)
reticularis
  formatio r.
reticulocyte
reticuloendothelial system
reticulonodular pattern
reticulosis
  polymorphic r.
reticulum
  endoplasmic r. (ER)
  rough endoplasmic r.
  sarcoplasmic r.
retinal
  r. artery occlusion
  r. vein occlusion
retinoblastoma
retinoid
retinol-binding protein (RBP)
RET proto-oncogene
retracted stoma
retractile
  r. concealed penis
  r. mesenteritis
  r. testis
retraction
retractor
  Army-Navy r.
  Aronson esophageal r.
  baby Balfour r.
  Balfour r.
  Balfour abdominal r.

Balfour self-retaining r.
Barr rectal r.
Beardsley esophageal r.
B.E. Glass abdominal r.
Berens esophageal r.
Bookwalter r.
Bookwalter-Goulet r.
Bookwalter-Hill-Ferguson
  rectal r.
Bookwalter ring r.
Bookwalter-St. Mark deep
  pelvic r.
Breisky-Navratil straight r.
Buie-Smith r.
Christie gallbladder r.
Collin abdominal r.
Collins intestinal r.
Crile angle r.
Deaver r.
Delaginiere abdominal r.
Denis Browne abdominal r.
Deucher abdominal r.
Doyen r.
Doyen abdominal r.
fan r.
fan elevator r.
fan-type laparoscopic r.
Farabeuf r.
Finochietto r.
fixed ring r.
Foerster abdominal ring r.
Forder r.
Foss bifid gallbladder r.
Foss biliary duct r.
Franz abdominal r.
Friedman perineal r.
gallows-type r.
Gelpi self-retaining r.
Gibson-Balfour abdominal r.
Gil-Vernet r.
Goelet r.
Goligher r.
Gosset appendectomy r.
Grant gallbladder r.
Greene r.
Greishaber self-retaining r.
hand-held r.
Harrington Deaver r.
Harrington splanchnic r.
Hill-Ferguson rectal r.
Hill rectal r.
Israel r.
Jansen r.

Johns Hopkins gallbladder r.
Kelly r.
Kelly abdominal r.
Kirschner abdominal r.
Kocher gallbladder r.
Lowsley r.
malleable r.
Mayo abdominal r.
Mayo-Adams appendectomy r.
McBurney r.
Mediflex-Gazayerli r.
metal bar r.
Mik r.
Mikulicz r.
Miller-Senn r.
Millin bladder r.
Moon rectal r.
Murphy gallbladder r.
Ochsner r.
Oettingen abdominal r.
Omnitract r.
O'Sullivan-O'Connor
    abdominal r.
Parker r.
Parks r.
Percy-Wolfson gallbladder r.
Polytrac Gomez r.
Pratt bivalve r.
Quervain abdominal r.
rake r.
Rehne abdominal r.
ribbon r.
Richards abdominal r.
Richardson r.
Richardson appendectomy r.
Rigby appendectomy r.
ring abdominal r.
Robin-Masse abdominal r.
Roux r.
Sawyer rectal r.
Scott r.
self-retaining r.
self-retaining ring r.
Senn r.
Senn-Kanavel r.
Smith-Buie rectal r.
Smith rectal r.

spoon r.
spring-wire r.
Stamey dorsal vein apical r.
T-bar r.
Tuffier abdominal r.
U.S. r.
vein r.
Volkmann rake r.
Walker gallbladder r.
Webb-Balfour abdominal r.
Weinberg vagotomy r.
Weitlaner r.
Wesson perineal r.
Wexler r.
Wilkinson abdominal r.
Wolfson gallbladder r.
Wylie splanchnic r.
Young prostatic r.
Yu-Holtgrewe prostatic r.
retransplantation
retreatment
    lithotripsy r.
retrieval balloon
retriever
    Entract stone r.
    Positrap r.
    snail-headed catheter r.
    stone r.
    three-pronged polyp r.
retrocecal
    r. abscess
    r. appendicitis
    r. appendix
retrocecalis tumor thrombus
retrocolic
    r. end-to-end
        pancreatojejunostomy
    r. end-to-side
        choledochojejunostomy
retroduodenal
    r. artery severance
    r. perforation
retroflexed
    r. cystoscopy sheath
    r. scope
    r. uterus
    r. view

R

NOTES

retroflexion
  endoscopic r.
retrogastric pseudocyst
retrograde
  r. amnesia
  r. balloon rupture
  r. cannulation
  r. cholangiography
  r. contrast study
  r. duodenogastroscopy (RDG)
  r. ejaculation
  r. fashion
  r. flow on barium enema
  r. genitography
  r. hernia
  r. intrarenal surgery
  r. intussusception
  r. occlusion balloon catheter
  r. pancreatocholangiography
  r. pancreatography
  r. pyelogram
  r. sphincterotomy
  r. technique
  r. ureteropyelogram
  r. urethrogram (RUG)
  r. urography
  r. vascularization of superior
    mesenteric artery
retrohepatic
  r. vena cava
retroileal
  r. appendicitis
  r. appendix
Retromax endopyelotomy stent
retropancreatic tunnel
retroperitoneal
  r. approach
  r. cavity
  r. cutaneous ureterostomy
  r. fibrosis
  r. fistula
  r. hernia
  r. lymphadenectomy
  r. neoplasm
  r. perforation
  r. pneumography
  r. region
  r. space
  r. tumor
retroperitoneal-iliopsoas abscess
retroperitoneoscopic vein ligature
retroperitoneoscopy
retroperitoneum

retroperitonitis
  idiopathic fibrous r.
retropneumoperitoneum
retropubic
  r. implant
  r. Lapides-Ball bladder neck
    suspension
  r. urethrolysis
  r. urethroscopy
retrorectal lymph node
retrosternal
  r. chest pain
  r. hernia
retroversion
retroverted uterus
retrovirus
  r. infection
retrusive meatus
rettgeri
  Proteus r.
  Providencia r.
return
  r. electrode monitor (REM)
  total predicted r.
Retzius
  space of R.
  R. space
  R. veins
REUS
  rectal endoscopic ultrasonography
reusable laparoscopic electrode
revascularization
  myocardial r.
  penile r.
  renal r.
revenge
  Montezuma r.
Reverdin abdominal spatula
reversal jejunoileal bypass surgery
reverse
  r. alpha sigmoid loop
  r. cystotome
  r. osmosis pump
  r. sigma penoscrotal
    transposition repair
  r. sphincterotome
  r. transcriptase (RT)
  r. transcriptase-polymerase
    chain reaction
  r. transcriptase reaction
  r. Trendelenburg position
reversed
  r. Mercedes Benz sign

r. peristalsis
r. reimplanted
    appendicocystostomy
reverse-dot hybridization
Rex-Cantli-Serege line
Reye syndrome
rhabdoid tumor
rhabdomyoblastic differentiation
rhabdomyolysis
    exertional r.
    hypoxia-induced r.
rhabdomyoma
rhabdomyosarcoma (RMS)
    alveolar r.
    paratesticular r.
    prostate r.
rhabdosphincter
    r. electromyography
    r. muscle
rHBcAg
    recombinant HBcAg
Rheaban
Rheomacrodex
rh-EPO
    recombinant human erythropoietin
rheumatica
    scarlatina r.
rheumatic disease
rheumatism
    palindromic r.
rheumatoid
    r. arthritis
    r. vasculitis
Rhizopus
    R. species
rhizotomy
    selective sacral r.
rhodamine
    alexandrite and r.
    r. 6G dye
    r. laser
    r. stain
rhonchus, pl. **rhonchi**
rho protein
RHV
    right hepatic vein

rhythm
    biphasic diurnal r.
    circadian r.
    gallop r.
    irregular r.
    paced r.
    r. strip
    ultradian r.
rhythmicity
    circadian r.
rhythmometry
    cosinor r.
RIA
    radioimmunoassay
RIA-KIT
RIBA
    recombinant immunoblot assay
    RIBA test
RIBA-2 test
ribbon
    iridium r.
    r. retractor
    r. stool
rib cutter
ribonuclease
    low-molecular weight protein r.
ribonucleic acid (RNA)
ribonucleoprotein (RNP)
riboprobe
    ^{35}S antisense fibronectin r.
ribose-1-phosphate
ribose-5-phosphate
ribosome
    free r.
rice-flour breath test
rice-fruit diet
rice-water stool
Richards abdominal retractor
Richardson
    R. appendectomy retractor
    R. procedure
    R. retractor
Richard Wolf video resectoscope
Richet fascia umbilicus
Richter hernia
Richter-Monroe line

R

NOTES

rickets
    celiac r.
    hypophosphatemic r.
Rickettsia conorii
Rider-Moeller glossitis
ridge
    interureteric r.
    rete r.
ridged-convoluted villus
Riedel lobe
Riepe-Bard gastric balloon
Rieux hernia
rifampicin
rifampin
rifamycin
rIFN-a
    recombinant interferon-alfa
Rigby appendectomy retractor
Righini procedure
right
    r. anterior pararenal space
    r. antero-oblique position
    r. colon
    r. colonic flexure
    r. gutter
    r. hepatic duct
    r. hepatic radicle
    r. hepatic vein (RHV)
    r. lobe
    r. lower quadrant (RLQ)
    r. ovarian vein syndrome
    r. upper quadrant (RUQ)
right-angle
    r.-a. clamp
    r.-a. electrode
    r.-a. lens
right-angled end-to-side anastomosis
right hepatic vein (RHV)
right-sided
    r.-s. clonus
    r.-s. lesion
rigid
    r. abdomen
    r. endoscope
    r. nephroscope
    r. proctoscopy
    r. proctosigmoidoscopy
    r. scoop
    r. sigmoidoscope
    r. ureteroscope
    r. ureteroscopy

rigidity
    abdominal r.
    board-like r.
    involuntary reflex r.
    nuchal r.
Rigiflator hand-held
inflation/deflation device
Rigiflex
    R. ABD balloon dilatation
      catheter
    R. achalasia balloon
    R. achalasia dilator
    R. balloon dilator
    R. biliary balloon dilatation
      catheter
    R. OTW balloon dilatation
      catheter
    R. TTS balloon
    R. TTS balloon dilatation
      catheter
    R. TTS balloon dilator
RigiScan
    R. device
    R. measurement
    R. penile tumescence and
      rigidity monitor
Rigler sign
Rigoflex esophageal TTS
rigor mortis
RIGS
    radioimmunoguided surgery
Riley-Day
    R.-D. syndrome
    R.-D. syndrome of familial
      dysautonomia
rim of fascia
ring
    A r.
    abdominal r.
    r. abdominal retractor
    anorectal r.
    apex of external r.
    B r.
    biofragmentable anastomotic r.
      (BAR)
    R. catheter
    confidence r.
    constriction r.
    distal esophageal r.
    elastic O r.
    esophageal r.
    esophageal A r.

esophageal B r.
esophageal contractile r.
esophageal mucosal r.
esophageal muscular r.
external r.
external inguinal r.
r. forceps
ilioinguinal r.
iliopsoas r.
inguinal r.
inositol r.
internal abdominal r.
internal inguinal r.
intrahaustral contraction r.
Kayser-Fleischer r.
lower esophageal r.
lower esophageal B r.
lower esophageal mucosal r.
Lyon r.
Maclet magnetic r.
mucosal r.
mucosal esophageal r.
muscular esophageal r.
Ochsner r.
Osbon pressure-point tension r.
pressure-point tension r.
pyloric r.
rust r.
Schatzki r.
Silastic r.
silicone elastomer r.
Smith r.
sphincter contraction r.
Ringer lactate
ringlike contractions
"ring-type" rigidity measuring device
Riopan
    R. Plus
    R. Plus 2
RIP
    respiratory inversion point
Ripstein
    R. anterior sling rectopexy
    R. procedure
    R. rectal prolapse operation

risk
    Goldman classification
      operative r.
    neoplasia r.
Ritalin
RiteBite biopsy forceps
RJL Model 10 bioelectrical impedance analyzer
RLP
    restriction fragment length polymorphism
RLQ
    right lower quadrant
RMS
    rhabdomyosarcoma
    RMS voltage
RNA
    ribonucleic acid
    albumin messenger RNA
    HCV RNA
      hepatitis C RNA detection
      hepatitis C virus RNA
    hepatitis C virus RNA (HCV RNA)
    IGF-1R RNA
    messenger RNA (mRNA)
    RNA probe
RNAse digestion
RNP
    ribonucleoprotein
Robbers forceps
Robengatope radioactive agent
Roberts
    R. esophagoscope
    R. folding esophagoscope
    R. oval esophagoscope
Roberts-Jesberg esophagoscope
Robertson
    R. sign
    R. TM urethroscope
Ro-Bile
Robin-Masse abdominal retractor
Robinow syndrome
Robinson catheter
Robinson-Kepler-Power water test

NOTES

Robinul
R. Forte
Roboprep G instrument
robotic-automated assist device
Robson
R. intestinal forceps
R. point
R. position
ROC
receiver-operating characteristic
Rocaltrol
Rocephin
Rochester-Carmalt forceps
Rochester gallstone forceps
Rochester-Mixter forceps
Rochester-Ochsner forceps
Rochester-Péan
R.-P. forceps
R.-P. hemostat
Rockey-Davis incision
rod
Biethium ostomy r.
colostomy r.
Gram-negative r.
ileostomy r.
Meckel r.
Reichmann r.
rod-lens system
rodless end-loop stoma
Rodney Smith biliary stricture
repair
Roeder
R. loop
R. loop knot
roentgen finding
roentgenography
Roger
R. reflex
R. syndrome
Rokitansky
R. disease
R. diverticulum
R. hernia
Rokitansky-Aschoff
R.-A. sinus
R.-A. sinus hyperplasia
Rokitansky-Cushing ulcer
Rokitansky-Kuster-Hauser syndrome
Rolaids
role
plasmid profile r.
roll
iliac r.

roller pump
rolling hiatal hernia
Romazicon
Rome criteria
roof
pseudoaneurysmal r.
Roosevelt clamp
rooting reflex
root mean square voltage
ROS
reactive oxygen species
rose
r. bengal sodium ^{131}I biliary
scan
r. bengal sodium ^{131}I
radioactive agent
r. bengal test
r. thorn ulcer
r. thorn ulcer of mucosa
rosebud stoma
Rosenbach-Gmelin test
Rosenbach sign
Rosenthal test
rosette
r. appearance of anus
Homer Wright r.
rosetted
Ross carbohydrate free (RCF)
Rosser crypt hook
Rossetti modification of Nissen
fundoplication
rotary shadowing electron
microscopy
rotating
r. endo-scissors
r. sphincterotome
rotation
external r.
internal r.
rotator
Jarit r.
rotavirus
r. diarrhea
r. gastroenteritis
r. infection
Rotazyme test
Roth
R. Grip-Tip suture guide
R. polyp retrieval net
Rotor syndrome
rotund abdomen
roughage
rough endoplasmic reticulum

round
    r. ligament
    r. ulcer
roundworm
route
    fecal-oral r.
    paracellular r.
routine neonatal circumcision
Roux
    R. limb
    R. limb emptying
    R. retractor
    R. stasis syndrome
Roux-en-Y, Roux-Y
    R.-e.-Y. anastomosis
    R.-e.-Y. biliary bypass with
    antrectomy
    R.-e.-Y. choledochojejunostomy
    R.-e.-Y. distal jejunoileostomy
    R.-e.-Y. esophagojejunostomy
    R.-e.-Y. gastric bypass
    R.-e.-Y. gastroenterostomy
    R.-e.-Y. gastrojejunostomy
    R.-e.-Y. hepaticojejunostomy
    R.-e.-Y. jejunal limb
    R.-e.-Y. limb enteroscopy
    R.-e.-Y. loop
    R.-e.-Y. loop of jejunum
    R.-e.-Y. operation
    R.-e.-Y. pancreaticojejunostomy
    R.-e.-Y. procedure
    R.-e.-Y. procedure with
    vagotomy
    R.-e.-Y. reanastomosis
    R.-e.-Y. reconstruction
Roux-en-Y-cyst-jejunostomy
Roux-gastric reflux
Roux-limb
    R.-l. stasis
Roux-Y (*var. of* Roux-en-Y)
Rovighi sign
Rovsing
    R. operation
    R. sign
Rowasa
    R. enema
roxatidine acetate

Roxicodone
Roxin
roxithromycin
RP
    restorative proctocolectomy
RP3 stain
RPC
    recurrent pyogenic
    cholangiohepatitis
RPF
    renal plasma flow
RPGN
    rapidly progressive
    glomerulonephritis
RPMI 1640 culture medium
RPN
    renal papillary necrosis
RPT
    rapid pull-through
        RPT technique
RR
    rate ratio
RRP
    radical retropubic prostatectomy
RS
    rehydrating solution
RSR
    rectosphincteric reflex
RT
    reverse transcriptase
RTA-I
    renal tubular acidosis I
RTFNA
    real-time fine-needle aspiration
rub
    friction r.
    peritoneal friction r.
    pleural r.
rubber
    r. band ligation
    r. band ligation of hemorrhoid
    r. band ligator (RBL)
    r. dam
rubber-shod clamp
rubella
rubeola

R

NOTES

**Rubin-Quinton small-bowel biopsy
 tube**
rubor
　dependent r.
rubra
　miliaria r.
Rubratope-57 radioactive agent
ructus
Rudd-Clinic
　R.-C. hemorrhoidal forceps
　R.-C. hemorrhoidal ligator
rufloxacin
RUG
　retrograde urethrogram
ruga, pl. **rugae**
rugal
　r. fold
　r. hypertrophy
　r. pattern
rugitus
rule
　Goodsall r.
rumble
rumbling
　r. bowel sounds
Rumel tourniquet
rumen
rumination
running suture
runny stool
"runs"
runting syndrome
Runyon group III mycobacteria
rupture
　acute hepatic r.
　duodenopancreat-
　　icocholedochal r.
　ERCP-induced splenic r.
　esophageal r.
　gastric r.
　hepatic r.
　hydatid cyst intra-hepatic r.
　Mallory-Weiss mucosal r.
　mesenteric r.

　penile r.
　renal allograft r.
　retrograde balloon r.
　splenic r.
　spontaneous r.
　traumatic r.
　umbilical hernia r.
　uterine r.
ruptured
　r. aneurysm
　r. appendix
　r. hepatic tumor
　r. peliotic lesion
　r. pseudoaneurysm
　r. sigmoid diverticulum
RUQ
　right upper quadrant
Rüsch stent
rush
　peristaltic r.'s
rushing
Russell
　R. gastrostomy kit
　R. peel-away sheath dilator
　R. percutaneous endoscopic
　　gastrostomy
　R. technique
　R. viper venom test
　R. viper venom time
Russian tissue forceps
rust ring
ruthenium red
RUV
　residual urine volume
Ruysch disease
RVR
　renal vascular resistance
RVRI
　renal vascular resistance index
R-wave triggering
RWG
　rye whole-grain
rye whole-grain (RWG)
Ryle tube

S
S. cell
S. neuron
S-100
S. immunohistochemical stain
S. protein
SAAG
serum-ascites albumin gradient
Saathoff test
saber stroke
Sabouraud glucose agar
sabre
coup de s.
en coup de s.
SAB reagent
saburra
saburral
sac
enterocele s.
fluid-filled s.
greater peritoneal s.
hernia s.
hernial s.
high ligation of hernia s.
indirect hernial s.
lesser peritoneal s.
peritoneal s.
wide-mouth s.
yolk s.
saccharin
Saccharomyces boulardii
Saccomanno
S. fixative
S. solution
saccular
s. aneurysm
s. colon
sacculation
tubular narrowing and s.
saccule
Sachs
S. solution
S. urethrotome
sack
entrapment s.
Sacks
S. QuickStick catheter
S. Single-Step catheter
Sacks-Vine
S.-V. feeding gastrostomy tube

S.-V. gastrostomy kit
S.-V. PEG system
S.-V. type PEG
sacral
s. edema
s. promontory
sacroabdominoperineal pull-through
sacrococcygeal
s. cyst
s. teratoma
sacrofixation operation
sacroiliitis
**sacrospinalis ligament vaginal
fixation**
**sacrospinous ligament vaginal
fixation**
sacrotuberous ligament
sacrum
SAD
sinoaortic denervation
s-adenosylmethione (SAM)
Saeed technique
**Safe and Dry panty and pad
system**
safe-gastrocutaneous fistulous tract
safe-tract
safety
s. pin ingestion
s. wire
saffron stain
SAGES
Society of American Gastrointestinal
Endoscoping Surgeons
saginata
Taenia s.
sagittal image
sago-grain stool
Sahli glutoid test
Sahli-Nencki test
Saint triad
s-albumin
Salem
S. duodenal sump tube
S. sump tube
salicylate
s. abuse
methyl s.
salicylazosulfapyridine
saline
s. cleansing enema

S

507

saline *(continued)*
  s. continence test
  s. cystometry
  s. flush
  half-normal s.
  heparinized s.
  hypertonic s.
  indigo-carmine-stained
    normal s.
  s. injection therapy
  isotonic s.
  s. load test
  phosphate-buffered s. (PBS)
  s. slush
  s. test
saline-epinephrine
  hypertonic s.-e.
saline-filled cholangiocatheter
saline-moistened sponge
saliva
  s. bicarbonate
  pooled s.
  s. substitute
salivarius
  Streptococcus s.
Salivart
salivary
  s. amylase
  s. epidermal growth factor
    (sEGF)
  s. epidermal growth factor-1
  s. gland enlargement
  s. gland scan
  s. hypersecretion
  s. mass
  s. tenderness
  s. testing
salivation
Salkowski-Schipper test
Salle procedure
Salmonella
  S. colitis
  S. enteritidis
  S. enteritidis orchitis
  S. food poisoning
  S. newport
  nontyphoidal *S.*
  S. typhi
  S. typhimurium
  S. typhimurium enterocolitis
  S. typhimurium R5
salmonellosis
  nontyphoidal s.

salmonicida
  Aeromonas s.
Salomon test
salpingitis
salpinx
salt
  bile s.'s
  bismuth s.
  s. consumption
  dihydroxy s.
  fura pentapotassium s.
  gold s.
  low s. (LNaCl)
  monohydroxy bile s.
  s. and pepper duodenal erosion
  trihydroxy s.
salt-losing nephritis
salt-sensitive hypertension
Saluron
Salutensin
salvage
  s. cystectomy
  s. cytology
  s. cytology technique
  s. prostatectomy
  s. surgery
  s. therapy
Salvati proctoscope
SAM
  s-adenosylmethione
sample
  arterial blood s.
  aspirated s.
  Bethesda System for
    cervicovaginal s.
  blood s.
  random stool s.
  stool s.
  urine s.
  venous blood s.
sampling
  s. gate
  mediastinal lymph node s.
  tissue s.
  transhepatic portal venous s.
Sam Roberts esophagoscope
sand
  hydatid s.
  urinary s.
sandbag
Sand-Eze EGD pillow
Sandhill-800 TDS chart recorder
Sandhill P32 pH antimony probe

Sandifer syndrome
Sandimmune
Sandostatin
Sandoz
S. Caluso 22F, 28F super
PEG
S. Caluso PEG gastrostomy
tube
S. 22F balloon replacement
tube
S. feeding/suction tube
sandwich
s. staghorn calculus therapy
s. therapy
sandy skin prepping paste
sanguineous
s. drainage
s. fluid
sanguis
Streptococcus s.
Sani Pads medicated cleansing pad
Sanorex
Sansert
Santiani-Stone classification
santonin test
Santorini
duct of S.
S. sphincter
S. venous plexus
Santorinicele
SAP
serum amyloid P
saphenofemoral junction
saphenous
saphrophytism
saponifiable fecal bile acid
saponification
saprophyticus
Staphylococcus s.
SAPS
single-action pumping system
saralasin
sarcoidosis
epididymal s.
hepatic s.
pancreatic s.
urethral s.

sarcoma
appendiceal Kaposi s.
botryoid s.
clear cell s.
Ewing s.
gastric s.
gastric Kaposi s.
gastrointestinal Kaposi s.
hemangioendothelial s.
intracolonic Kaposi s.
Ito cell s.
Kaposi s. (KS)
Kupffer cell s.
lipoblastic s.
osteogenic s.
vasoablative endothelial s.
(VABES)
sarcomatoid squamous cell
carcinoma
sarcoplasmic reticulum
Sarfeh principle
Sarns Siok II blood pump
SART
standard acid reflux test
satellite lesion
satiety
early s.
Satinsky clamp
Satric-500
satriuresis
saturation
arterial s.
s. index (SI)
oxygen s.
percent transferrin s.
transferrin s.
saturnine colic
saturnism
saucerization
saucerized biopsy
Saundby test
Saunders disease
sausage digits
Savary
S. bougie
S. bronchoscope
complete S.

S

NOTES

Savary *(continued)*
   S. dilator
   S. tapered thermoplastic dilator
Savary-Gilliard
   S.-G. metal olive
   S.-G. over-the-wire dilator
   S.-G. Silastic flexible bougie
   S.-G. wire-guided bougie
Savary-Miller
   S.-M. criteria
   S.-M. II grade
Saver
   Cell S.
sawtooth
   s. appearance sign
   s. irregularity of bowel
     contour
Sawyer
   S. rectal retractor
   S. rectal speculum
S-B
   Sengstaken-Blakemore
   S-B tube
SBE
   small bowel enteroscopy
SBFT
   small-bowel follow-through
s-bilirubin
SBO
   small-bowel obstruction
SBP
   spontaneous bacterial peritonitis
SBPN
   simultaneous bilateral percutaneous
     nephrolithotomy
SBT
   skin bleeding time
SC
   secretory component
   subcutaneous
   sulfur colloid
   ^{99m}Tc SC
scale
   Charrière s.
   children's coma s.
   ECOG performance status s.
   Glasgow coma s.
   Goldberg Anorectic Attitude s.
   gray s.
   Karnofsky performance
     status s.
   Kodsi s.
   Lanza s.

   Likert s.
   Madsen-Iversen s.
scalloped bowel lumen
scalpel
   s. blade
   harmonic s.
   ultrasonic s.
scan
   bone s.
   colloid shift on liver-spleen s.
   CT s.
   dimercaptosuccinic acid
     renal s.
   dimethyl iminodiacetic acid s.
   DISIDA s.
   dual-energy CT s.
   esophageal transit s.
   gallbladder s.
   gallium s.
   gastric emptying s.
   gastroesophageal reflux s.
   GI bleeding s.
   hepatic blood pool s.
   hepatobiliary s.
   HIDA s.
   Hybritech PSA s.
   indium 64-labeled white blood
     cell s.
   indium leukocyte s.
   intercostal s.
   iodine s.
   isotope renal s.
   isotopic s.
   isotropic s.
   liver-spleen s.
   Meckel s.
   monoclonal antibody
     scintigraphic s.
   MRI s.
   nuclear bleeding s.
   nuclear isotope s.
   nuclear medicine s.
   peritoneovenous shunt
     patency s.
   PIPIDA s.
   radioisotope s.
   radionuclide s.
   renal s.
   rose bengal sodium ^{131}I
     biliary s.
   salivary gland s.
   SPECT s.
   sulfur colloid liver s.

tagged red blood cell
bleeding s.
^{99m}Tc-DMSA s.
^{99m}Tc-DTPA renal s.
TcHIDA s.
^{99m}Tc HMPAO-labeled
leukocyte s.
^{99m}Tc IDA s.
^{99m}Tc MDP nuclear isotope
bone s.
^{99m}Tc pertechnetate s.
^{99m}Tc RBC bleeding s.
^{99m}Tc sulfur colloid s.
technetium s.
technetium-labeled autologous
red blood cell s.
technetium-labeled red blood
cell s.
technetium-99m
diethylenetriamine pentaacetic
acid s.
technetium-99m IDA s.
technetium radionuclide s.
transabdominal s.
transrectal s.
transvesical s.
UJ13A nuclear isotope bone s.
ultrasound s.
scan-directed biopsy
scanner
Bruel-Kjaer s.
conventional static s.
high-resolution real-time s.
Kretz Combison 330
ultrasound s.
Kretz 311 ultrasound s.
linear convex array s.
Lunar DPX total-body s.
7.5 MHz sector s.
MKII automated s.
Tesla GE Signa whole
body s.
scanning
captopril-DTPA s.
s. electron microscope
s. electron microscopy
fluorescent gene s.

s. force microscopy (SFM)
iodine hippurate s.
radioisotope s.
transrectal ultrasound s.
(TRUS)
scaphoid abdomen
scar
Billroth II anastomotic s.
chest tube s.
episiotomy s.
s. formation
iridectomy s.
railroad track s.'s
sternotomy s.
thoracotomy s.
s. tissue reaction
Scardino
S. flap
S. vertical flap pyeloplasty
scarified duodenum
scarlatina rheumatica
scarlatiniform rash
Scarpa
S. fascia
S. triangle
scarring
gastrostomy s.
local s.
postdystrophic s.
postnecrotic s.
scatoma
scattered fluorescein
scattering
scavenger
free radical s.
hydroxyl radical s.
SCC
squamous cell carcinoma
S-CCK-Pz
secretin-cholecystokinin-
pancreatozymin
S-CCK-Pz stimulation
S-CCK-Pz test
SCD MaleFactor Pak
SCFA
short-chain fatty acid
Schatzki ring

NOTES

S

Schaumann body
Scheffe-F test
Schiff
   S. stain
   S. test
Schilling test
Schindler
   S. esophagoscope
   S. peritoneal forceps
   S. semiflexible gastroscope
Schistosoma
   S. haematobium
   S. mansoni
schistosomal liver disease
schistosomiasis
   Asiatic s.
   hepatic s.
   intestinal s.
   s. japonica, Japanese s.
   s. mansoni, Manson s.
   s. mekongi
   Oriental s.
Schmidt diet
Schneider stent
Schnidt
   S. gall duct forceps
   S. thoracic forceps
Schoemaker
   S. anastomosis
   S. gastroenterostomy
   S. procedure
Schoenberg intestinal forceps
Schuchardt relaxing incision
Schwann
   S. cell
   S. cell lipidosis
schwannian spindle cell
schwannoma
   penile s.
Schwartz
   S. method
   S. test
SCI
   spinal cord injury
sciatica
sciatic hernia
SCID
   severe combined immunodeficiency
scintigraph
scintigraphic
   s. balloon
   s. balloon topography

   s. diagnosis
   s. reflux
scintigraphy
   aberrations by s.
   adrenal s.
   dimercaptosuccinic acid s.
    (DMSA scintigraphy)
   direct vesicoureteral s. (DVS)
   DMSA s.
    dimercaptosuccinic acid
    scintigraphy
   gastroesophageal s.
   hepatobiliary s.
   OctreoScan s.
   OncoScint colorectal/ovarian
    carcinoma localization s.
    (OncoScint CR/OV)
   per-rectal portal s.
   quantitative hepatobiliary s.
    (QHS)
   radioisotope s.
   radionuclide s.
   renal gallium 67 s.
   ^{99m}Tc pertechnetate s.
   technetium-99m red cell s.
γ-scintillation camera
scintillation vial
scintiphotosplenoportography
scintiscan
   biliary s.
   false-positive s.
   gastroesophageal s.
scirrhous
   s. adenocarcinoma
   s. carcinoma
   s. lesion
scirrhousness
scissors
   Buie rectal s.
   Busch umbilical s.
   cold s.
   curved Mayo s.
   s. dissection
   dissection s.
   Doyen abdominal s.
   electrosurgical s.
   electrosurgical curved s.
   endoscopic s.
   hook s.
   insulated curved s.
   insulated straight s.
   Kelly fistula s.
   Mayo s.

meatotomy s.
Metzenbaum s.
Miller rectal s.
Nelson s.
Nu-Tip laparoscopic s.
Panzer gallbladder s.
Penn umbilical s.
Potts s.
Potts-Smith s.
Pratt s.
Pratt rectal s.
Snowden-Pencer s.
strabismus s.
Strulle s.
Super-cut s.
surgical s.
suture s.
Sweet esophageal s.
Thorek-Feldman gallbladder s.
Thorek gallbladder s.
umbilical s.
Vezien abdominal s.
Westcott s.
scissor-valve
Quinton single port s.-v.
Scivoletto test
sclera, pl. **sclerae**
anicteric s.
icteric s.
nonicteric s.
scleral icterus
scleroderma
s. bowel disease
esophageal s.
s. of esophagus
sclerohyaline wall
Scleromate
S. sclerosant
sclerosant
absolute alcohol s.
bucrylate s.
s. dosage
esophageal variceal s.
ethanolamine oleate s.
s. injection
Krazy Glue s.
latex s.

morrhuate s.
polidocanol s.
Scleromate s.
sodium tetradecyl sulfate s.
s. solution
Sotradecol s.
thrombin-Keflin-sotredochal s.
variceal s.
sclerose
sclerosing
s. adenosis
s. agent
s. cholangitis
s. hepatic carcinoma (SHC)
s. peritonitis
s. solution
s. therapy
sclerosis
alcohol s.
biliary s.
central hyaline s.
endoscopic s.
endoscopic injection s.
esophageal variceal s.
focal s.
gastric s.
hepatic s.
hepatoportal s.
injection s.
laser s.
multiple s.
nuclear s.
progressive systemic s. (PSS)
systemic s.
tuberous s.
variceal s.
sclerosus
lichen s.
sclerotherapist
sclerotherapy
s. complication
endoscopic s.
endoscopic injection s. (EIS)
endoscopic retrograde s.
endoscopic variceal s.
esophageal variceal s.
fiberoptic injection s. (FIS)

S

NOTES

sclerotherapy *(continued)*
    hemorrhoidal s.
    injection s.
    intravariceal s.
    low-volume s.
    s. needle
    paravariceal s.
    prophylactic s.
    ultra-low-volume s.
    variceal s.
sclerotic
    s. atrophy
    s. stomach
scolex, pl. **scoleces**
scoliosis
scoop
    Desjardins gallbladder s.
    Ferguson gallstone s.
    gallbladder s.
    Klebanoff gallstone s.
    malleable s.
    Mayo common duct s.
    Mayo gallstone s.
    Moore gallstone s.
    Moynihan gallstone s.
    rigid s.
scope
    baby s.
    retroflexed s.
    torquing of s.
Scopinaro pancreaticobiliary bypass
scopolamine
S-cord
Score
    International Prostate
      Symptom S. (IPSS)
score
    APACHE-II s.
    Baylor bleeding s.
    Beppu s.
    Boyarsky BPH symptom s.
    Child-Pugh s.
    fibrin s.
    Gleason s.
    hostility s.
    International Prognostic
      Index s.
    Karnofsky s.
    Knodell s.
    symptom s.
Scott
    S. AMS inflatable penile
    prosthesis

    S. jejunoileal bypass
    S. operation
    S. retractor
"scotty dog" graft
SCP
    squamous cell papilloma
SCr
    serum creatinine
sCR1
Scrapie protein
s-creatinine
screen
    ENA s.
screening
    cancer s.
    colon cancer s.
    colonoscopy s.
    s. cystometry
    endocrine s.
scrota (*pl. of* scrotum)
scrotal
    s. agenesis
    s. encroachment
    s. hernia
    s. mass
    s. pain
    s. pouch operation
    s. pouch orchiopexy
    s. tenderness
    s. violation
scrotectomy
    total s.
scroti
    elephantiasis s.
scrotitis
scrotocele
scrotoplasty
scrotoscopy
scrotum, pl. **scrota, scrotums**
    acute s.
    bifid s.
    lymph s.
    watering-can s.
scrub
    Betadine s.
    pHisoHex s.
Scudder
    S. intestinal clamp
    S. intestinal forceps
Scultetus position
scybalous
    s. stool
scybalum, pl. **scybala**

SDB
sleep-disordered breathing
SDH
sorbitol dehydrogenase
succinate dehydrogenase activity
SDH enzyme
SDS
sodium dodecyl sulfate
sea anemone ulcer
sea-blue histiocyte syndrome
seal
fibrin s.
Karaya 5 s.
Sears Wee Alert
sebaceum
adenoma s.
SEC
superficial esophageal carcinoma
secalin
secondary
s. achalasia
s. amyloidosis
s. bacterial peritonitis
s. biliary cirrhosis
s. biliary fibrosis
s. cholangitis
s. closure
s. contraction
s. incontinence
s. jejunal ulcer
s. megaureter
s. metastatic carcinoma
s. peristaltic wave
s. pseudo-obstruction syndrome
s. renal calculus
s. surgery
s. suture
s. syphilis
s. volvulus
second-generation
s.-g. enzyme immunoassay
(EIA-2)
s.-g. recombinant immunoblot
assay
second generation lithotriptor
second-line drug

second-look
s.-l. laparotomy
s.-l. operation
secosteroid hormone
secretagogue
luminal s.
secreted
regulated upon activation,
normal T cell expressed
and s. (RANTES)
secretin
s. provocation test
s. stimulation
s. stimulation test
secretin-CCK stimulation test
**secretin-cholecystokinin-
pancreatozymin (S-CCK-Pz)**
s.-c.-p. stimulation
Secretin-Ferring
**secretin-glucagon-vasoactive intestinal
peptide family**
**secretin-pancreozymin stimulation
test**
secretion
acid s.
basal s.
basal acid s.
biliary cholesterol s.
gastric s.
hydrochloric acid s.
idiopathic gastric acid s.
intrinsic factor s.
Leydig cell s.
macromolecular s.
meal-stimulated s.
meal-stimulated pancreatic s.
medication-associated
suppression of gastric s.
mucoid s.
pepsin s.
physiologic role in acid s.
renin s.
toxin-mediated intestinal s.
secretions
expressed prostatic s. (EPS)
secretory
s. coil

NOTES

secretory *(continued)*
  s. component (SC)
  s. diarrhea
  s. IgA (sIgA)
  s. immunoglobulin A
  s. product
  s. reflex
section
  abdominal s.
  distal shave s.
  frozen s.
  Giemsa-stained s.
  perineal s.
  permanent s.
  renal histologic s.'s
  ultrathin araldite s.
sectioning
  "thin shave" s.
sector
  7.5 MHz s. scanner
Sectral
sedation
  benzodiazepine conscious s.
  conscious s.
  meperidine conscious s.
  midazolam conscious s.
sedation-induced hypoventilation
sedative
  anxiolytic s.
sediment
  nephritic s.
  urinary s.
sedimentation
  Ficoll-Hypaque gradient s.
sedoanalgesia
seed
  iridium s.
  mustard s.
seeding
  instrument-tract s.
  malignant s.
  needle-tract s.
  peritoneal s.
  tumor s.
seg
  segmented neutrophil
sEGF
  salivary epidermal growth factor
segment
  Ask-Upmark renal s.
  demucosalized augmentation
  with gastric s. (DAWG)

ileocecal s.
vaterian s.
segmental
  s. appendicitis
  s. change
  s. colonic adenomatous
    polyposis syndrome
  s. colonic resection
  s. colonic tuberculosis
  s. enteritis
  s. glomerulosclerosis
  s. ischemic colitis
  s. liver graft
  s. testicular infarction
segmentary pancreatitis
segmentation movement
segmentectomy of liver
segmented neutrophil (seg)
Segura-Dretler laser basket
SeHCAT
  selenium-labeled homocholic acid
    conjugated with taurine
  SeHCAT test
Seidlitz powder
Seitzinger tripolar cutting forceps
seizure disorder
Sekomic SS-100F recorder
^{75}Se-labeled bile acid test
Seldinger
  S. cystic duct catheterization
  S. needle
  S. technique
selection
  patient s.
selective
  s. cannulation
  s. catheterization
  s. ductal cannulation
  s. intestinal decontamination
    (SID)
  s. left gastric arteriography
  s. mesenteric angiography
  s. proximal vagotomy (SPV)
  s. sacral rhizotomy
  s. targeting
selective endothelin A
selectivity
  charge s.
selenite
  insulin-transferrin-sodium s.
**selenium-labeled homocholic acid
  conjugated with taurine
  (SeHCAT)**

selenomethionine radioactive agent
self-antigen
self-bougienage
> s.-b. treatment

self-catheterization
self-expandable
> s.-e. metal stent
> s.-e. stainless steel braided
>   endoprosthesis

self-expanding
> s.-e. biliary metal stent
> s.-e. coil stent
> s.-e. metallic stent (SEMS)

self-induced
> s.-i. purging
> s.-i. vomiting

self-injection therapy
self-MHC
self-monitoring
> nocturnal tumescence s.-m.

self-obturation
> intermittent s.-o.

self-poisoning
self-retaining
> s.-r. catheter
> s.-r. coil stent
> s.-r. retractor
> s.-r. ring retractor

self-tightening slip knot
Seltzer
> Bromo S.

SELU
> seromuscular enterocystoplasty lined
>   with urothelium

semantic conditioning
Semb ligature carrier
semen
semielemental
> s. diet
> s. enteral feeding

semiellipsoid
semiflexible endoscope
semiformed stool
Semilente insulin
semilunar-shaped fold
seminal
> s. tract washout

s. vesical cyst
> s. vesicle
> s. vesicle aspiration

seminiferous
seminoma
> anaplastic s.
> testicular s.

seminomatous
semioblique position
semi-open hemorrhoidectomy
semipedunculated lesion
semiquantitative agglutination
> **SERA-TEK Ames**

semirigid
> s. endoscope
> s. fiber optic ureteroscope
> s. Nottingham introducer
> s. sigmoidoscope

semisolid stool
Semken tissue forceps
SEMS
> self-expanding metallic stent

senescent cell
Sengstaken-Blakemore (S-B)
> S.-B. esophageal balloon
> S.-B. method
> S.-B. tamponade
> S.-B. tube
> S.-B. tube insertion

senna
> extractum s.

Senn-Kanavel retractor
Senn retractor
Senokot-S
Senokot X-Prep
Sensa
> Hemoccult S.

sensation
> esophageal globus s.
> foreign body s.
> rectal s.
> S. Short Throw snare
> threshold of rectal s.

sensitive and specific ELISA
sensitivity
> anaphylactoid food s.
> culture and s. (C&S)

NOTES

sensitivity *(continued)*
    gluten s.
    interpersonal s.
    penile s.
    soy protein s.
sensor
    bladder pressure s.
    FiberOptic s.
    manometric s.
sensorium change
Sensor Medics pressure transducer
sensory
    s. finding
    s. loss
    s. neuron
    s. receptor
    s. urgency
sentinel
    s. clot
    s. fold
    s. hyperplastic polyp
    s. loop
    s. node
    s. pile
    s. tag
sentry system
separator
    Benson pylorus s.
Sephacryl S-300 HR gel
Sepharose
    S. 4B-coupled-protein-A column
    Protein A S.
sepsis
    anorectal s.
    biliary s.
    Gram-negative s.
    Gram-positive s.
    intra-abdominal s. (IAS)
    pancreatic s.
    post-rubber band s.
    staph s.
septa *(pl. of* septum)
septal hematoma
Septata intestinalis
septate vagina
septectomy
septic
    s. cholangitis
    s. shock
    s. wound
septicemia
Septisol
Septopal beads

Septra
    S. DS
septum, pl. septa
    deviated s.
    interhaustral s.
    pancreaticobiliary s.
    perforated nasal s.
    urethrovaginal s.
sequela, pl. sequelae
sequence
    adenoma-carcinoma s.
    adenomatous polyp-cancer s.
    contrast-enhanced fast s. (CE-FAST)
    dysplasia-to-carcinoma s.
    esophageal manometric s. (EMS)
    FLASH pulse s.
    genomic s.
    leucine zipper s.
    metaplasia-dysplasia-carcinoma s.
    papilloma-carcinoma s.
    phasic wave s.
sequence-sequence oligonucleotide hybridization
sequencing
    s. analysis
    molecular cloning and s.
sequential
    s. motility
    s. multiple analyzer (SMA)
    s. quadruple drug regimen
    s. video converter
sequestration
    fluid s.
sera *(pl. of* serum)
SERAFLO blood line
Serentil
serial
    s. cholangiogram
    s. dilutions
serial 7s
series
    Gastrografin GI s.
    motor meal barium GI s.
    upper GI s.
serine
    s. protease
    s. protease-activated prorenin
seroconversion
    s. rate

**Serodia (β HIV, β HTLV-1)
commercial kit**
seroepidemiological study
seroepidemiology
serologic
s. diagnosis
s. marker
s. test
serology
specific anti-Hp s.
seromuscular
s. colocystoplasty
s. enterocystoplasty lined with urothelium (SELU)
s. intestinal patch graft
s. layer
s. Lembert suture
seromyotomy
laparoscopic s.
seronegative polyarthritis
seroprevalence
s. rate
seroprotection
serosa
cecal s.
gastric s.
serosal
s. blood vessel
s. surface
s. tear
serosanguineous
s. drainage
s. fluid
serositis
uremic s.
serotonergic type 3 receptor
serotonin (5-HT)
s. antagonist
s. antagonist treatment
s. cell
serum s.
serotoninergic neuron
serous
s. diarrhea
s. membrane
Serpasil
Serpasil-Esidrix

serpiginous
s. microcystic duct
s. ulcer
s. ulceration
Serratia
S. liquefaciens
S. marcescens
serrefine clamp
Sertina
Sertoli
S. cell secretory function
S. cell tumor
Sertoli-cell-only syndrome
Sertoli-Leydig cell
serum, pl. sera
s. albumin
s. alpha$_1$-protease inhibitor
s. ammonia
s. amylase
s. amylase test
s. amyloid P (SAP)
s. amyloid P component
s. bile acid measurement
s. bilirubin
s. calcitonin
s. calcium concentration
calibrator s.
s. carotene
s. ceruloplasmin
s. cholesterol
s. cholinesterase activity
s. concentration
s. creatinine (SCr)
s. elastase 1
s. electrophoresis
familial nephritis s.
s. ferritin
fetal calf s.
s. gastrin
s. gastrin level
s. glutamic-oxaloacetic transaminase (SGOT)
s. glutamic-oxaloacetic transaminase (SGOT)
s. glutamic-pyruvic transaminase (SGPT)
s. γ-glutamyltransferase

NOTES

serum *(continued)*
   s. haptoglobin
   heat-inactivated fetal calf s.
   s. hepatitis
   s. interleukin-2
   s. interleukin-6
   s. iron test
   s. lipase
   s. marker
   s. nephritis
   s. noradrenaline
   s. PGI
   s. phospholipid
   s. protein
   s. protein test
   s. RIBA-2 test
   s. serotonin
   s. testosterone
   s. transferrin
   s. triglyceride
   s. uric acid
   s. virus antibody
serum-ascites albumin gradient (SAAG)
serum glutamic-pyruvic transaminase (SGPT)
Serutan
servo-mechanism sphincter
sessile
   s. adenoma
   endoscopic s.
   s. lesion
   s. nodular carcinoma
   s. polyp
set
   Coloplast ostomy irrigation s.
   Conseal ostomy irrigation s.
   Criticare HN-Isocal tube feeding s.
   Dansac ostomy irrigation s.
   dilating s.
   ELIMINATOR nasal biliary catheter s.
   Freiburg biopsy s.
   French introducer s.
   Heyer-Schulte Small-Carrion sizing s.
   Hulbert endo-electrode s.
   introducer s.
   Jeffrey introducer s.
   mandril s.
   over-the-wire s.

   s. point theory
   United Ostomy irrigation s.
   urology s.
Sethotope radioactive agent
seton
   s. management
   Penrose s.
   silk s.
Seton treatment of high anal fistula
setophobia
severance
   retroduodenal artery s.
severe
   s. combined immunodeficiency (SCID)
   s. erosive esophagitis
   s. gastritis
   s. macrovesicular steatosis
   s. pain
   s. reflux esophagitis
Severity
   Crohn Disease Endoscopic Index of S. (CDEIS)
sex
   s. hormone binding globulin (SHBG)
   phenotypic s.
sextant technique
sexual
   s. differentiation
   s. evaluation
   s. function
   s. rehabilitation
sexually
   s. related intestinal disease
   s. transmitted disease (STD)
Seyd-Neblett perineal template
SF
   sucrose-free
   Isomil SF
SF-9 baculovirus-insect cell system
SFM
   scanning force microscopy
Sgambati reaction test
SGOT
   serum glutamic-oxaloacetic transaminase
   SGOT test
SGP-2
   sulfated glycoprotein-2

SGPT
    serum glutamic-pyruvic
      transaminase
    SGPT test
SH2
    src-homology 2
SH2-binding domain
shadow
    dumbbell-shaped s.
    obliteration of psoas s.
    psoas s.
shadowing
    hyperechoic s.
shaft
    Eder-Puestow dilator s.
shaggy tumor
shaker
    Dubrof s.
sham
    s. feeding test
    s. injection
    s. surgery
Shambaugh fistula hook
shape
    s. memory alloy (SMA)
    s. memory alloy stent
shaped
    olive s.
Sharing
    United Network for Organ S.
      (UNOS)
shark
    s. fin papillotome
    s. tooth forceps
sharp
    s. dissection
    s. spoon
sharp-edged
    s.-e. orifice
    s.-e. tip
Sharpoint
    S. cutting instrument
    S. microsuture
shave biopsy
SHBG
    sex hormone binding globulin

SHC
    sclerosing hepatic carcinoma
sheath
    Amplatz s.
    anterior rectus s.
    fibrous s.
    nephroscope s.
    overtube s.
    peel-away s.
    perivascular s.
    posterior rectus s.
    quill s.
    rectus s.
    resectoscope s.
    retroflexed cystoscopy s.
    Teflon s.
    Universal s.
    uretero-renoscope procedure s.
    ureteroscope s.
    Waldeyer s.
    working s.
sheathed
    s. cytology brush
    s. flexible sigmoidoscope
shedding
    virus s.
sheet
    Dacron-impregnated Silastic s.
shelf
    Blumer rectal s.
    mesocolic s.
    rectal s.
shell vial culture
shelving edge of Poupart ligament
shepherd's hook catheter
shield
    Active Living incontinence s.
    Fuller rectal s.
    syringe s.
shift
    fluid s.
    mediastinal s.
shifting dullness
shiga-like toxin
Shigella
    S. colitis
    S. dysenteriae

NOTES

Shigella (continued)
    S. dysentery
    S. *flexneri*
    S. *sonnei*
shigelloides
    Plesiomonas s.
shigellosis
shim
    step-up s.
Shiner tube
Shirodkar cervical cerclage
shock
    hypovolemic s.
    s. liver
    s. number
    s. patient
    septic s.
    s. wave
    s. wave lithotripsy, s.-wave
      lithotripsy
    s. wave lithotriptor
    s. wave treatment
Shoemaker intestinal clamp
Shohl solution
short
    s. band stenosis
    s. incubation hepatitis
short-bowel syndrome
short-chain fatty acid (SCFA)
short-dwell hypertonic exchange
short-gut syndrome
short-segment lesion
shot
    flat low-angle s. (FLASH)
shotty lymph node
shoulder
    s. girdle
    s. shrug
Shouldice inguinal herniorrhaphy
shrapnel-induced
    s.-i. biliary obstruction
    s.-i. obstructive jaundice
shrug
    shoulder s.
shrunken liver
shunt
    Al-Ghorab modification s.
    angiographic portacaval s.
    arteriovenous s.
    AV shunt
    biliopancreatic s.
    Brescia-Cimino s.
    Buselmeier s.

    cavernospongiosum s.
    cerebral fluid s.
    congenital portacaval s.
    Cordis-Hakim s.
    Denver s.
    Denver peritoneovenous s.
    distal splenorenal s. (DSRS)
    Drapanas s.
    end-to-side portacaval s.
    esophageal s.
    extrahepatic s.
    gastric venacaval s.
    gastrorenal s.
    Gott s.
    Hashmat s.
    Hashmat-Waterhouse s.
    hepatofugal arterioportal s.
    hepatofugal porto-systemic
      venous s.
    Hyde s.
    s. index via the inferior
      mesenteric vein (SI-I)
    s. index via the superior
      mesenteric vein (SI-S)
    intrahepatic s.
    intrahepatic artery-systemic s.
    jejunoileal s.
    LeVeen ascites s.
    LeVeen peritoneal s.
    LeVeen peritoneovenous s.
    Linton s.
    mesocaval s.
    mesocaval H-graft s.
    mesocaval interposition s.
    pentose phosphate s.
    peritoneal-atrial s.
    peritoneocaval s.
    peritoneojugular s.
    peritoneovenous s. (PVS)
    portacaval s.
    portal-systemic s.
    portasystemic s.
    portopulmonary s.
    proximal splenorenal s.
    radiologic portacaval s.
    side-to-side s.
    small-bowel s.
    splenorenal s.
    splenorenal bypass s.
    transhepatic portacaval s.
    transjugular intrahepatic
      portosystemic s. (TIPS)

transjugular intrahepatic
portosystemic stent s. (TIPSS)
s. tubing
ventriculoperitoneal s.
vesicoamniotic s.
Warren splenorenal s.
Winter s.
shunting
arterioportal vein s. (APS)
intrapulmonary s.
portosystemic s. (PSS)
surgical portosystemic s.
shunt-like pore
Shwachman-Diamond syndrome
Shwachman syndrome
SI
saturation index
SI of bile
sialic acid residue
sialoadenectomy
sialoglycoprotein
sialomucin
sialorrhea
sialyl
s. Lewis A
s. Lewis A antigen
s. residue
sialylated
s. derivative
s. lacto-N-fucopentaose
sialylation
sibling
HLA-identical s.
SIBO
small intestinal bacterial overgrowth
sicca
cholera s.
s. syndrome
sicchasia
sickle
s. cell anemia
s. cell disease
sickling
erythrocyte s.
sickness
black s.
Indian s.

Jamaican vomiting s.
milk s.
motion s.
Sickness Impact profile
SID
selective intestinal decontamination
Side-Fire laser
sideropenic dysphagia
siderotic splenomegaly
side-to-side
s.-t.-s. anastomosis
s.-t.-s. shunt
side-viewing
s.-v. endoscope
s.-v. fiberoptic or video
duodenoscope
s.-v. fiberscope
sidewall
pelvic s.
Siegel-Cohen dilating catheter
Sielaff gastroscope
Siemens
S. Endo-P endodrectal
transducer
S. Lithostar
S. Lithostar Plus System C
lithotriptor
S. lithotriptor
S. MRI unit
S. Somatom DRH CT analyzer
S. Somatom DRH CT analyzer
unit
S. Sonoline ultrasonography
sieving
dextran s.
s. effect
s. function
Keller hydrodynamic hypothesis
of s.
s. of solid food
sIgA
secretory IgA
sigma
s. rectum pouch
s. type I
sigmoid
s. colon

S

NOTES

sigmoid *(continued)*
s. colon carcinoma
s. colon volvulus
s. curve
s. cystoplasty
s. disease
s. diverticulitis
s. diverticulum
s. enterocystoplasty
s. flexure
s. fold
s. loop
s. loop reduction
s. neobladder
s. rectum pouch
s. ulcer
s. volvulus
sigmoidectomy
sigmoid-end colostomy
sigmoid-loop rod colostomy
sigmoidocystoplasty
sigmoidopexy
endoscopic s.
sigmoidoscope
adult s.
American ACMI (S3565, TX-915) flexible fiberoptic s.
disposable sheathed flexible s.
fiberoptic s.
flexible s.
Fujinon s.
Fujinon PRO-PC flexible fiberoptic s.
Fujinon SIG-EK-series flexible fiberoptic s.
Fujinon SIG-E-series flexible fiberoptic s.
Fujinon SIG-ET-series flexible fiberoptic s.
Lloyd-Davis s.
Olympus CF-L-series flexible s.
Olympus CF-OSF-series flexible s.
Pentax FS-series flexible fiberoptic video s.
Reichert FLPS-series flexible fiberoptic s.
Reichert MH-series flexible fiberoptic s.
Reichert MS-series flexible fiberoptic s.

Reichert SC-series flexible fiberoptic s.
rigid s.
semirigid s.
sheathed flexible s.
Vision System s.
VSI 2000 s.
Welch Allyn flexible s.
sigmoidoscopy
fiberoptic s.
flexible s.
s. table
sigmoidotomy
sigmoidovesical fistula
sign
Aaron s.
Babinski s.
Ballance s.
barber pole s.
Battle s.
beading s.
blue dot s.
Blumberg s.
bowler hat s.
Boyce s.
Brudzinski s.
Carnett s.
chain-of-lakes s.
Chilaiditi s.
Christmas tree s.
Claybrook s.
cobblestoning s.
Cole s.
colon cut-off s.
comb-like redness s.
comet s.
Courvoisier s.
Cruveilhier s.
Cullen s.
cushion s.
double-bubble duodenal s.
double duct s.
Duroziez s.
Federici s.
flapping tremor s.
Fraley s.
Gilbert s.
Gowers s.
Grey Turner s.
Grocco s.
guarding s.
Guyon s.
Hampton s.

Henning s.
Horn s.
Howship-Romberg s.
iliopsoas s.
inverted-V s.
Kantor s.
Kehr s.
Kernig s.
Klemm s.
Lennhoff s.
s. of Leser-Trelal
Leser-Trelat s.
liver flap s.
lollipop tree s.
malignant meniscus s.
McBurney s.
McCormack gastric mucosal s.
McCort s.
meniscus s.
moulage s.
multiple concentric ring s.
Murphy s.
obturator s.
peritoneal s.
pillow s.
Prehn s.
pruning s.
pseudocholangiocarcinoma s.
pseudoparallel channel s.
psoas s.
puddle s.
pyloric string s.
rat-tail s.
RCS s.
rebound s.
red-color s. (RCS)
red ring s.
reversed Mercedes Benz s.
Rigler s.
Robertson s.
Rosenbach s.
Rovighi s.
Rovsing s.
sawtooth appearance s.
Sister Mary Joseph s.
snow-white duodenum s.
Stierlin s.

Stransky s.
Strauss s.
string s.
string of pearl s.
Sumner s.
Terry fingernail s.
tethered-bowel s.
thread and streaks s.
thumbprinting s.
Toma s.
Trimadeau s.
Troisier s.
Turner s.
vital s.
white nipple s.

signal
β-actin mRNA s.
s. transduction process
transmembrane s.

signal-to-cutoff ratio
signal-transduction pathway
signet-ring
s.-r. cell
s.-r. cell carcinoma

significance
visible vessel s.

SI-I
shunt index via the inferior
mesenteric vein

Silastic
S. catheter
S. collar-reinforced stoma
S. indwelling ureteral stent
S. ring
S. silo reduction of
gastroschisis
S. sling
S. stent

Silber technique
silent
s. abdomen
s. aspiration
s. auto-nephrectomy
s. gallstone
s. stone
s. thrombosis

NOTES

S

silicone
- s. donut prosthesis
- s. elastomer band
- s. elastomer ring
- s. elastomer ring vertical gastroplasty (SRVG) particulate s.
- s. pressure sensor device
- s. rubber Dacron-cuffed catheter
- s. sizer

silicone-coated
- s.-c. metallic self-expanding stent
- s.-c. stent

Silitek Uropass stent

silk
- s. ligature
- s. pop-off suture
- s. seton
- s. suture
- s. traction suture

Silon
- S. tent
- S. tent for gastroschisis

silver
- s. catheter
- s. cell
- s. clip
- s. probe
- s. stool

silver-coated stent
Silverman-Boeker needle
Silverman needle
SIM
  small intestine mesentery
Simeco
simethicone
  aluminum hydroxide, magnesium hydroxide, and s. calcium carbonate and s.
Similac PM 60/40 low-iron formula
Simplastic catheter
simple
- s. cold storage preservation
- s. mechanical obstruction

simplex
  exulceratio s.
  herpes s.
simplified nocturnal home hemodialysis (SNHHD)
Simpson endoscope

Sims
- S. position
- S. rectal speculum

simultaneous
- s. bilateral extracorporeal shock wave
- s. bilateral percutaneous nephrolithotomy (SBPN)
- s. pancreas-kidney (SPK)
- s. urethral cystometry
- s. waves

simvastatin
sincalide
Sinemet
sinensis
  Clonorchis s.
Sinequan
Singer-Blom endoscopic tracheoesophageal puncture technique
single
- s. β-actin mRNA species
- s. cell keratinization
- s. contrast radiography
- s. lens reflex (SLR)
- s. loop tourniquet
- s. lumen
- s. pigtail stent
- s. potential analysis of cavernous electrical
- s. potential analysis cavernous electrical activity (SPACE)
- s. stapling
- s. strand conformation polymorphism analysis

single-action pumping system (SAPS)
single-channel
- s.-c. in vivo light dosimeter
- s.-c. wire-guided sphincterotome

single-color direct immunofluorescence study
single-contrast barium enema
single-dose I.V. Timentin
single-drug therapy
single-fiber
- s.-f. EMG electrode
- s.-f. needle electromyography

single-lens reflex camera
single-nephron GFR
single-parameter
- s.-p. DNA
- s.-p. DNA analysis

single-photon emission computerized
  tomography (SPECT)
single-puncture laparoscopy
single-stage total proctocolectomy
single-stripe colitis (SSC)
Singley intestinal forceps
Singoserp
Singular Oval polypectomy snare
singultus
"sink-trap" malformation
sinoaortic
  s. baroreceptor
  s. denervation (SAD)
sinogram
sinography
  catheter s.
sinus
  anal s.
  s. bradycardia
  coronary s.
  perineal s.
  pilonidal s.
  pyriform s.
  renal s.
  Rokitansky-Aschoff s.
  subpubic s.
  s. tachycardia
  s. tenderness
  s. tract
  urachal s.
  urogenital s.
sinusoid
  erectile s.
  hepatic s.'s
  liver s.
sinusoidal
  s. capillary pressure
  s. endothelium
  s. endothelium cornucopia
  s. fibrosis
  s. lymphocyte
sinusoid-lining cell
siphonage
Sipple syndrome
Sippy
  S. diet
  S. esophageal dilator

SI-S
  shunt index via the superior
    mesenteric vein
Sister
  S. Mary Joseph nodule
  S. Mary Joseph lymph node
  S. Mary Joseph sign
site
  bleeding s.
  crypt-villus s.
  endoscopic biopsy s.
  entry s.
  estrogen binding s. (EBS)
  exit s.
  genomic s.
  injection s.
  internal ribosome entry s.
    (IRES)
  lymphoid aggregates at
    mucosal s.
  stoma s.
site-specificity
sitosterolemia
situ
  adenocarcinoma in s.
  carcinoma in s. (CIS)
  in s.
situs
  s. inversus
  s. inversus viscerum
sitz bath
Siurala classification
six-wire spiral tip Segura basket
size
  enlarged uterine s.
  inoculum s.
  large needle s.
  spot s.
  uterine s.
sizer
  silicone s.
Sjögren syndrome (SS)
SJS
  Stevens-Johnson syndrome
skatole
Skelaxin
skeletal muscle disease

S

NOTES

skeletonize
Skene duct
skin
  anicteric s.
  s. atrophy
  s. bleeding time (SBT)
  s. crease
  s. dimpling
  dry s.
  s. graft neovagina
  icteric s.
  jaundiced s.
  s. knife
  s. lines
  nonicteric s.
  ostomy s.
  peristomal s.
  s. staple
  s. stapling
  s. tag
  s. tube
  s. turgor
  s. xanthoma
skin-CNS-bladder reflex
skinfold thickness test
skinny
  s. Chiba needle
  s. needle
skinny-needle biopsy
skip
  s. area
  s. lesion
ski position
Skirrow
  S. agar plate
  S. medium
SL20
  Storz Modulith S.
SLA
  soluble liver antigen
SLC
  sodium-lithium countertransporter
SLE
  systemic lupus erythematosus
sleep apnea syndrome
sleep-disordered breathing (SDB)
sleeve
  s. advancement
  Dent s.
  ileal s.
  laparoscopic trocar s.
  s. technique

Watzki s.
Williams overtube s.
sleeve-type circumcision
slide
  gelatin-subbed s.
  guaiac-impregnated s.
  Hemoccult Sensa s.
  poly-L-lysine-coated glass s.
  s. system
slide-by view
sliding
  s. esophageal hiatal hernia
  s. filament model of
    contraction
  s. hiatal hernia
  s. tube
sling
  intestinal s.
  s. muscle fiber
  puboprostatic s.
  puborectalis s.
  pubourethral s.
  pubovaginal s.
  Raz 4-corner vaginal wall s.
  rectus fascial s.
  Silastic s.
  suburethral s.
"sling and blanket" technique
sling-ring complex
slipped
  s. Nissen fundoplication
  s. Nissen repair
slipper-tipped guidewire
slit
  Cheatle s.
  dorsal s.
  s. lamp
  s. pore length density
SLM-8000 fluorescence
  spectrophotometer
Slo-Bid
slotted
  s. anoscope
  s. instrument
  s. nerve clamp
  s. speculum
sloughed papilla
sloughing of mucosa
slow
  s. bilirubin glucuronidation
    phenotype
  s. colonic transit
  S. Fe

s. phasic contraction
s. transit constipation
s. twitch striated muscle fiber
s. wave
Slow-K
slow-twitch oxidative
SLR
single lens reflex
SLT contact MTRL laser
sludge
biliary s.
gallbladder s.
slurry of stool
slush
ice s.
saline s.
SMA
sequential multiple analyzer
shape memory alloy
smooth muscle antibody
SMA formula
SMA spiral stent
small
s. bowel
s. bowel enteroscopy (SBE)
s. dissecting sponge
s. granule cell
s. intestinal bacterial
overgrowth (SIBO)
s. intestinal Crohn disease
s. intestinal infarction
s. intestinal membrane
s. intestinal stenosis
s. intestinal ulcer
s. intestinal villus
s. intestine
s. intestine leiomyosarcoma
s. intestine mesentery (SIM)
s. intestine trauma
s. noncleaved-cell lymphoma
s. polyp removal
small-bowel
s.-b. biopsy
s.-b. enema
s.-b. enteroclysis
s.-b. follow-through (SBFT)
s.-b. infarct

s.-b. meal
s.-b. obstruction (SBO)
s.-b. shunt
s.-b. tube
Small-Carrion penile prosthesis
small-cell tumor
small-diameter endosonographic
instrument
small-droplet fatty liver
smaller gauge needle
SmallHand polpypectomy snare
small-stomach syndrome
SMA-portogram
SMART
sperm micro-aspiration retrieval
technique
SMAS
superior mesenteric artery syndrome
Smead-Jones closure
smear
KOH s.
Pap s.
potassium hydroxide s.
smegma
smegmatis
smelling
foul s.
"smiley face" knotting technique
smiling incision
Smith
S. method of silver staining
S. rectal retractor
S. ring
S. test
Smith-Boyce operation
Smith-Buie rectal retractor
Smith-Hodge pessary
smithii
Methanobrevibacter s.
Smith-Lemli-Opitz syndrome
smoker's
s. palate
s. tongue
smooth
s. diet
s. muscle
s. muscle antibody (SMA)

S

NOTES

smooth *(continued)*
   s. muscle isoform actin
   s. muscle motilin receptor
   s. muscle relaxant
   s. tissue forceps
smooth-muscle immunological study
SMV
   superior mesenteric vein
   SMV thrombosis
SMX/TMP
   sulfamethoxazole and trimethoprim
snail-headed catheter retriever
snake-skin mucosal pattern
snap
   s. gauge
   s. gauge band
   s. gauge test
snap-frozen biopsy
Snap-Gauge
Snap-It lubricating jelly
snare
   Captiflex polypectomy s.
   Captivator polypectomy s.
   s. cautery
   coaxial s.
   colorectal s.
   crescent s.
   diathermal s.
   Douglas rectal s.
   s. electrocoagulation
   electrosurgical s.
   endoscopic s.
   s. excision biopsy
   Frankfeldt rectal s.
   hexagon s.
   incarcerated s.
   lasso s.
   long-nose retriever s.
   s. loop biopsy
   Norwood rectal s.
   open electrocautery s.
   oval s.
   polypectomy s.
   Profile pediatric
     polypectomy s.
   rectal s.
   Sensation Short Throw s.
   Singular Oval polypectomy s.
   SmallHand polpypectomy s.
   standard endoscopy
     polypectomy s.
   UroSnare cystoscopic tumor s.

   Weston rectal s.
   wire s.
SNHHD
   simplified nocturnal home
   hemodialysis
Snowden-Pencer scissors
Snow procedure
snow-white duodenum sign
SNP
   sodium nitroprusside
SNS
   sympathetic nervous system
SO
   sphincter of Oddi
soak
   perianal s.
soapsuds enema (SSE)
Soave
   S. endorectal pull-through
   S. operation
sobria
   Aeromonas s.
Society of American Gastrointestinal
  Endoscoping Surgeons (SAGES)
sock
   polytetrafluoroethylene s.
SOD
   sphincter of Oddi dysfunction
   superoxide dismutase
Soda
sodium
   acyclovir s.
   s. azide
   s. balance
   s. bicarbonate
   brequinar s.
   s. butyrate concentration
   cefazolin s.
   ceftriaxone s.
   s. chloride
   s. citrate
   s. citrate and potassium citrate
     mixture
   s. cromoglycate
   dantrolene s.
   s. deoxycholate
   s. diatrizoate with Menoquinon
   diclofenac s.
   docusate s.
   s. dodecylsulfate
   s. dodecyl sulfate (SDS)
   s. electrolyte
   epoprostenol s.

estramustine phosphate s.
s. exchange
s. fluorescein (NaF)
s. flux
fractional excretion of s.
(FENa)
s. homeostasis
s. iodipamide
s. iodipamide contrast medium
s. iothalamate
low s. (LNa)
s. meclofenamate
s. meclofenamate-induced
esophageal ulcer
mesalamine s.
s. methylglucamine diatrizoate
s. morrhuate
s. morrhuate injection
naproxen s.
s. nitroprusside (SNP)
olsalazine s.
oxychlorosene s.
pentosan polysulfate s.
s. phosphate
s. phosphate-based laxative
(NaP)
s. picosulfate
s. pump
renal s.
s. restriction
s. retention
subactam s.
s. taurocholate
s. tauroglycocholate
s. tetradecyl injection
s. tetradecyl sulfate
s. tetradecyl sulfate sclerosant
s. transport
tyropanoate s.
sodium-linked process
sodium-lithium countertransporter
(SLC)
Soehendra
S. catheter dilator
S. catheter system
S. dilating catheter

S. stent extractor
S. stent retrieval device
soft
s. abdomen
s. bland diet
s. diet
s. food dysphagia
S. Guard XL Skin Barrier
Modane S.
s. stool
s. tissue
s. tissue mass
s. tissue stranding
s. x-ray film
softener
stool s.
SofTouch vacuum erection device
soft-tipped wire guide
software
CODAS s.
Cytologic s.
Medtrax urology s.
t-EASE s.
soilage
peritoneal s.
soiling
colostomy s.
solar fever
Solcia classification
solder
laser tissue welding s.
solid
s. bolus challenge
s. egg white meal
s. emptying
s. food
s. food digestion
s. food dysphagia
s. sphere test
s. tumor
solid-phase
s.-p. extraction chromatography
s.-p. radioimmunoassay
solid-state
s.-s. esophageal manometry
catheter
s.-s. pressure transducer

S

NOTES

solitarius
    nucleus tractus s.
solitary
    s. hepatic cyst
    s. kidney
    s. rectal ulcer syndrome
      (SRUS)
    s. testis
    s. ulcer
    s. ulcer syndrome
solium
    Taenia s.
SoloPass Percuflex biliary stent
SOLO-Surg Colo-Rectal self-
  retaining retractor system
solubility
solubilization
Solu-Biloptin
    S.-B. contrast medium
soluble liver antigen (SLA)
soluble recombinant complement
  receptor 1
Solu-Medrol
    pulsed S.-M.
solute
    s. equilibrium
    s. transport
solution
    AIO parenteral s.
    amino acid-based dialysate s.
    Aminofusin L Forte amino
      acid s.
    BA-EDTA s.
    balanced electrolyte s.
    Balance lavage s.
    Belzer s.
    Belzer UW liver
      preservation s.
    bile acid-EDTA solution
    Block-Ace s.
    Bouin s.
    Bouin fixative s.
    Bretschneider histidine
      tryptophan s.
    buffer s.
    Cidex activated dialdehyde s.
    Cidex Plus s.
    Collins s.
    Collins indigo carmine s.
    Collins intracellular
      electrolyte s.
    colonic lavage s.
    commercial dialysis s. (CDS)

Delflex peritoneal dialysis s.
Denhardt s.
3,3-diaminobenzidine
  tetrahydrochloride s. (DAB)
diphosphate buffer s.
Domeboro s.
Earle s.
electrolyte flush s.
electrolyte-polyethylene glycol
  lavage s.
Euro-Collins s.
formaldehyde s.
FreAmine amino acid s.
Gastrolyte oral s.
gelatine Hank buffered s.
  (GHBSS)
GoLYTELY s.
Hank balanced salt s. (HBSS)
Hank buffer s.
HepatAmine amino acid s.
HEPES s.
Hollande s.
HSE s.
s. hybridization RNAse
  protection assay
hypertonic saline-epinephrine s.
  (HSE)
iced lactated Ringer s.
inulin s.
Krebs s.
Krebs-Ringer s.
lactated Ringer s.
lavage s.
Liposyn II fat emulsion s.
Lugol iodine s.
Lytren electrolyte s.
Mayer-hematoxylin s.
Mefoxin-saline s.
900 mOsmolar amino acid-
  glucose s. (P-900)
mucolytic-antifoam s.
normal saline s.
Pedialyte RS electrolyte s.
perfusate s.
phosphate buffered saline s.
physiologic salt s. (PSS)
podofilox s.
polyethylene glycol
  electrolyte s.
polyethylene glycol electrolyte
  lavage s. (PEG-ELS)
probenecid-containing s.
rehydrating s. (RS)

Resol electrolyte s.
Saccomanno s.
Sachs s.
sclerosant s.
sclerosing s.
Shohl s.
Soyalac fat emulsion s.
Suby G s.
Synthamin amino acid s.
taurocholate s.
Tolerex feeding s.
Travamulsion fat emulsion s.
University of Wisconsin s.
UW s.
Vamin amino acid s.
warm saline s.
whole-gut lavage s.
Y-type Dianeal peritoneal
    dialysis s.
solution-diluted India ink
Solutrast 300 contrast
Soluvite
solvent
s. infusion
stone s.
SOM
somatostatin
sphincter of Oddi manometry
Soma
somatic
s. allelic deletion
s. growth
s. pain
s. teniasis
somatization
somatointestinal reflex
somatomedin C
Somatome DRG CT technique
somatostatin (SOM, SS)
s. analog octreotide
s. analogue therapy
antral s.
s. cell
s. infusion therapy
^{125}I-Tyr1-s.
s. mRNA-D-cell density ratio
s. mRNA level

s. peptide
s. prevention
s. receptor (SSR)
s. therapy
somatostatin-14
somatostatin-28
somatostatinoma
s. syndrome
somatropin injection
Somogyi
S. unit
S. units to measure amylase
sonde enteroscope
Sonicath endoluminal ultrasound
    catheter
Sonne dysentery
sonnei
Shigella s.
Sonnenberg classification
Sonoblate ablation device
Sonocath ultrasound probe
sonoelasticity imaging
sonogram
fatty meal s. (FMS)
transverse s.
sonographic
s. gallstone pattern
s. pattern
sonography
colonic transabdominal s.
    (CTAS)
color-coded Doppler s.
color-coded duplex s.
3-D s.
endoureteral ultrasound s.
gray scale s.
high frequency s.
high resolution endoluminal s.
    (HRES)
renal s.
transabdominal hydrocolonic s.
transrectal s.
sonography-guided aspiration
sonoguided biopsy
Sonoline SI-200/250 ultrasound
    imaging system

S

NOTES

Sonotrode
    S. channel
    S. lithotriptor
sono-urethrography
Sony Promavica still capture device
SOP
    sphincter of Oddi pressure
sorbitol
    s. dehydrogenase (SDH)
sore
    canker s.
    pressure s.
Soreson pressure transducer
sorter
    fluorescence-activated cell s.
      (FACS, FACScan)
SOS
    Surgitek One-Step
soterenol
Sotradecol
    S. sclerosant
sound
    absent bowel s.'s
    active bowel s.'s
    apical s.
    auscultation of bowel s.'s
    auscultatory s.
    Béniqué s.
    bowel s.'s
    breath s.
    bronchial s.
    Campbell s.
    common duct s.
    crescendoing bowel s.
    Davis interlocking s.
    diminished bowel s.'s
    distant heart s.
    esophageal s.
    extra heart s.
    Greenwald s.
    gurgling bowel s.'s
    high-pitched bowel s.'s
    hyperactive bowel s.'s
    hypoactive bowel s.'s
    Jewett s.
    Klebanoff common duct s.
    Le Fort s.
    low-pitched bowel s.'s
    McCrea s.
    musical bowel s.'s
    normoactive bowel s.'s
      (NABS)
    positive bowel s.'s

    quiet bowel s.'s
    rumbling bowel s.'s
    succussion s.
    tinkling bowel s.'s
    Van Buren s.
    Walther s.
sour
    s. brash
    s. stomach
source
    discrete bleeding s.
    endoscopic light s.
    xenon light s.
Southern
    S. blot
    S. blot analysis
    S. blot hybridization
Souttar tube
soya-induced enteropathy
Soyalac
    S. fat emulsion solution
    S. formula
soy-based formula
soy protein sensitivity
SP
    substance P
S/P
    status post
SPACE
    single potential analysis cavernous
    electrical activity
space
    anorectal s.
    Bogros s.
    Bowman s.
    dead s.
    deep postanal anorectal s.
    s. of Disse
    Disse s.
    extravascular s.
    intercellular s.
    intercostal s.
    intersphincteric s.
    intersphincteric anorectal s.
    ischiorectal s.
    ischiorectal anorectal s.
    Kiernan s.
    Lesgaft s.
    perianal s.
    perianal anorectal s.
    perisinusoidal s.
    peritoneal s.
    preperitoneal s.

presacral s.
retroperitoneal s.
s. of Retzius
Retzius s.
right anterior pararenal s.
subhepatic s.
subperitoneal s.
subphrenic s.
subumbilical s.
suprahepatic s.
supralevator s.
supralevator anorectal s.
supraomental s.
Traube semilunar s.

space-occupying
    s.-o. disease
    s.-o. lesion

span
    hepatic s.
    levator s.
    liver s.

spansule
Sparine
sparing
    rectal s.

spark-gap shock wave generator
sparteine
spasm
    acid-provoked s.
    cervical s.
    cricopharyngeal s.
    diffuse esophageal s. (DES)
    esophageal s.
    fecal paradoxical
      puborectalis s.
    muscle s.

spasmodic stricture
Spasmolin
spasmolytic
Spasmophen
spastic
    s. bowel syndrome
    s. colon
    s. constipation
    s. esophagus
    s. gait
    s. ileus

s. motor disorder
s. paraparesis
s. pelvic floor syndrome

spatial change
spatula
    Davis s.
    electrosurgical s.
    Haberer abdominal s.
    Pucci-Seed s.
    Reverdin abdominal s.
    s. tip laparoscopic electrode
    Tuffier abdominal s.

spatulation
    graft s.
    ureteral s.

Spearman
    S. rank
    S. rank correlation
    S. test

specialized columnar epithelium
species
    gastrin mRNA s.
    G3PDH mRNA s.
    reactive oxygen s. (ROS)
    single β-actin mRNA s.

species
    Cryptosporidium s.
    Cunninghamella s.
    Cyclospora s.
    Microsporium s.
    Rhizopus s.
    Vibrionaceae s.

specific
    s. activity
    antigen s.
    s. anti-Hp serology
    s. gastritis
    s. oligonucleotide

specificity
specimen
    cytologic s.
    intraurethral swab s.
    paraffin-embedded s.
    yarn-collected s.

speck
    hemorrhagic s.

S

NOTES

SPECT
single-photon emission computerized
tomography
SPECT scan
spectinomycin
spectometry
time-of-flight mass s.
(TOFMS)
spectral
s. analysis
s. broadening
Spectramed transducer
spectrometer
liquid scintillation s.
spectrometry
gas isotope ratio mass s.
spectrophotometer
atomic absorbance s.
Genetics Systems microplate
reader s.
Hitachi F-2000 fluorescence s.
Model IL 750, AA s.
Perkin-Elmer model 5000
atomic absorption s.
reflectance s.
SLM-8000 fluorescence s.
spectrophotometric analysis
spectrophotometry
endoscopic reflectance s.
reflectance s.
spectroscopy
Fourier transform infrared s.
(FTIR)
gas chromatography/mass s.
(GC/MS)
infrared s.
magnetic resonance s.
Model 3-60 mass s.
phosphorous-31 magnetic
resonance s.
speculum
Barr rectal s.
Barr-Shuford rectal s.
beveled s.
Bodenhammer rectal s.
Brinkerhoff rectal s.
Chelsea-Eaton anal s.
Cook rectal s.
Czerny rectal s.
David rectal s.
Hinkle-James rectal s.
Hirschmann s.
Kelly rectal s.

Killian rectal s.
Martin-Davis rectal s.
Mathews rectal s.
Pennington rectal s.
Pratt s.
Pratt rectal s.
rectal s.
Sawyer rectal s.
Sims rectal s.
slotted s.
Vernon-David rectal s.
speech
garbled s.
speedbander
multishot s.
Speed Lok soft stent
Spence procedure
Spencer disease
Spenco padding
sperm
s. aspiration
s. cryopreservation
extracted ductal s.
s. immunobead coincubation
s. micro-aspiration retrieval
technique (SMART)
microsurgical extraction of
ductal s. (MEDS)
s. yield
spermatic
s. cord
s. cord torsion
s. fistula
s. vein ligation
s. vesicle
spermatocele
spermatocelectomy
spermatocyst
spermatogenic arrest
spermatogonia
spermatogram
spermatorrhea
spermatozoa
acrosome-reacted s.
disordered acrosome reaction
of s.
spermicidal jelly
spermicide
sperm-immunobead binding
spermine
s. NONOate
polyamine s.
spermolith

spheroplast
mycobacterial s.
sphincter
AMS 700-series double-cuff
Silastic artificial urinary s.
AMS 800-series double-cuff
Silastic artificial urinary s.
anal s.
anal ileostomy with
preservation of s.
anorectal s.
artificial s.
artificial urinary s.
s. atony
biliary s.
Boyden s.
cardiac s.
cardioesophageal s.
choledochal s.
s. contraction ring
cricopharyngeal s.
double-cuff urinary s.
s. dysfunction
s. EMG
esophageal s.
external anal s. (EAS)
external rectal s.
s. function
gastroesophageal s.
Giordano s.
Hydroflex s.
hypertensive lower
esophageal s.
Hyrtl s.
ileocecal s.
incompetent s.
inguinal s.
internal s.
internal anal s. (IAS)
internal rectal s.
intrinsic striated s.
lower esophageal s. (LES)
Lütkens s.
Nélaton s.
neo-anal s.
O'Beirne s.
s. of Oddi (SO)

s. of Oddi dysfunction (SOD)
s. of Oddi homogenate
s. of Oddi manometry (SOM)
s. of Oddi pressure (SOP)
pancreatic duct s.
pancreaticobiliary s.
pharyngoesophageal s.
prepyloric s.
pyloric s.
s. reaction
s. reconstruction
rectal s.
s. repair
Santorini s.
servo-mechanism s.
stomach s.
striated s.
threshold of internal s.
s. tone
upper esophageal s. (UES)
Wirsung s.
sphincteral achalasia
sphincterectomy
endoscopic s.
sphincteric
s. construction
s. disobedience syndrome
s. mechanism
s. squeeze
sphincteroplasty
pancreatic s.
transduodenal s.
sphincterotome
bipolar s.
Bitome bipolar s.
Cotton s.
Demling-Classen s.
double-channel s.
ERCP s.
Fluorotome double-lumen s.
kneedle-knife s.
long-nosed s.
needle-knife s.
needle-tipped s.
Olympus s.
open s.
precut s.

NOTES

S

sphincterotome *(continued)*
   reverse s.
   rotating s.
   single-channel wire-guided s.
   Ultratome double lumen s.
   Ultratome XL triple-lumen s.
   Wilson-Cook double-channel s.
   wire-guided s.
sphincterotomy
   s. basket
   biliary s.
   Doubilet s.
   endoscopic s. (ES)
   endoscopic pancreatic duct s.
   Erlangen pull-type s.
   external s.
   Geenen s.
   internal s.
   Mulholland s.
   needle-knife s.
   pancreatic duct s.
   Parks partial s.
   retrograde s.
   s. stenosis
   transduodenal s.
   transendoscopic s.
   transurethral s.
   urethral s.
sphingomyelin
spiculations on colon
spicule
   bony s.
spicules in profile
spider
   s. angioma
   arterial s.
   colonic arterial s.
   s. nevus
   s. telangiectasia
spigelian hernia
spike
   s. burst on electromyogram of colon
   s. potential
spike-burst electrical activity
spiking fever
spillage
   fecal s.
   tumor s.
   s. of tumor cells
spina bifida
spinach stool

spinal
   s. cord compression
   s. cord injury (SCI)
   s. cord necrosis
   s. dysraphism
   s. fluid finding
   s. hemangioblastoma
spindle
   s. cell
   s. colonic groove
Spinelli biopsy needle
spinobulbar-spinal micturition reflex
spinous
   s. aspect
   s. process
   s. tenderness
spiral
   s. bacterium
   s. CT
   s. CT technique
   intraprostatic s.
   s. tip catheter
   s. valve
spiralis
   Trichinella s.
spirillar dysentery
spirochetal dysentery
spirochete
   intestinal s.
spirochetosis
spirometry
   incentive s.
Spironazide
spironolactone
   hydrochlorothiazide and s.
Spirozide
Spivack valve
SPK
   simultaneous pancreas-kidney
   SPK transplantation
splanchnectopia
splanchnemphraxis
splanchnic
   s. AV fistula
   s. blood flow
   s. capillary pressure
   s. hyperemia
   s. nerve
   s. primary afferent
   s. vasoconstriction
   s. vein
splanchnicectomy
   chemical s.

splanchnicus
    Bacteroides s.
splanchnocele
splanchnodiastasis
splanchnolith
splanchnopathy
splanchnoptosis, splanchnoptosia
splanchnotomy
splanchnotribe
splash
    succussion s.
S-plasty
spleen
    s. index
    murine s.
    s. tip
splenalgia
splenectomy
    incidental s.
splenic
    s. abscess
    s. agenesis syndrome
    s. angiogram
    s. anlage
    s. arterial embolization
    s. artery
    s. atrophy
    s. AV fistula
    s. avulsion
    s. capillary hemangiomatosis
    s. capsule
    s. dullness
    s. flexure
    s. flexure carcinoma
    s. flexure colonoscopy
    s. flexure syndrome
    s. function
    s. hilum
    s. injury
    s. notch
    s. penetration
    s. pulp
    s. rupture
    s. tissue
    s. trauma
    s. vein
    s. vein obstruction (SVO)

    s. vein thrombosis
    s. venous blood flow
splenobronchial fistula
splenocolic ligament
splenodynia
splenogastric omentum
splenography
splenomegaly, splenomegalia
    congenital s.
    congestive s.
    Egyptian s.
    fibrocongestive s.
    Gaucher s.
    hemolytic s.
    infectious s.
    infective s.
    myelophthisic s.
    siderotic s.
    spodogenous s.
    tropical s.
splenopancreatic ligament
splenopathy
splenoportal hypertension
splenoportography
splenorenal
    s. angle
    s. bypass
    s. bypass shunt
    s. ligament
    s. recess
    s. shunt
    s. venous anastomosis
splenorrhaphy
splenosis
splice-cite mutation
splicing
    alternate mRNA s.
splinting of abdomen
split
    s. cuff nipple technique
    s. ileostomy
    s. overtube
    s. renal function
    s. renal function test
    s. and roll technique
    s. sheath introducer
split-beam coupler for TURP

S

NOTES

split-liver transplant
splitter
    Syn-Optics video image s.
split-thickness skin graft
SPN
    support parenteral nutrition
spodogenous splenomegaly
spondylitis
    ankylosing s.
sponge
    absorbable s.
    absorbable gelatin s.
    cherry s.
    s. count
    s. dissector
    Endozime s.
    fibrin s.
    s. forceps
    gauze s.
    gelatin s.
    Ivalon s.
    laparotomy s.
    Lapwall laparotomy s.
    peanut s.
    polyvinyl alcohol s.
    Prosthex s.
    saline-moistened s.
    small dissecting s.
    s. stick
    Weck-cel s.
Spongel
spongiofibrosis
spongioplasty
spongiosa
spongiosal
spongiosi
    tunica albuginea corporis s.
spongiositis
spontaneous
    s. ascites filtration
    s. bacterial peritonitis (SBP)
    s. cystometry
    s. cyst reabsorption
    s. dialytic ultrafiltration
    s. dissection
    s. partial elimination
    s. passage
    s. penile ischemic necrosis
    s. regression
    s. rupture
spoon
    s. forceps
    gall duct s.

Mayo common duct s.
    s. retractor
    sharp s.
    s. tip laparoscopic electrode
    Volkmann pancreatic
        calculus s.
Sporacidin disinfectant
sporadic visceral myopathy
sporazoites
spore
    fungal s.
sporocyst
sporotrinichosis
sporulation
    coccidian s.
spot
    central s.
    cherry-red s. (CRS)
    cold s.
    cotton-wool s.
    DeMorgan s.
    epigastric s.
    Fordyce s.
    gastric red s.
    hematocystic s. (HCS)
    hot s.
    hyperechoic s.
    Koplik s.
    mongolian s.
    s. size
spout
    ileal s.
SPP
    stannous pyrophosphate
    ^{99m}Tc SPP
Spratt curette
spray
    DDAVP nasal s.
spray-fixed
spraying
    dye s.
spreader
    meatal s.
    pyloric s.
spreading fistulation
spring
    s. loaded type biopsy
        instrument
    s. wire coil
spring-loaded biopsy gun
spring-wire retractor
Sprinz-Dubin syndrome
Sprinz-Nelson syndrome

sprue
    celiac s.
    collagenous s.
    nontropical s.
    subclinical s.
    tropical s.
SPT
    station pull-through
    SPT technique
spuria
    hemospermia s.
spurting blood
sputum, pl. **sputa**
    s. aerogenosum
    green s.
SPV
    selective proximal vagotomy
SQMP
    subcutaneous morphine pump
squamocolumnar mucosal junction
squamous
    s. cell
    s. cell cancer
    s. cell carcinoma (SCC)
    s. cell papilloma (SCP)
    s. epithelium
squeeze
    hot s.
    phasic fluctuation on s.
    s. pressure
    s. pressure profile of anal
      sphincter test
    sphincteric s.
src-homology 2 (SH2)
src-homology 2 domain
src phosphorylation
SRH
    stigmata of recent hemorrhage
SRUS
    solitary rectal ulcer syndrome
SRVG
    silicone elastomer ring vertical
      gastroplasty
SS
    Sjögren syndrome
    somatostatin
    Uroplus SS

Ssabanejew-Frank gastrostomy
SSC
    single-stripe colitis
SSE
    soapsuds enema
SSE2-L electrosurgical unit
S-shaped
    S.-s. body
    S.-s. ileal pouch-anal
      anastomosis
    S.-s. pouch
    S.-s. reservoir
SSI
    symptom severity index
SSR
    somatostatin receptor
stab
    s. incision
    s. wound
stability
    detrusor s.
    structural s.
stabilizer
stable face
stab-wound drain
staccato voiding
stack of coins appearance
Stadol
stage
    s. B carcinoma
    s. C2
    s. C carcinoma
    Dukes s.
    Hoehn and Yahr s.
    s. III papillary serous
      cystadenocarcinoma
    morphologic s.
    post-TNM s. (I, II, III, IV)
    Tanner s.
staged orchiopexy
stage-specific embryonic antigen
staghorn
    s. calculus
    s. stone
staging
    Ann Arbor cancer s.
    Boden-Gibb tumor s.

S

NOTES

staging *(continued)*
 s. of cancer
 clinicopathologic s.
 neoplasm s.
 s. operation
 operative s.
 primary gastric lymphoma s.
 Stanford s.
 TNM system for tumor s.
 transrectal s.
 transrectal ultrasound s.
 tumor s.
stagnant
 s. bile
 s. loop syndrome
 s. syndrome
stain
 19A2 s.
 acid-Schiff s.
 Alcian blue s.
 anti-Schiff s.
 argentaffin s.
 azan s.
 Bryan-Leishman s.
 Congo red s.
 Diff-Quik s.
 eosin s.
 esterase s.
 Fite s.
 Fontana-Masson s.
 Genta s.
 Giemsa s.
 Glaxo s.
 Gram s.
 Grimelius silver s.
 Grocott methenamine silver s.
 Hale colloidal iron s.
 Hansel s.
 H&E s.
 hematoxylin s.
 hematoxylin and eosin s.
 immunocytochemical s.
 immunohistochemical s.
 immunoperoxidase s.
 indigo carmine s.
 Jones s.
 Kossa s.
 lead citrate s.
 Lendrum s.
 Lugol solution s.
 Mallory-Azan s.
 Martius scarlet blue s.
 Masson trichrome s.

 Mayer acid alum
  hematoxylin s.
 May-Grünwald-Giemsa s.
 methylene blue s.
 NADPH diaphorase s.
 oil red O s.
 Orcein s.
 Papanicolaou s.
 PAS s.
 periodic acid-Schiff s.
 periodic acid Schiff-Alcian
  blue combination s. (PAS-
  AB)
 Perls s.
 peroxidase s.
 rhodamine s.
 RP3 s.
 saffron s.
 Schiff s.
 S-100 immunohistochemical s.
 Steiner s.
 Sudan black B fat s.
 sulfated mucin s.
 toluidine blue s.
 trichrome s.
 uranyl acetate s.
 van Gieson s.
 von Kossa s.
 Warthin-Starry silver s.
 Wright s.
 Wright-Giemsa s.
 Ziehl-Neelsen s.
staining
 Berlin blue s.
 cytokeratin s.
 ethidium bromide s.
 Feulgen s.
 Grimelius s.
 immunohistochemical s.
 immunoperoxidase s.
 lectin s.
 MIB-1 s.
 p53 nuclear s.
 Smith method of silver s.
 Steiner modification of
  Warthin-Starry s.
 vimentin s.
 vital s.
stainless steel suture
stairstep air/fluid levels
stalk
 polyp s.

Stamey
- S. colosuspension
- S. dorsal vein apical retractor
- S. Malecot catheter
- S. needle suspension
- S. open tip ureteral catheter
- S. procedure
- S. test
- S. tube
- S. urethropexy

Stamey-Martius procedure

Stamm
- S. gastroplasty
- S. gastrostomy
- S. gastrostomy tube

stammering
- s. of the bladder

stand
- Mayo s.

standard
- s. acid reflux test (SART)
- s. colonoscope
- s. duodenoscope
- s. endoscopy polypectomy snare
- s. ERCP catheter
- s. fatty meal
- s. radioenzymatic method

Stanford
- S. radical retropubic prostatectomy
- S. staging

stannous pyrophosphate (SPP)

stanolone

stanozolol

staph sepsis

Staphylococcus
- S. aureus
- coagulase-negative S.
- S. epidermidis
- S. food poisoning
- S. saprophyticus
- S. viridans

staple
- s. line dehiscence
- metallic s.
- skin s.

stapled strictureplasty

stapler
- anvil portion of EEA s.
- Autosuture s.
- CEEA s.
- circular s.
- Cobe s.
- double-headed P190 s.
- EEA s.
- EEA AutoSuture s.
- end-end s.
- Endo-Babcock s.
- EndoGIA (30, 60) s.
- Endopath (30, 60) s.
- GIA s.
- hernia s.
- ILA surgical s.
- intraluminal s. (ILS)
- LDS s.
- linear s.
- PI90 double-headed s.
- PI surgical s.
- Proximate flexible linear s.
- Proximate intraluminal s.
- TA30 s.
- TA55 s.
- TA90-BN s.

stapling
- gastric s.
- single s.
- skin s.
- surgical s.

starch
- s. blocker
- s. granulomatous peritonitis
- wheat s.

Starck dilator

star construction test

stasis, pl. **stases**
- antral s.
- bile s.
- biliary s.
- s. cirrhosis
- s. esophagitis
- fecal s.
- s. gallbladder
- gallbladder s.

S

NOTES

stasis *(continued)*
  gastric s.
  ileal s.
  intestinal s.
  s. liver
  pelvicaliceal s.
  postgastrectomy s.
  postsurgical gastric s.
  Roux-limb s.
  s. syndrome
  s. ulceration
state
  gradient-recalled acquisition in
    a steady s. (GRASS)
  hypercoagulable s.
  hypermetabolic s.
  hypogonadal s.
  proteinuric s.
State end-to-end anastomosis
Statham
  S. external transducer
  S. P23 strain gauge
static
  s. closure pressure
  s. cystogram
  s. cytophotometry
  s. image DNA cytometry
station
  s. pull-through (SPT)
  s. pull-through esophageal
    manometry technique
station-pull-through technique
statistics
  nonparametric Wilcoxon s.
status
  s. evaluation
  fertility s.
  Karnofsky performance s.
  nutritional s.
  s. post (S/P)
  ureteroenteric s.
Stat-View
  S.-V. computer program
Stauffer syndrome
stay suture
STD
  sexually transmitted disease
STDS
  stone-tissue detection-system
steady pain
steakhouse syndrome
steal
  arterial s.

steam autoclave
stearrhea
steatohepatitis
  non-alcoholic s.
steatohepatomegaly
steatorrhea
  biliary s.
  idiopathic s.
  intestinal s.
  pancreatic s.
steatosis
  drug-induced s.
  hepatic s.
  microvesicular s.
  severe macrovesicular s.
  toxic s.
steerable cystoscopy
Steers replicator
stegnosis
stegnotic
Steigmann-Goff
  S.-G. endoscopic ligator kit
  S.-G. endoscopic ligature
    overtube
Steiner
  S. modification of Warthin-
    Starry staining
  S. stain
Steinert disease
Stein-Leventhal syndrome
Steinmann intestinal forceps
steinstrasse
Stelazine
stellate cell
Stemetic
stemline
  DNA s.
stenosis, pl. stenoses
  ampullary s.
  anal s.
  anorectal s.
  antral s.
  aortic s.
  aortic valvular s.
  atherosclerotic s.
  atherosclerotic renal artery s.
  benign s.
  benign papillary s.
  choledochoduodenal
    junctional s.
  congenital s.
  congenital hypertrophic
    pyloric s.

congenital pyloric s.
distal esophageal s.
duodenal s.
esophageal s.
hypertrophic pyloric s.
ileoureteric s.
infantile hypertrophic pyloric s.
infundibulopelvic s.
malignant s.
meatal s.
pancreaticojejunostomy s.
papillary s.
preputial s.
pyloric s.
radiation s.
rectal s.
renal artery s.
short band s.
small intestinal s.
sphincterotomy s.
stomal s.
s. of TIPS
transplant renal artery s.
(TRAS)
ureteroileal s.
vesicoureteric s.

stenotic
s. lesion
s. stoma

stent
Amsterdam biliary s.
Amsterdam-type biliary s.
Angiomed blue s.
Angiomed Puroflex s.
antibiotic-coated s.
antireflux double-J s.
ASI prostatic s.
Beamer ejection s.
Beamer injection s.
biliary s.
Black Beauty ureteral s.
Braun s.
Carson internal/external
endopyelotomy s.
C-Flex Amsterdam s.
C-Flex ureteral s.
coil s.

common bile duct s.
conventional s.
Cook s.
Cotton-Huibregtse double
pigtail s.
Cotton-Leung biliary s.
Cysto Flex s.
double-J s.
double-J Surgitek catheter s.
double-J ureteral s.
double pigtail s.
Elastalloy esophageal s.
ELIMINATOR biliary s.
ELIMINATOR pancreatic s.
encrustation of s.
Endocoil esophageal s.
endoscopic s.
endoscopic biliary s.
Entract s.
EsophaCoil self-expanding
esophageal s.
esophageal s.
esophageal Strecker s.
expandable esophageal s.
(EES)
expandable intrahepatic
portacaval shunt s.
expandable metallic s.
Fader Tip s.
Fader Tip ureteral s.
Firlit-Kluge s.
French s.
French double-J ureteral s.
Gianturco s.
Gianturco metal urethral s.
Gianturco-Rosch self-expandable
Z-stent s.
Gibbon indwelling ureteral s.
Greenen pancreatic s.
helical-ridged ureteral s.
Heyer-Schulte s.
Huibregtse biliary s.
Hydromer coated
polyurethane s.
Hydro Plus s.
s. incrustation
intracholedochal s.

S

NOTES

stent *(continued)*
intraesophageal s.
intraluminal Silastic
esophageal s.
intraprostatic s.
iridium-192-loaded s.
J-Maxx s.
Lubri-flex ureteral s.
magnetic internal ureteral s.
Mardis soft s.
Memotherm s.
mesh s.
metal s.
metallic biliary s.
Metal Z s.
Microvasive s.
Multi-Flex s.
nitinol s.
Palmaz s.
Palmaz balloon-expandable s.
pancreatic s.
pancreatic duct s.
s. patency
Percuflex Amsterdam s.
Percuflex biliary s.
Percuflex endopyelotomy s.
Percuflex Plus ureteral s.
percutaneous s.
pigtail s.
pigtail biliary s.
polyethylene s.
Prostacoil s.
Prostakath urethral s.
prostatic s.
recanalization of clogged
biliary s.
Retromax endopyelotomy s.
Rüsch s.
Schneider s.
self-expandable metal s.
self-expanding biliary metal s.
self-expanding coil s.
self-expanding metallic s.
(SEMS)
self-retaining coil s.
shape memory alloy s.
Silastic s.
Silastic indwelling ureteral s.
silicone-coated s.
silicone-coated metallic self-
expanding s.
Silitek Uropass s.
silver-coated s.

single pigtail s.
SMA spiral s.
SoloPass Percuflex biliary s.
Speed Lok soft s.
straight s.
Strecker s.
Surgitek s.
Surgitek Tractfinder ureteral s.
Surgitek Uropass s.
thermoexpandable s.
s. through wire mesh
technique
Titan s.
titanium urethral s.
transhepatic biliary s.
transpapillary cystopancreatic s.
transpapillary insertion of self-
expanding biliary metal s.
T-tube s.
Ultraflex esophageal s.
Ultraflex Microvasive s.
Ultraflex nitinol expandable
esophageal s.
uncoated mesh s.
Universal s.
ureteral s.
Uro-Guide s.
UroLume prostate s.
Urosoft s.
Urospiral urethral s.
U-tube s.
s. and vent system
Wallstent s.
whistle s.
Wilson-Cook s.
Wilson-Cook French s.
Z s.
Zimmon biliary s.
stent-induced pneumoperitoneum
stenting
biliary s.
s. catheter
endoscopic s.
endoscopic pancreatic s. (EPS)
endoscopic papillotomy and s.
endoscopic retrograde biliary s.
pancreatic transpapillary s.
tumor s.
ureteral s.
stentography
stepladder incision technique
steppage gait
stepper

stepping reflex
step-up shim
step-wise regression analysis
steradian
Sterapred
stercolith
stercoraceous
    s. vomiting
    s. vomitus
stercoral
    s. abscess
    s. appendicitis
    s. diarrhea
    s. fistula
    s. ulcer
    s. ulceration
stercoralis
    Strongyloides s.
stercoroma
stercorous
stercus
stereognost-3-α enzymatic test
sterile
    s. dressing
    s. pancreatic necrosis
    s. peritonitis
sterility
    aspermatogenic s.
    dysspermatogenic s.
    normospermatogenic s.
sterilization
    ETO s.
    gas s.
sterilize
sterilized
    autoclave s.
Steris automatic reprocessor
steri-stripped
    s.-s. incision
Steri-Strips
sternocleidomastoid
sternotomy
    s. scar
sternum
    bowed s.
steroid
    anabolic s.

    s. foam enema
    high-dose pulse s.
    s. moiety
    s. resistant idiopathic nephrosis
    s. responsive pancolitis
    s. sensitive/dependent idiopathic
      nephrosis
    s. therapy
steroid-dependent
    s.-d. Crohn disease
    s.-d. diet
steroid-induced azoospermia
steroid-refractory
    s.-r. Crohn disease
    s.-r. diet
steroid-resistant nephrotic syndrome
sterol
Stetten intestinal clamp
Stevens-Johnson syndrome (SJS)
Stewart crypt hook
Stewart-Treves syndrome
stick
    sponge s.
    s. tie
Stiegmann-Goff
    S.-G. Clearvue endoscopic
      ligator
    S.-G. technique
    S.-G. variceal ligator
Stierlin sign
Stifcore transbronchial aspiration
   needle
stiffening tube
stiff-man syndrome
stigma, pl. **stigmata**
stigmata
    Turner s.
still camera
Stille
    S. elevator
    S. gallstone forceps
Stille-Barraya intestinal forceps
Stilphostrol
stimulant laxative
stimulated
    s. gastric secretion test
    s. gracilis neosphincter

S

NOTES

stimulated *(continued)*
  s. gracilis neosphincter
    technique
  s. release
stimulation
  adenyl cyclase s.
  anal electrical s.
  anocutaneous s.
  antigen s.
  central vagal nerve s.
  electrogalvanic s. (EGS)
  s. fork
  gastric electrical s.
  hilum s.
  interferon-gamma s.
  intraoperative cavernous
    nerve s.
  intravaginal electrical s.
  mitogenic s.
  nociceptive s.
  pelvic s.
  s. probe
  S-CCK-Pz s.
  secretin s.
  secretin-cholecystokinin-
    pancreatozymin s.
  s. test
  transcutaneous electrical
    nerve s. (TENS)
  transurethral electrical
    bladder s. (TEBS)
  vagal s.
  vaginal electrical s.
stimulator
  EGS Model 100
    electrogalvanic s.
  electrogalvanic s.
  Grass Model S9 s.
  Nicolet SM-300 s.
  URYS 800 nerve s.
stimulus
  external s.
  mitogenic s.
  symbolic s.
stipules
stirrups
  pediatric s.
stitch
  baseball s.
  Connell s.
  inter-symphyseal s.
  marker s.

  tagging s.
  tilt s.
St. Mark pudendal electrode
stochastic knotting
stoichiometry
  coupling s.
Stokvis test
Stoller scoring system
Stoll test
stoma, pl. **stomas, stomata**
  abdominal s.
  anastomotic s.
  Benchekroun s.
  bowel s.
  concealed umbilical s.
  diverting s.
  dusky s.
  end s.
  end-loop s.
  gastrointestinal s.
  Gomez horizontal gastroplasty
    with reinforced s.
  ileostomy s.
  Laws gastroplasty with Silastic
    collar-reinforced s.
  loop s.
  maturing the s.
  Mitrofanoff s.
  nippled s.
  permanent s.
  prolapsed s.
  retracted s.
  rodless end-loop s.
  rosebud s.
  Silastic collar-reinforced s.
  s. site
  stenotic s.
  ureteral s.
  ureteric s.
stomach
  aberrant umbilical s.
  s. ache
  acid-suppressed s.
  anacidic s.
  angulus of s.
  antrum of s.
  bilocular s.
  butterflies in the s.
  s. calculus
  cardia of s.
  cardiac s.
  cascade s.
  cirrhosis of s.

Dieulafoy vascular
  malformation of the s.
distal blind s.
dumping s.
functional disorder s.
greater curvature of s.
hourglass s.
insufflation of s.
intrathoracic s.
s. lavage
leather-bottle s.
mucous lake of the s.
s. neoplasm
s. pump
s. reefing
sclerotic s.
sour s.
s. sphincter
succussion splash over the s.
thoracic s.
trifid s.
s. tube
upset s.
upside down s.
watermelon s. (WS)
water-trap s.

stomachalgia
stomachodynia
Stomahesive
  S. Paste
  S. skin barrier wafer
  S. Wafer
stomal
  s. bag
  s. duskiness
  s. invagination
  s. prolapse
  s. stenosis
  s. ulcer
stoma-like channel
stomas (*pl. of* stoma)
stomata (*pl. of* stoma)
Stomate
  S. decompression tube
  S. extension tube

stomatitis
  aphthous s.
  herpetic s.
stomatoscopy
  diagnostic fiberoptic s.
stone
  ampullary s.
  s. basket
  s. and basket impaction
  bile duct s.
  biliary tract s.
  bilirubinate s.
  black faceted s.
  black pigment s.
  bladder s.
  brown pigment s.
  s. burden
  calcium s.
  calcium bilirubinate s.
  calcium oxalate s.
  calcium oxalate dihydrate s.
  calcium oxalate monohydrate s.
  carbonate apatite s.
  cholesterol s.
  S. clamp applier
  s. comminution
  common bile duct s.
  common duct s.
  complex s.
  s. cup
  cystic duct s.
  cystine s.
  s. disease
  endoscopic duct s.
  endoscopic extraction pancreatic
    duct s.
  s. extraction
  extraction bile duct s.
  extraction pancreatic s.
  s. forceps
  s. formers
  s. fragmentation
  gallbladder s.
  s. granuloma
  s. granuloma formation
  hyperoxaluric s.
  impacted s.

S

NOTES

stone *(continued)*
    impacted ampullary s.
    s. impaction
    s. impactor
    S. intestinal clamp
    intrahepatic s.
    intraluminal s.
    kidney s.
    large common duct s.
    s. maturation
    metabolic s.
    mulberry s.
    multiple s.
    noncalcified s.
    nonstruvite s.
    pancreatic s.
    pancreatic duct s.
    pelvic s.
    periureteral s.
    renal s.
    residual s.
    s. retrieval balloon
    s. retrieval basket
    s. retriever
    silent s.
    s. solvent
    staghorn s.
    struvite s.
    s. surgery
    ureteral s.
    urinary s.
stone-free
    s.-f. rate
stone-grasping forceps
Stone-Holcombe intestinal clamp
stone-holding basket forceps
StoneRisk
    S. citrate test
    S. cystine test
    S. diagnostic monitoring kit
    S. diagnostic profile
    S. diagnostic test
stone-tissue
    s.-t. detection-system (STDS)
    s.-t. recognition system (STR)
StoneTrack
stool
    acholic s.
    bilious s.
    black tarry s.
    blood admixed with s.
    blood on surface of s.
    blood passed with s.

blood-streaked s.
bloody s.
brown s.
bulky s.
butter s.
clay-colored s.
Clinitest-negative s.
Clinitest-positive s.
s. color
continent of s.
s. culture
currant jelly s.
s. cytotoxin test
dark s.
diarrhea s.
s. electrolyte
s. electrolyte test
s. elimination
s. evacuation
fatty s.
floating s.
foamy s.
formed s.
foul-smelling s.
frank blood in s.
frequency of s.
Gram stain of s.
green s.
guaiac-negative s.
guaiac-positive s.
hard s.
heme-negative s.
heme-positive s.
impacted s.
s. incontinence
lienteric s.
liquid s.
loose s.
mahogany-colored s.
malodorous s.
maroon-colored s.
melenic s.
mucoid s.
mucous s.
mushy s.
nonbloody s.
s. for occult blood
oily s.
s. osmolality test
s. osmotic gap
s. osmotic gap test
s. for ova and parasites
pale s.

palpable s.
passage of s.
pea soup s.
pelleted s.
pencil-like s.
pipestem s.
rabbit s.
reducing substance in s.
residual s.
s. retention
ribbon s.
rice-water s.
runny s.
sago-grain s.
s. sample
scybalous s.
semiformed s.
semisolid s.
silver s.
slurry of s.
soft s.
s. softener
spinach s.
straining at s.
tarry black s.
Trélat s.'s
undigested food in s.
unformed s.
watery s.
Wright stain of s.
stooling
stop-cock
three-way s.-c.
storage
cold s.
hypothermic s.
store
hepatic glycogen s.
liver iron s.
liver protein s.
Storz
S. cystoscope
S. esophagoscope
S. minilaparoscope
S. Modulith SL20
S. Monolith lithotriptor

S. multifunction valve
trocar/cannula system
S. nephroscope
S. panendoscope
S. resectoscope
S. 27022 SK ureteroscope
S. syringe
S. urethrotome
STR
stone-tissue recognition system
strabismus scissors
straight
s. Maryland forceps
s. mosquito clamp
s. stent
straightening maneuver
strain
Cowan I s.
eubacterial s.
s. gauge transducer
metronidazole-resistant s.
Statham P23 s. gauge
straining
s. at stool
defecatory s.
excessive s.
strand
fibrin s.
stranding
fascial s.
mesenteric s.
pericholecystic s.
soft tissue s.
strangulated
s. bowel
s. bowel obstruction
s. hemorrhoid
s. hernia
s. viscus
strangulation necrosis
stranguria
strangury
Stransky sign
strap
Montgomery abdominal s.'s
Strassburg test
Stratagene SCS-96 thermocycler

S

NOTES

stratum malpighii
Strauss sign
strawberry
   s. gallbladder
   s. hemangioma
straw-colored
   s.-c. ascites
   s.-c. fluid
streak
   erythematous s.
   s. gonad
   lymphangitic s.
   s. ovary
stream
   curve of s.
Strecker stent
Strelinger colon clamp
strength
   artery weld s.
   hemostatic bond s.
   masseter s.
   tensile s.
strep
   streptococcus
   anhemolytic strep
   beta-hemolytic strep
   hemolytic strep
   nonhemolytic strep
streptavidin
   peroxidase-conjugated s.
streptavidin-biotin peroxidase
   complex (SAB reagent)
streptococcal esophagitis
Streptococcus
   S. agalactiae
   S. bovis
   S. bovis endocarditis
   S. faecalis
   S. pyogenes
   S. salivarius
   S. sanguis
streptococcus (strep)
   alpha-hemolytic s.
   group B s. (GBS)
streptokinase
Streptomyces misakiensis
streptomycin
streptozocin
streptozotocin
streptozotocin-induced diabetes
   mellitus

stress
   s. erosion
   s. erythrocytosis
   s. gastritis
   s. incontinence
   s. lesion
   s. protein
   surgical s.
   s. ulcer
   s. ulceration
   s. ulcer hemorrhage
   s. ulcer prophylaxis
   s. urethral pressure profile
   s. urinary incontinence (SUI)
stress-induced gastric ulceration
stress-related
   s.-r. erosive syndrome
   s.-r. mucosal injury
Stresstein liquid feeding
stretch receptor
stria, pl. striae
striated
   s. muscle innervation
   s. sphincter
stricture
   anal s.
   anastomotic s.
   annular esophageal s.
   antral s.
   benign s.
   benign bile duct s.
   benign biliary s.
   bile duct s.
   biliary s.
   biliary tract s.
   bulbomembranous s.
   bulbourethral s.
   cicatricial s.
   colorectal s.
   contractile s.
   corrosive esophageal s.
   diaphragm-like s.
   distal esophageal s.
   ductal s.
   esophageal s.
   extrahepatic biliary s.
   filiform s.
   hourglass s.
   Hunner s.
   intestinal s.
   intrahepatic biliary s.
   irritable s.

longitudinal esophageal s.
malignant s.
nonsteroidal anti-inflammatory
  drug-induced intestinal s.
pancreatic duct s.
peptic s.
peptic esophageal s.
postoperative s.
s. prophylaxis
pyloric s.
rectal s.
recurrent s.
reflux-related s.
spasmodic s.
ureteral s.
ureterocolic s.
ureteroileal s.
urethral s.
vesicouretral anastomotic s.
strictured esophagus
strictureplasty (SXPL)
Finney s.
stapled s.
stricturoplasty
Thal s.
stricturotomy
endoscopic s.
stridor
string
s. guideline
s. of pearl sign
s. sign
swallowed s.
s. test
string method for treatment of
penile incarceration
strip
Bio-Gen urine test s.
s. biopsy
s. biopsy resection technique
DisIntek reagent s.
ganglion-free muscle s.
Pyloritek reagent s.
s. resection
rhythm s.

stripe
s. interstitial fibrosis
properitoneal flank s.
stripping
mucosal s.
stroke
saber s.
stroma, pl. stromata
fibroelastic connective tissue s.
fibrous s.
hyalinized s.
s. ovarii
stromal tumors of unknown
malignant potential (STUMP)
Strongyloides
S. *stercoralis*
strongyloidiasis
strongyloma
strontium-89 chloride
structural
s. fatigue
s. stability
structure
biliary s.
cord s.
ductular s.
glandular s.
insular s.
malignant nuclear s.
mixed s.
nociceptive s.
trabecular s.
undifferentiated s.
Strulle scissors
struma
Hashimoto s.
s. ovarii
strut
Mersilene s.
struvite
s. calculus
s. crystal formation
s. stone
STS lithotripsy system
stuartii
Providencia s.
Stucker bile duct dilator

NOTES

S

studding
  omental s.
  peritoneal s.
Studer
  S. bladder substitute
  S. pouch procedure
  S. reservoir urinary diversion
study
  A28 immunological s.
  antegrade contrast s.
  anti-DNA immunological s.
  anti-ENA immunological s.
  anti-hepatitis A-IgM
    immunological s.
  antinuclear antibody
    immunological s.
  anti-SSA immunological s.
  anti-SSB immunological s.
  barium s.
  bead chain s.
  B_{12} immunological s.
  bulb tip retrograde s.
  Candida immunological s.
  C3 immunological s.
  cinefluorographic s.
  circulating immunocomplexes
    immunological s.
  colonic transit s.
  colorectal physiologic s.
  diuretic renal quantitative
    camera s.
  DNCB immunological s.
  ESR immunological study
    immunological s.
  flow cytometric s.
  gene-blotting s.
  HBeAg immunological s.
  HBsAg immunological s.
  hematologic s.
  HLA typing immunological s.
  IgA immunological s.
  IgG immunological s.
  IgM immunological s.
  immunological s.
  Intergroup
    Rhabdomyosarcoma S. (IRS)
  isotope s.
  kinetic gallbladder s.
  light micrographic s.
  manometric s.
  marker transit s.
  mitochondrial immunological s.
  molecular s.

  nuclear-tagged red blood cell
    bleeding s.
  peak urinary flow s.
  phenotypic s.
  polarographic s.
  positive secretin stimulation s.
  PPD immunological s.
  pressure s.
  pressure-flow
    electromyography s.
  radiological s.
  radionuclide transit s.
  rectosphincter manometric s.,
    rectosphincteromanometric s.
  retrograde contrast s.
  seroepidemiological s.
  single-color direct
    immunofluorescence s.
  smooth-muscle
    immunological s.
  The National Cooperative
    Dialysis S.
  Treponema
    immunofluorescence s.
  T-tube s.
  twenty-four-hour intraesophageal
    pH s.
  upper gastrointestinal barium
    roentgenographic s.
  urodynamic flow s.
  videofluoroscopic swallow s.
  videofluorourodynamic s.
  voiding s.
STUMP
  stromal tumors of unknown
    malignant potential
stump
  appendiceal s.
  blind s.
  dehiscence of cystic s.
  duodenal s.
  funicular s.
  gastric s.
  s. invagination
  s. ligation
  rectal s.
stuporous
Sturge-Weber syndrome
stuttering
  s. priapism
  urinary s.
  s. urination
S-type amylase

Stypven time test
subactam sodium
subacute
    s. abscess
    s. fatty liver of pregnancy
    s. hepatic necrosis
    s. hepatitis
    s. necrosis
    s. nonspecific peritonitis
subareolar
subcapsular
    s. hematoma
    s. hemorrhage
    s. hepatic abscess
subcarinal node
subcecal appendix
subcholangiopancreatoscope
subcitrate
    colloidal bismuth s. (CBS)
subclavian
    s. catheter
    s. vein
    s. vein catheterization
subclinical
    s. hepatitis
    s. sprue
subconjunctival hemorrhage
subcoronal hypospadias
subcostal
    s. flank incision
    s. incision
    s. margin
    s. port
    s. transperitoneal incision
subcu
    subcutaneous
subcutaneous (SC, subcu, subq)
    s. EGF
    s. emphysema
    s. fat
    s. layer
    s. morphine pump (SQMP)
    s. tissue
    s. urinary diversion
subcuticular suture
subdeterminant
    hepatitis B surface antigen s.

subdiaphragmatic abscess
subendoscope
subepithelial hemorrhage
subfertile
subfraction
    uremic serum s.
subfulminant liver failure
subglottic lesion
subhepatic
    s. abscess
    s. area
    s. space
subinguinal
    s. microsurgical
        varicocelectomy
    s. varicocelectomy
subjective vertigo
submassive necrosis
submucosa
submucosal
    s. calculus
    s. dissection
    s. gastric hemorrhage
    s. ileal lipoma
    s. lesion
    s. mass
    s. plexus
    s. tattoo
    s. Teflon injection
    s. thickening
    s. upper gastrointestinal tract
        lesion
    s. vaginal muscle
    s. vaginal smooth
        musculofascial layer
    s. vascular dilation
    s. venous plexus
    s. wound
submuscular
subparta
    ileus s.
subperitoneal
    s. appendicitis
    s. space
subphrenic
    s. abscess
    s. space

S

NOTES

subpubic sinus
subq
subcutaneous
Subrini penile prosthesis
subsalicylate
bismuth s.
subsegmentectomy
hepatic s.
subserosal
s. disease
s. layer
subserous tunnel
substaging
pathologic s.
substance
s. abuse
caustic s.
hepatic stimulatory s. (HSS)
noncholecystokinin s.
substance K
substance P (SP)
substance S
substitute
ileal orthotopic bladder s.
low pressure bladder s.
olestra fat s.
saliva s.
Studer bladder s.
substitution
bladder s.
substrate
copolymerized s.
subsymphyseal epispadias
subtotal
s. colectomy
s. gastrectomy
s. gastric exclusion
s. pancreatectomy
subtraction angiography
subtrigonal
subtunical venule
subtype
HBsAg s.
subtyping
HLA-DR2 s.
subumbilical space
β-subunit
transmembrane β-s.
suburethral
s. rectus fascial sling
procedure
s. sling
s. sling procedure

suburothelial
s. infiltrative cancer
s. nerve plexus
s. vascular bed
subvesical duct
subxiphoid
Suby G solution
subzonal insemination (SUZI)
succinate
chloromyceth sodium s.
s. dehydrogenase activity
(SDH)
succinylcholine
succorrhea
succulent mesenteric lymph node
succuss
succussion
hippocratic s.
s. sound
s. splash
s. splash over the stomach
sucker
tonsil s.
sucralfate
s. retention enema
s. therapy
sucrase-isomaltase
sucrose
sucrose-free (SF)
suction
s. biopsy
bulb s.
continuous NG s.
s. cylinder
s. drain
s. drainage
flexible dental s.
s. foot pedal
Gomco s.
lavage and s.
low intermittent s.
nasogastric s.
NG s.
s. pump
s. tip
s. tube
Wangensteen s.
suction-coagulator
Cameron-Miller s.-c.
suctioning
intermittent s.
Sudan black B fat stain

**Suda (type I, II, III) classification
 of papilla**
sudden onset of pain
Sudeck point
sugar
 s. oxime
 s. test
sugar-free
 Citrucel s.-f.
Sugiura
 S. esophageal variceal
 transection
 S. procedure
SUI
 stress urinary incontinence
suite
 endoscopy s.
sulbactam
sulciolar gastric mucosa
sulcus
 coronal s.
sulfa
sulfacytine
sulfadiazine
Sulfamethoprim
sulfamethoxazole
 s. and phenazopyridine
 trimethoprim s.
 trimethoprim and s.
 (TMP/SMX)
 s. and trimethoprim
 (SMX/TMP)
sulfasalazine
 s. enema
sulfasoxazole
sulfate
 atropine s.
 barium s.
 dehydroepiandrosterone s.
 (DHAS)
 ferrous s.
 gentamicin s.
 hyoscyamine s.
 protamine s.
 quinidine s.
 sodium dodecyl s. (SDS)

 sodium tetradecyl s.
 tetradecyl s.
sulfated
 s. glycoprotein-2 (SGP-2)
 s. mucin stain
Sulfatrim DS
sulfhydryl
sulfisoxazole
 s. and phenazopyridine
sulfolithocholylglycine
sulfolithocholyltaurine
sulfonamide
sulfonate
 mercaptoethane s.
sulfone
 s. syndrome
sulfoxide
 dimethyl s. (DMSO)
sulfur
 s. amino acid metabolism
 s. colloid (SC)
 s. colloid liver scan
sulfuric acid
sulglycotide
sulindac
sulmarin
sulphydryl donor
sulpiride
summer diarrhea
Sumner sign
sump
 s. drain
 s. nasogastric tube
 s. syndrome
 s. ulcer
Sumycin
superantigens
Super-Bright microsphere
SuperChar
Super-cut scissors
superfibronectin
superficial
 s. bladder cancer
 s. esophageal carcinoma (SEC)
 s. fluorescein
 s. gastric carcinoma
 s. gastritis

S

NOTES

superficial *(continued)*
  s. inguinal pouch
  s. linear ulcer
  s. trigonal muscle
  s. tumor
superimposed alcoholic hepatitis
superinfection
  delta hepatitis s.
  hepatitis D s.
superior
  s. mesenteric angiography
  s. mesenteric arteriogram
  s. mesenteric artery
  s. mesenteric artery syndrome
    (SMAS)
  s. mesenteric vein (SMV)
  s. mesenterorenal bypass
  s. mesenterorenal bypass
    technique
  s. pubic ramotomy
  s. rectal vein
  s. rectal venous plexus
supernatant
superoxide
  s. dismutase (SOD)
  s. production
  s. radical
supersaturated bile
superselective
  s. arteriography
  s. vagotomy
supination
supine position
supplement
  caloric s.
  Casec calcium s.
  Dent s.
  food s.
  keto acid-amino acid s.
  Polycose glucose s.
  protein s.
  Travasorb MCT s.
supplementation
  calcium s.
  dietary s.
  fish oil s.
  prostaglandin s.
  vitamin D s.
support
  artificial hepatic s.
  bladder s.
  emotional s.
  nutritional s.

  s. parenteral nutrition (SPN)
  psychological s.
  psychosexual s.
suppository
  B&O s.
  rectal s.
  vaginal s.
suppression
  acid s.
  cell-mediated s.
  immune s.
  s. treatment
suppressor T cell
suppuration
suppurativa
  hidradenitis s.
suppurative
  s. appendicitis
  s. appendix
  s. cholangitis
  s. nephritis
supraceliac
  s. aorta
supraclavicular
supracolic compartment
supradiaphragmatic
supraduodenal approach
Supra-Foley catheter
supragastric bursoscopy
supraglottic squamous cell
  carcinoma
suprahepatic
  s. caval cuff
  s. space
  s. vena cava
suprahilar disease
supralevator
  s. anorectal space
  s. pelvic exenteration
  s. perirectal abscess
  s. space
supraomental space
suprapapillary Roux-en-Y
  duodenojejunostomy
supraprostatectomy
suprapubic
  s. cystotomy
  s. cystotomy tract urethral
    atresia
  s. lithotomy
  s. port
  s. prostatectomy
  s. region

suprarenal
    s. Greenfield filter
    s. impression
suprarenalectomy
suprasphincteric fistula
supravaterian duodenum
supravesical urinary diversion
suramin
SureBite biopsy forceps
Sure-Cut biopsy needle
Sureseal pressure bandage
Suretys
    S. incontinence briefs
    S. pants
    S. panty system
surface
    cholesterolosis of mucosal s.
    colonic mucosal s.
    s. cooling
    s. cooling technique
    s. electrode
    s. epithelium
    s. nodularity
    s. nodule
    serosal s.
    s. thermometer
    ventral s.
surface-to-volume ratio
Surfak
Sur-Fit
    S.-F. Mini pouch
    S.-F. Pouch cover
    S.-F. Stoma cap
Surgenomic endoscope
Surgeons
    Society of American
    Gastrointestinal
    Endoscoping S. (SAGES)
surgeon's knot
surgery
    anorectal s.
    antireflux s.
    bariatric s.
    bench s.
    colorectal s.
    concomitant antireflux s.
    cytoreductive s.

    dialysis access s.
    extracorporeal s.
    gastric bypass s.
    intestinal s.
    jejunoileal bypass s.
    laser s.
    minimal access s.
    nephron-sparing s.
    nonbench s.
    parenchymal sparing s.
    pelvic colonic s.
    penile venous ligation s.
    portal-systemic shunt s.
    primary perineal hypospadias s.
    radical s.
    radioimmunoguided s. (RIGS)
    rectovaginal s.
    retrograde intrarenal s.
    reversal jejunoileal bypass s.
    salvage s.
    secondary s.
    sham s.
    stone s.
    telerobotic assisted
      laparoscopic s.
    transsexual s.
    urologic s.
    vascular s.
    weight reduction s.
surgical
    s. abdomen
    s. cystgastrostomy
    s. decompression
    s. drain
    s. drape
    s. extirpation
    s. flap
    s. incision
    s. loupe
    s. portosystemic shunting
    s. scissors
    s. stapling
    s. stress
    s. therapy
    s. vagotomy
Surgicel gauze
Surgilube lubricant

S

NOTES

Surgi-PEG replacement gastrostomy feeding system
Surgitek
  S. button
  S. catheter
  S. Flexi-Flate II penile implant
  S. graduated cystocope GC-16
  S. graduated cystoscope
  S. One-Step (SOS)
  S. One-Step percutaneous
    endoscopic gastrostomy
  S. stent
  S. Tractfinder ureteral stent
  S. Uropass stent
Surgitite ligating loop
Surgiwip suture ligature
surreptitious vomiting
surrogate marker
surveillance
  endoscopic s.
  s. protocol
survey
  metabolic bone s.
survival
  graft s.
  mean allograft s. (MAS)
  s. rate
Susano
suspension
  barium s.
  bladder neck s.
  charcoal s.
  colloidal bismuth s.
  extraperitoneal laparoscopic
    bladder neck s. (ELBNS)
  Gittes-Loughlin bladder neck s.
  nystatin s.
  OK432 streptococcal s.
  oral barium s.
  Pereyra bladder neck s.
  Raz bladder neck s.
  Raz four-quadrant s.
  Raz needle s.
  Raz urethral s.
  retropubic Lapides-Ball bladder
    neck s.
  Stamey needle s.
  urethral s.
suspensory bandage
Sustacal
  S. HC liquid feeding
  S. pudding
Sustagen liquid feeding

suture
  absorbable s.
  Albert s.
  anastomotic s.
  anchoring s.
  Appolito s.
  approximation s.
  atraumatic s.
  Bell s.
  bolster s.
  s. bridge
  buried s.
  button s.
  cardinal s.
  chain s.
  chromic s.
  chromic catgut s.
  chromic gut s.
  circular s.
  Connell s.
  continuous s.
  corner s.
  cotton s.
  Cushing s.
  s. cutter
  Czerny s.
  Czerny-Lembert s.
  Dacron s.
  dermal s.
  Dexon s.
  Dupuytren s.
  Ethibond s.
  Ethiflex s.
  everting s.
  s. fatigue
  figure-of-eight s.
  furrier s.
  Gambee s.
  Gély s.
  s. granuloma
  s. guide
  Gussenbauer s.
  Halsted s.
  heavy silk s.
  hemostatic s.
  horizontal mattress s.
  Horsley s.
  interrupted s.
  intracuticular s.
  intradermal s.
  inverting s.
  Jobert de Lamballe s.
  Kessler-Kleinert s.

Lembert s.
Lembert inverting
  seromuscular s.
s. ligated
s. ligature
s. line
s. line dehiscence
locking s.
lock-stitch s.
loop s.
s. material
mattress s.
Mersilene s.
Monocryl s.
monofilament s.
monofilament nylon s.
nonabsorbable s.
over-and-over s.
Parker-Kerr s.
PDS s.
PDS Vicryl s.
pericostal s.
Perma-hand silk s.
plain catgut s.
plain gut s.
s. plication
plication s.
Polydek s.
polydioxanone s.
polyglactin s.
polyglecaprone 25 s.
polyglycolic acid s.
polyglyconate s.
polypropylene s.
pop-off s.
primary s.
Prolene s.
pursestring s.
quilted s.
reinforcing s.
relaxation s.
retention s.
running s.
s. scissors
secondary s.
seromuscular Lembert s.
silk s.

silk pop-off s.
silk traction s.
stainless steel s.
stay s.
subcuticular s.
swaged-on s.
Teflon-coated Dacron s.
Tevdek s.
Ti-Cron s.
Tom Jones s.
traction s.
transition s.
Tycron s.
s. ulcer
vascular s.
vertical mattress s.
whipstitch s.
Z s.
sutureless
  s. bowel anastomosis
  s. colostomy closure
suture-release needle
SUZI
  subzonal insemination
SVO
  splenic vein obstruction
SVRI
  systemic vascular resistance index
swaged needle
swaged-on
  s.-o. needle
  s.-o. suture
swallow
  barium s.
  dry s.
  Gastrografin s.
  Hypaque s.
  ice-water s.
  modified barium s. (MBS)
  water-soluble contrast
    esophageal s.
  wet s.
swallowed string
swallowing
  air s.
  s. center

S

NOTES

swallowing *(continued)*
four phases of s.
s. mechanism
Swan-Ganz pulmonary artery catheter
swan-neck
s.-n. catheter
s.-n. Coil-Cath catheter
s.-n. deformity
s.-n. Missouri catheter
s.-n. pediatric Coil-Cath catheter
sweating
gustatory s.
sweat test
Sween
S. Cream
S. Micro Guard cream
S. Micro Guard powder
S. Prep
Sween-A-Peel skin barrier
sweep
duodenal s.
Sweet esophageal scissors
swelling
cell s.
external s.
lysosomal s.
popliteal s.
testicular s.
uvular s.
Swenson
S. abdominal pull-through
S. papillotome
swim-up processing
Swiss Lithoclast
"Swiss roll" embedding technique
switch
duodenal s.
optical s.
swollen
s. tongue
s. turbinate
Swyer syndrome
SXPL
strictureplasty
Sydney
S. classification of gastritis
S. System
S. system gastritis classification
Syllact
Syllamalt
sylvian fistula

symbolic stimulus
symmetric face movement
Symmetry endo-bipolar generator
sympathetic
s. chain
s. nervous system (SNS)
s. nervous system activity
s. projection
s. response to vasodilation
s. sphincter constrictor reflex
symphyseal bar
symphysis
pubic s.
s. pubis
symptom
alcohol-induced gastrointestinal s.
chronic functional gastrointestinal s.
s. control
head s.
s. index
intradialytic s.
irritative s.
postcibal s.
prodromal s.
s. score
s. sensitivity index
s. severity index (SSI)
target s.
symptomatic
s. fluid gain
s. gallstone
s. varicocele
symptomatology
chronic functional s.
symptom-free
Syms tractor
Synalar
synaptic transmission
synaptogenesis
synchondroseotomy
SYNCHRON CX-5, CX-7
automated analyzer
synchronous
s. adenomas
s. bladder reconstruction
s. inferior cavography
s. lesion
s. neonatal torsion
s. polyp
s. superior cavography
s. urinary tract infection

syncope
defecation s.
Synder drain
syndrome
abdominal muscle deficiency s.
acquired immunodeficiency s.
(AIDS)
acute flank pain s.
Addison s.
adrenogenital s.
adult respiratory distress s.
afferent loop s.
Alagille s.
Alcock s.
Allen-Masters s.
Alport s.
anorexia-cachexia s.
anterior abdominal wall s.
anterior cord s.
anterior rib impingement s.
anticardiolipin antibody s.
anti-müllerian derivative s.
antiphospholipid s.
Apert s.
apple-peel bowel s.
Arias s.
Asherson s.
asplenia s.
autoimmune deficiency s.
bacterial overgrowth s.
Banti s.
Barrett s.
Bartter s.
basal cell nevus s.
Bassen-Kornzweig s.
Bearn-Kunkel-Slater s.
Beckwith-Wiedemann s.
Behçet s.
bent nail s.
Bernard-Sergent s.
Bernard-Soulier s.
Bessauds-Hilmand-Augier s.
blind loop s.
blue diaper s.
blue rubber-bleb nevus s.
blue rubber nevus s.
Boerhaave s.

Bouveret s.
bowel bypass s.
Brennemann s.
brown bowel s. (BBS)
Budd-Chiari s.
Bürger-Grütz s.
buried bumper s.
Burnett s.
cafe coronary s.
Canada-Cronkhite s.
cancer family s.
carcinoid s.
Caroli s.
Carpenter s.
Carter-Horsley-Hughes s.
cast s.
cauda equina s.
caudal regression s.
cerebrohepatorenal s.
CHARGE s.
Chilaiditi s.
cholestatic s.
chronic intestinal ischemic s.
chronic intestinal pseudo-
obstruction s.
Clarke-Hadfield s.
Cohen s.
colonic pseudo-obstruction s.
colonic solitary ulcer s.
colorectal cancer s.
Conn s.
constipation predominant
irritable bowel s.
Courvoisier-Terrier s.
couvade s.
Cowden s.
CREST s.
Cri-du-Chat s.
Crigler-Najjar s.
Cronkhite-Canada s.
CRST s.
Cruveilhier-Baumgarten s.
Cushing s.
Danbolt-Closs s.
Dejerine-Sottas s.
Denys-Drash s.
descending perineum s.

NOTES

563

syndrome *(continued)*
dialysis disequilibrium s.
dialysis encephalopathy s.
diencephalic s.
DiGeorge s.
Down s.
Drash s.
Dubin-Johnson s.
Dubin-Sprinz s.
dumping s.
Eagle-Barrett s.
Edwards s.
Ehlers-Danlos s.
encephalotrigeminal s.
eosinophilic gastroenteritis s.
familial polyposis s.
Fancon-De Toni-Debre s.
Fanconi s.
Felty s.
female urethral s.
Fitz-Hugh and Curtis s.
Flood s.
flu-like s.
Fraley s.
frequency-urgency-pain s.
functional bowel s.
Gardner s. (GS)
gas-bloat s.
gastrointestinal
  immunodeficiency s.
gastrojejunal loop
  obstruction s.
GAVE s.
gay bowel s.
Gee-Herter-Heubner s.
Gianotti-Crosti s.
Gilbert s.
glucagonoma s.
Goodpasture s.
Gopalan s.
Gorlin s.
Gorlin basal cell nevus s.
Guillain-Barré s.
Hadefield-Clarke s.
Hadju-Cheney acroosteolysis s.
Hanot-Chauffard s.
Hartnup s.
HELLP s.
hematuria-dysuria s.
hemolytic-uremic s. (HUS)
hepatorenal s.,
  hepatonephoric s. (HRS)

hereditary flat adenoma s.
  (HFAS)
Hermansky-Pudlak s.
Heyde s.
Hinman s.
Hinman-Allen s.
Horner s.
Howel-Evans s.
hypertensive lower esophageal
  sphincter s.
iatrogenic immunodeficiency s.
idiopathic hypereosinophilic s.
  (IHES)
idiopathic nephrotic s.
ileocecal s.
impaired regeneration s. (IRS)
infantile nephrotic s.
inflammatory bowel s. (IBS)
inhibitory s.
inspissated bile s.
inspissated sump s.
irritable bowel s. (IBS)
irritable colon s.
irritable gut s.
isolated retained antrum s.
Ivemark s.
Jadassohn s.
Jamaican vomiting s.
jejunal s.
Job s.
Joubert s.
Kallmann s.
Katayama s.
Kawasaki s.
Kearns-Sayre s. (KSS)
Klinefelter s.
Koenig s.
Koro s.
Korsakoff s.
Kunkel s.
Ladd s.
late dumping s.
Laubry-Soulle s.
Laurence-Moon-Bardet-Biedl s.
Laurence-Moon-Biedl s.
Lesch-Nyhan s.
levator s.
levator ani s.
locker room s.
Lucey-Driscoll s.
Lyell s.
lymphadenopathy s. (LAS)
lymphoproliferative s.

Lynch s.
Lynch s. I
Lynch s. II
Mad Hatter s.
Maffucci s.
malabsorption s.
maldigestion/absorption s.
malignant B-cell s.
malignant carcinoid s.
Mallory-Weiss s.
Mallory-Weiss mucosal s.
Marfan s.
massive bowel resection s.
Mayer-Rokitansky s.
Meckel-Gruber s.
meconium plug s.
megacystic s.
megacystis-megaureter s.
megacystitis-microcolon-intestinal
  hypoperistalsis s.
megasigmoid s.
Meigs s.
Melkersson-Rosenthal s.
MEN s.
MEN I s.
metastatic carcinoid s.
microscopic colitis s.
milk-alkali s.
mind-bladder s.
minimal-change nephrotic s.
minimal-lesion nephrotic s.
Mirizzi s.
Mosse s.
mucocutaneous pigmentation of
  Peutz-Jeghers s.
Muir-Torre s.
müllerian duct derivation s.
multiple endocrine neoplasia s.
  (MENS)
multiple hamartoma s.
myoclonus-opsoclonus s.
narcotic bowel s.
nephritic s.
nephrotic s.
Neu-Laxova s.
neurocutaneous s.
Noonan s.

obesity hypoventilation s.
  (OHS)
Ochoa s.
Ogilvie s.
Oldfield s.
Osler-Weber-Rendu s.
ovarian hyperstimulation s.
ovarian overstimulation s.
ovarian remnant s.
ovarian vein s.
overlap s.
pancreatic cholera s.
pancreaticohepatic s.
paraneoplastic s.
Paterson-Brown-Kelly s.
Paterson-Kelly s.
Pearson marrow-pancreas s.
pelvic floor s.
Pento-X s.
pericolic membrane s.
perihepatitis s.
persistent müllerian duct s.
Peutz-Jeghers s.
pharyngeal pouch s.
Plummer-Vinson s.
Polhemus-Schafer-Ivemark s.
POLIP s.
polyposis s.
polysplenia s.
postcholecystectomy s. (PCS)
postcolonoscopy distention s.
postfundoplication s.
postgastrectomy s.
postpolypectomy coagulation s.
post-thrombotic s.
postvagotomy s.
Potter s.
Prader-Willi s.
primary antiphospholipid s.
s. of primary biliary cirrhosis
primary pseudo-obstruction s.
prune-belly s.
pseudo-obstruction s.
pseudopancreatic cholera s.
puborectalis s.
Rapunzel s.
Reichmann s.

S

NOTES

syndrome *(continued)*
Reiter s.
renal Fanconi-like s.
Rendu-Olser-Weber s.
respiratory distress s.
restless leg s.
retained antrum s.
Reye s.
right ovarian vein s.
Riley-Day s.
Robinow s.
Roger s.
Rokitansky-Kuster-Hauser s.
Rotor s.
Roux stasis s.
runting s.
Sandifer s.
sea-blue histiocyte s.
secondary pseudo-obstruction s.
segmental colonic adenomatous
  polyposis s.
Sertoli-cell-only s.
short-bowel s.
short-gut s.
Shwachman s.
Shwachman-Diamond s.
sicca s.
Sipple s.
Sjögren s. (SS)
sleep apnea s.
small-stomach s.
Smith-Lemli-Opitz s.
solitary rectal ulcer s. (SRUS)
solitary ulcer s.
somatostatinoma s.
spastic bowel s.
spastic pelvic floor s.
sphincteric disobedience s.
splenic agenesis s.
splenic flexure s.
Sprinz-Dubin s.
Sprinz-Nelson s.
stagnant s.
stagnant loop s.
stasis s.
Stauffer s.
steakhouse s.
Stein-Leventhal s.
steroid-resistant nephrotic s.
Stevens-Johnson s. (SJS)
Stewart-Treves s.
stiff-man s.
stress-related erosive s.

Sturge-Weber s.
sulfone s.
sump s.
superior mesenteric artery s.
  (SMAS)
Swyer s.
Takayasu s.
terminal reservoir s.
testicular feminization s.
tethered-cord s. (TCS)
Thorn s.
three week sulfasalazine s.
Torres s.
toxic shock s.
transurethral resection s.
tremor-nystagmus-ulcer s.
triad s.
Trousseau s.
TUR s.
Turcot s.
Turner s.
urethral s.
urethritis s.
urge s.
urofacial s.
vanished testis s.
vanishing bile duct s.
vascular steal s.
VATER s.
Verner-Morrison s.
Vinson s.
von Hippel-Lindau s.
vulvar vestibulitis s.
wasting s.
watery diarrhea s.
Watson-Alagille s.
Welt s.
Wermer s.
Wernicke s.
Wernicke-Korsakoff s.
Wiskott-Aldrich s.
Wolfram s.
Youssef s.
ZE s.
Zellweger s.
Zieve s.
Zollinger-Ellison s. (ZES)
synechia, pl. **synechiae**
synechiae
penile s.
synectenterotomy
Synectics
S. computer program

S.-Dantec Flo-Lab II
  uroflowmeter
S.-Dantec UD1000
  uroflowmeter
S. 6000 digital pH-meter
  meter
synergism
  in vitro s.
Synergist vacuum erection device
synergy
Syn-Optics video image splitter
synovial fluid
Synthamin amino acid solution
synthase
  citrate s.
  nitric oxide s. (iNOS, NOS)
synthesis
  albumin s.
  collagen s.
  DNA s.
  focal collagen s.
  hepatocyte protein s.
  hormone-stimulated cAMP s.
  impaired lecithin s.
  mucosal prostaglandin s.
  prostaglandin s.
  protein s.
synthesizer
  deoxyribonucleic acid s.
synthetase
  nitric oxide s.
synthetic
  s. 5-channel, water-perfused
    motility catheter
  s. mesh
  s. vascular graft
**Synthetics dual-channel, solid state
  digitrapper**
Synthroid
syphilis
  gastric s.
  primary s.
  secondary s.
  tertiary s.
syphilitic
  s. gastritis
  s. hepatitis

syringe
  Arrow Raulerson s.
  Asepto irrigation s.
  aspiration s.
  Fortuna s.
  LeVeen s.
  LeVeen inflation s.
  Lewy s.
  Luer-Lok s.
  motor s.
  Neisser s.
  piston-type s.
  s. shield
  Storz s.
  Toomey s.
  tuberculin s.
  Wolff s.
syrosingopine
syrup
  Calcidrine s.
  ipecac s.
system
  Abbott Lifeshield needleless s.
  Advantx digital s.
  AJCC/UICC staging s.
  alimentary s.
  Alliance integrated inflation s.
  Amplatz TractMaster s.
  anomalous arrangement of
    pancreaticobiliary ductal s.
    (AAPBDS)
  antigen-antibody s.
  Arndorfer capillary perfusion s.
  Arndorfer pneumohydraulic
    capillary infusion s.
  Arrow UserGard injection
    cap s.
  ASAP Stacker automated
    multi-sample biopsy s.
  autonomic nervous s. (ANS)
  Balthazar grading s.
  Bard Urolase fiber laser s.
  Baxter Interline IV s.
  Beamer injection stent s.
  Bergkvist grading s.
  BICAP hemostatic s.
  Bitome bipolar s.

S

NOTES

system *(continued)*
B-lymphocyte s.
Bookwalter retractor s.
Boyarsky symptom scoring s.
Bruel-Kjaer 1846 ultrasound s.
Can-Opt dual lumen ERCP s.
Cell Analysis s. (CAS)
Cell Soft s.
central nervous s. (CNS)
classification s.
Clave needleless s.
close suction drainage s.
coculture s.
collecting s.
collection s.
Comhaire grading s.
computer-aided diagnostic s.
computer-controlled sedation
infusion s.
computerized image analysis s.
Conseal one-piece continent
colostomy s.
contact-tip laser s.
Contrajet ERCP contrast
delivery s.
core-cut s.
COSTART s.
C-Trak surgical guidance s.
cytochrome P450 s.
Dantec 12-channel Urocolor
Video s.
Dantec Etude s.
Dantec Menuet s.
data aquisition s.
digestive s.
Digitrapper Mark II pH
monitoring s.
DIONEX 2000 s.
DNA Sequencing S.
Doppler Quantum color
flow s.
double-antibody sandwich s.
Drake-Willock delivery s.
Drake-Willock peritoneal
dialysis s.
drug carrier s.
Dual-Port s.
ductal s.
Dukes staging s.
Dumon-Gilliard
endoprosthesis s.
EdGr s.
Edmondson grading s.

e10 electrosurgery s.
endocrine s.
endoscopic s.
enteric nervous s. (ENS)
ErecAid vacuum s.
fiberTome s.
Fisher Capillary S.
free-beam laser s.
French Pharmacovigilance s.
Fresenius volumetric dialysate
balancing s.
Fujinon SP-501 sonoprobe s.
Fujinon video endoscopy s.
GastrograpH ambulatory pH
monitoring s.
Gleason staging s.
Grabstald (Memorial) staging s.
hemi-Kock s.
high-affinity, low-capacity s.
high-affinity, sodium-dependent
phosphate transport s.
H+/K+ ATPase enzyme s.
human cytochrome P-450
enzyme s.
hydraulic capillary infusion s.
Hydra Vision IV urology s.
illumination s.
immune s.
Impact lithotriptor s.
IMx PSA s.
InjecAid s.
Innova home incontinence
therapy s.
integrated automatic stone-tissue
detection s.
intensified radiographic
imaging s. (IRIS)
International Biomedical Mode
745-100 microcapillary
infusion s.
intrarenal collecting s.
Ivac Needleless IV S.
Jackson staging s.
Jewett-Whitmore Cancer
Staging S.
Johns Hopkins prostate cancer
grading s.
Joyce-Loebl Magiscan image
analysis s.
Kleinert Safe and Dry panty
and pad s.
Kretz ultrasound s.
Laparolift s.

laparoscopic retraction s.
Laser CHRP rigid fiber
  scope s.
Lorad StereoGuide prone breast
  biopsy s.
low-affinity, high-capacity s.
low-compliance perfusion s.
low-pressure venous s.
Madsen-Iversen scoring s.
Mayo grading s.
mechanical assist s.
Mediflex MD-7 endoscopic
  video s.
Medstone IRIS s.
Medstone STS lithotripsy s.
Menuet Compact
  urodynamics s.
Menuet urodynamics s.
MetaFluor s.
Microvasive Ultraflex
  esophageal stent s.
mitochondrial ethanol
  oxidase s.
MOP-Videoplan
  morphometric s.
Morganstern
  aspiration/injection s.
Mui Scientific pressurized
  capillary infusion s.
Mycotrim triphasic culture s.
myeloperoxidase-H2O2-halide s.
NA+-linked cotransport s.
NA+ transport s.
needleless s.
Olympus CLV-series
  fiberoptic s.
Olympus endoscopy s. (OES)
Olympus EVIS color computer
  chip s.
Olympus OSP fluorescence
  measuring s.
Olympus video endoscopy s.
Olympus video urology
  procedure s.
Omni-LapoTract support s.
One Action, Stent
  Introduction S. (OASIS)

optical s.
optical multichannel analyzer s.
Ortho Diagnostic S.
O'Sullivan scoring s.
Palco enuretic alarm s.
pancreaticobiliary ductal s.
pelvicaliceal s.
Performa ultrasound s.
pneumohydraulic capillary
  infusion s.
Polachrome 35-mm slide s.
portal venous s.
Prempree modification
  staging s.
probenecid-inhibited organic
  anion transport s.
Proscan ultrasound imaging s.
Prostathermer prostatic
  hyperthermia s.
Pugh-Child scoring s.
Ranson grading s.
R&D S.
Redy hemodialysis s.
Relay suture delivery s.
renal kallikrein-kinin s.
renal preservation perfusion s.
renin-aldosterone s.
renin-angiotensin s. (RAS)
renin-angiotensin-aldosterone s.
  (RAAS, RAS)
reproductive s.
reticuloendothelial s.
rod-lens s.
Sacks-Vine PEG s.
Safe and Dry panty and
  pad s.
sentry s.
SF-9 baculovirus-insect cell s.
single-action pumping s.
  (SAPS)
slide s.
Soehendra catheter s.
SOLO-Surg Colo-Rectal self-
  retaining retractor s.
stent and vent s.
Stoller scoring s.

S

NOTES

system *(continued)*
stone-tissue recognition s.
(STR)
Storz multifunction valve
trocar/cannula s.
STS lithotripsy s.
Suretys panty s.
Surgi-PEG replacement
gastrostomy feeding s.
Sydney S.
sympathetic nervous s. (SNS)
testosterone transdermal s.
Top Notch automated
biopsy s.
Tricomponent Coaxial S.
(TCS)
triple-lumen perfused
catheter s.
Ultrabag S.
UltraPak enteral closed
feeding s.
Ultra Twin bag s.
Ultra Y-set s.
United States Renal Data S.
(USRDS)
Universal sheath s.
urocyte diagnostic cytometry s.
Uro-jet delivery s.
Uro-Pak s.
Urotract x-ray s.
Urovision ultrasound
imaging s.
VET-CO vacuum s.
Visick gastric cancer
grading s.
Visick grading s.

Vision Sciences VSI 2000
flexible sigmoidoscope s.
Welch Allyn video
endoscopy s.
Whitmore-Jewitt prostate cancer
classification s.
Wolf delivery s.
wolffian müllerian ductal s.
Y-set s.
Z-stent esophageal
endoprosthesis s.
systematic sextant biopsy
systemic
s. amyloidosis
s. arterial pressure
s. effect
s. endotoxemia
s. hypertension
s. hypotension
s. lupus erythematosus (SLE)
s. lupus erythematosus
vasculitis
s. MAP
s. mast cell disease
s. mastocytosis
s. mercury intoxication
s. sclerosis
s. vascular resistance
s. vascular resistance index
(SVRI)
s. venodilation
systolic
s. click
s. murmur
Systral
Szabo test

T

T cell
T cell-specific protein
T connector
T effector cell
T lymphocyte
T tube
T tubogram
TA30 stapler
TA55 stapler
TA90-BN stapler
TAA
   tumor-associated antigen
table
   Dornier Urotract cysto t.
   floating t.
   Gerhardt t.
   lithotripsy t.
   Maquet endoscopy t.
   sigmoidoscopy t.
   Urodiagnost x-ray t.
tablet
   Asacol delayed-release t.
   Dairy-Ease chewable t.
   delayed-release t.
   Nullo deodorant t.'s
   wax-matrix t.
TAC
   total abdominal colectomy
tachycardia
   sinus t.
   ventricular t.
tachygastria
tachykinin
tachykinin-bombesin family
tachyoddia contractions
tachypnea
tacked down
tacrolimus
tactile probe
tactor
Tactyl 1 glove
tadpole-like appearance
TAE
   total abdominal evisceration
   transcatheter arterial embolization
Taenia
   T. saginata
   T. solium

taenia (*var. of* tenia)
   t. mesocolica
   t. omentalis
   t. strip of soft tissue
   t.'s of Valsalva
tag
   edematous t.
   external skin t.
   hemorrhoidal t.
   H-shaped tilt t.
   perianal skin t.
   perineal skin t.
   sentinel t.
   skin t.
TAG-72 glycoprotein
Tagamet
   T. HB
tagged red blood cell bleeding scan
tagging stitch
tail of pancreas
TA instrument
Tait law
Takayasu
   T. arteritis
   T. disease
   T. syndrome
takedown
   bilateral ureterostomy t.
   colostomy t.
   t. of colostomy
   t. of pelvic sling procedure
taking down of adhesions
TAL
   thick ascending limb
talc embolus
talin
TALT
   testicular adrenal-like tissue
Tamm-Horsfall
   T.-H. mucoprotein (THM)
   T.-H. protein
tamoxifen
tampon
   Corner t.
   t. tube
tamponade, tamponage
   balloon t.
   balloon tube t.
   esophageal balloon t.
   esophagogastric t.

571

tamponade *(continued)*
    esophagogastric balloon t.
    (EGBT)
    ferromagnetic t.
    Sengstaken-Blakemore t.
    tract t.
tamponing, tamponment
Tanagho
    T. bladder flap urethroplasty
    T. bladder neck reconstruction
tandem
    t. colonoscopy (TC)
    T.-ERA PSA immuenzymetric
    assay
    t. PSA assay
    t. PSA test
    T.-R assay kit
    T.-R PSA assay
    T. thin-shaft transureteroscopic
    balloon dilatation catheter
    T. XL triple-lumen ERCP
    cannula
tangential
    t. biopsy
    t. colonic submucosal injection
Tangier disease
tangle of hemorrhoidal veins
Tanner
    T. operation
    T. stage
tannex
    bisacodyl t.
tannic acid
tantalum-182
TAP
    T. gene
tap
    abdominal t.
    t. 2 peptide transporter gene
    peritoneal t.
    t. water enema
tape
    adhesive t.
    appendectomy t.
    Cath-Secure t.
    circular t.
    laparotomy t.
    Mersilene t.
    Montgomery t.
    polyester-reinforced Dacron t.
    umbilical t.

tapered
    t. needle
    t. rubber bougie
tapered-tip hydrophilic-coated push
    catheter
taper-tip catheter
tapeworm
    beef t.
    Cestoda t.
    fish t.
    pork t.
Taq polymerase
tarda
    porphyria cutanea t. (PCT)
tardive
    forme t.
target
    t. cell
    t. lesion
    t. localization
    t. symptom
targeting
    selective t.
tarry black stool
tartrate
    metoprolol t.
taste perversion
tattoo
    colonic t.
    colonoscopic t.
    endoscopic t.
    endoscopic four-quadrant t.
    India ink t.
    submucosal t.
tattooing
    four-quadrant t.
taurine
    t. cotransporter (TCT)
    t. cotransporter mRNA
    selenium-labeled homocholic
    acid conjugated with t.
    (SeHCAT)
taurocholate
    sodium t.
    t. solution
taurocholic acid
tauroglycocholate
    sodium t.
taurolithocholate
taxis
Taylor
    T. gastric balloon
    T. gastroscope

T-bar retractor
TBI
    total body irradiation
TBM
    thin basement membrane
TBMD
    thin basement membrane disease
TBN
    total body nitrogen
TBW
    total body water
TC
    tandem colonoscopy
    therapeutic concentrate
    transhepatic cholangiography
Tc
    technetium
⁹⁹ᵐTc, Tc-99m
    technetium-99m
        ⁹⁹ᵐTc albumin colloid
        ⁹⁹ᵐTc albumin microsphere
        ⁹⁹ᵐTc DMSA
        ⁹⁹ᵐTc-DMSA scan
        ⁹⁹ᵐTc-DPTA
            technetium-99m
                diethylenetriamine penta-
                ascetic acid
        ⁹⁹ᵐTc DTPA aerosol
        ⁹⁹ᵐTc-DTPA renal scan
        ⁹⁹ᵐTc GHP
        ⁹⁹ᵐTc HDP
        ⁹⁹ᵐTc HIDA
        ⁹⁹ᵐTc HMPAO-labeled
        leukocyte scan
        ⁹⁹ᵐTc IDA scan
        ⁹⁹ᵐTc-labeled Amberlite pellet
        ⁹⁹ᵐTc labeled stannous
        methylene diphosphonate
        ⁹⁹ᵐTc lidofenin
        ⁹⁹ᵐTc MAA
        ⁹⁹ᵐTc-MAA
            technetium-99m
                macroaggregated albumin
        ⁹⁹ᵐTc-MAG-3 isotope
        ⁹⁹ᵐTc MDP
        ⁹⁹ᵐTc MDP nuclear isotope
        bone scan

        ⁹⁹ᵐTc medronate
        ⁹⁹ᵐTc pentetic acid
        ⁹⁹ᵐTc pertechnetate scan
        ⁹⁹ᵐTc pertechnetate scintigraphy
        ⁹⁹ᵐTc PIPIDA
        ⁹⁹ᵐTc polyphosphate
        ⁹⁹ᵐTc PYP
        ⁹⁹ᵐTc RBC bleeding scan
        ⁹⁹ᵐTc SC
        ⁹⁹ᵐTc sodium pertechnetate
        ⁹⁹ᵐTc SPP
        ⁹⁹ᵐTc sulfur colloid scan
        ⁹⁹ᵐTc tin colloid
TCA
    tricarboxylic acid
    trichloroacetic acid
    trihydrocoprostanic acid
TCCA
    transitional cell cancer of the bladder
Tc DTPA, I125 Iodothalamate
T-cell
    T-c. adhesion
    T-c. crossmatch
    T-c. cytotoxic therapy
    T-c. depletion by elutriation
    T-c. epitope
    T-c. line
    T-c. lymphoma
    T-c. receptor (TCR)
    T-c. second messengers
T-cell-dependent mechanism
TcHIDA scan
Tc-99m (*var. of* ⁹⁹ᵐTc)
T-C needle holder
TCR
    T-cell receptor
TCS
    tethered-cord syndrome
    Tricomponent Coaxial System
⁹⁹ᵐTc-SC
    technetium-99m sulfur colloid
Tc-sulfur colloid
TCT
    taurine cotransporter
        TCT mRNA
TDU
    time domain ultrasound

T

NOTES

TDX fluorescent polarization immunoassay
TE
   tracheoesophageal
TEA
   tetraethylammonium
tear
   capsular t.
   diastatic serosal t.
   t. duct
   esophageal t.
   gastric t.
   Mallory-Weiss t.
   mesenteric t.
   mucosal t.
   pharyngoesophageal t.
   serosal t.
teardrop poikilocyte
tearing
   t. pain
   t. through
t-EASE software
TEBS
   transurethral electrical bladder stimulation
TEC
   transpapillary endoscopic cholecystotomy
Technescan, TechneScan
   T. MAG-3
technetium (Tc)
   t. radionuclide scan
   t. scan
technetium-labeled
   t.-l. autologous red blood cell scan
   t.-l. red blood cell scan
technetium-99m (^{99m}Tc, Tc-99m)
   t. diethylenetriamine pentaacetic acid scan
   t. diethylenetriamine penta-ascetic acid (^{99m}Tc-DPTA)
   t. IDA scan
   t. macroaggregated albumin (^{99m}Tc-MAA)
   t. mercaptoacetythiglycine isotope
   t. pertechnetate
   t. pyrophosphate-tagged RBC
   t. red cell scintigraphy
   t. sulfur colloid (^{99m}Tc-SC)
   t. Tc-99m iminodiacetic acid
   t. Tc-99m tin colloid (^{99m}Tc tin colloid)
technique
   abdominal pressure t.
   anthrone colorimetric t.
   antireflux ureteral implantation t.
   autosuture t.
   balloon-catheter and basket-retrieval t.
   Barcat t.
   Belt t.
   bench surgical t.
   bladder neck preserving t.
   blind t.
   Brackin t.
   Campbell t.
   Cape Town t.
   capsule flap t.
   cavernosal alpha blockade t.
   cell separation t.
   cephalo-trigonal t.
   clam-shell t.
   closed tubule fixation t.
   Coffey t.
   Cohen cross-trigonal t.
   continuous pull-through t.
   Coomassie brilliant blue t.
   cup-patch t.
   Davis t.
   Deisting t.
   Denis Browne urethroplsty t.
   de novo needle knife t.
   double-balloon t.
   double-folded cup-patch t.
   double-staple t.
   dufourmentel t.
   Eisenberger t.
   en bloc t.
   end-to-side vasoepididymostomy t.
   enuresis alarm t.
   esophageal banding t.
   extra-anatomical renal revascularization t.
   extraction balloon t.
   extravesical ureteral reimplantation t.
   finger fracture t.
   first-line screening t.
   flap t.
   flip-flap t.

flow microsphere florescent immunoassay t.
Gaur balloon distension t.
Gil-Vernet t.
Gittes t.
Glenn-Anderson t.
Goldschmiedt t.
gold seed implantation t.
Goodwin t.
Goodwin-Hohenfellner t.
Goodwin-Scott t.
Graves t.
gravimetric t.
Grimelius t.
guidewire and mini-snare t.
Hale colloidal iron t.
Hartmann reconstruction t.
Hauri t.
Higgins t.
hippuran clearance t.
histocytochemical t.
Hofmeister t.
hot biopsy t.
immunoperoxidase staining t.
^{111}In-leukocyte t.
intradermal tattooing t.
invagination t.
Jaboulay-Doyen-Winkleman t.
Jones-Politano t.
Keystone t.
King t.
Kock t.
laparoscopic colposuspension t.
laser welding t.
lateral bending t.
lateral window t.
Lazarus-Nelson t.
Leach t.
Leadbetter modification t.
Leadbetter tunneling t.
LeDuc t.
Lich t.
Lich extravesical t.
Lich-Gregoire t.
3-loop t.
Marlex plug t.
Masson trichrome staining t.

Mathieu t.
Meares-Stamey t.
membrane catheter t.
Menghini t.
Michal II t.
microtransducer t.
micro-tubulotomy t.
Mitrofanoff t.
Mitrofanoff continent urinary diversion t.
modified Cantwell t.
modified Hassan open t.
modified Sacks-Vine push-pull t.
Moh microsurgery t.
morcellation t.
muscle-splitting t.
nasovesicular catheter t.
needle-knife t.
Norfolk t.
onlay t.
onlay-tube-onlay urethroplasty t.
Orandi t.
orbital exenteration gastroscopic access t.
over-the-wire t.
Palomo t.
Paquin t.
patch t.
pelviscopic clip ligation t.
perfusion hypothermia t.
Pólya t.
Ponsky t.
Ponsky pull or guidewire insertion t.
prograde t.
pull-through t.
push t.
push-pull T t.
quadrant sampling t.
Quantikine quantitative immunoenzymatometric sandwich t.
Quartey t.
rapid pull-through esophageal manometry t.
reconstruction t.

T

NOTES

575

technique *(continued)*
relaxation t.
retrograde t.
RPT t.
Russell t.
Saeed t.
salvage cytology t.
Seldinger t.
sextant t.
Silber t.
Singer-Blom endoscopic
tracheoesophageal puncture t.
sleeve t.
"sling and blanket" t.
"smiley face" knotting t.
Somatome DRG CT t.
sperm micro-aspiration
retrieval t. (SMART)
spiral CT t.
split cuff nipple t.
split and roll t.
SPT t.
station-pull-through t.
station pull-through esophageal
manometry t.
stent through wire mesh t.
Stiegmann-Goff t.
stimulated gracilis
neosphincter t.
strip biopsy resection t.
superior mesenterorenal
bypass t.
surface cooling t.
"Swiss roll" embedding t.
Thomas t.
Thompson t.
tube-within-tube t.
turn-and-suction t.
Turnbull t.
turn and suction biopsy t.
two-layer open t.
Ussing chamber t.
ventral bending t.
videofluoroscopic t.
video transurethral resection t.
Vim-Silverman t.
Warwick and Ashken t.
Wickham t.
xenon-washout t.
Young t.
Young-Dees t.
technology
endoscopic t.

fiberoptic instrument t.
polymerase chain reaction t.
Technomed Sonolith 3000
lithotriptor
teeth
carious t.
full-surface micro mesh t.
interdigitating t.
TEF
tracheoesophageal fistula
Teflon
T. catheter
T. ERCP cannula
T. injector
T. nasobiliary drain
T. nasobiliary tube
T. sheath
T. sling rectopexy
T. tube
Teflon-coated
T.-c. Dacron suture
T.-c. guidewire
Tegaderm dressing
Tegretol
Tektronix digital oscilloscope
telangiectasia
calcinosis cutis, Raynaud
phenomenon, esophageal
motility disorder,
sclerodactyly, and t. (CREST)
calcinosis cutis, Raynaud
phenomenon, sclerodactyly,
and t. (CRST)
duodenal t.
gastrointestinal t.
hepatic t.
hereditary hemorrhagic t.
(HHT)
Osler-Weber-Rendu t.
radiation t.
spider t.
t. syndrome
telangiectatic
t. angioma
t. vessel
Telepaque contrast medium
telerobotic assisted laparoscopic
surgery
telescope
forward-viewing t.
t. heater

Hopkins t.
Wolff t.
teletherapy
orthovoltage t.
television
t. camera
t. monitor
t. photography
Telfa dressing
Teline
telopeptide
TEM
transanal endoscopic microsurgery
transmission electron microscopy
TEM transanal endoscopy
Temaril
temazepam
temperature
core t.
hand t.
laser t.
template
Mick prostate t.
Seyd-Neblett perineal t.
Tempo
temporary
t. end colostomy
t. enteroscope
t. loop ileostomy
temporomandibular arthritis
TEN
total enteral nutrition
Vivonex TEN
Tena pouch
Tenascin
tenascin
Tenckhoff
T. catheter
T. 2-cuff catheter
T. peritoneal catheter
tender
t. liver
t. thyroid
tenderness
adnexal t.
ballottement t.

bony t.
cervical motion t.
costochondral t.
costovertebral angle t. (CVAT)
diffuse t.
exquisite t.
facial t.
focal t.
frontal t.
localizing t.
palpation t.
paracervical t.
percussion t.
point t.
popliteal t.
rebound t.
rectal t.
salivary t.
scrotal t.
sinus t.
spinous t.
thyroid t.
uterine t.
tendon
conjoined t.
tenesmic
tenesmus
rectal t.
Tenex
tenia, taenia, pl. **teniae**
t. coli
t. libera
t. omentalis
teniamyotomy
teniasis
somatic t.
teniposide (VM-26)
Ten-K
Tenoretic
Tenormin
TENS
transcutaneous electrical nerve
stimulation
tense ascites
tensile strength
Tensilon test

T

NOTES

tension
t. pneumoperitoneum
t. pneumothorax
tension-free anastomosis
tent
Silon t.
tenting
baseline t.
Tenuate
Tepanil
Tepoxalin
teratoca
teratogenesis
medication t.
teratogenic medicine
teratoma
benign cystic t.
gastric t.
sacrococcygeal t.
testicular t.
t. testicular cancer
teratospermia
terazosin
terbutaline
t. hepatitis
teres
ligamentum t.
terfenadine
terlipressin
terminal
t. anuria vesical dialysis
t. bile duct
t. colostomy
t. hematuria
t. ileal disease
t. ileal pouch
t. ileal resection
t. ileitis
t. ileostomy
t. ileum
t. ileum intubation (TII)
t. ileus
t. inner medullary collecting
duct
t. reservoir syndrome
terminus
amino t.
duodenal t.
intrapapillary t.
terodiline
terrifying pain
Terry fingernail sign

tertiary
t. contraction
t. radicle
t. syphilis
tertium
Clostridium t.
Terumo
T. dialyzer
T. Glidewire
T. guidewire
T. hydrophilic guidewire
Terumo/Meditech guidewire
**Terumo-Radiofocus hydrophilic
polymer-coated guidewire**
terzosin
Tesberg esophagoscope
Tesla
T. GE Signa whole body
scanner
T. Signa MR imager
test
acid clearance t. (ACT)
acid hemolysis t.
acidification of stool t.
acid perfusion t.
acid reflux t.
Albarran t.
alkaline phosphatase t.
alkalinization t.
Allen t.
ALT t.
Ames t.
aminopyrine breath t.
angiotensin II infusion t.
anorectal t.
anti-SLA t.
Apt-Downey alkali
denaturation t.
argentaffin reaction t.
artificial erection t.
AST t.
ASTRA profile t.
β_2 t.
Baermann stool t.
balloon expulsion t.
basal secretory flow rate t.
belt t.
bentiromide t.
bentonite flocculation t.
Bernstein acid perfusion t.
betazole stimulation t.
bile acid breath t.
bile acid tolerance t.

bile solubility t.
bilirubin t.
binder t.
Bio-Enzabead t.
Bio-Gen urine t. strip
Biotel home screening t.
BioWhittaker assay t.
bolus challenge t.
Bonney t.
Bors ice water t.
Bourne t.
Boyle and Goldstein saline t.
Bozicevich t.
t. breakfast
breath t.
breath hydrogen t.
breath pentane t.
Breslow-Day t.
brushing urea breath t.
BSFR t.
BSP t.
BT-PABA t.
CA 19-9 t.
calcium infusion t.
Campylobacter t. (CLOtest)
Campylobacter-like organism t.
 (CLOtest)
cancelling A's t.
captopril t.
carbon 14 urea breath t.
carbon-14 urinary excretion t.
Casoni skin t.
^{13}C-bicarbonate breath t.
CBP t.
C-cholyl-glycine breath t.
CEA t.
cephalin-cholesterol
 flocculation t.
^{14}C-glycocholate breath t.
C-glycocholic acid breath t.
chew-and-spit t.
Chiron RIBA HCV t.
Chi-square t.
cholecystokinin t.
C of Hosmer-Lemeshow
 ratio t.
citrate t.

C-lactose t.
Clinitest stool t.
clonidine suppression t.
CO_2 breath t.
Cochran-Mantel-Haenszel t.
Cohen t.
cold-stress t.
colonic transit t.
Coloscreen Self-t.
complement fixation t.
complete blood count t.
copper-binding protein t.
cornflake esophageal motility t.
cough stress t.
Cox-Mantel t.
CP t.
creatinine t.
C&S t.
CSF glutamine t.
^{14}C-triolein breath t.
culture and sensitivity t.
C-urea breath t. (UBT)
deferoxamine mesylate
 infusion t.
Desican t.
dexamethasone suppression t.
diabetes home screening t.
differential renal function t.
differential ureteral
 catheterization t.
dilute Russell viper venom t.
 (DRVVT)
t. dinner
direct immunobead t.
direct immunofluorescence t.
 (DIF-test)
Doppler flow t. (DFT)
duodenal secretin t. (DST)
D-xylose absorption t.
edrophonium t.
Einhorn string t.
Eitest MONO P-II t.
Ektachem slide t.
ELISA t.
ELISA-I t., ELISA-1 t.
ELISA-II t., ELISA-2 t.
ELISA-III t., ELISA-3 t.

T

NOTES

test *(continued)*
Enzygnost antiHIV 1+2 t.
Enzymun t.
erythrocyte sedimentation
rate t.
esophageal acid infusion t.
esophageal function t.
FDL t.
fecal alpha₁antitrypsin t.
fecal fat t.
fecal leukocyte count t.
fecal occult blood t. (FOBT)
fingerprick latex
agglutination t.
Fisher exact probability t.
Fisher two-tailed exact t.
Fishman-Doubilet t.
FlexSure HP t.
fluorescein dilaurate t.
fluorescein string t.
Fouchet t.
Francis t.
GAP t.
gastric accommodation t.
gastric emptying t.
gastric secretory t.
gastrin stimulation t.
Gastroccult t.
GGT t.
Ghedini-Weinberg serologic t.
Glahn t.
Glazyme APF-EIA-TEST t.
glucose t.
Glucose analyzer II t.
glutamine t.
Gluzinski t.
glycopyrrolate t.
glycyltryptophan t.
Gmelin t.
graded esophageal balloon
distention t.
Graham t.
Gram stain of stool t.
Grassi t.
Gross t.
guaiac t.
Guenzberg t.
Ham t.
Hamel t.
Hanger t.
Harrison spot t.
hatching t.
Hay t.

H2 breath t.
HCV EIA 20 t.
hepatitis C virus enzyme
immunoassay
HCV ELISA t.
Hematest t.
HemaWipe t.
Hemoccult t.
Hemoccult II t.
Hemoccult Sensa t.
HemoQuant fecal blood t.
HemoSelect t.
Hepaplastin t.
Herzberg t.
Histalog stimulation t.
histamine t.
Hollander t.
home screening t.
HomeSelect t.
24-hour ambulatory pH t.
72-hour fecal fat t.
24-hour gastric acidity t.
Howard t.
hpfast rapid urease t.
5-HT t.
human lymphocyte
chromosomal aberration t.
Hunt t.
Huppert t.
hydrochloric acid t.
hydrogen breath t.
ice water t.
ICG t.
iliopsoas t.
immunological fecal occult
blood t. (IFOBT)
independent-t t.
[111]indium-labeled autologous
leukocyte t.
intraductal secretin t. (IDST)
intraesophageal acid t.
intraesophageal pH t.
intravenous secretin t.
Inutest t.
invasive diagnostic t.
Jacoby t.
Jatrox *Helicobacter pylori* t.
Javorski t.
Jolles t.
Kapsinow t.
Kashiwado t.
Kato t.
Kelling t.

Kinberg t.
Krokiewicz t.
Kruskal-Wallis t.
lactose breath hydrogen t.
lactose tolerance t.
lactulose hydrogen breath t.
LAP t.
Lapides t.
last-generation serologic
  ELISA t.
latex fixation t.
LDH t.
Leo t.
leucine aminopeptidase t.
levulose t.
Ligat t.
lipase t.
litmus milk t.
liver function t. (LFT)
log-rank t.
Lundh t.
Lüttke t.
Macdonald t.
Machado-Guerreiro t.
MacLean t.
magnetic susceptibility t.
Maly t.
Mann-Whitney t.
Mann-Whitney rank sum t.
Mantel-Haenszel t.
Mardi t.
Marechal-Rosen t.
Marshall t.
Marshall-Bonney t.
Marshall-Marchetti t.
Masset t.
McNemar ascites t.
t. meal
measurement t.
Meltzer-Lyon t.
methyl red t.
metyrapone stimulation t.
Mitscherlich t.
Mohr t.
monoethyl glycine xylidide
  liver function t.
morphine-neostigmine t.

Moynihan t.
Myers-Fine t.
Mylius t.
Nakayama t.
Nardi t.
N-benzoyl-L-tyrosyl-P-
  aminobenzoic acid
  excretion t.
NBT-PABA t.
Neukomm t.
nitrogen partition t.
noninvasive diagnostic t.
Normotest t.
number connection t.
obturator t.
one-hour office pad t.
one-minute endoscopy room t.
Oresus Potentest t.
PABA t.
Palmer acid t. for peptic ulcer
palmin t., palmitin t.
pancreatic secretory t.
PAP t.
Pap t.
PAS t.
peak secretory flow rate t.
Pearson $\chi 2$ t.
pentagastrin gastric secretory t.
pentagastrin infusion t.
pentagastrin provocative t.
pentagastrin stimulated
  analysis t.
Peptavlon stimulation t.
percutaneous pressure ureteral
  perfusion t.
perineal nerve terminal motor
  latency t.
periodic acid-Schiff t.
peritoneal equilibration t.
  (PET)
Pettenkofer t.
Phadebas angiotensin-I t.
phenoltetrachlorophthalein t.
phentolamine t.
physiologic reflux t. (PRT)
POA t.

NOTES

test *(continued)*
postage stamp penile tumescence t.
postcoital t.
posthoc t.
provocative t.
PSFR t.
psychometric t.
pudendal nerve terminal motor latency t.
PyloriScreen t.
Q-tip t.
qualitative fecal fat t.
quantitative fecal fat t.
Quick t.
Quidel-Quick-Vue H. pylori t.
Quinlan t.
Rabuteau t.
radioallergosorbent t. (RAST)
rapid serum amylase t.
rapid urease t.
Rapoport t.
reducing substances t.
Rehfuss t.
Reitan trail making t.
Reitman-Frankel t.
RIBA t.
RIBA-2 t.
rice-flour breath t.
Robinson-Kepler-Power water t.
rose bengal t.
Rosenbach-Gmelin t.
Rosenthal t.
Rotazyme t.
Russell viper venom t.
Saathoff t.
Sahli glutoid t.
Sahli-Nencki t.
saline t.
saline continence t.
saline load t.
Salkowski-Schipper t.
Salomon t.
santonin t.
Saundby t.
S-CCK-Pz t.
Scheffe-F t.
Schiff t.
Schilling t.
Schwartz t.
Scivoletto t.
secretin-CCK stimulation t.

secretin-pancreozymin stimulation t.
secretin provocation t.
secretin stimulation t.
SeHCAT t.
^{75}Se-labeled bile acid t.
serologic t.
serum amylase t.
serum iron t.
serum protein t.
serum RIBA-2 t.
Sgambati reaction t.
SGOT t.
SGPT t.
sham feeding t.
skinfold thickness t.
Smith t.
snap gauge t.
solid sphere t.
Spearman t.
split renal function t.
squeeze pressure profile of anal sphincter t.
Stamey t.
standard acid reflux t. (SART)
star construction t.
stereognost-3-α enzymatic t.
stimulated gastric secretion t.
stimulation t.
Stokvis t.
Stoll t.
StoneRisk citrate t.
StoneRisk cystine t.
StoneRisk diagnostic t.
stool cytotoxin t.
stool electrolyte t.
stool osmolality t.
stool osmotic gap t.
Strassburg t.
string t.
Stypven time t.
sugar t.
sweat t.
Szabo t.
tandem PSA t.
TIBC t.
tilt t.
TMT t.
Töpfer t.
Torquay t.
total fecal weight t.
total iron binding capacity t.
Trail t.

trail making t. (TMT)
transferrin t.
transmucosal electrical
  potential t.
triceps skinfold thickness t.
triolein C 14 breath t.
Trousseau t.
Tukey t.
Tuttle t.
twelve-hour home pad t.
two-stage triolein t.
two-tailed Fisher t.
two-tailed McNemar t.
t. type
Tyson t.
Udranszky t.
Uffelmann t.
Ultzmann t.
urea nitrogen t.
urease t.
Urecholine supersensitivity t.
uric acid t.
van den Bergh t.
ViraPap HPV dot blot
  hybridization t.
vitamin B_{12} absorption t.
Voges-Proskauer t.
von Jaksch t.
Wagner t.
washout t.
water-gurgle t.
water recovery t.
water-sipping t.
water-soluble contrast
  esophageal swallow t.
whiff t.
Whipple t.
Whipple triad t.
Whitaker pressure-perfusion t.
Wilcoxon-Gehar t.
Wilcoxon matched-pairs signed-
  rank t.
Wilcoxon rank sum t.
Winckler t.
Witz t.
Woldman t.
Wolff-Junghans t.

Woolf t.
x2 t.
xylose absorption t.
xylose tolerance t.
Yang Pros-Check PSA t.
Zappacosta t.

testalgia
testectomy
testes (*pl. of* testis)
testicle
  cryptorchid t.
testicular
  t. adrenal-like tissue (TALT)
  t. adrenal rest
  t. androgen-binding protein
  t. carcinoma
  t. descent
  t. feminization syndrome
  t. implant
  t. lymphoma
  t. mass
  t. pain
  t. prosthesis
  t. seminoma
  t. swelling
  t. teratoma
  t. torsion
  t. tubular adenoma
testing
  anorectal physiology t.
  histocompatibility t.
  lactose hydrogen breath t.
  (LHBT)
  penile injection t.
  physiology t.
  salivary t.
  urea breath t.
  viability t.
testis, pl. **testes**
  abdominal t.
  appendix t.
  t. cancer
  cryptorchid t.
  descensus aberrans t.
  descensus paradoxus t.
  dystopia transversa externa t.
  dystopia transversa interna t.

NOTES

T

testis *(continued)*
  ectopia t.
  t. ectopia
  ectopic t.
  high t.
  inverted t.
  irritable t.
  mediastinum t.
  mottled t.
  movable t.
  obstructed t.
  peeping t.
  t. redux
  retained t.
  rete t.
  retractile t.
  solitary t.
  torsion t.
  torsion of t.
  tunica albuginea t.
  undescended t.
testitis
Testoderm
testopathy
testosterone
  basal t.
  t. cyprionate
  t. enanthate
  t. repressed prostate message-2
    (TRPM-2)
  serum t.
  t. transdermal system
  t. transdermal therapy
Test-Size orchidometer
test-yolk buffer cryopreservation
  agent
tetanus globulin
tetany
  gastric t.
tether circulating leukocyte
tethered-bowel sign
tethered-cord
  t.-c. release
  t.-c. syndrome (TCS)
tethering
  t. of mucosa
Tetracap
tetrachloride
  carbon t.
tetracycline
  bismuth, metronidazole, t.
    (BMT)
  t. HCl

tetradecapetide
tetradecyl sulfate
tetradotoxin
tetraethylammonium (TEA)
Tetragastrin-NS
tetrahydrocannabinol (THC)
tetrahydrochloride
  3',3-diaminobenzidine t.
tetrahydrozoline
tetralogy
  Fallot t.
Tetram
tetramethyl a⁻ɴɪ ɪonium chloride
tetrapalmitate
  maltose t.
tetraplegia
tetrodotoxin (TTX)
  TTX t.
tetroxide
  osmium t.
Tevdek suture
Texas
  T. style two-piece catheter
  T. trauma
texture
  heterogeneous t.
  homogeneous t.
T-fastener
  Brown-Mueller T.-f.
TGE
  transgastrostomic enteroscopy
TGF-β
  transforming growth factor β
TGF
  transforming growth factor
  tubuloglomerular feedback
  human recombinant TGF
TGF-α
  transforming growth factor α
TGF-β1
  transforming growth factor-β1
  TGF-β1 gene
TGF-β2
  transforming growth factor-β2
TGF-β3
  transforming growth factor-β3
TGHA
  thyroglobulin antibody
Thal
  T. esophageal stricture repair
  T. esophagogastroscopy
  T. esophagogastrostomy
  T. fundic patch operation

T. fundoplasty
T. stricturoplasty
T-half emptying
thalidomide
Thalitone
thallium-201
thallium poisoning
thamuria
thaw-mount radioautography
THC
  tetrahydrocannabinol
  transhepatic cholangiography
THE
  transhepatic embolization
Thiersch-Duplay repair
thenar eminence
theophylline
  t. clearance
  t. ethylenediamine
  t. level
  t. olamine enema
  t. toxicity
theory
  overflow t.
  set point t.
Thephorin
TheraCys
Theradex
Theralax
therapeutic
  t. angiography
  t. colonoscopy
  t. concentrate (TC)
  t. duodenoscope
  t. laparoscopy
  t. side-viewing duodenoscope
  t. upper endoscopy
  t. value
therapy
  ablative laser t.
  acid-suppression t.
  adjuvant drug t.
  adrenalin injection t.
  alpha interferon t.
  amoxicillin-tinidazole-
    ranitidine t.
  amphotericin B t.

androgen ablation t. (AAT)
androgen deprivation t.
antibiotic t.
anticholinergic medicine t.
anticoagulation t.
antilymphocyte t.
antimicrobial t.
antireflux t.
antisecretory t.
argon laser t.
autolymphocyte t.
Aza-Pred t.
balloon t.
balloon photodynamic t.
bile acid t.
biologic t.
biologic response modifier t.
bismuth-free triple t.
bubble t.
buprenorphine narcotic
  analgesic t.
chemoradiation t.
cholestyramine t.
clarithromycin triple t.
coagulative laser t.
combined chemoradiation t.
conformal radiation t.
continuous renal replacement t.
  (CRRT)
corticosteroid t.
cytokine t.
cytolytic t.
diclofenac analgesic t.
dilation t.
diltiazem t.
doxycycline-metronidazole-
  bismuth subcitrate triple t.
drug t.
endocrine t.
endoscopic t.
endoscopic hemostatic t.
endoscopic injection t.
endoscopic laser t.
endoscopic pancreatic t.
enterostomal t. (ET)
erythropoietin t.
esophageal photodynamic t.

T

NOTES

585

therapy *(continued)*
    ethanol injection t.
    external beam radiation t.
    external vacuum t.
    fluid replacement t.
    flutamide t.
    foscarnet t.
    gamma globulin t.
    gene-transfer t.
    H2-antagonist t.
    heater probe t.
    hemofiltration t. (HFT)
    hormonal t.
    H2-receptor antagonist t.
    immunomodulatory t.
    immunosuppressive t.
    injection t.
    instillation t.
    interferon t.
    International Association for
        Enterostomal T.
    interstitial photodynamic t.
    intracavernous t.
    intracavernous injection t.
    intracavitary radiation boost t.
    intracorporeal injection t.
    IV fluid t.
    ketoprofen analgesic t.
    laser t.
    medical t.
    methyl-tert-butyl ether t.
        (MTBE therapy)
    monoclonal antibody t.
    morphine narcotic analgesic t.
    MTBE t.
        methyl-tert-butyl ether therapy
    Nd:YAG laser t.
    neodymium:YAG laser t.
    nutritional t.
    omeprazole t.
    omeprazole-clarithromycin-
        amoxicillin t.
    palliative t.
    pancreatic enzyme
        replacement t.
    pancreatic intraluminal
        radiation t.
    PEI t.
        percutaneous ethanol injection
            therapy
    penile injection t.
    penile vein occlusion t.
    percutaneous embolization t.
    percutaneous ethanol
        injection t. (PEI therapy)
    phosphate binder t.
    photodynamic t. (PDT)
    photoradiation t.
    physiologic testosterone-
        replacement t.
    placebo t.
    polidocanol injection t.
    polyestradiol phosphate t.
    postoperative anticoagulation t.
    posttransplant
        immunosuppression t.
    preventive intravesical t.
    proton pump inhibition t.
    quadruple t.
    quatro t.
    radiation t.
    ranitidine t.
    rehydration t.
    renal replacement t.
    rescue t.
    saline injection t.
    salvage t.
    sandwich t.
    sandwich staghorn calculus t.
    sclerosing t.
    self-injection t.
    single-drug t.
    somatostatin t.
    somatostatin analogue t.
    somatostatin infusion t.
    steroid t.
    sucralfate t.
    surgical t.
    T-cell cytotoxic t.
    testosterone transdermal t.
    thermal t.
    three-dimensional conformal
        radiation t.
    thrombolytic t.
    transcatheter arterial
        embolization t.
    transurethral collagen
        injection t.
    triple t. (TT)
    tumor t.
    ultrasound-guided shock
        wave t.
    valproic acid t.
TheraSeed
Therasonics lithotriptor

Therma Jaw disposable hot biopsy forceps
thermal
  t. burn
  t. therapy
thermally active method
Thermex-II transurethral prostate heating device
thermobaric footprint
thermocoagulation
  heat probe t.
  KeyMed heater probe t.
  laser t.
thermocoagulator
  Olympus CD-Z-series heat probe t.
thermocycler
  Stratagene SCS-96 t.
thermo-disinfector
  endoscopic t.-d.
thermoexpandable stent
ThermoFlex thermotherapy unit
thermogenesis
thermography
  Primus transrectal t.
thermomechanical
thermometer
  air t.
  alcohol t.
  Celsius t.
  centigrade t.
  Fahrenheit t.
  gas t.
  oral t.
  rectal t.
  surface t.
thermoreceptor
thermotherapy
  microwave t.
  transurethral microwave t. (TUMT)
  water-induced t. (WIT)
Thermovac tissue pulverizer
thetaiotaomicron
  Bacteroides t.
thiabendazole
thiamine deficiency

thiazide
  t. diuretic
thiazide-induced hyponatremia
thick
  t. adhesion
  t. ascending limb (TAL)
  t. bile
thickened
  t. gallbladder wall
  t. nail
thickening
  apical t.
  mediastinal t.
  plaque-like t.
  submucosal t.
  wall t.
thickness
  esophageal wall t. (EWT)
  mucous gel t.
  triceps skinfold t.
thick-walled gallbladder
Thiersch
  T. anal incontinence operation
  T. procedure
  T. tube
Thiersch-Duplay
  T.-D. proximal tube procedure
  T.-D. tube graft
  T.-D. urethroplasty
thiethylperazine
thigh graft arteriovenous fistula
thihexinol
thin
  t. adhesion
  t. basement membrane (TBM)
  t. basement membrane disease (TBMD)
thin-layer chromatography (TLC)
thin-needle percutaneous cholangiogram
"thin shave" sectioning
thin-walled gallbladder
thiocyanate
  guanidine t.
thiol
  exogenous t.
  t. intermediate

T

NOTES

Thiola
Thioplex
thiopropazate
thioridazine
　　t. hydrochloride
Thiosulfil
thiotepa
thiothixene
thiourea-resorcinol method
thiphenamil
third generation lithotriptor
thirst fever
Thiry fistula
Thiry-Vella fistula (TVF)
THM
　　Tamm-Horsfall mucoprotein
Thomas technique
Thompson
　　T. capsule flap pyeloplasty
　　T. procedure
　　T. technique
thoracic
　　t. aortic pathology
　　t. aortorenal bypass
　　t. esophagus
　　t. fistula
　　t. inlet
　　t. kidney
　　t. stomach
thoracoabdominal
　　t. collateral vein
　　t. esophagogastrectomy
　　t. extrapleural approach
　　t. incision
　　t. intrapleural approach
　　t. retroperitoneal
　　　lymphadenectomy
thoracolaparotomy
thoracotomy
　　esophagectomy with t.
　　t. scar
Thorazine
Thorek
　　T. gallbladder forceps
　　T. gallbladder scissors
Thorek-Feldman gallbladder scissors
Thorek-Mixter gallbladder forceps
thorium
　　colloidal t.
　　t. dioxide
Thorn syndrome
Thorotrast contrast medium
thread-locking device

thread and streaks sign
threadworm
thready pulse
three-armed basket forceps
three-dimensional conformal
　　radiation therapy
three-drug regimen
three-finger grip
three-loop ileal pouch
three-pronged
　　t.-p. grasper
　　t.-p. grasping forceps
　　t.-p. polyp retriever
three-quarter circle electrode
three-way
　　t.-w. irrigating catheter
　　t.-w. stop-cock
three week sulfasalazine syndrome
threonine
threshold
　　t. of internal sphincter
　　pH t.
　　t. of rectal sensation
thrill
thrive
　　failure to t.
thrombectomy
thrombi (pl. of thrombus)
thrombin
　　t.-antithrombin III
　　bovine t.
　　t.-Keflin-sotredechol
　　t.-Keflin-sotredochal sclerosant
　　topical bovine t.
thrombin-antithrombin III complex
Thrombinar
thrombocytopenia
　　heparin-induced t. (HIT)
thrombocytopenic purpura
thrombocytosis
thromboelastography
thromboembolic
　　t. disease
　　t. event
thromboendarterectomy
　　renal t.
Thrombogen
thrombolytic
　　t. agent
　　t. therapy
Thrombomodulin
thrombophlebitis

thrombosed
t. external hemorrhoid
t. internal and external hemorrhoid
thrombosis
arterial t.
bilateral renal vein t.
bland t.
glomerular microvascular t.
hepatic vein t.
inferior vena cava t.
intracapillary t.
intravascular t.
mesenteric arterial t.
mesenteric venous t.
nonocclusive mesenteric t.
peripheral venous t.
portal vein t. (PVT)
renal vein t.
silent t.
SMV t.
splenic vein t.
venous t.
thrombospondin
thrombotic
t. microangiopathy
t. thrombocytopenic purpura (TTP)
thromboxane
thromboxane A$_2$
thrombus, pl. thrombi
bile t.
mural t.
retrocecalis tumor t.
through
tearing t.
through-the-scope (TTS)
t.-t.-s. balloon
t.-t.-s. balloon dilation
t.-t.-s. balloon removal
t.-t.-s. bougie
t.-t.-s. dilation
t.-t.-s. dilator
t.-t.-s. injection needle
thrush
oral t.

thumbprinting
t. of mucosa
t. sign
thymic
t. EC
t. hypoplasia
thymidine
thymidine-labeling index
thymocyte NA+/H+ exchanger
thymosin
thymus
thymus-derived
t.-d. cell
t.-d. lymphocyte
thyreoideus impar plexus
thyroglobulin antibody (TGHA)
thyroid
t. autoimmunity
t. disease
t. hormone
t. hormone serum concentration
medullary carcinoma of t. (MCT)
t. microsomal antibody
t. nodule
tender t.
t. tenderness
thyroiditis
autoimmune t.
Hashimoto t.
thyroid-stimulating hormone level
thyromegaly
thyrotoxicosis
thyrotropin-releasing hormone
thyroxine
free t. (FT4)
TI
tubulointerstitial
TIBC
total iron binding capacity
TIBC test
ticarcillin
ticklish
Ti-Cron suture
ticrynafen-induced jaundice
tidal drainage

T

NOTES

tie
free t.
stick t.
Tycron t.
tie-over dressing
Tigan
tight
t. abdomen
t. adhesion
t. Nissen repair
tight-junction protein
TII
terminal ileum intubation
TIL
tumor infiltrating lymphocytes
tilt
t. stitch
t. test
Timberlake obturator
time
abdominopelvic orocecal
transit t.
activated partial
thromboplastin t.
activated thromboplastin t.
bleeding t.
calyceal filling t.
clotting t.
coagulation t.
cold ischemia t. (CIT)
colonic transit t.
dextrinizing t.
t. domain ultrasound (TDU)
doubling t.
duration t.
esophageal transit t.
explosive doubling t.
gastric bleeding t. (GBT)
gastric emptying t.
gastric transit t.
mean input t. (MIT)
mean resistance t. (MRT)
mean transit t.
nucleation t. (NT)
orocecal transit t. (OCTT)
partial thromboplastin t. (PTT)
pH holding t.
post-UUO t.
preservation t.
pro-t.
prothrombin time
prothrombin t. (pro-time, PT)

prothrombin time/partial
thromboplastin t. (PT/PTT)
PSA doubling t.
radionuclide esophageal
emptying t.
Russell viper venom t.
skin bleeding t. (SBT)
transit t.
warm ischemia t.
time-activity curve
Timecaps
Levsinex T.
time/concentration curve
time-dependent variable
Timentin
double-dose I.V. T.
single-dose I.V. T.
time-of-flight mass spectometry
(TOFMS)
timer
video t.
Tim knot
timolol
TIMP (-1, -2, -3)
tissue metalloproteinase
TIN
tubulointerstitial nephritis
tincture
t. of belladonna
t. of benzoin
Tindal
tinidazole
tinkling bowel sounds
tiopronin
tip
Buie rectal suction t.
Buie suction t.
filiform t.
Frazier suction t.
open end flo-thru radiopaque t.
papillary t.
sharp-edged t.
spleen t.
suction t.
tulip t.
vessel t.
TIPS
transjugular intrahepatic
portosystemic shunt
occlusion of TIPS
TIPS procedure
stenosis of TIPS

TIPSS
  transjugular intrahepatic
    portosystemic stent shunt
tissue
  acinar t.
  adipose t.
  ampullary granulation t.
  t. approximation
  chromaffin t.
  cicatricial t.
  t. coagulation
  connective t.
  cryostat t.
  t. culture
  t. culture assay
  t. cushion
  extraperitoneal t.
  exuberant granulation t.
  fatty t.
  fibroadipose t.
  fibroelastic t.
  fibrous t.
  t. forceps
  formalin-fixed t.
  t. fusion
  gastrointestinal-associated
    lymphoid t. (GALT)
  t. glue
  gut-associated lymphoid t.
    (GALT)
  hilar structure scar t.
  t. kallikrein
  lipoma-like t.
  lipomatous t.
  t. metalloproteinase (TIMP (-1, -
    2, -3))
  t. morcellator
  mucosa-associated lymphoid t.
    (MALT)
  t. necrosis
  necrotic t.
  neoplastic t.
  nonviable t.
  paracancerous t.
  paraffin-embedded t.
  parenchymal t.
  penoid t.

  periadvential t.
  perinephric t.
  periprostatic t.
  t. plasminogen activator (TPA)
  t. polypeptide antigen
  redundant sac t.
  t. renewal
  t. resistance
  t. sampling
  soft t.
  t. spectrum analyzer TS-200
  splenic t.
  subcutaneous t.
  taenia strip of soft t.
  T. Tek-II cryostat
  testicular adrenal-like t.
    (TALT)
tissue-specific gene expression
**tissue-type plasminogen activator (t-
  PA)**
Titan
  T. endoprosthesis
  T. stent
titanium
  t. clip
  t. urethral stent
titanous chloride
titer
  anti-HSV IgM Ab t.
  antineutrophil cytoplasmic
    antibody t.
  antistreptolysin-O t.
  ELISA t.
  end-point dilution t.
  IgM-HEV antibody t.
  viral serologic t.
Titralac Plus
TLA
  transperitoneal laparoscopic
    adrenalectomy
TLC
  thin-layer chromatography
TLN
  transperitoneal laparoscopic
    nephrectomy
**T-lymphocyte-mediated cytotoxic
  reaction**

T

NOTES

TMP/SMX
  trimethoprim and sulfamethoxazole
  trimethoprim/sulfamethoxazole
  lomefloxacin TMP/SMX
TMT
  trail making test
  TMT test
TNF
  tumor necrosis factor
  TNF α-gene
TNFα
  tumor necrosis factor α
TNF-α assay
TNM
  T. carcinoma classification
  T. classification of carcinoma
  T. system for tumor staging
TNTC
  too numerous to count
tobramycin
tocodynamometer
  guard-ring t.
  Nihon t.
Tocosamine
Todd cirrhosis
TOFMS
  time-of-flight mass spectometry
Tofranil
Tofranil-PM
toilet
  peritoneal t.
tolazoline
  t. hydrochloride
tolbutamide-induced cholestasis
Toldt
  line of T.
  white line of T.
tolerance
  glucose t.
  oral t.
Tolerex
  T. feeding solution
Tolmetin
tolnaftate
toluidine
  t. blue
  t. blue stain
Toma sign
Tomenius gastroscope
Tom Jones suture
Tomocat
tomodensitometric examination

tomography
  computed t. (CT)
  computerized t. (CT)
  contrast-enhanced computed t.
  single-photon emission
    computerized t. (SPECT)
  ultrafast computerized t.
Tomudex
tone
  anal sphincter t.
  bowel t.
  cardiac sympathovagal t.
  lower esophageal sphincter t.
  renal vascular t.
  sphincter t.
tongs
tongue
  bifid t.
  black hairy t.
  t. deviation
  fissured t.
  geographic t.
  hairy t.
  t. movement
  mucosal t.
  smoker's t.
  swollen t.
tongue-shaped villus
tonic
  t. contraction
  t. neck
Tonkaflo pump
tonometry
tonsil
  t. clamp
  t. forceps
  orange-colored t.
  t. sucker
tonsillar enlargement
tonsillectomy
Toomey syringe
too numerous to count (TNTC)
toothed tissue forceps
TOPA
  topical oropharyngeal anesthesia
Töpfer test
topical
  t. anesthesia
  t. anesthetic
  t. antibiotic
  t. betamethasone
  t. bovine thrombin

t. oropharyngeal anesthesia
(TOPA)
t. treatment
t. Xylocaine
**topical oropharyngeal anesthesia
(TOPA)**
topic effect
Topicort
**Top Notch automated biopsy
system**
topogram
balloon t.
topography
scintigraphic balloon t.
topotecan
topromide
Toradol
Torbot faceplate
Torecan
Torek
T. operation
T. orchiopexy
Toronto-Western catheter
Torquay test
torque
translation of t.
t. wire
torquing of scope
torrential hemorrhage
Torres syndrome
torsemide
torsion
adnexal t.
t. of appendage
biliary tract t.
extravaginal t.
gallbladder t.
t. of gallbladder
intravaginal t.
penile t.
perinatal t.
spermatic cord t.
synchronous neonatal t.
testicular t.
t. of testis
t. testis
torso crease

torticollis
tortuous
t. esophagus
t. venous ectasia
Torulopsis
T. glabrata
torulopsis infection
torus palatinus
Toshiba
T. ERVF 1A video floppy
recorder
T. micro-endoprobe
T. Sal 38B real-time
ultrasonography
T. Sonolayer SSA250A
transrectal ultrasonography
T. TCE-M-series colonoscope
T. video endoscope
Totacillin
total
t. abdominal colectomy (TAC)
t. abdominal evisceration
(TAE)
t. bilateral vagotomy
t. bilirubin
t. body irradiation (TBI)
t. body nitrogen (TBN)
t. body water (TBW)
t. bowel rest
t. colonoscopy
t. cystectomy
t. enteral nutrition (TEN)
t. fecal weight test
t. gastrectomy
t. gastric wrap
t. glutathione content
t. hematuria
t. hemolytic complement
t. infarction
t. internal reflection
t. iron binding capacity
(TIBC)
t. iron binding capacity test
t. lymphocyte (TTL)
t. pancreatectomy
t. parenteral alimentation
t. parenteral nutrition (TPN)

NOTES

total *(continued)*
  t. pelvic exenteration
  t. perineal prostatectomy
  t. predicted return
  t. prostatoseminal vesiculectomy
  t. protein
  t. protein concentration
  t. scrotectomy
  t. slit pore length
  t. transurethral resection of prostate (T-TURP)
total enteral nutrition (TEN)
total iron binding capacity (TIBC)
totalis
  varicosis coli t.
totally stapled restorative proctocolectomy (TSRPC)
touch
  t. cytology
Touch preparation
Touhy-Borst connector
tourniquet
  double loop t.
  Dupuytren t.
  Gill renal t.
  t. occlusion
  Rumel t.
  single loop t.
towel clip
toxemia
  hepatic t.
  t. of pregnancy
toxic
  t. cirrhosis
  t. colitis
  t. diarrhea
  t. dilation of colon
  t. gastritis
  t. glomerulopathy
  t. hepatitis
  t. megacolon
  t. metabolite
  t. shock syndrome
  t. steatosis
toxicity
  acute hepatic t.
  aluminum t.
  ammonia t.
  chloroform t.
  chlorzoxazone t.
  cyclosporine t.
  direct tubular t.
  octreotide-induced hepatic t.

  progressive t.
  protein-mediated tubular t.
  renal t.
  theophylline t.
  vitamin A t.
toxicosis
toxicum
  erythema t.
toxigenic bacterium
toxin
  t. A
  t. assay
  botulinum t.
  cholera t.
  t. exposure
  industrial t.
  occupational t.
  shiga-like t.
  vacA t.
toxin-mediated intestinal secretion
toxins
  Coley t.
toxocariasis
Toxoplasma gondii
toxoplasmosis
TPA
  12-O-tetradecanoylphorbol-13-acetate
  tissue plasminogen activator
    phorbol ester TPA
      phorbol ester 12-O-tetradecanoylphorbol-13-acetate
t-PA
  tissue-type plasminogen activator
TPH
  transrectal prostatic hyperthermia
TPN
  total parenteral nutrition
trabecular
  t. bone fracture
  t. structure
trabecular/sinusoidal pattern
trabeculated bladder
trabeculation
Trabucco double balloon catheter
trace-gas analysis
tracer
  focal accumulation of t.
tracheal deviation
trachelocystitis
tracheoesophageal (TE)

t. fistula (TEF)
t. junction
tracheostomy
trachomatis
    Chlamydia t.
tracing
    Narco Bio-Systems MMS 200
    physiograph t.
Tracker catheter
tracks
    radial suture t.
tract
    alimentary t.
    biliary t.
    digestive t.
    t. dilation
    fistulous t.
    gastrointestinal t. (GIT)
    genitourinary t.
    GI t.
    hepatic outflow t.
    ileal inflow t.
    ileal outflow t.
    infected t.
    intestinal t.
    intramural fistulous t.
    needle t.
    oro-respiratory t.
    outflow t.
    pancreaticobiliary t.
    perineal sinus t.
    portal t.
    safe-gastrocutaneous fistulous t.
    sinus t.
    t. tamponade
    T-tube t.
    upper gastrointestinal t.
traction
    cephalad t.
    t. diverticulum
    t. suture
tractor
    Lowsley t.
    Syms t.
    Young prostatic t.
trafficking
    membrane t.

trail
    t. making test (TMT)
Trail test
training
    pelvic muscle t.
    pubococcygeal muscle t.
trait
    X-linked recessive t.
Tral
tramazoline
tram-line calcification
Trandate
tranexamic acid
tranquilizer
transabdominal
    t. hydrocolonic sonography
    t. repair
    t. scan
transaminase
    glutamate pyruvate t. (GLPT)
    glutamic-oxaloacetic t. (GOT)
    glutamic-pyruvic t. (GPT)
    serum glutamic-oxaloacetic t.
    (SGOT)
    serum glutamic-pyruvic t.
    (SGPT)
transampullary
transanal
    t. endoscopic microsurgery
    (TEM)
    t. endoscopic microsurgical
    resection
transarterial
    t. embolization
    t. perfusion cooling
trans-blotting cell
transcapillary
    t. diffusion
    t. escape rate
    t. hydrostatic pressure gradient
transcarbamylase
    heterozygous ornithine t.
    (HOTC)
transcatheter
    t. arterial embolization (TAE)
    t. arterial embolization therapy
    t. embolotherapy

T

NOTES

transcatheter *(continued)*
  t. hepatic arterial embolization
  t. perfusion
  t. splenic arterial embolization
  (TSAE)
  t. treatment
  t. variceal embolization
transcriptase
  avian myeloblastosis virus
  reverse t.
  t. polymerase chain reaction
  assay
  reverse t. (RT)
transcription factor AP1
transcutaneous
  t. biopsy
  t. electrical nerve stimulation
  (TENS)
  t. nerve
  t. registration
  t. sonogram endoscope
  t. ultrasonography
  t. ultrasound
  t. ultrasound imaging
Transderm-Nitro
transducer
  antral pressure t.
  Bruel-Kjaer axial t.
  electromagnetic flow t.
  Elema-Siemens AB pressure t.
  Gould pressure t.
  linear array t.
  linear 35-Mhz t.
  LSC 7000 curved array t.
  3.5-10 MHz curved array t.
  Nellcor Durasensor adult
  oxygen t.
  P23b Statham pressure t.
  piezoelectric t.
  pressure t.
  Sensor Medics pressure t.
  Siemens Endo-P endodrectal t.
  solid-state pressure t.
  Soreson pressure t.
  Spectramed t.
  Statham external t.
  strain gauge t.
  transrectal multiplane 3-
  dimensional t.
  ultrasound t.
  volume displacement t.
transductal cystodigestive diversion

transduction
  downstream signal t.
  receptor and signal t.
transduodenal
  t. approach
  t. drainage
  t. endoscopic decompression
  t. sphincteroplasty
  t. sphincterotomy
transection
  t. and devascularization
  operation
  esophageal t.
  Sugiura esophageal variceal t.
transendoscopic
  t. electrocoagulation
  t. laser photocoagulation
  t. sphincterotomy
transesophageal
  t. endoscopy
  t. ligation
  t. ligation of varix
transfer
  t. dysfunction
  t. dysphagia
  gamete intrafallopian t. (GIFT)
  unidirectional t.
transferase
  aspartate t.
  choline acetyl t. (ChAT)
  gamma-glutamyl t. (GGT)
  glucuronyl t.
  glutathione t.
  phenylethylamine N-methyl t.
  (PNMT)
transferrin
  t. saturation
  serum t.
  t. test
transformary mass
transformation
  blastoid t.
  Eadie-Hofstee t.
  giant cell t. (GCT)
  neoplastic t.
  nodular t.
transforming
  t. growth factor (TGF)
  t. growth factor α (TGF-α)
  t. growth factor β (TGF-β)
  t. growth factor-β1 (TGF-β1)
  t. growth factor-β2 (TGF-β2)
  t. growth factor-β3 (TGF-β3)

transfuse
transfusion
    autologous t.
    blood t.
    donor-specific t. (DST)
    intraoperative t.
    intraoperative autologous t.
    peritoneal t.
    platelet t.
    postoperative t.
    postoperative autologous t.
    type-specific blood t.
transfusion-associated hepatitis
transfusion-related chronic liver
  disease
transgastric
    t. cholangiogram
    t. drainage
    t. esophageal bougienage
    t. fine-needle-aspiration biopsy
    t. ligation
    t. plication
transgastrostomic enteroscopy (TGE)
transglomerular hydrostatic
  filtration pressure
transglutaminase
trans-Golgi network
transhepatic
    t. antegrade biliary drainage
      procedure
    t. biliary drainage
    t. biliary stent
    t. cholangiogram
    t. cholangiography (TC, THC)
    t. embolization (THE)
    t. portacaval shunt
    t. portal venous sampling
    t. portography
    t. vascular resistance
transhiatal blunt esophagectomy
transient
    t. cholangitis
    t. gastroparesis
transileostomy manometry
transilluminate
transillumination

transilluminator
    UV t.
transistor
    ion-sensitive field effect t.
transit
    gastrointestinal t.
    mean colonic t. (MCT)
    slow colonic t.
    t. time
transitional
    t. cell
    t. cell cancer of the bladder
      (TCCA)
    t. cell carcinoma
    t. epithelium
    t. zone
    t. zone biopsy
transition suture
transitory block
transjugular
    t. intrahepatic portosystemic
      shunt (TIPS)
    t. intrahepatic portosystemic
      stent shunt (TIPSS)
    t. liver biopsy
    t. portal venography
translation of torque
translumbar inferior vena cava
  catheter
transluminal
    t. ultrasonography
transmembrane
    t. electrical potential difference
    t. hydraulic pressure
    t. protein
    t. signal
    t. β-subunit
transmesenteric plication
transmission
    blood-borne t.
    t. electron microscopy (TEM)
    fecal t.
    fecal-oral t.
    horizontal t.
    oral t.
    synaptic t.
    vertical t.

T

NOTES

transmitter
  NANC inhibitory t.
  nonadrenergic noncholinergic
    inhibitory t.
transmucosal electrical potential test
transmural
  t. approach
  t. burn
  t. colitis
  t. drainage
  t. fibrosis
  t. hydrostatic pressure gradient
  t. ileocolitis
transnasal
  t. bile duct catheterization
  t. endoscopy
  t. pancreatico-biliary drain
Transorb-HN
Transorb-STD
transpapillary
  t. approach
  t. biopsy
  t. cannulation
  t. catheterization
  t. cystopancreatic stent
  t. drain
  t. drainage
  t. endoscopic cholecystotomy
    (TEC)
  t. endoscopic endoprosthesis
  t. insertion of self-expanding
    biliary metal stent
transparent elastic band ligating
device
transpeptidase
  gamma-glutamyl t. (GGTP)
  glutamyl t. (GTP)
transperineal
  t. palladium 103
  t. seed implant
transperitoneal
  t. laparoscopic adrenalectomy
    (TLA)
  t. laparoscopic nephrectomy
    (TLN)
  t. laparoscopic
    nephroureterectomy
transplant
  acute rejection of liver t.
  allogenic kidney t.
  cadaveric t.
  cadaveric renal t.

  heart t.
  heart-kidney t.
  hypercholesterolemic cadaveric
    renal t.
  kidney t.
  liver t.
  living donor t.
  t. nephrectomy
  orthotopic liver t. (OLT)
  pancreas-kidney t.
  t. rejection
  renal t.
  t. renal artery stenosis (TRAS)
  split-liver t.
transplantation
  anhepatic stage of liver t.
  bone marrow t. (BMT)
  heart t.
  hepatocyte t.
  kidney t.
  liver t.
  organ t.
  orthotopic t.
  orthotopic liver t. (OLT)
  pancreaticoduodenal t.
  piggyback liver t.
  renal t.
  SPK t.
  xenograft t.
transplantectomy
transplanted cancer
transport
  cation t.
  fluid t.
  lymphatic t.
  nephron t.
  peritoneal membrane t.
  peritoneal solute t.
  sodium t.
  solute t.
  urine t.
transporter
  glucose t.
  low-affinity t.
  polarized glucose t.
transposition
  buttonhole preputial t.
  gastric t.
  gluteus maximus t.
  penoscrotal t.
transpubic incision
transpyloric tube

transrectal
t. multiplane 3-dimensional transducer
t. probe
t. prostatic hyperthermia (TPH)
t. scan
t. sonography
t. staging
t. ultrasonography (TRUS)
t. ultrasound
t. ultrasound-guided-sextant biopsy
t. ultrasound scanning (TRUS)
t. ultrasound staging
transscrotal
transseptal orchiopexy
transsexual
t. surgery
transsexualism
transsphincteric anal fistula
transthoracic
t. esophagectomy
t. resection of esophageal carcinoma
transthyretin
transudative ascites
transureteroureteral anastomosis
transureteroureterostomy (TUU)
transurethral
t. ablative prostatectomy
t. balloon dilation
t. collagen injection therapy
t. electrical bladder stimulation (TEBS)
t. evaporation of prostate (TUEP)
t. grooving of prostate
t. incision of prostate (TUIP)
t. laser incision of the prostate
t. microwave thermotherapy (TUMT)
t. needle ablation (TUNA)
t. prostatectomy
t. rectal ultrasound (TRUS)
t. resection (photometer, TUR,

TUR-Cue photometer, TUR-Cue photometer)
t. resection (of) bladder tumor (TURBT)
t. resection of prostate (TURP)
t. resection syndrome
t. sphincterotomy
t. ultrasound (TRUS)
t. ultrasound-guided laser-induced prostatectomy
t. unroofing
t. ureterorenoscopy (URS)
t. vaporization of prostate (TUVP)
transurothelial permeability
transvaginal
t. Burch procedure
t. urethrolysis
transvenous
t. liver biopsy
t. perfusion
transversalis fascia
transverse
t. colectomy
t. colon
t. colostomy effluent
t. duodenotomy
t. image
t. incision
t. loop
t. process
t. resection
t. semilunar skin incision
t. sonogram
t. testicular ectopia
t. umbilical line
t. view
transverse-loop rod colostomy
transversostomy
transvesical scan
transwell
cell culture t.
Tranxene
tranylcypromine
trap
Endodynamics suction polyp t.
trapezoid method

T

NOTES

trapping
    penoscrotal t.
TRAS
    transplant renal artery stenosis
Tratner catheter
Traube semilunar space
trauma
    autoerotic rectal t.
    bile duct t.
    blunt t.
    blunt abdominal t.
    blunt liver t.
    blunt pancreatic t.
    colorectal t.
    diaphragmatic hernial t.
    duodenal t.
    esophageal t.
    external t.
    foreign body t.
    t. of gallbladder
    gallbladder t.
    gastric t.
    hepatic t.
    homosexual rectal t.
    iatrogenic t.
    iatrogenic pancreatic t.
    liver t.
    pancreatic t.
    penetrating t.
    penetrating abdominal t.
    penetrating pancreatic t.
    perineal impact t.
    rectal t.
    renal t.
    small intestine t.
    splenic t.
    Texas t.
TraumaCal enteral feeding
Traum-Aid HBC enteral feeding
traumatic
    t. appendicitis
    t. corporeal veno-occlusive
      dysfunction
    t. diaphragmatic hernia
    t. grasping forceps
    t. inflammation
    t. lesion
    t. locking grasper
    t. masturbation
    t. orchitis
    t. proctitis
    t. renal mass
    t. rupture

Travamulsion fat emulsion solution
Travasol amino acid
Travasorb
    T. Hepatic Diet
    T. HN powdered feeding
    T. MCT liquid feeding
    T. MCT supplement
    T. Renal Diet
    T. STD liquid feeding
travelers'
    t. chemoprophylaxis
    t. diarrhea
tray
    Urine Meter Foley t.
trazodone
treatment
    acorn t.
    adjuvant t.
    alpha interferon t.
    alternate-day t.
    amoxicillin/omeprazole t.
    anabolic steroid t.
    anoplasty t.
    anti-*Helicobacter pylori* t.
    behavioral t.
    t. channel
    cholecystectomy t.
    chronic anoplasty t.
    corticosteroid t.
    dialytic t.
    elemental diet t.
    endoscopic t.
    esophageal dilation t.
    t. failure
    famotidine maintenance t.
    foscarnet t.
    Gelfoam particles transarterial
      embolization t.
    glucocorticoid t.
    interferon t.
    intracavernosal injection t.
    intralesional t.
    lipiodol transarterial
      embolization t.
    maintenance t.
    mercury bougienage t.
    mitomycin transarterial
      embolization t.
    t. morbidity
    neoadjuvant antiandrogenic t.
    oxandrolone t.
    photocoagulation t.
    prophylactic t.

prophylactic antibiotic t. (PAT)
prostatic thermal t.
t. protocol
rectovaginal surgical t.
self-bougienage t.
serotonin antagonist t.
shock wave t.
suppression t.
topical t.
transcatheter t.

tree
biliary t.
cannulation of the biliary t.
hepatobiliary t.
phylogenetic t.

trefoil
t. deformity
t. peptide

trehalose

Treitz
T. hernia
ligament of T.

Trélat stools

tremor
resting t.

tremor-nystagmus-ulcer syndrome

trench nephritis

Trendelenburg
T. gait
T. position

Trental

Treponema
T. immunofluorescence study
T. pallidum

tretinoin

TRI
intracytoplasmic tuboreticular
inclusion
tubuloreticular inclusion

triad
Charcot t.
Dieulafoy t.
hepatic t.
portal t.
radiographic t.
Saint t.

t. syndrome
Whipple t.

triaditis
portal t.

trial
clinical t.
direct current electrotherapy t.
Prostate Cancer Intervention
Versus Observation T.
(PCIVOT)

triamcinolone

Triaminicin

triamterene
hydrochlorothiazide and t.

triangle
Calot t.
cardiohepatic t.
Charcot t.
cystohepatic t.
digastric t.
femoral t.
Grynfeltt t.
Henke t.
Hesselbach t.
inguinal t.
Labbe t.
Lesgaft t.
Livingston t.
lumbocostoabdominal t.
mesenteric t.
Petit t.
Scarpa t.

triangular ligament

triangulation stapling method

triazolam

triazoles

tricarboxylic acid (TCA)

triceps
t. skinfold thickness
t. skinfold thickness test

Trichinella spiralis

trichinelliasis

trichinellosis

trichiniasis

trichinosis

NOTES

trichiura
  Trichuris t.
trichlorethylene
trichlormethiazide
trichloroacetic acid (TCA)
trichobezoar
trichocyst
trichomonal balanitis
trichomonas
Trichomonas vaginalis
trichomoniasis
  vaginal t.
trichophagia
trichophytobezoar
Trichosporon beigelli
trichrome
  Masson t.
  t. stain
trichuriasis
Trichuris trichiura
tricitrate
trick
  Hafter diet t.
trickle perfusion
Tricomponent Coaxial System
  (TCS)
tricyclamol
tricyclic
  t. antidepressant
tridecapeptide
tridihexethyl
  t. chloride
Tridrate bowel prep
trifid stomach
trifluoperazine
triflupromazine
trifurcation variant
trigeminy
triggering
  R-wave t.
triglyceride
  t. enzyme deficiency
  long-chain t. (LCT)
  medium-chain t. (MCT)
  serum t.
  VLDL t.
triglycyl-lycine vasopressin
trigonal
  t. plate
trigone
  deep t.
trigonitis
trihexyphenidyl

trihydrate
  amoxicillin t.
trihydrocoprostanic acid (TCA)
trihydroxy salt
triiodobenzene
Trilafon
trilobar
  t. hyperplasia
  t. hypertrophy
Trilogy low profile balloon
  dilatation catheter
Trimadeau sign
Trimedyne Optilase 1000 device
trimeprazine
trimer
trimetaphan
trimethidinium
trimethobenzamide
trimethoprim
  sulfamethoxazole and t.
    (SMX/TMP)
  t. and sulfamethoxazole
    (TMP/SMX)
  t. sulfamethoxazole
trimethoprim-sulfamethoxazole
  t.-s. DS
trimethoprim/sulfamethoxazole
  (TMP/SMX)
trimethylsilyl ether
trimetrexate
Trimox
Trimpex
Trinalin
trinitrate
  glyceryl t. (GTN)
Trinsicon
triolein C 14 breath test
triphasic cystometric curve
triphosphatase
  adenosine t. (ATPase)
triphosphate
  adenosine t. (ATP)
  guanosine t. (GTP)
  inositol t.
1,4,5-triphosphate
  inositol -t. (IP3)
triple
  t. intussusception
  t. lobe hepatectomy
  t. loop pouch
  t. therapy (TT)
triple-lumen
  t.-l. manometry catheter

t.-l. perfused catheter system
t.-l. Sengstaken-Blakemore tube
triplet
neurofilament protein t.
triplication
tripod
t. grasping forceps
tripotassium dicitrato bismuthate
tripsinization
triptorelin
tri-radiate cecal fold
tris
tris(hydroxymethyl)aminomethane
trisegmentectomy
Tris HCl
tris(hydroxymethyl)aminomethane
(tris)
trisilicate
aluminum hydroxide and
magnesium t.
trismus presentation
Triton tumor
trocar
accessory t.
Campbell t.
conical t.
Cook urological t.
t. cystostomy
ensheathing t.
Ethicon t.
gallbladder t.
Landau t.
Ochsner gallbladder t.
Origin t.
pyramidal t.
trochanter
troglitazone
Troisier sign
tromethamine
carboprost t.
ketorolac t.
Tronolane
trophic change
tropical
t. calcific pancreatitis
t. diarrhea
t. hyphemia

t. splenomegaly
t. sprue
tropicalis
Candida t.
tropomyosin
troponin
Trousseau
T. esophageal bougie
T. syndrome
T. test
Troutman rectus forceps
TRPM-2
testosterone repressed prostate
message-2
Tru-Cut
T.-C. biopsy
T.-C. biopsy needle
T.-C. needle
T.-C. needle biopsy
trumpet
nasal t.
truncal
t. vagotomy
t. vagotomy and
gastroenterostomy
t. vagotomy and pyloroplasty
truncus
bicarotid t.
trunk
celiac t.
lumbosacral t.
portal t.
TRUS
transrectal ultrasonography
transrectal ultrasound scanning
transurethral rectal ultrasound
transurethral ultrasound
truss
Tru Taper Ethalloy needle
Tru-Trax
Trypan blue-stained cell
Trypanosoma cruzi
trypanosomiasis
American t.
trypsin
bovine t.
t. inhibitor

T

NOTES

trypsinogen
tryptic soy broth
tryptophan
t. metabolism
TS-200
tissue spectrum analyzer T.
TSAE
transcatheter splenic arterial
embolization
TSC
tuberous sclerosis complex
TSRPC
totally stapled restorative
proctocolectomy
TT
triple therapy
TT-3 needle
TTC
T-tube cholangiogram
TTL
total lymphocyte
TTP
thrombotic thrombocytopenic
purpura
TTS
through-the-scope
TTS balloon dilation
TTS dilator
Rigoflex esophageal TTS
T-tube
T.-t. cholangiogram (TTC)
T.-t. drain
T.-t. drainage
French T.-t.
T.-t. stent
T.-t. study
T.-t. tract
T.-t. tract
choledochofiberoscopy
T.-t. tract choledochoscopy
T-TURP
total transurethral resection of
prostate
TTX
tetrodotoxin
TTX tetrodotoxin
tuaminoheptane
tubal
t. ectopic pregnancy
t. infertility
t. ligation
tube
Abbott t.

Abbott-Miller t.
Abbott-Rawson double-lumen
gastrointestinal t.
Anderson gastric t.
Argyle chest t.
Argyle-Salem sump t.
ascites drainage t.
aspiration and dissection t.
Aspisafe nasogastric t.
Atkinson silicone rubber t.
Axiom double sump t.
Baker intestinal
decompression t.
Baker jejunostomy t.
Bard gastrostomy feeding t.
Bard PEG t.
Blakemore t.
Blakemore-Sengstaken t.
Bower PEG t.
Boyce modification of
Sengstaken-Blakemore t.
Broncho-Cath double-lumen
endotracheal t.
Buie rectal suction t.
Caluso PEG gastrostomy t.
Cantor t.
cast-like t.
t. cecostomy
Celestin t.
Celestin esophageal t.
Celestin latex rubber t.
chest t.
Compat feeding t.
conical centrifuge t.
Cope loop nephrostomy t.
Corpak feeding t.
Corpak weighted-tip, self-
lubricating t.
cuffed endotracheal t.
cystostomy t.
t. decompression
decompression t.
Dennis t.
Dennis intestinal t.
Dobbhoff feeding t.
Dobbhoff gastric
decompression t.
Dobbhoff PEG t.
double-lumen t.
drainage t.
Dreiling t.
dual percutaneous
gastrostomy t.

Dumon-Gilliard prosthesis
pushing t.
Edlich gastric lavage t.
endoscopic t.
endoscopic gastrostomy t.
endothelial t.
endotracheal t.
ENDO-Tube nasal jejunal
feeding t.
t. enlargement
enteroclysis t.
t. enteroscope
EntriStar feeding t.
EntriStar polyurethane PEG t.
Eppendorf t.
ESKA-Buess esophageal t.
esophageal t.
Ewald t.
fallopian t.
feeding t.
t. feeding
feeding gastrostomy t.
Flexiflo Inverta-Peg t.
Flexiflo stoma creator t.
Flexiflo tungsten-weighted
feeding t.
Flexiflo Versa-PEG t.
four-lumen t.
Frazier suction t.
Frederick-Miller t.
gastric aspiration t.
gastric augment and single
pedicle t. (GASP)
gastric lavage t.
gastrostomy t.
Glasser gastrostomy t.
Gomco suction t.
Gott t.
t. graft
guttered T t.
Haldane-Priestly t.
Har-el pharyngeal t.
Harris t.
Hodge intestinal
decompression t.
insertion t.
jejunal feeding t.

jejunostomy t.
Kangaroo gastrostomy t.
Kaslow intestinal t.
Keofeed feeding t.
Killian suction t.
large-bore gastric lavage t.
t. leakage
Lepley-Ernst t.
Levin t.
Linton-Nachlas t.
long intestinal t.
Malecot gastrostomy t.
Malecot nephrostomy t.
marked t.
Medena t.
mediastinal t.
Medina t.
Medoc-Celestin pulsion t.
mercury-weighted t.
metal-weighted Silastic
feeding t.
MIC gastrostomy t.
t. migration
Mik gastrostomy t.
Miller-Abbott t.
Miller-Abbott intestinal t.
Minnesota t.
modified Minnesota t.
Montgomery salivary bypass t.
Moss t.
Moss gastrostomy t.
Moss Mark IV t.
Mousseau-Barbin prosthetic t.
myringotomy t.
nasobiliary t.
nasocystic drainage t.
nasoduodenal feeding t.
nasoenteric t.
nasoenteric feeding t.
nasogastric t. (NGT)
nasogastric feeding t.
nasoileal t.
nasojejunal t.
nasojejunal feeding t.
negative pressure t.
negative pressure-controlled t.
nephrostomy t.

T

NOTES

tube *(continued)*
nephrotomy t.
NJ feeding t.
Nuport PEG t.
Nyhus-Nelson gastric
  decompression and jejunal
  feeding t.
Olympus one-step button
  gastrostomy t.
orogastric Ewald t.
oropharyngeal t.
t. overgrowth
Paul-Mixter t.
pediatric feeding t.
pediatric nasogastric t.
Pedi PEG t.
Pee Wee low profile
  gastrostomy t.
PEG t.
PEG-400 t.
PEJ t.
percutanoue endoscopic
  placement of jejunal t.
photomultiplier t.
pigtail nephrostomy t.
t. placement
pleural t.
polyethylene t.
Poole suction t.
post-pyloric feeding t.
Procter-Livingstone t.
pusher t.
Quinton t.
rectal t.
Rehfuss stomach t.
t. removal
t. replacement
Replogle t.
Rubin-Quinton small-bowel
  biopsy t.
Ryle t.
Sacks-Vine feeding
  gastrostomy t.
Salem duodenal sump t.
Salem sump t.
Sandoz Caluso PEG
  gastrostomy t.
Sandoz 22F balloon
  replacement t.
Sandoz feeding/suction t.
Sengstaken-Blakemore t.
Shiner t.
skin t.

sliding t.
small-bowel t.
Souttar t.
Stamey t.
Stamm gastrostomy t.
stiffening t.
stomach t.
Stomate decompression t.
Stomate extension t.
suction t.
sump nasogastric t.
T t.
tampon t.
Teflon t.
Teflon nasobiliary t.
Thiersch t.
transpyloric t.
triple-lumen Sengstaken-
  Blakemore t.
Vivonex Moss t.
Wangensteen suction t.
Willscher t.
Wilson-Cook nasobiliary t.
Wilson-Cook NJFT-series
  feeding t.
Wookey skin t.
woven dacron t.
Wurbs-type nasobiliary t.
Yankauer suction t.
tubed
t. free skin graft
t. groin flap
t. urethroplasty
tube-fed patient
tubeless lithotriptor
tubercle
pubic t.
tubercular involvement
tuberculin syringe
tuberculocele
tuberculosis
  Mycobacterium t.
tuberculosis
colonic t.
duodenal t.
esophageal t.
gastric t.
ileocecal t.
intestinal t.
miliary t.
peritoneal t.
t. polyp

renal t.
segmental colonic t.
tuberculous
  t. enteritis
  t. esophagitis
  t. gastritis
  t. infectious esophagitis
  t. peritonitis
tuberosity
  ischial t.
tuberous
  t. sclerosis
  t. sclerosis complex (TSC)
tube-within-tube technique
tubing
  t. clamp
  large-bore Tygon t.
  polyvinyl t.
  shunt t.
  Tygon venovenous bypass t.
  Y-connecting t.
tubogram
  T t.
tubular
  t. atrophy
  t. basement membrane
  t. carcinoma
  t. cell desquamation
  t. colonic duplication
  t. damage
  t. duplication
  t. epithelial cell
  t. epithelial cell injury
  t. excretory mass
  t. iron accumulation
  t. ischemia
  t. morphologic injury
  t. narrowing and sacculation
  t. necrosis
  t. polyp
  t. reabsorption of phosphorus
  t. regeneration
  t. resorption
  t. vertical gastroplasty
tubularized
  t. bladder neck reconstruction
  t. cecal flap

tubule
  collecting t.
  distal t. (DT)
  distal convoluted t.
  epididymal t.
  epithelium-lined t.
  human proximal t. (HPT)
  isolated cortical t. (ICT)
  nonischemic t.
  proximal t. (PT)
  proximal convoluted t. (PCT)
  proximal straight t. (PST)
  renal t.
tubuli (*pl. of* tubulus)
tubulitis
tubulocystic
tubulogenesis
  vitronectin inhibiting HGF-
    induced t.
tubulogenic
tubuloglomerular
  t. feedback (TGF)
Tubuloglomerular Feedback
  Mechanism
tubulointerstitial (TI)
  t. disease
  t. fibrosis
  t. injury
  t. nephritis (TIN)
  t. nephropathy
tubulointerstitium
tubulointestinal nephritis
tubulopathy
  cyclosporine t.
tubuloreticular inclusion (TRI)
tubulotoxic effect
tubulovillar lesion
tubulovillous
  t. adenoma
  t. polyp
tubulus, pl. tubuli
tubus digestorius
tuck
  dorsal tunical t.
Tucker
  T. esophagoscope
  T. spindle-shaped dilator

T

NOTES

Tucks ointment
TUEP
  transurethral evaporation of prostate
Tuffier
  T. abdominal retractor
  T. abdominal spatula
tuft
  glomerular t.
  vascular t.
TUIP
  transurethral incision of prostate
Tukey test
tulip tip
tumefaction
  mesenteric t.
tumescence
  nocturnal t.
  nocturnal penile t. (NPT)
tumor
  abdominal desmoid t.
  t. ablation
  Abrikosov t.
  adenomatoid t.
  adnexal t.
  ampullary t.
  anaplastic t.
  anaplastic Wilms t.
  t. angiogenesis
  angiomatoid t.
  benign t.
  bifurcation t.
  bilateral renal t.
  biliary tract t.
  bladder t.
  bleeding t.
  brain t.
  burned-out t.
  Buschke-Löwenstein t.
  t. cachexia
  carcinoid t.
  Castleman t.
  celiac t.
  t. cell
  t. cell lysis
  chromophobe cell t.
  core of t.
  debulking of t.
  desmoid t.
  diploid t.
  ductectatic t.
  duodenal t.
  embryonal t.
  encapsulated carcinoid t.

  t. encapsulation
  epithelial t.
  esophageal t.
  extracapsular t.
  fecal t.
  focal t.
  foci of t.
  gastric carcinoid t.
  gastrin-secreting non-beta islet
    cell t.
  gastroenteropancreatic t.
  germ cell t.
  glomus t.
  t. grading
  granular cell t. (GCT)
  granulosa cell t.
  Grawitz t.
  gritty t.
  hepatic t.
  hypersecreting t.
  t. infiltrating lymphocytes
    (TIL)
  t. infiltration
  interstitial cell t. of testis
  intra-abdominal desmoid t.
  intraductal mucin-producing t.
  intraparenchymal t.
  islet cell t.
  juxtaglomerular apparatus t.
  Klatskin t.
  Krukenberg t.
  Leydig cell t.
  t. location
  lymphoid t.
  malignant mesenchymal t.
  t. marker
  MCF-7 t.
  mediastinal t.
  metachronous t.
  mixed germ cell-sex cord
    stromal t.
  mucin-hypersecreting t.
  mucinous cystic t.
  mucinous pancreatic t.
  mucin-producing t.
  myogenic t.
  t. necrosis
  t. necrosis factor (TNF)
  t. necrosis factor α (TNFα)
  t. necrosis factor-α assay
    (TNF-α assay)
  neuroendocrine t.
  neurogenic t.

nonaneuploid t.
non-B islet cell t.
noninvasive t.
nonseminomatous t.
nonseminomatous germ cell t.
pancreatic islet cell t.
paraumbilical vein t. (PUVT)
parenchymal t.
periampullary t.
periampullary duodenal t.
pituitary t.
polypoid t.
prepubertal testicular t. (PPTT)
primitive neuroectodermal t.
 (PNET)
t. probe
Recklinghausen t.
rectal carcinoid t. (RCT)
renin secreting juxtaglomerular
 cell t.
retroperitoneal t.
rhabdoid t.
ruptured hepatic t.
t. seeding
Sertoli cell t.
shaggy t.
small-cell t.
solid t.
t. spillage
t. staging
t. stenting
superficial t.
t. suppressor gene
t. therapy
transurethral resection (of)
 bladder t. (TURBT)
Triton t.
ureteral t.
urethral t.
urothelial t.
t. vaccine
vasoactive intestinal
 polypeptide t. (VIPoma)
villous t.
virilizing t.
Wilms t.

yolk sac t.
Zollinger-Ellison t.
tumor-associated antigen (TAA)
tumorigenesis
 t. activity
tumorigenic
tumorlet
 Wilms t.
tumorous pseudopodia
Tums
TUMT
 transurethral microwave
 thermotherapy
TUNA
 transurethral needle ablation
tunable
 t. dye laser lithotripsy
 t. pulsed dye laser
tunic
 t. cyst
 epididymal t.
tunica
 t. albuginea
 t. albuginea corporis spongiosi
 t. albuginea corporum
 cavernosorum
 t. albuginea ovarii
 t. albuginea testis
 t. muscularis
 t. propria
 t. replacement
 t. vaginalis
 t. vaginalis blanket wrap
tunnel
 t. creation
 t. disease
 extravesical seromuscular t.
 t. infection
 retropancreatic t.
 subserous t.
 ureteral t.
 t. vision
 Witzel feeding jejunostomy t.
tunneler
 Davol t.
Tuohy-Borst adaptor

T

NOTES

609

TUR
transurethral resection
TUR syndrome
video monitored TUR
Turapy device
turbid
t. bile
t. peritoneal fluid
turbinate
swollen t.
TURBT
transurethral resection (of) bladder
tumor
turbulent flow
Turcot syndrome
TUR-Cue photometer
transurethral resection
turgescence
penile t.
turgor
skin t.
turista
turn-and-suction technique
Turnbull
T. colostomy
T. end-loop ileostomy
T. multiple ostomy operation
T. technique
Turner
T. sign
T. stigmata
T. syndrome
Turner-Warwick
T.-W. inlay
T.-W. needle
turn and suction biopsy technique
TURP
transurethral resection of prostate
direct-beam coupler for TURP
split-beam coupler for TURP
turpentine enema
turpette
Turrell-Wittner rectal forceps
Tuttle test
TUU
transureteroureterostomy
TUVP
transurethral vaporization of prostate
TVF
Thiry-Vella fistula
TVP
T-wave
flipped T.-w.

Tween 20
twelve-hour home pad test
twenty-four-hour intraesophageal pH
study
twin pulse shock wave release
twisted β-pleated sheet fibril
two-channel endoscope
two-dimensional flow cytometric
analysis
two-finger grip
two-layer
t.-l. anastomosis
t.-l. enteroenterostomy
t.-l. open technique
two-loop J-shaped ileal pouch
two-piece ostomy pouch
two-stage
t.-s. repair
t.-s. triolein test
two-step
Aztec t.-s.
t.-s. orchiopexy
two-tailed
t.-t. Fisher test
t.-t. McNemar test
two-wing Malecot drain
TxA2 receptor antagonist
Tycron
T. suture
T. tie
Tygon venovenous bypass tubing
Tylenol
Tylosis palmaris et plantaris
Tylox
tymazoline
tympanites
false t.
uterine t.
tympanitic
t. abdomen
t. dullness
tympany
abdominal t.
Type
T. 1 autoimmune hepatitis
T. III glycogenosis
type
t. A gastritis
t. 2 autoimmune hepatitis
t. B antral gastritis
t. B gastritis
blood t.
t. C cirrhosis

chronic-continuous t.
diffuse vasculitis of
  polyarteritis nodosa t.
DR2 1501 HLA-DRB tissue t.
DR2 1502 HLA-DRB tissue t.
DR2 1601 HLA-DRB tissue t.
DR2 1602 HLA-DRB tissue t.
DR1 HLA-DRB tissue t.
DR2 HLA-DRB tissue t.
DR3 HLA-DRB tissue t.
DR4 HLA-DRB tissue t.
DR7 HLA-DRB tissue t.
DR9 HLA-DRB tissue t.
DRw8 HLA-DRB tissue t.
DRw10 HLA-DRB tissue t.
DRw11 HLA-DRB tissue t.
DRw12 HLA-DRB tissue t.
DRw13 HLA-DRB tissue t.
DRw14 HLA-DRB tissue t.
t. I familial
  hyperlipoproteinemia
t. II cryoglobulinemia
t. II diabetes mellitus
t. II familial
  hyperlipoproteinemia
t. III cholangiocarcinoma
t. III collagen
t. III familial
  hyperlipoproteinemia
t. III incontinence
t. I mesangiocapillary
  glomerulonephritis
t. IV amyloidosis
t. IV collagen
t. IV familial
  hyperlipoproteinemia
phage t.
t. 0 stress urinary incontinence
test t.
t. V familial
  hyperlipoproteinemia
type-1 plasminogen activator
  inhibitor (PAI-1)
type-2 plasminogen activator
  inhibitor (PAI-2)
type-C ulcer

typed blood
type-D ulcer
type-specific blood transfusion
typhi
  Salmonella t.
typhimurium
  Salmonella t.
typhlectasis
typhlectomy
typhlenteritis
typhlitis
typhlodicliditis
typhloempyema
typhlolithiasis
typhlomegaly
typhlonous debris
typhlopexy, typhlopexia
typhlorrhaphy
typhlostenosis
typhlostomy
typhlotomy
typhloureterostomy
typhoid
  abdominal t.
  t. fever
typing
  HLA t.
  HLA-DR t.
  HLA-DR DNA t.
tyramine
tyremesis
tyropanoate
  t. contrast medium
  t. sodium
tyrosine
  t. kinase activity
  t. kinase growth factor
    receptor
  peptide t.
  t. phosphorylation
  t. protein kinase
tyrosinemia
  hereditary t.
tyrosis
Tyshak catheter
Tyson test

T

NOTES

U

U pouch
U pouch construction

UA

urinalysis

UBM

urothelial basement membrane

UBT

C-urea breath test

UC

ulcerative colitis

UCB

unconjugated bilirubin

UCHL-1 monoclonal antibody

UDC

ursodeoxycholate

UDCA

ursodeoxycholic acid

UDP

uridine 5'-diphosphate
uridine 5'-diphosphate

Udranszky test

UES

upper esophageal sphincter

UESR

upper esophageal sphincter
relaxation

UF

ultrafiltration

Uffelmann test

UGI

upper gastrointestinal
UGI angiomata
UGI endoscope
UGI endoscopy

UGIB

upper gastrointestinal bleeding

UICC tumor classification

UJ13A nuclear isotope bone scan

ulcer

acid peptic u.
active duodenal u.
agranulocytic u.
amebic u.
anastomotic u.
anastomotic/stomal u.
anterior duodenal u.
anterior wall antral u.
antral u.
antroduodenal u.

aphthoid u.
aphthous u.
apical duodenal u.
Barrett u.
u. base
bear claw u.
u. bed
benign u.
benign gastric u.
bleeding u.
Bouveret u.
bulbar peptic u.
cecal u.
cervical u.
chronic u.
CMV-related u.
coalescent u.
collar-button-like u.
colonic u.
colorectal u.
corneal u.
u. crater
Crohn duodenal u.
Cruveilhier u.
Curling u.
Cushing u.
cysteamine-induced duodenal u.
decubitus u.
Dieulafoy u.
distention u.
drug-induced u.
duodenal u. (DU)
u. duodenum
elusive u.
esophageal u.
Fenwick-Hunner u.
focal colonic mucosal u.
gastric u.
gastroduodenal double u.
general peptic u.
giant peptic u.
greater curvature u.
healed u.
herpetic u.
Hunner u.
idiopathic esophageal u. (IEU)
indolent radiation-induced
rectal u.
intractable u.
jejunal u.

U

ulcer *(continued)*
juxtapyloric u.
kissing u.
Kocher u.
lesser curvature u.
linear u.
malignant u.
Mann-Williamson u.
marginal u.
Martorell hypertensive u.
minute bleeding mucosal u.
mucosal gastric u.
nonhealing u.
open u.
oral u.
penetrating u.
peptic u.
perforated acid peptic u.
perforated peptic u.
perforating u.
perineal u.
phantom u.
postbulbar duodenal u.
posterior duodenal u.
postligation u.
postsurgical recurrent u.
prepyloric u.
prepyloric gastric u.
punched-out u.
punctate u.
pyloric channel u.
rake u.
rectal u.
recurrent u.
refractory duodenal u.
reserpine-induced u.
Rokitansky-Cushing u.
rose thorn u.
round u.
sea anemone u.
secondary jejunal u.
serpiginous u.
sigmoid u.
small intestinal u.
sodium meclofenamate-induced esophageal u.
solitary u.
stercoral u.
stomal u.
stress u.
sump u.
superficial linear u.

suture u.
type-C u.
type-D u.
vaginal u.
u. vessel
V-shaped u.
u. with heaped up edges
ulcerating
u. adenocarcinoma
u. carcinoma
ulceration
anal u.
anastomotic u.
ASA-induced gastric u.
CMV-associated u.
CMV-induced esophageal u.
collar-button u.
duodenal u.
esophageal u.
gastric u.
labial u.
necrotic u.
patchy colonic u.
radiation-induced u.
serpiginous u.
stasis u.
stercoral u.
stress u.
stress-induced gastric u.
ulcerative
u. colitis (UC)
u. enteritis
u. esophagitis
u. gastritis
u. lymphoma
u. proctitis
ulcer-like dyspepsia
ulcero-erosive disease
ulcerogenic
u. fistula
ulcer-prone personality
Ulex europeus I antigen
ulnar deviation
UltimaBloc
ultra
u. high-magnification endoscopy
U. Twin bag system
U. Y-set system
Ultrabag System
ultradian rhythm
ultrafast computerized tomography
Ultrafem pants

ultrafiltrate
glomerular u.
ultrafiltration (UF)
u. coefficient
continuous arteriovenous u.
(CAVU)
dialytic u. (DU)
extracorporeal u. (ECU)
glomerular u.
u. hemodialyzer
spontaneous dialytic u.
Ultraflex
U. esophageal prosthesis
U. esophageal stent
U. Microvasive stent
U. nitinol expandable
esophageal stent
UltraKlenz skin cleanser
Ultralente insulin
Ultraline
U. laser
Lasersonic ACMI U.
ultra-low-volume sclerotherapy
**UltraPak enteral closed feeding
system**
Ultrase
U. MT12
ultrasonic
u. aspirator and dissector
u. diagnosis
u. dissector
u. fragmentation
u. lithotresis
u. lithotripsy
u. lithotriptor
u. lithotriptor probe
U. oscillating bur
u. scalpel
ultrasonics
ultrasonographic finding
ultrasonography
abdominal u.
B-mode u.
color Doppler u.
Doppler u.
endoluminal u.
endoluminal rectal u. (ELUS)

endoscopic u. (EUS)
endoscopic color Doppler u.
endoscopic Doppler u.
gray scale u.
high-resolution 25-megahertz u.
intraductal u. (IDUS)
intrarectal u.
penile duplex u.
pharmaco-duplex u.
real-time u.
rectal endoscopic u. (REUS)
Siemens Sonoline u.
Toshiba Sal 38B real-time u.
Toshiba Sonolayer SSA250A
transrectal u.
transcutaneous u.
transluminal u.
transrectal u. (TRUS)
ultrasound
abdominal u.
compression u. (CUS)
endoluminal u.
endorectal u. (ERUS)
u. endoscope
endoscopic u.
u. gastrointestinal fiberscope
gray scale u.
intraductal u. (IDUS)
laparoscopic u. (LUS)
power Doppler u.
pulsed Doppler u.
real-time u.
real-time gallbladder u.
u. scan
time domain u. (TDU)
transcutaneous u.
u. transducer
transrectal u.
transurethral u. (TRUS)
transurethral rectal u. (TRUS)
u. wand
ultrasound-assisted
u.-a. PEG placement
u.-a. percutaneous endoscopic
gastrostomy
ultrasound-guided
u.-g. biopsy

NOTES

U

ultrasound-guided *(continued)*
  u.-g. laser
  u.-g. shock wave therapy
ultrastructural basket-weave change
ultrathin
  u. araldite section
  u. pancreatoscope
Ultratome
  U. double lumen
    sphincterotome
  U. XL triple-lumen
    sphincterotome
ultratome
ultraviolet irradiation
Ultravist 300
Ultrex
  U. cylinder
  U. Plus penile prosthesis
Ultroid
Ultzmann test
umbilical
  u. artery
  u. cord
  u. fissure
  u. fistula
  u. granuloma
  u. hernia
  u. hernia rupture
  u. ligament
  u. port
  u. port grasper
  u. scissors
  u. tape
  u. vein
  u. vein catheterization
  u. vein recanalization
umbilicated angioma
umbilication
umbilicus
  everted u.
  Richet fascia u.
umbrella
  Mobin-Uddin u.
UMCL
  upper midclavicular line
Unasyn
UNaV
  urinary sodium excretion
unbanded gastroplasty
uncinate
  u. process
  u. process of pancreas
uncoated mesh stent

unconjugated
  u. bilirubin (UCB)
  u. hyperbilirubinemia
undecapeptide
  amino-terminal u.
underactivity
  detrusor u.
underfilling
  arterial u.
undersurface of liver
underwater spark gap
undescended testis
undifferentiated
  u. adenoma
  u. cell
  u. embryonal sarcoma of liver
  u. structure
undigested food in stool
undiversion
  urinary u.
unequal calf diameter
unformed stool
unicentricity
unicornuate uterus
unidirectional transfer
Uni-Flate 1000 penile prosthesis
uniformis
  Bacteroides u.
unilateral
  u. nephrectomy
  u. periorbital emphysema
  u. renal hypoplasia
  u. renin production
  u. subcostal incision
  u. ureteral obstruction (UUO)
unilobular cirrhosis
unilocular cyst
uninhibited
  u. neurogenic bladder
  u. overactive bladder
union
  anomalous pancreaticobiliary
    ductal u. (APBDU)
uni-planar imaging
unipolar
  u. glass electrode
  u. neuron
unit
  amylase u.
  arbitrary u. (AU)
  Bovie electrocoagulation u.
  Cameron-Miller
    electrocoagulation u.

Century bicarbonate dialysis control u.
colony forming u. (CFU)
crypt-villus u.
densitometric u.
Diasonics DRF ultrasound u.
electrosurgical u. (ESU)
Erbotom F2 electrocoagulation u.
GPL u.
Grass Model SIU5A stimulation isolation u.
Hounsfield u.
image-processing u.
Karmen u.
KeyMed u.
5-15 King Armstrong u.
OSMO reverse osmosis u.
Proscan ultrasound u.
QAD-1 sonography u.
real-time sonographic u.
Siemens MRI u.
Siemens Somatom DRH CT analyzer u.
Somogyi u.
SSE2-L electrosurgical u.
ThermoFlex thermotherapy u.
UroCystom u.
Valleylab SSE-2 cautery u.
Unitary inflatable penile prosthesis
United
U. Bongort Life-style pouch
U. Max-E drainable pouch
U. Network for Organ Sharing (UNOS)
U. Ostomy Association (UOA)
U. Ostomy irrigation set
U. Skin Prep
U. States Renal Data System (USRDS)
U. Surgical Bongort Life-style pouch
U. Surgical Convex insert
U. Surgical Featherlite ileostomy pouch
U. Surgical Hypalon faceplate
U. Surgical Seal Tite gasket

U. Surgical Shear Plus drainable pouch
U. Surgical Soft & Secure pouch
U. XL 14 skin barrier
units of packed red blood cells (UPRBC)
univariate
u. analysis
Universal
U. esophagoscope
U. gastroscope
U. sheath
U. sheath system
U. stent
University
U. of Wisconsin (UW)
U. of Wisconsin fluid
U. of Wisconsin solution
UNOS
United Network for Organ Sharing
unreconstructable obstructive azoospermia
unrelenting
u. diarrhea
u. pain
unrelieved pain
unremitting pain
unresectable
u. hepatocellular carcinoma
unroofing
transurethral u.
unsex
unsporulated coccidian
unstable
u. bladder
u. urethra
unsteady gait
untethering procedure
UOA
United Ostomy Association
Uosm
urine osmolarity
UPJ
ureteropelvic junction
U pouch

U

NOTES

upper
- u. alimentary endoscopy
- u. endoscopy and colonoscopy
- u. esophageal sphincter (UES)
- u. esophageal sphincter relaxation (UESR)
- u. gastrointestinal (UGI)
- u. gastrointestinal angiomata
- u. gastrointestinal barium roentgenographic study
- u. gastrointestinal bleeding (UGIB)
- u. gastrointestinal endoscopy
- u. gastrointestinal panendoscopy
- u. gastrointestinal tract
- u. GI endoscope
- u. GI hemorrhage
- u. GI series
- u. GI tract foreign body
- u. midclavicular line (UMCL)
- u. tract disease

UPRBC
- units of packed red blood cells

up-regulation

upset stomach

upside down stomach

upstream pancreatic duct

upstroke
- delayed u.

uptake
- glucose u.
- hepatic u.
- [3H]thymidine u.

URA
- urethral resistance factor

Urabeth tabs

urachal
- u. abscess
- u. cyst
- u. disorder
- u. diverticulum
- u. fistula
- u. sinus

urachus
- patent u.

uranyl
- u. acetate
- u. acetate stain

Urapine

urate
- u. crystal
- u. nephropathy

urea
- u. breath testing
- hepatic u.
- u. hydrolysis
- u. kinetics
- Kt/V u.
- u. nitrogen test
- u. permeability
- u. reduction ratio

urea-derived cyanate

ureahydrochloride
- quinine u.

urea-impermeable membrane

urealyticum
- *Ureaplasma u.*

Ureaplasma
- *U. urealyticum*
- *U. urethritis*

urease
- mucosal u.
- u. test

urea-splitting organism

urecchysis

Urecholine
- U. supersensitivity test

uredema

Urelief

uremia

uremic
- u. acidosis
- u. breath
- u. cardiomyopathy
- u. colitis
- u. gastrointestinal lesion
- u. PMN
- u. serositis
- u. serum subfraction

ureolyticus
- *Bacteroides u.*

ureter
- ectopic u.
- impassable u.
- u. implantation
- intramural u.

ureteral
- u. atony
- u. augmentation
- u. bladder augmentation
- u. carcinoma
- u. catheterization
- u. colic
- u. ectopia
- u. encasement

u. endoscopic disconnection
u. injury
u. meatotomy
u. obstruction
u. occlusion balloon catheter
u. orifice
u. patch procedure
u. pressure
u. reimplantation
u. spatulation
u. split cuff nipple
u. stent
u. stenting
u. stent placement
u. stoma
u. stoma removal
u. stone
u. stricture
u. tumor
u. tunnel
ureteralgia
uretercystoscope
ureterectasia
ureterectomy
distal u.
ureteric
u. bud
u. obstruction
u. retrieval net
u. stoma
ureteritis
ureterocalicostomy
ureterocele
ectopic u.
ureterocelorraphy
ureterocervical
ureterocolic
u. fistula
u. stricture
ureterocolonic anastomosis
ureterocolostomy
ureterocutaneous fistula
ureterocystanastomosis
ureterocystoplasty
ureterocystoscope
ureterocystostomy
ureteroendoscopy

ureteroenteric
u. status
ureteroenterostomy
ureterogram
bulb-tipped retrograde u.
ureterography
ureterohydronephrosis
ureteroileal
u. anastomosis
u. stenosis
u. stricture
ureteroileocecoproctostomy
ureteroileoneocystostomy
ureteroileostomy
Bricker u.
ureteroileourethral anastalsis
ureterolith
ureterolithiasis
ureterolithotomy
laparoscopic u.
ureterolysis
combined u.
extravesical u.
intravesical u.
Lich-Gregoire u.
Pacquin u.
Politano-Leadbetter u.
Ureteromat
ureteroneocystostomy
u. herniation
reoperative u.
ureteroneopyelostomy
ureteronephrectomy
ureteropelvic
u. fungus ball
u. junction (UPJ)
u. junction obstruction
ureteroplasty
ileal patch u.
ureteroproctostomy
ureteropyelitis
ureteropyelogram
retrograde u.
ureteropyelography
ureteropyeloneostomy
ureteropyelonephritis
ureteropyelonephrostomy

U

NOTES

ureteropyeloplasty
ureteropyeloscope
ureteropyeloscopy
  flexible u.
ureteropyelostomy
ureteropyosis
ureterorectostomy
ureterorenal reflux
ureterorenoscope
uretero-renoscope procedure sheath
ureterorenoscopy
  transurethral u. (URS)
ureterorrhagia
ureterorrhaphy
ureteroscope
  Circon-ACMI (MR-6, MR-
    9) u.
  flexible u.
  Micro-6 u.
  offset lens u.
  Panoview rod-lens u.
  rigid u.
  semirigid fiber optic u.
  u. sheath
  Storz 27022 SK u.
  Wolf u.
  working port u.
ureteroscopy
  rigid u.
ureterosigmoid
  u. anastomosis
ureterosigmoidostomy
  ileocecal u.
  Maydl u.
ureterostegnosis
ureterostenoma
ureterostenosis
ureterostoma
ureterostomy
  cutaneous u.
  cutaneous loop u.
  Davis intubated u.
  high-loop cutaneous u.
  low-loop cutaneous u.
  retroperitoneal cutaneous u.
ureterotome
  optical u.
ureterotomy
  Davis intubated u.
  intubated u.
ureterotrigonoenterostomy
ureterotubal anastomosis

ureteroureteral
  u. anastomosis
ureteroureterostomy
ureterouterine
  u. fistula
ureterovaginal
  u. fistula
ureterovesical junction (UVJ)
ureterovesical obstruction
ureterovesicostomy
urethra
  accessory phallic u.
  anterior u.
  AS 800 male bulbous u.
  bulbomembranous u.
  devastated u.
  fixed drain pipe u.
  intrinsic striated muscle of
    the u.
  membranous u.
  penile u.
  posterior u.
  prostatic u.
  unstable u.
urethrae
  bulbus u.
  compressor u.
urethral
  u. atresia
  u. carcinoma
  u. caruncle
  u. closure mechanism
  u. closure pressure profile
  u. dilation
  u. diverticulectomy
  u. diverticulum
  u. electrical conductance
  u. hematuria
  u. hypermobility
  u. obstruction
  u. occlusion
  u. plate
  u. plug
  u. pressure
  u. pressure measurement
  u. pressure profile
  u. prolapse
  u. pseudotumor
  u. resistance
  u. resistance factor (URA)
  u. sarcoidosis
  u. sphincterotomy
  u. sphincter recruitment reflex

u. stricture
u. suspension
u. syndrome
u. tumor
u. vein
urethralgia
urethralis
crista u.
urethrameter
urethrascope
urethratresia
urethrectomy
urethremorrhagia
urethremphraxis
urethreurynter
urethrin
urethrism, urethrismus
urethritis
acute u.
chlamydia u.
hypoestrogenic u.
mycoplasma u.
nongonococcal u.
u. syndrome
Ureaplasma u.
urethrobalanoplasty
urethrocavernous fistula
urethrocecal anastomosis
urethrocele
urethrocystitis
urethrocystometrography
urethrocystometry
urethrocystopexy
urethrocystoplasty
urethrocystorectometry
urethrocystoscopy
urethrodetrusor facilitative reflex
urethrodynia
urethrogram
retrograde u. (RUG)
urethrograph
urethrography
urethrohymenal fusion
urethrolysis
retropubic u.
transvaginal u.
urethrometer

urethropelvic ligament
urethropexy
Gittes u.
Lapides-Ball u.
Marshall-Marchetti-Krantz u.
Stamey u.
urethrophraxis
urethrophyma
urethroplasty
Cantwell-Ransley u.
Cecil u.
modified Young u.
onlay island flap u.
pedicle flap u.
Tanagho bladder flap u.
Thiersch-Duplay u.
tubed u.
urethrorectal fistula
urethrorrhagia
urethrorrhaphy
urethrorrhea
urethroscope
Robertson TM u.
urethroscopic
urethroscopy
retropubic u.
urethrospasm
urethrosphincteric
u. guarding reflex
u. inhibitory reflex
urethrostaxis
urethrostenosis
urethrostomy
perineal u.
urethrotome
u. knife
Otis u.
Sachs u.
Storz u.
urethrotomy
direct vision internal u.
(DVIU)
endoscopic optical u.
external u.
internal u.
perineal u.

U

NOTES

urethrovaginal
 u. fistula
 u. septum
urethrovesicopexy
Urex
URF-P2 choledochoscope
urge
 u. to defecate
 u. incontinence
 u. syndrome
urgency
 defecatory u.
 u. incontinence
 motor u.
 sensory u.
 urinary u.
uric
 u. acid
 u. acid calculus
 u. acid infarct
 u. acid level
 u. acid lithiasis
 u. acid nephropathy
 u. acid test
uricosuric
Uricult
uridine
 u. 5'-diphosphate (UDP)
 u. phosphorylase
 u. rescue
Uridium
uridyltransferase
 galactose-1-phosphate u.
Urifon-Forte
Urigen
Uri-Kit culture kit
Urimar-T
urinal
 condom u.
 "Millie" female u.
 Uro-Tex McGuire male u.
 URSEC u.
urinalysis (UA)
 u. dipstick
urinary
 u. acidity
 u. amylase
 u. ascites
 u. bladder
 u. calculus
 u. cast
 u. catecholamines
 u. catheterization

 u. cGMP level
 u. chloride excretion
 u. continence
 u. cyclic AMP
 u. cyst
 u. diversion
 u. excretion
 u. exertional incontinence
 u. extravasation
 u. extraversion
 u. fistula
 u. frequency
 u. incontinence
 u. kallikrein excretion
 u. lithogenesis
 u. marker protein
 u. 3-methylhistidine
 u. obstruction
 u. protein excretion
 u. retention
 u. sand
 u. sediment
 u. sodium excretion (UNaV)
 u. stone
 u. stress incontinence
 u. stuttering
 u. tract disease
 u. tract infection (UTI)
 u. trypsin inhibitor
 u. umbilical fistula
 u. undiversion
 u. urea nitrogen excretion
 (UUN)
 u. urgency
urinary diversion
 ileocolonic pouch u. d.
 Le Bag u. d.
urination
 stuttering u.
urine
 barium sediment in u.
 u. bilirubin
 concentrated u.
 u. culture
 dark u.
 dark concentrated u.
 u. dipstick
 u. electrophoresis
 U. Meter Foley tray
 u. osmolality
 u. osmolarity (Uosm)
 residual u.
 u. sample

u. transport
u. urea nitrogen (UUN)
u. urobilinogen
urinoma
Urised
Urisedamine
Urispas
Uri-Three culture kit
Uritrol
Urizole
uroanthelone
Urobak
urobilinogen
fecal u.
urine u.
Urobiotic
Uro-Bond skin adhesive
Urocam video camera
Urocath external catheter
urocele
urocheras
urochesia
Urocit
Urocit-K
Urocystin
urocystitis
UroCystom unit
urocyte diagnostic cytometry system
UROD
uroporphyrinogen decarboxylase
UroDIAGNOST
Urodiagnost x-ray table
urodilatin
urodynamic
u. catheter
u. dysfunction
u. flow study
u. obstruction
urodynamics
ambulatory u.
Menuet Compact u. system
Menuet u. system
urodynia
urodysfunction
uroedema
uroenterone

uroepithelial glycoid receptor
urofacial syndrome
uroflow
u. index
peak u.
uroflowmeter
Dantec Urodyn 1000 u.
Drake u.
Etude cystometer u.
Synectics-Dantec Flo-Lab II u.
Synectics-Dantec UD10000 u.
uroflowmetry
home u.
urogastrone
urogenital
u. diaphragm
u. fistula
u. sinus
u. sphincter muscle
Urogesic
Urografin
U. 290 contrast medium
urogram
excretory u.
intravenous u. (IVU)
urograph
Disa 5500 u.
urography
antegrade u.
cystoscopic u.
excretory u. (EU, EXU)
intravenous u.
retrograde u.
Uro-Guide stent
Uro-jet delivery system
urokinase
u. plasminogen activator
Uro-KP-Neutral
UROLAB Janus II
Urolab Janus System III
Urolase
CR Bard U.
U. laser
U. neodymium:YAG laser fiber
Urolene Blue
urolith

U

NOTES

urolithiasis
  asymptomatic u.
  recurrent calcium u. (RCU)
urolithic
urolithology
urologic, urological
  u. surgery
  u. system cancer
urologist
urology
  perinatal u.
  u. set
UroLume
  U. Endourethral Wallstent
    prosthesis
  U. prostate stent
  U. urethral prosthesis
  U. Wallstent
Uro-Mag
Uromat
  U. dilation
UroMax II high-pressure balloon catheter
uromodulin gene
uronate
  glycosaminoglycans u. (GAGUA)
  macromolecular u. (MMUA)
uroncus
uronephrosis
uronic acid-rich protein
Uro-Pak system
uropathogen
uropathy
  chronic obstructive u.
  congenital u.
  obstructive u.
  positional obstructive u.
uroplania
Uroplus
  U. DS
  U. SS
uropontin
uroporphyrinogen decarboxylase (UROD)
uropsammus
Uroqid-Acid
uroradiology
Uro-San Plus external catheter
uroscheocele
uroschesis
urosepsis
uroseptic

UroSnare cystoscopic tumor snare
Urosoft stent
Urospiral urethral stent
urostomy
Uro-Tex McGuire male urinal
urothelial
  u. basement membrane (UBM)
  u. carcinoma
  u. dysplasia
  u. tumor
urothelium
  seromuscular enterocystoplasty lined with u. (SELU)
Urotract x-ray system
Urotrol
uroureter
Urovac bladder evacuator
Urovision
  U. ultrasound imaging system
Urovist
  U. Cysto
  U. Meguluine
  U. Sodium 300
urp
urpiness
urpy
URS
  transurethral ureterorenoscopy
URSEC urinal
ursodeoxycholate (UDC)
ursodeoxycholic acid (UDCA)
ursodiol
urticaria
  u. pigmentosa
  u. pigmentosa with systemic mastocytosis
urticarial
  u. fever
  u. reaction
URYS 800 nerve stimulator
u-shaped skin flap
USRDS
  United States Renal Data System
U.S. retractor
Ussing
  U. chambers
  U. chamber technique
uteri
  descensus u.
uterine
  u. colic
  u. enlargement
  u. fibroid

u. rupture
u. size
u. tenderness
u. tympanites
utero
hydronephrosis in u.
uterolysis
laparoscopic u.
uteroscope
Circon-ACMI u.
uterus
anteflexed u.
anteverted u.
bicornuate u.
double u.
duplicate u.
pregnant u.
retroflexed u.
retroverted u.
unicornuate u.
U-test
Mann-Whitney U.-t.
UTI
urinary tract infection
utricle
prostatic u.

utriculitis
utriculocele
U-tube stent
U-turn maneuver
UUN
urinary urea nitrogen excretion
urine urea nitrogen
UUO
unilateral ureteral obstruction
Uv
microvolt
uveitis
UV-Flash ultraviolet germicidal exchange device
UVJ
ureterovesical junction
UV-linked
UV transilluminator
uvular
u. deviation
u. swelling
UW
University of Wisconsin
UW solution

NOTES

U

V33W high density endocavity probe
V8 protease
VAB
  Velban, actinomycin-D, and bleomycin
VABES
  vasoablative endothelial sarcoma
VAB-II
  Velban, actinomycin-D, bleomycin, and platinum
VAB-VI
  cyclophosphamide, Velban, actinomycin-D, bleomycin, and platinum
VAC
  vincristine, Adriamycin, and cyclophosphamide
vacA toxin
vaccine
  BCG v.
  hepatitis A v.
  hepatitis B v.
  hepatitis B virus v. (HBVV)
  irradiated tumor v.
  mucosal v.
  OraVax v.
  tumor v.
  yeast-recombinant hepatitis B v.
vacuolar
  v. H+-ATPase
  v. type protein pump immunocytochemistry
vacuolating cytotoxin
vacuole
  pinocytosis v.
vacuolization
  isometric tubular v.
Vacutainer
  V. bag
  V. bottle
vacuum
  v. constriction device (VCD)
  v. constriction erection
  v. entrapment device
  v. erection device (VED)
  v. extraction device
  v. tumescence device

VAD
  vincristine, doxorubicin and dexamethasone
vagal stimulation
vagina
  atrophic v.
  high-ending v.
  passage of flatus per v.
  septate v.
vaginal
  v. atresia
  v. bleeding
  v. cone biopsy
  v. construction
  v. cuff cellulitis
  v. cutback
  v. discharge
  v. electrical stimulation
  v. eversion
  v. fistula
  v. fistula cup
  v. foreign body
  v. inflammation
  v. lithotomy
  v. mass
  v. mucosa
  v. needle suspension procedure
  v. suppository
  v. trichomoniasis
  v. ulcer
  v. vesicostomy
  v. wall approach
  v. wall sling procedure
vaginalis
  Gardnerella v.
  processus v.
  Trichomonas v.
  tunica v.
vaginalitis
vaginoplasty
  cutback type v.
  posterior flap v.
vaginosis
  bacterial v.
vaginourethroplasty
vagosympathetic balance
vagotomy
  v. and antrectomy with gastroduodenostomy
  bilateral v.

V

vagotomy *(continued)*
   highly selective v.
   laparoscopic v.
   laser laparoscopic v.
   medical v.
   parietal cell v. (PCV)
   proximal gastric v. (PGV)
   v. and pyloroplasty
   Roux-en-Y procedure with v.
   selective proximal v. (SPV)
   superselective v.
   surgical v.
   total bilateral v.
   truncal v.
vagus nerve
Valethamate
valine
Valium
vallecula, pl. **valleculae**
vallecular
   v. dysphagia
   v. pooling
Valleylab
   V. SSE-2 cautery unit
   V. SSE2L generator
Valpin
Valpin 50
valproate
valproic
   v. acid
   v. acid therapy
Valsalva
   V. leak point pressure concept
   V. maneuver
   V. ratio
   taeniae of V.
Valtrac BAR
value
   F v.
   predictive v.
   reference v.'s
   therapeutic v.
valve
   v. ablation
   anal v.
   v. of Bauhin
   Benchekroun hydraulic v.
   Benchekroun ileal v.
   v. bladder
   blunting of v.
   competent v.
   competent ileocecal v.
   failed nipple v.

   v. of Guerin
   Holter v.
   v. of Houston
   ileal nipple v.
   ileocecal v.
   incompetent v.
   incompetent ileocecal v.
   LeVeen v.
   lipomatous ileocecal v.
   Lopez enteral v.
   Mitrofanoff v.
   nipple v.
   nonintussuscepted v.
   posterior urethral v. (PUV)
   v. prolapse
   rectal v.
   spiral v.
   Spivack v.
valved voice prosthesis
valves of Kerckring
valvulae conniventes
valvular heart disease
Vamin amino acid solution
van
   V. Bogaert disease
   V. Buren disease
   V. Buren sound
   V. de Kramer fecal fat procedure
   v. den Bergh test
   V. Hees index
   v. Sonnenberg drain
   v. Sonnenberg gallbladder catheter
   v. Sonnenberg sump drain
Vanceril inhaler
Vancocin
   V. HCl
vancomycin
   v. hydrochloride
vancomycin/nalidixic acid agar
van Gieson stain
vanillacetic acid (VLA)
vanillylmandelic acid (VMA)
vanished testis syndrome
vanishing
   v. bile duct syndrome
   v. gonad
Vansil
Vantin
vaporization
   Contact Laser v.
   laser v.

VaporTrode
 V. electrode
Varco gallbladder forceps
variability
variable
 v. nuclear crowding
 time-dependent v.
variance
 analysis of v. (ANOVA)
Varian model 3600 gas
 chromatography
variant
 trifurcation v.
variation
 coefficient of v.
 phasic-free tone v.
variceal
 v. band ligation
 v. bleeding
 v. column
 v. decompression
 v. hemorrhage
 v. ligator
 v. pressure
 v. sclerosant
 v. sclerosis
 v. sclerotherapy
 v. sclerotherapy in esophagus
 v. size inclusion criteria
 v. wall
varicella-zoster
 v.-z. infection
 v.-z. virus (VZV)
varices (*pl. of* varix)
 blue v.
 common bile duct v.
 duodenal v.
 ectopic v.
 endoscopic band ligation of v.
 esophageal v.
 familial colonic v.
 gallbladder v.
 gastric v.
 idiopathic v.
 obliterated v.
 v. on varix
 paraesophageal v.

varicocele
 symptomatic v.
varicocelectomy
 laparoscopic v.
 microsurgical inguinal v.
 subinguinal v.
 subinguinal microsurgical v.
varicole
varicosclerant
Varicoscreen
varicosis coli totalis
varicosity
Variject needle
varioliform
 v. gastritis
 v. gastritis or gastropathy
varioliformis
 gastritis v.
variolosa
 orchitis v.
varix, pl. **varices**
 actively bleeding v.
 alcoholic v.
 anorectal v.
 bar-type esophageal v.
 colonic v.
 downhill esophageal v.
 duodenal v.
 EEA stapling of v.
 esophageal v.
 esophagogastric v.
 fundal v.
 gastric v.
 ileal v.
 v. ligation
 mesenteric v.
 Okuda transhepatic obliteration
  of v.
 paraesophageal v.
 percutaneous transhepatic
  obliteration of esophageal v.
 peristomal v.
 radius of v.
 rectal v.
 rectosigmoid v.
 transesophageal ligation of v.
 varices on v.

V

NOTES

vasa
    v. recta
    v. vasorum
vasa deferentia (*pl. of* vas deferens)
Vas-Cath
vascular
    v. abnormality
    v. access
    v. access failure
    v. anastomosis
    v. bruits
    v. cachexia
    v. cirrhosis
    v. clamp
    v. collateral network
    v. complication
    v. compromise
    v. disease
    v. ectasia
    v. hemangioma
    v. injury
    v. insufficiency
    v. invasion
    v. laceration
    v. laceration repair
    v. lesion
    v. malformation
    v. pattern
    v. pedicle
    peripheral v.
    v. permeability factor (VPF)
    v. permeation of tumor cell
    v. plasminogen activator (v-PA)
    v. plexus
    v. rejection
    v. renal mass
    v. smooth muscle
    v. smooth muscle cell (VSMC)
    v. steal syndrome
    v. surgery
    v. suture
    v. tuft
vasculature
    preglomerular v.
    v. responsiveness
vasculitic
    v. lesion
    v. neuropathy
vasculitis
    allergic v.
    extrarenal v.
    necrotizing v.
    necrotizing bowel v.
    renal v.
    rheumatoid v.
    systemic lupus erythematosus v.
    visceral v.
vasculogenic impotence
vasculopathy
    acute renal transplant v.
    noncerebral v.
    portal hypertensive intestinal v. (PHIV)
vas deferens, pl. **vasa deferentia**
vasectomy
    no-scalpel v.
Vaseline gauze
vasitis
vasoablative endothelial sarcoma (VABES)
vasoactive
    v. drug
    v. intestinal peptide (VIP)
    v. intestinal peptide distribution
    v. intestinal polypeptide (VIP)
    v. intestinal polypeptide binding
    v. intestinal polypeptide immunoreactivity (VIP-IR)
    v. intestinal polypeptide tumor (VIPoma)
    v. peptide-cytokine interaction
vasoconstriction
    afferent arteriolar v.
    baroreceptor-mediated mesenteric arterial v.
    radiocontrast-induced renal v.
    reflex splanchnic v.
    splanchnic v.
vasocutaneous fistula
vasodilation
    endothelium-dependent v.
    v. of portasystemic collateral
    renal v.
    sympathetic response to v.
vasodilator
    renal v.
vasoepididymostomy
vasoformative
vasography
vasoligation
vasomotor disorder
vaso-orchidostomy

vasopressin
    arginine v. (AVP)
    1-deamino-8-d-arginine v.
    v. infusion
    triglycyl-lycine v.
    v. with nitroglycerin
vasopressin-induced cAMP
vasorelaxation
vasorum
    vasa v.
vasosection
vasospasm
vasostomy
Vasotec
vasotomy
vasovagal reflex
vasovasostomy
vasovesiculectomy
vaso-vesiculography
Vasoxyl
vas recta
Vater
    ampulla of V.
    invaginating ampulla of V.
    papilla of V.
vaterian segment
VATER syndrome
vault
    rectal v.
VBG
    vertical banded gastroplasty
VCA
    anti-viral capsid antigen
VCD
    vacuum constriction device
        Dacomed Catalyst VCD
        Mentor-Piston VCD
        Mentor Response VCD
        Mentor-Touch VCD
        Mission VED VCD
        Osbon ErecAid VCD
        Pos-T-Vac VCD
VCG
    voiding cystogram
VCR
    vincristine

VCUG
    voiding cystourethrogram
Vd
    volume of distribution
vector
    amplitude-acrophase v.
    bacterial v.
VED
    vacuum erection device
Veetids
vegetans
    pyostomatitis v.
vegetarian diet
vegetative lesion
veil
    Jackson v.
vein
    aberrant obturator v.
    arcuate v.
    azygos v.
    cavernous v.
    cavernous transformation of the
      portal v. (CTPV)
    deep dorsal v.
    dilated v.
    external spermatic v.
    extrahepatic portal v.
    gastric v.
    gonadal v.
    gubernacular v.
    hepatic v.
    iliac v.
    inferior mesenteric v. (IMV)
    inferior rectal v.
    internal pudendal v.
    left hepatic v. (LHV)
    middle hepatic v. (MHV)
    middle rectal v.
    North American Medical
      Incorporated deep dorsal v.
    omental v.
    pancreaticoduodenal v.
    paraumbilical v.
    v. patch
    peripheral acinar v.
    peritoneal v.
    portal v. (PV)

V

NOTES

vein *(continued)*
    renal v.
    v. retractor
    Retzius v.'s
    right hepatic v. (RHV)
    shunt index via the inferior mesenteric v. (SI-I)
    shunt index via the superior mesenteric v. (SI-S)
    splanchnic v.
    splenic v.
    subclavian v.
    superior mesenteric v. (SMV)
    superior rectal v.
    tangle of hemorrhoidal v.'s
    thoracoabdominal collateral v.
    umbilical v.
    urethral v.
Velban
Velban, actinomycin-D, and bleomycin (VAB)
Velban, actinomycin-D, bleomycin, and platinum (VAB-II)
Vella fistula
velocity
    angular v.
    v. measurement
    prostate-specific antigen v. (PSAV)
Velosef
Velpeau hernia
vena, gen. and pl. **venae**
    v. cava
    v. cavography
venacavaplasty
    face-a-face v.
venacavogram
venae (*gen. and pl. of* vena)
venereal
    v. disease
    v. proctocolitis
    v. wart
venereum
    lymphogranuloma v. (LGV)
veneris
    mons v.
venodilation
    nitrate-induced v.
    systemic v.
venogenic impotence
venogram
    hepatic v.

    weeping willow appearance on v.
venography
    hepatic v.
    pedal control v.
    transjugular portal v.
veno-occlusive
    v.-o. disease (VOD)
    v.-o. dysfunction
    v.-o. liver disease
venoperitoneostomy
venosum
    ligamentum v.
venous
    v. blood sample
    v. circulation
    v. hum
    v. invasion
    v. leak impotence
    v. outflow obstructive disease
    v. pattern
    v. pooling
    v. thrombosis
    v. web
    v. web disease
venovenous
    v. continuous hemodialysis
    v. hemodialysis
venter propendens
ventilation
    mechanical v.
venting percutaneous gastrostomy (VPG)
Ventolin
ventral
    v. bending technique
    v. bud
    v. chronic calcific pancreatitis
    v. hernia
    v. herniorrhaphy
    v. surface
ventricle
ventricular tachycardia
ventriculoperitoneal shunt
ventrocystorrhaphy
ventroscopy
ventrotomy
ventrum penis flap
venule
    collecting v.
    hepatic v.
    portal v.
    subtunical v.

VePesid
vera
 hemospermia v.
 polycythemia v.
verapamil
Veratrum alkaloids
Veress
 V. cannula
 V. needle
verge
 anal v.
veritas
 in vivo v.
vermicular
 v. colic
 v. movement
vermicularis
 Enterobius v.
vermiform
 v. appendix
 v. body
verminous ileus
Vermox
Verner-Morrison syndrome
Vernon-David rectal speculum
verruca vulgaris
verruciform xanthoma
verrucous
 v. carcinoma
 v. gastritis
Versabran
 Modane V.
Versa-PEG gastrostomy kit
VersaPulse Select laser
Versed
vertex
vertical
 v. banded gastroplasty (VBG)
 v. mattress suture
 v. midline incision
 v. ring gastroplasty (VRG)
 v. Silastic ring gastroplasty
 v. transmission
vertigo
 gastric v.
 objective v.
 subjective v.

verumontanum
very
 v. late activation (VLA)
very-low-calorie diet (VLCD)
very-low-density
 v.-l.-d. lipoprotein (VLDL)
 v.-l.-d. lipoprotein cholesterol
vesicae
 ectopia v.
vesical
 v. calculus
 v. compliance
 v. diverticulectomy
 v. diverticulum
 v. exstrophy
 v. external sphincter
 dyssynergia (VSD)
 v. fibrosis
 v. fistula
 v. hematuria
 v. lithotomy
 v. neck resistance
vesical-sacral-sphincter loop
Vesica percutaneous bladder neck
 suspension kit
vesicle
 brush-border membrane v.
 (BBMV)
 endocytotic v.
 v. hernia
 seminal v.
 spermatic v.
vesico-acetabular fistula
vesicoamniotic shunt
vesicoanal reflex
vesicocele
vesicoclysis
vesicocolic fistula
vesicocutaneous fistula
vesicoenteric fistula
vesicofixation
vesicoileal reflux
vesicointestinal fistula
vesicolithiasis
vesicomyectomy
vesicomyotomy
vesico-ovarian fistula

V

NOTES

633

vesicorectal fistula
vesicorectostomy
vesicosalpingovaginal fistula
vesicosigmoidostomy
vesicosphincteric dyssynergia
vesicostomy
    cutaneous v.
    preputial continent v.
    vaginal v.
vesicotomy
vesicoureteral
    v. reflux (VUR)
vesicoureteric
    v. reflux
    v. stenosis
vesicourethral anastomosis
vesicouretral anastomotic stricture
vesicouterine fistula
vesicovaginal
    v. fistula
    v. Holter
vesicovaginorectal fistula
vesicovaginostomy
vesiculectomy
    prostatoseminal v.
    total prostatoseminal v.
vesiculitis
vesiculobullous disorder
vesiculogram
vesiculography
vesiculoprostatitis
vesiculotomy
Vespore disinfectant
Vesprin
Vess chair
vessel
    accessory v.
    blood v.
    capsular blood v.
    chyliferous v.
    v. dilator
    dysmorphic v.
    ectatic v.
    gastroepiploic blood v.
    hypoplastic blind-ending
     spermatic v.'s
    ileal blood v.
    ileocolic v.
    lacteal v.
    lymphatic v.
    mesocolonic v.
    nonbleeding visible v. (NBVV)
    replaced hepatic v.

    serosal blood v.
    telangiectatic v.
    v. tip
    ulcer v.
    visible v.
    visible ulcer v.
vestibule
    laryngeal v.
vest-over-pants
    v.-o.-p. hernial repair
    v.-o.-p. herniorrhaphy
VET-CO vacuum system
Vezien abdominal scissors
V-flap meatoplasty
Vα gene
Vβ gene
viability
    intestinal v.
    v. testing
vial
    Port-A-Germ anaerobic
     transport v.
    scintillation v.
Vibramycin
Vibrio
    V. cholerae
    V. fetus infection
    V. infection
    V. parahaemolyticus
    V. vulnificus
Vibrionaceae species
Vickers M85a microdensitometer
Vicodin
viculin
vidarabine
video
    v. colonoscope
    v. densitometry
    v. duodenoscope
    v. endoscope
    v. endoscopy
    v. esophagoscopy
    v. monitor
    v. monitored TUR
    v. pressure flow
    electromyography
    v. processor
    v. push enteroscope
    v. recorder
    v. small bowel enteroscopy
    v. timer
    v. transurethral resection
    technique

videocolonoscope
EVE Fujinon v.
videocystourethrography
videoelectroscope
Fujinon CEG-FP-series v.
videoendoscope
double-channel v.
Olympus GIF-series v.
Olympus GIF-series double-
channel therapeutic v.
Olympus GIF-SQ-series v.
Olympus GIF-T-series v.
videoendoscopy
videoesophagram
videofluoroscopic
v. swallow study
v. technique
videofluorourodynamic study
Video Image Processor model 450
videoproctography
videosigmoidoscope
videourodynamic
v. evaluation
view
en face v.
longitudinal v.
postevacuation v.
retroflexed v.
slide-by v.
transverse v.
vigorous achalasia
villi (*pl. of* villus)
villiformity
villoglandular
v. adenoma
v. polyp
villous
v. atrophy
v. colorectal adenoma
v. epithelium
v. polyp
v. tumor
villus, pl. **villi**
colonic v.
duodenal v.
finger-like v.
intestinal v.

jejunal v.
leaf-like v.
ridged-convoluted v.
small intestinal v.
tongue-shaped v.
vimentin staining
Vim-Silverman
V.-S. biopsy needle
V.-S. needle
V.-S. technique
V.-S. technique for liver
biopsy
vinblastine
**vinblastine, actinomycin D, and
bleomycin (mini-VAB)**
Vincent curtsy
vincristine (VCR)
v., Adriamycin, and
cyclophosphamide (VAC)
v., doxorubicin and
dexamethasone (VAD)
**Vindelov method flow cytometry
analysis**
Vinson syndrome
Viokase
violaceous
violation
scrotal v.
violet
gentian v.
violin-string adhesion
VIP
vasoactive intestinal peptide
vasoactive intestinal polypeptide
voluntary interruption of pregnancy
VIP antiserum
VIP-IR
vasoactive intestinal polypeptide
immunoreactivity
VIPoma
vasoactive intestinal polypeptide
tumor
VIP-secreting neuronoma
Virag
V. injector
V. operation

V

NOTES

viral
- v. cholangitis
- v. colitis
- v. cystitis
- v. diarrhea
- v. dysentery
- v. enteritis
- v. gastritis
- v. gastroenteritis
- v. hemorrhagic fever
- v. hepatitis
- v. hepatitis marker
- v. hepatitis type A
- v. hepatitis type B
- v. inclusion body
- v. infection
- v. membrane fusion
- v. replication
- v. serologic titer

ViraPap HPV dot blot hybridization test
Virchow sentinel node
Virchow-Troisier node
viremia
- hepatitis C v.

virgin lymphocyte
viridans
- *Staphylococcus v.*

virilizing tumor
Virilon
virological
virology
virtual focus shock wave
virucidal agent
virulent diarrhea
virus
- adeno-associated v. (AAV)
- antibody to hepatitis C v. (anti-HCV)
- antibody to hepatitis D v. (anti-HDV)
- delta v.
- dengue v.
- Epstein-Barr v. (EBV)
- esophageal condyloma v.
- Hanta v.
- Hawaii v.
- v. hepatitis
- hepatitis A v. (HAV)
- hepatitis B v. (HBV)
- hepatitis B-like DNA v.
- hepatitis C v. (HCV)
- hepatitis D v. (HDV)
- hepatitis delta v. (HDV)
- hepatitis E v. (HEV)
- herpes simplex v. (HSV)
- human immunodeficiency v. (HIV)
- human T-cell leukemia v. of type I (HTLV-I)
- influenza v.
- live attenuated v.
- Marburg v.
- molluscum contagiosum v. (MCV)
- mother-to-infant transmission of hepatitis C v.
- neutropic v.
- Norwalk v.
- v. shedding
- varicella-zoster v. (VZV)

virus-like
- v.-l. action (VLA)
- v.-l. particle (VLP)

viscera (*pl. of* viscus)
visceral
- v. arteriography
- v. dysfunction
- v. hyperalgesia
- v. ischemia
- v. larva migrans
- v. leishmaniasis
- v. neuropathy
- v. pain
- v. peritoneum
- v. traction reflex
- v. vasculitis

visceralgia
visceromegaly
visceromotor
visceroparietal
visceroptosis, visceroptosia
viscerosensory reflex
viscerotomy
viscerotrophic
viscerotropic
viscerum
- situs inversus v.

viscid bile
viscidosis
viscoelastic
- v. collagen fiber
- v. gel

viscoelasticity
viscometer

viscosity
    plasma v.
viscous
    v. bile
    v. lidocaine
    v. lidocaine premedication
    v. Xylocaine gargle
viscus, pl. **viscera**
    abdominal v.
    hollow v.
    intra-abdominal v.
    intraperitoneal v.
    intraperitoneal v. rupture
    perforated v.
    strangulated v.
visible
    v. abdominal distention
    v. peristalsis
    v. ulcer vessel
    v. vessel
    v. vessel significance
visibly normal
Visicath endoscope
Visick
    V. dysphagia classification
    V. gastric cancer grading
    system
    V. grading system
vision
    direct v.
    V. Sciences VSI 2000 flexible
    sigmoidoscope system
    V. System EndoSheath
    V. System sigmoidoscope
    tunnel v.
Visken
Vistaril
visual
    v. endoscopically controlled
    laser
    v. evoked potential
    v. laser ablation
    v. laser ablation of prostate
    (VLAP)
    v. laser assisted prostatectomy
    (VLAP)
visualization

Vital
    V. feeding
vital
    v. sign
    v. staining
vitamin
    v. A toxicity
    v. B_{12}
    v. B_{12} absorption test
    v. B_{12} malabsorption
    v. D deficiency
    v. D-dependent calbindin-D9k
    v. D supplementation
    fat-soluble v.
    v. K2
    water-soluble v.
Vitaneed feeding
vitelline
    v. duct
    v. duct anomaly
vitellointestinal cyst
vitro
    in v.
vitronectin inhibiting HGF-induced
  tubulogenesis
Vivactil
vividialysis
vividiffusion
vivo
    ex v.
    in v.
Vivonex
    V. HN powdered feeding
    V. Moss tube
    V. TEN
    V. TEN feeding
VLA
    vanillacetic acid
    very late activation
    virus-like action
VLAP
    visual laser ablation of prostate
    visual laser assisted prostatectomy
VLCD
    very-low-calorie diet
VLDL
    very-low-density lipoprotein

NOTES

VLDL *(continued)*
    VLDL cholesterol
    VLDL triglyceride
VLP
    virus-like particle
VM-26
    teniposide
VMA
    vanillylmandelic acid
VMC
    von Meyenburg complex
vocal cord
VOD
    veno-occlusive disease
Voges-Proskauer test
voice restoration
voiding
    alarm clock v.
    v. cystogram (VCG)
    v. cystometrography
    v. cystometry
    v. cystourethrogram (VCUG)
    v. diary
    dysfunctional v.
    v. flow rate
    fractionated v.
    incomplete v.
    orthotopic v.
    reflex v.
    staccato v.
    v. study
    v. urethral pressure
       measurements (VUPP)
vol
    volume
volar
Volkmann
    V. pancreatic calculus spoon
    V. rake retractor
    V. spoon for pancreatic
       calculus
volmar
voltage
    RMS v.
    root mean square v.
voltage-gated channel
Voltaren
volume (vol)
    bladder v.
    v. displacement transducer
    v. of distribution (Vd)
    drain v.
    emptying delta v.

    v. expansion
    extracellular fluid v.
    fiber bundle v. (FBV)
    gastric v.
    intraperitoneal v.
    liver v.
    mean corpuscular v. (MCV)
    mean renal v.
    v. overload
    PET dialysate v.
    prostatic v.
    renal v.
    v. replacement
    residual urine v. (RUV)
    weight-based peritoneal
       exchange v.
voluminous hiatus hernia
voluntary
    v. guarding
    v. interruption of pregnancy
       (VIP)
volvulated
volvulus
    cecal v.
    colonic v.
    gastric v.
    idiopathic v.
    intestinal v.
    mesenteroaxial gastric v.
    organoaxial gastric v.
    v. reduction
    secondary v.
    sigmoid v.
    sigmoid colon v.
vomica
vomicus
vomiting
    bilious v.
    v. center
    chemotherapy-induced v.
    concealed v.
    cyclic v.
    cyclical v.
    dry v.
    epidemic v.
    episodic v.
    erotic v.
    fecal v.
    hysterical v.
    intractable v.
    ipecac-induced v.
    metabolic derangement from v.
    nausea and v. (N&V)

nervous v.
periodic v.
perioperative v.
pernicious v.
persistent v.
postoperative v.
postprandial v.
post-tussive v.
profuse v.
projectile v.
psychogenic v.
recurrent bouts of v.
retention v.
self-induced v.
stercoraceous v.
surreptitious v.
winter v.
vomition
vomitive
vomitory
vomiturition
vomitus
Barcoo v.
bile-stained v.
black v.
bloody v.
bright red v.
coffee-grounds v.
v. cruentes
feculent v.
v. marinus
v. niger
nonbilious v.
stercoraceous v.
von, Von
V. Andel dilating catheter
v. Gierke disease
V. Haberer-Finney anastomosis
V. Haberer gastroenterostomy
v. Hanseman cell
v. Hippel-Lindau cerebellar
hemangioblastomatosis
v. Hippel-Lindau disease
v. Hippel-Lindau syndrome
v. Jaksch test
v. Kossa stain
v. Kupffer cell

v. Meyenburg complex (VMC)
V. Petz suturing apparatus
v. Recklinghausen disease
v. Recklinghausen
neurofibromatosis
v. Rokitansky disease
v. Willebrand factor
v. Willebrand disease
Vp-16
v-PA
vascular plasminogen activator
VPF
vascular permeability factor
VPG
venting percutaneous gastrostomy
VPI
Coloscreen VPI
VPI nonadhesive open-end
pouch
V/Q mismatch
VRG
vertical ring gastroplasty
VSD
vesical external sphincter
dyssynergia
V-shaped ulcer
VSI 2000 sigmoidoscope
VSMC
vascular smooth muscle cell
VTC biliary catheter
VTU-1 vacuum erection device
vulgaris
acne v.
pemphigus v.
verruca v.
vulgaris
Proteus v.
vulgatus
Bacteroides v.
vulnificus
Vibrio v.
vulva
vulvar
v. carcinoma
v. vestibulitis syndrome
vulvovaginal candidiasis

V

NOTES

VUPP
    voiding urethral pressure
      measurements
VUR
    vesicoureteral reflux

Vygon Nutricath S catheter
V-Y plasty
VZV
    varicella-zoster virus

Wacker Sil-Gel 604 silicone cement
wafer
    Stomahesive W.
    Stomahesive skin barrier w.
Wagner test
Waldenström macroglobulinemia
Waldeyer
    W. fascia
    W. sheath
Walker gallbladder retractor
walking stick phenomenon
wall
    abdominal w.
    anterior abdominal w.
    bowel w.
    capillary w.
    colonic w.
    esophageal w.
    gallbladder w.
    glomerular capillary w. (GCW)
    midabdominal w.
    pharyngeal w.
    posterior abdominal w.
    sclerohyaline w.
    thickened gallbladder w.
    w. thickening
    variceal w.
Wallstent
    W. delivery device
    W. endoprosthesis
    W. esophageal prosthesis
    W. stent
    UroLume W.
Walsh radical retropubic
   prostatectomy
Walther
    W. dilator
    W. sound
wand
    ultrasound w.
wandering
    w. gallbladder
    w. liver
Wangensteen
    W. drain
    W. drainage
    W. suction
    W. suction apparatus
    W. suction tube

Wappler
    W. cystoscope with microlens
      optics
    W. cystourethroscope
    W. microlens cystourethroscope
warfarin
warfarin-associated subcapsular
   hematoma
warm
    w. ischemia time
    w. saline solution
Warren splenorenal shunt
wart
    anal w.
    cervical w.
    exophytic w.
    genital w.
    intra-anal w.
    perianal w.
    venereal w.
Warthin-Starry silver stain
Warwick and Ashken technique
washer
    Olympus Europe ETD
      automated endoscope w.
washing
    bladder w.
    w. catheter
washout
    w. cannula
    w. factor
    high rectal w.
    mucosal w.
    seminal tract w.
    w. test
wastage
    pregnancy w.
wastebasket
    w. diagnosis
    w. pouchitis
waste nitrogen excretion
wasting
    muscle w.
    renal sodium w.
    w. syndrome
water
    w. brash
    contamination of w.
    w. cushion lithotriptor
    w. cystometry

W

water *(continued)*
  w. displacing balloon
  fecal contamination of w.
  w. immersion
  w. loading
  w. pot perineum
  w. probe
  w. recovery test
  w. soluble contrast enema
  total body w. (TBW)
water-gurgle test
water-induced thermotherapy (WIT)
water-infusion esophageal
  manometry catheter
watering-can
  w.-c. perineum
  w.-c. scrotum
watermelon
  w. cecum
  w. rectum
  w. stomach (WS)
Water Pik
  endoscopic W.P.
watershed area
water-sipping test
water-soluble
  w.-s. bilirubin
  w.-s. contrast esophageal
    swallow
  w.-s. contrast esophageal
    swallow test
  w.-s. contrast medium
  w.-s. vitamin
Waterston method
water-trap stomach
watery
  w. diarrhea
  w. diarrhea, hypokalemia,
    achlorhydria (WDHA)
  w. diarrhea syndrome
  w. stool
Watson
  W. capsule
  W. capsule biopsy
Watson-Alagille syndrome
wattage
Watzki sleeve
Waugh-Clagett
  pancreaticoduodenostomy
wave
  abdominal fluid w.
  extracorporeal shock w.
  fluid w.

  focused shock w.
  mechanical stress w.
  peristaltic w.
  primary peristaltic w.
  real focus shock w.
  secondary peristaltic w.
  shock w.
  simultaneous bilateral
    extracorporeal shock w.
  slow w.
  virtual focus shock w.
waveform
  blend w.
  coag w.
  cut w.
  electrical w.
  low-pulsatility arterial w.
waveguide
  quartz w.
wavelength
waves
  clustered w. (CW)
  clustered jejunal w.
  propulsive w.
  simultaneous w.
Wavicide disinfectant
wax-matrix
  w.-m. slow-release form
  w.-m. tablet
wax-tipped bougie
WBC
  white blood cell
  WBC bands
  WBC basos
  WBC blasts
  WBC differential
  elevated WBC count
  WBC immature forms
  WBC leukocytes
  WBC lymphocytes
  WBC monocytes
  WBC neutrophils
WD
  Whipple disease
  Wilson disease
WDHA
  watery diarrhea, hypokalemia,
    achlorhydria
  WDHA syndrome
WDPM
  well-differentiated papillary
    mesothelioma

weakness
  extremity w.
  proximal muscle w.
weaning brash
web
  duodenal w.
  esophageal w.
  hepatic w.
  intestinal w.
  mucosal w.
  postcricoid w.
  venous w.
Webb-Balfour abdominal retractor
webbed penis
webbing
  penoscrotal w.
Weber-Christian disease
Weck
  W.-cel sponge
  W. clip
  W. high flow laparator
weddellite calculus
wedge
  w. hepatic biopsy
  w. pressure
  w. resection
wedged hepatic venous pressure (WHVP)
weeping willow appearance on venogram
Weerda endoscope
Wegener granulomatosis
Weibel-Palade granule
Weigert-Meyer law
weighing
  gravimetric w.
weight (wt)
  dry w.
  Femina vaginal w.
  w. gain
  ideal body w. (IBW)
  kidney w. (KW)
  w. loss
  w. loss with hyperphagia
  molecular w. (mol wt)
  w. reduction surgery

weight-based peritoneal exchange volume
Weight Watchers diet
Weinberg
  W. modification of pyloroplasty
  W. pyloroplasty
  W. vagotomy retractor
Weiss reaction
Weitlaner retractor
Welch
  W. Allyn flexible sigmoidoscope
  W. Allyn video colonoscope 8451
  W. Allyn video endoscope
  W. Allyn video endoscopy system
welchii
  Clostridium w.
weld
  laser tissue w.
welding
  chromophore enhanced laser w.
  laser w.
  laser tissue w.
well-differentiated
  w.-d. adenoma
  w.-d. papillary mesothelioma (WDPM)
Wells posterior rectopexy
Welt syndrome
Werdnig-Hoffman disease
Wermer syndrome
Wernicke
  W. encephalopathy
  W. syndrome
Wernicke-Korsakoff syndrome
Wesson perineal retractor
Westcott scissors
Western
  W. blot analysis
  W. blotting
  W. diet
Weston rectal snare

W

NOTES

Westphal
  W. gall duct forceps
  W. hemostat
Westphal-Strümpell disease
wet
  w. colostomy
  w. swallow
Wexler retractor
Wharton duct
wheal
wheat
  w. gluten
  w. starch
Wheelhouse operation
"w" hernia
whewellite calculus
whiff test
Whip
  Maalox W.
Whipple
  W. disease (WD)
  W. operation
  W. pancreatectomy
  W. pancreaticoduodenectomy
  W. pancreaticoduodenostomy
  W. procedure
  W. resection
  W. test
  W. triad
  W. triad test
whipstitch
  w. suture
whipworm
  w. infection
whispered pectoriloquy
whistle stent
whistle-tip catheter
Whitaker
  W. hook
  W. pressure-perfusion test
white
  w. atrophy
  w. bile
  w. blood cell (WBC)
  w. blood cell cast
  w. blood cell count
  w. line
  w. line of Toldt
  w. nipple sign
  w. patch
Whitehead
  W. classification

  W. deformity
  W. operation
Whitmore
  W. bag
  W. classification prostate
    cancer
Whitmore-Jewitt prostate cancer
  classification system
WHO
  World Health Organization
  WHO gastric carcinoma
    classification
whole
  w. blood
  w. body cooling
whole-blood trough level
whole-cell oxygen consumption
whole-grain
  rye w.-g. (RWG)
whole-gut
  w.-g. irrigation
  w.-g. lavage solution
whole-kidney fractional excretion
WHVP
  wedged hepatic venous pressure
Wickham technique
wide
  w. albumin gradient ascites
  w. elliptical anastomosis
wide-angled loupe
wide-mouth sac
widening
  mediastinal w.
width
  red cell distribution w. (RDW)
Wilcoxon
  W. matched-pairs signed-rank
    test
  W. rank sum test
Wilcoxon-Gehar test
wild-type
  p53 w.-t.
Wilkie disease
Wilkins-Chilgren agar
Wilkinson abdominal retractor
Williams
  W. intestinal forceps
  W. needle
  W. overtube sleeve
  W. varices injection overtube
Willis
  antrum of W.

W. pancreas
W. pouch
Willscher
W. catheter
W. tube
Wilms
W. tumor
W. tumorlet
Wilpowr
Wilson-Cook
W.-C. dilating balloon
W.-C. double-channel
sphincterotome
W.-C. endoprosthesis
W.-C. esophageal balloon
W.-C. feeding tube kit
W.-C. fine-needle-aspiration
catheter
W.-C. French stent
W.-C. gastric balloon
W.-C. mechanical lithotriptor
W.-C. nasobiliary tube
W.-C. NJFT-series feeding tube
W.-C. papillotome
W.-C. plastic prosthesis
W.-C. prosthesis introducer
W.-C. Protector guidewire
W.-C. stent
W.-C. THSF-series guidewire
W.-C. Tracer guidewire
Wilson disease (WD)
Wiltek papillotome
Winckler test
window
gastric w.
mesenteric w.
peritoneal w.
zinc selenide w.
windowed esophageal balloon
windows of Deaver
winged
w. catheter
w. steel needle
WinGel
wings
glans w.

Winslow
foramen of W.
W. pancreas
winter
w. acidosis
w. gastroenteritis
W. procedure
W. shunt
w. vomiting
wire (*See also* guidewire)
Birtcher Hyfricator cautery w.
bypass w.
cesium-137 w.
cutting w.
diathermy w.
Extra Stiff Amplatz w.
glide w.
^{192}Ir w.
J w.
memory w.
nitinol w.
safety w.
torque w.
wire-guided
w.-g. balloon-assisted
endoscopic biliary stent
exchange
w.-g. hydrostatic balloon
w.-g. J-tube
w.-g. metal spiral retrieval
device
w.-g. placement
w.-g. polyvinyl bougie
w.-g. sphincterotome
Wire-Wrap
wiring
jaw w.
Wirsung
duct of W.
W. sphincter
Wirthlin splenorenal clamp
Wiskott-Aldrich syndrome
WIT
water-induced thermotherapy
Witzel
W. duodenostomy
W. enterostomy catheter

W

NOTES

Witzel *(continued)*
    W. feeding jejunostomy tunnel
    W. gastrostomy
    W. jejunostomy
Witz test
Woldman test
Wolf
    W. delivery system
    W. lithotrite
    W. percutaneous universal
      nephroscope
    W. Piezolith 2300 lithotripsy
      device
    W. Piezolith 2300 lithotriptor
    W. resectoscope
    W. rigid panendoscope
    W. Sonolith lithotriptor
    W. ureteroscope
Wolff
    W. syringe
    W. telescope
wolffian
    w. duct
    w. müllerian ductal system
Wolff-Junghans test
Wolf-Henning gastroscope
Wolf-Knittlingen gastroscope
Wolfler gastroenterostomy
Wolfram syndrome
**Wolf-Schindler semiflexible
gastroscope**
Wolfson
    W. gallbladder retractor
    W. intestinal clamp
Wolinella
Wolman
    W. disease
    W. xanthomatosis
Wood lamp
Woodward
    W. esophagogastroscopy
    W. esophagogastrostomy
Wookey skin tube
wool ball
Woolf
    W. method
    W. test
working
    w. port ureteroscope
    w. sheath
workstation
    Dornier MFL 5000
    urological w.

    DynaCell motility morphometry
      measurement w.
World Health Organization (WHO)
worm
    bilharzial w.
    bladder w.
    kidney w.
wound
    anal w.
    w. approximation
    aseptic w.
    w. closure
    w. dehiscence
    w. drainage
    w. healing
    w. infection
    open w.
    penetrating w.
    septic w.
    stab w.
    submucosal w.
woven dacron tube
wrap
    gastric fundus w.
    Kerlix w.
    Nissen fundoplication w.
    rectus fascial w.
    total gastric w.
    tunica vaginalis blanket w.
Wright
    W. stain
    W. stain of stool
Wright-Giemsa stain
writer
    laser w.
writing
    xanthography-yellow w.
WS
    watermelon stomach
W-shaped
    W.-s. forceps
    W.-s. ileal pouch-anal
      anastomosis
    W.-s. pouch
wt
    weight
    mol wt
      molecular weight
Wurbs-type nasobiliary tube
Wyamine
Wyanoids

Wylie
    W. hypogastric clamp
    W. splanchnic retractor

Wymox

W

x2 test
Xa
> factor Xa

Xanax
xanthelasma
xanthine
> x. oxidase
> x. oxidation

xanthogranulomatous
> x. cholecystitis
> x. cystitis
> x. pyelonephritis (XGP)

xanthography-yellow writing
xanthoma
> bladder x.
> x. cell
> gastric x.
> planar x.
> skin x.
> verruciform x.

xanthomatosis
> biliary x.
> biliary hypercholesterolemia x.
> cerebrotendinous x.
> familial hypercholesteremic x.
> Wolman x.

Xc
> reactance

Xc/R
> reactance and resistance
> Xc/R ratio

xenograft transplantation
xenon
> x. lamp
> x. light source

xenon-washout technique
xenoreactive antibody
xerophthalmia
xerostomia
XGP
> xanthogranulomatous pyelonephritis

XIa
> factor XIa

XIIa
> factor XIIa

XIII
xiphisternum
xiphoid
> x. appendix
> x.-to-pubis midline abdominal
> incision
> x.-to-umbilicus incision

XL
> Procardia XL

XL1-Blue cell
X-linked
> X.-l. infantile
> agammaglobulinemia
> X.-l. recessive nephrolithiasis
> (XRN)
> X.-l. recessive trait

XM-50 Dialow membrane
X-Prep
> X.-P. bowel prep
> Senokot X.-P.

XQ video instrument
x-ray
> x.-r. analysis
> x.-r. diffractometry

XRN
> X-linked recessive nephrolithiasis

XX male mosaicism
xylene
Xylocaine
> X. jelly
> topical X.
> X. topical anesthetic

xylometazoline
xylose
> x. absorption test
> x. tolerance test

xyphoid

X

YAG
  yttrium, aluminum, garnet
    YAG 1064
    YAG laser
    Laserscope YAG 1064
Yang
  Y. needle
  Y. polyclonal assay
  Y. Pros-Check PSA assay
  Y. Pros-Check PSA test
  Y. PSA radioimmunoassay
Yangtze Valley fever
Yankauer
  Y. esophagoscope
  Y. suction tube
yarn-collected specimen
Yates correction
Y chromosome
Y-connecting tubing
90Y-CYT-356
yeast balanitis
yeast-recombinant hepatitis B
  vaccine
Yellolax
yellow
  y. atrophy of the liver
  y. nodule
  y. phosphorus hepatotoxicity
Yeoman rectal biopsy forceps
Yeoman-Wittner rectal forceps
Yersinia
  Y. enterocolitica
  Y. enterocolitica colitis
  Y. pseudotuberculosis
yersiniasis
yersiniosis
yield
  sperm y.
Yocon
yohimbine
  y. HCl
  y. hydrochloride

Yohimex
yolk
  y. sac
  y. sac carcinoma
  y. sac tumor
Young
  Y. cystoscope
  Y. intestinal forceps
  Y. needle holder
  Y. prostatic retractor
  Y. prostatic tractor
  Y. technique
  Y. type epispadias repair
Young-Dees
  Y.-D. bladder neck
    reconstruction
  Y.-D. operation
  Y.-D. procedure
  Y.-D. technique
Young-Dees-Leadbetter
  Y.-D.-L. bladder neck
    reconstruction
  Y.-D.-L. operation
Youssef syndrome
yo-yo weight fluctuation
  phenomenon
Y-port connector
Y-set system
Y-shaped incision
yttrium-90
yttrium, aluminum, garnet (YAG)
Y-type Dianeal peritoneal dialysis
  solution
Yu-Holtgrewe prostatic retractor
Y-V
  Y.-V. anoplasty
  Y.-V. plasty
YY
  beta-endorphin peptide Y.
    (PYY)
  peptide Y. (PYY)

Y

Z
Z line
Z stent
Z suture
Zachary Cope-DeMartel clamp
Zahn
anomaly of Z.
Z. infarct
Zamboni fixative
zamifenicin
Zanosar
Zanoterone
Zantac
Z. EFFERdose
Z. GELdose
Zappacosta test
Zaroxolyn
ZE
Zollinger-Ellison
ZE Caps
ZE syndrome
Zebra exchange guidewire
Zebrax
Zeiss
Z. IDO3 phase-contrast
microscope
Z. morphomate M30
Z. S9 electron microscope
Zellweger syndrome
Zenker
Z. diverticulum
Z. pouch
zenobiotic glutathione conjugate
Zeppelin clamp
ZES
Zollinger-Ellison syndrome
Zestril
Zeta probe nylon filter
Ziehl-Neelsen stain
Zieve syndrome
zileuton
Zimmon
Z. biliary stent
Z. papillotome/sphincterotome
zinc
z. colic
z. selenide window
zipper
leucine z.
Zipser penile clamp

Zixoryn
Z-line
Z-Med catheter
Zocor
Zoladex
Z. implant
Zolicef
Zollinger-Ellison (ZE)
Z.-E. syndrome (ZES)
Z.-E. tumor
zomepirac
zona
z. glomerulosa
z. pellucida (ZP)
zonal gastritis
zona pellucida (ZP)
zone
abdominal z.
anal transition z.
border z.
high pressure z. (HPZ)
hyperemic border z.
portal z.
transitional z.
Zoon
balanitis of Z.
Z. erythroplasia
zoster
herpes z.
Zovirax
ZP
zona pellucida
Z-plasty
Z-stent
Z.-s. esophageal endoprosthesis
system
Gianturco Z.-s.
Gianturco-Rosch biliary Z.-s.
Z-test
Z-type deformity
Zyderm
Zygomycetes
zygomycosis
Zyloprim
Zymase
zymogen granule
zymogenic cell
zymosan
opsonized z.
Zypan

Z

ZZ phenotype · **ZZ phenotype**

ZZ phenotype

Appendix 1
Anatomical Illustrations

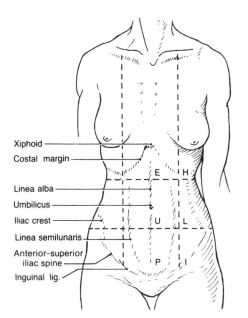

Xiphoid

Costal margin

Linea alba

Umbilicus

Iliac crest

Linea semilunaris

Anterior-superior iliac spine

Inguinal lig.

Figure 1. *Abdomen divided by regions.* A, Left and right hypochondriac (H), lateral (L), and inguinal (I) regions with medial epigastric (E), umbilical (U), and pubic (P) regions. Prominent landmarks and surface features are indicated. From April EW. Anatomy, 2nd ed. Baltimore: Williams & Wilkins, 1990.

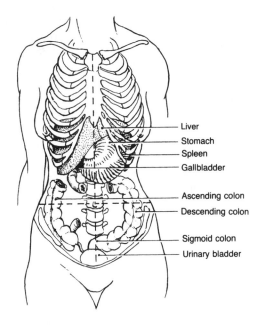

Liver

Stomach

Spleen

Gallbladder

Ascending colon

Descending colon

Sigmoid colon

Urinary bladder

Figure 2. *Abdomen divided by quadrants.* Left and right upper and lower quadrants are depicted with the principal underlying structures. From April EW. Anatomy, 2nd ed. Baltimore: Williams & Wilkins, 1990.

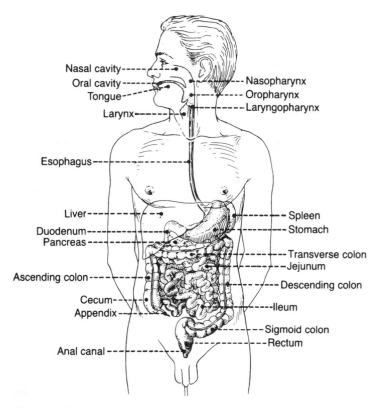

Figure 3. *Diagram of the digestive system.* From Chung KW. Gross anatomy, 2nd ed. Baltimore: Williams & Wilkins, 1991.

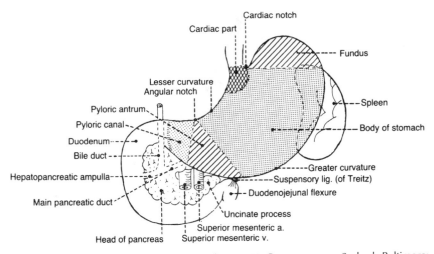

Figure 4. *Stomach and duodenum.* From Chung KW. Gross anatomy, 2nd ed. Baltimore: Williams & Wilkins, 1991.

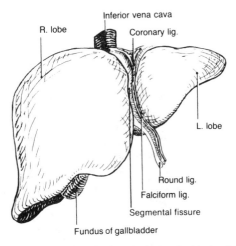

Figure 5. *Liver.* The anterior surface of the liver is depicted with the right and left lobes separated by the falciform ligament. From April EW. Anatomy, 2nd ed. Baltimore: Williams & Wilkins, 1990.

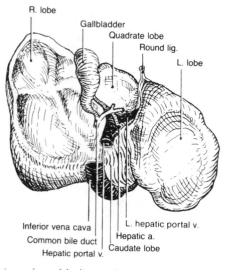

Figure 6. *Liver.* The inferior surface of the liver is shown with the left, right, quadrate, and caudate lobes as well as the gallbladder located between the right and quadrate lobes. From April EW. Anatomy, 2nd ed. Baltimore: Williams & Wilkins, 1990.

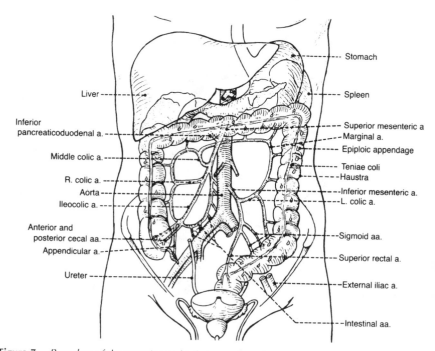

Figure 7. *Branches of the superior and inferior mesenteric arteries.* From Chung KW. Gross anatomy, 2nd ed. Baltimore: Williams & Wilkins, 1991.

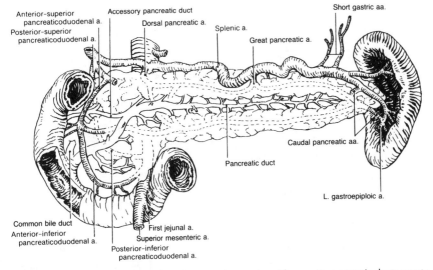

Figure 8. *Pancreas and spleen.* The primary and secondary (if present) pancreatic ducts empty into the descending portion of the duodenum. The pancreas receives its blood supply from the branches of the celiac and superior mesenteric arteries. The spleen receives a profuse blood supply from the splenic branch of the celiac artery. From April EW. Anatomy, 2nd ed. Baltimore: Williams & Wilkins, 1990.

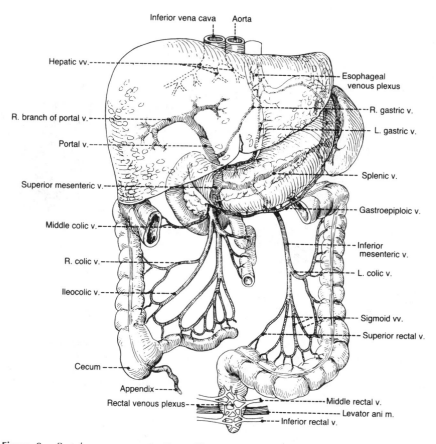

Figure 9. *Portal venous system.* From Chung KW. Gross anatomy, 2nd ed. Baltimore: Williams & Wilkins, 1991.

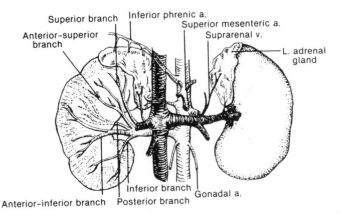

Figure 10. *Blood supply and venous drainage of the kidneys and adrenal glands.* The five segmental arteries of the right kidney are shown as are the three arteries supplying the right adrenal gland. The venous drainage of the left kidney and adrenal gland is depicted on the opposite side. From April EW. Anatomy, 2nd ed. Baltimore: Williams & Wilkins, 1990.

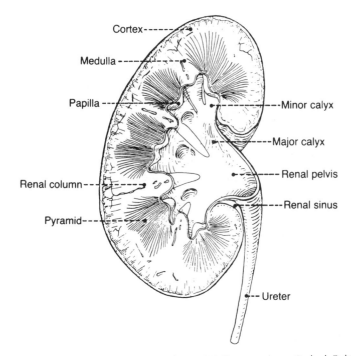

Figure 11. *Frontal section of the kidney.* From Chung KW. Gross anatomy, 2nd ed. Baltimore: Williams & Wilkins, 1991.

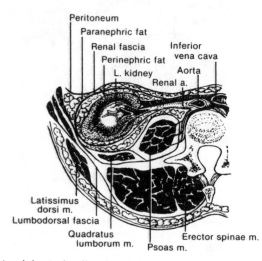

Figure 12. *Posterior abdominal wall and renal fascia.* From April EW. Anatomy, 2nd ed. Baltimore: Williams & Wilkins, 1990.

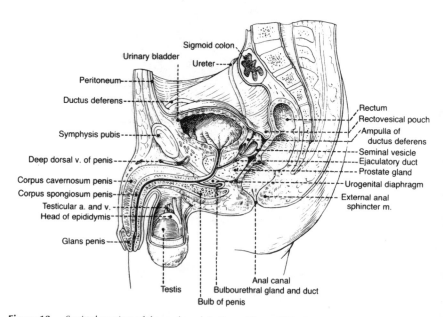

Figure 13. *Sagittal section of the male pelvis.* From Chung KW. Gross anatomy, 2nd ed. Baltimore: Williams & Wilkins, 1991.

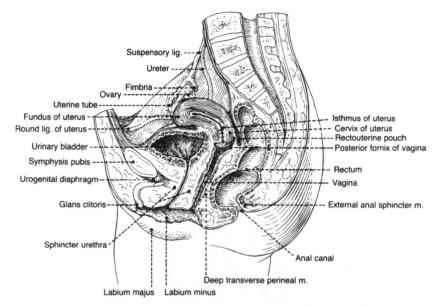

Figure 14. *Sagittal section of the female pelvis.* From Chung KW. Gross anatomy, 2nd ed. Baltimore: Williams & Wilkins, 1991.

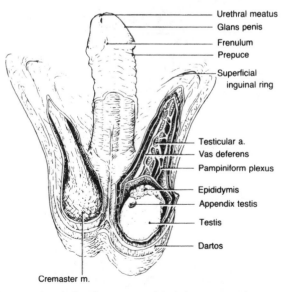

Figure 15. *Male external genitalia.* The contents of the left scrotum and spermatic cord are indicated. From April EW. Anatomy, 2nd ed. Baltimore: Williams & Wilkins, 1990.

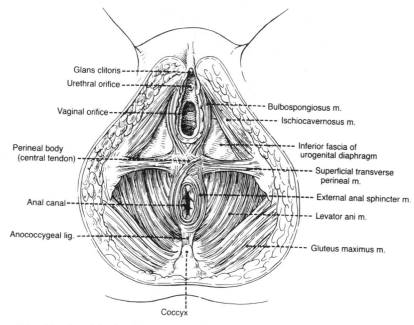

Figure 16. *Muscles of the female perineum.* From Chung KW. Gross anatomy, 2nd ed. Baltimore: Williams & Wilkins, 1991.

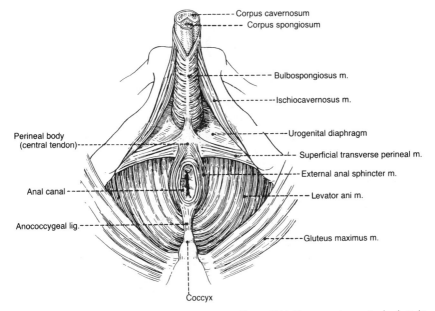

Figure 17. *Muscles of the male perineum.* From Chung KW. Gross anatomy, 2nd ed. Baltimore: Williams & Wilkins, 1991.

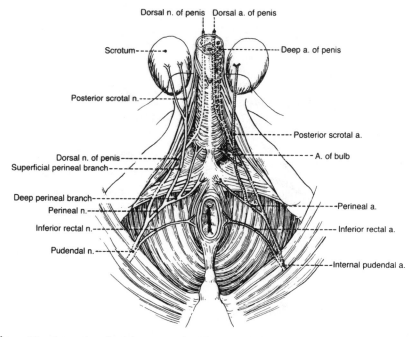

Figure 18. *Internal pudendal artery and pudendal nerve and branches.* From Chung KW.
Gross anatomy, 2nd ed. Baltimore: Williams & Wilkins, 1991.

Drug Names by Indication

Ascites

Aldactone
Aquatensen
Aquazide-H
bendroflumethiazide
bumetanide
Bumex
chlorothiazide
chlorthalidone
Demadex injection
Demadex Oral
Diaqua
Diucardin
Diurigen
Diuril
Edecrin Oral
Edecrin Sodium injection
Enduron
Esidrix
ethacrynic acid
Ezide
furosemide
hydrochlorothiazide
Hydro-Diuril
hydroflumethiazide
Hydro-Par
Hydro-T
Hygroton
indapamide
Lasix injection
Lasix Oral
Lozol
Metahydrin
methyclothiazide
metolazone
Mictrin
Mykrox
Naqua
Naturetin
Oretic

polythiazide
Renese
Saluron
spironolactone
Thalitone
torsemide
trichlormethiazide
Zaroxolyn

Bacillary Dysentery

Achromycin V Oral
ampicillin
Bactrim
Bactrim DS
Cipro injection
Cipro Oral
ciprofloxacin hydrochloride
Cotrim
Cotrim DS
co-trimoxazole
enoxacin
Floxin injection
Floxin Oral
lomefloxacin hydrochloride
Marcillin
Maxaquin Oral
norfloxacin
Noroxin Oral
Nor-tet Oral
ofloxacin
Omnipen
Omnipen-N
Panmycin Oral
Penetrex Oral
Polycillin
Polycillin-N
Principen
Robitet Oral
Septra
Septra DS
Sulfamethoprim

Sulfatrim
Sulfatrim DS
Sumycin Oral
Teline Oral
Tetracap Oral
tetracycline
Tetralan Oral
Tetram Oral
Totacillin
Totacillin-N
Uroplus DS
Uroplus SS

Bacteroides Fragilis Infection

amoxicillin and clavulanic acid
ampicillin and sulbactam
Augmentin
bacampicillin hydrochloride
cefmetazole sodium
Cefotan
cefotetan disodium
cefoxitin sodium
chloramphenicol
Chloromycetin
Cleocin HCl
Cleocin Pediatric
Cleocin Phosphate
clindamycin
Flagyl Oral
imipenem/cilastatin
Mefoxin
Metro I.V. injection
metronidazole
piperacillin sodium and tazobactam
    sodium
Primaxin
Protostat Oral
Spectrobid
ticarcillin and clavulanic acid
Timentin
Unasyn
Zefazone
Zosyn

Bacteroides Other Than Fragilis Infection

ampicillin
ampicillin and sulbactam
bacampicillin hydrochloride
cefmetazole sodium
Cefotan
cefotetan disodium
cefoxitin sodium
chloramphenicol
Chloromycetin
Cleocin HCl
Cleocin Pediatric
Cleocin Phosphate
clindamycin
Flagyl Oral
imipenem/cilastatin
Marcillin
Mefoxin
Metro I.V. injection
metronidazole
Mezlin
mezlocillin sodium
Omnipen
Omnipen-N
penicillin g, parenteral, aqueous
Pfizerpen injection
piperacillin sodium
piperacillin sodium and tazobactam
    sodium
Pipracil
Polycillin
Polycillin-N
Primaxin
Principen
Protostat Oral
Spectrobid
ticarcillin and clavulanic acid
Timentin
Totacillin
Totacillin-N
Unasyn
Zefazone
Zosyn

Behçet Syndrome
azathioprine
chlorambucil
cyclophosphamide
cyclosporine
Cytoxan injection
Cytoxan Oral
Deltasone Oral
Imuran
Leukeran
Liquid Pred Oral
Meticorten Oral
Neoral Oral
Neosar injection
Orasone Oral
Prednicen-M Oral
prednisone
Sandimmune injection
Sterapred Oral

Bowel Cleansing
Alphamul
castor oil
Co-Lav
Colovage
CoLyte
Emulsoil
Evac-Q-Mag
Fleet Enema
Fleet Flavored Castor Oil
Fleet Phospho-Soda
Go-Evac
GoLytely
magnesium citrate
Neoloid
NuLYTELY
OCL
polyethylene glycol-electrolyte solution
Purge
sodium phosphate

Bowel Sterilization
Achromycin V Oral
E.E.S. Oral

E-Mycin Oral
Eryc Oral
EryPed Oral
Ery-Tab Oral
Erythrocin Oral
erythromycin
Flagyl Oral
Ilosone Oral
metronidazole
Mycifradin Sulfate Oral
Neo-fradin Oral
neomycin sulfate
Neo-Tabs Oral
Nor-tet Oral
Panmycin Oral
PCE Oral
Protostat Oral
Robitet Oral
Sumycin Oral
Teline Oral
Tetracap Oral
tetracycline
Tetralan Oral
Tetram Oral

Campylobacter Jejuni Infection
Achromycin V Oral
amoxicillin and clavulanic acid
Augmentin
Bio-Tab Oral
chloramphenicol
Chloromycetin
Cipro injection
Cipro Oral
ciprofloxacin hydrochloride
Cleocin HCl
Cleocin Pediatric
Cleocin Phosphate
clindamycin
Doryx Oral
Doxy Oral
Doxychel injection
Doxychel Oral

doxycycline
E.E.S. Oral
E-Mycin Oral
enoxacin
Eryc Oral
EryPed Oral
Ery-Tab Oral
Erythrocin Oral
erythromycin
Floxin injection
Floxin Oral
Garamycin Ophthalmic
gentamicin sulfate
Ilosone Oral
Jenamicin injection
lomefloxacin hydrochloride
Maxaquin Oral
Monodox Oral
norfloxacin
Noroxin Oral
Nor-tet Oral
ofloxacin
Panmycin Oral
PCE Oral
Penetrex Oral
Robitet Oral
Sumycin Oral
Teline Oral
Tetracap Oral
tetracycline
Tetralan Oral
Tetram Oral
Vibramycin injection
Vibramycin Oral
Vibra-Tabs

Candidiasis (Oropharyngeal)

amphotericin B
clotrimazole
Diflucan injection
Diflucan Oral
fluconazole
Fungizone
Fungizone Intravenous

ketoconazole
Lotrimin
Mycelex
Mycostatin Oral
Nilstat Oral
nystatin
Nystat-Rx
Nystex Oral
O-V Staticin Oral/Vaginal

Carcinoid (Intestinal Tract)

Cosmegen
dacarbazine
dactinomycin
DTIC-Dome
Nizoral Oral
octreotide acetate
Sandostatin
streptozocin
Zanosar

Carcinoma (Bladder)

Adriamycin PFS
Adriamycin RDF
Adrucil injection
Bacillus Calmette-Guérin (BCG) Live
carboplatin
cisplatin
doxorubicin hydrochloride
Efudex Topical
etoposide
Fluoroplex Topical
fluorouracil
mitomycin
Mutamycin
Paraplatin
Platinol
Platinol-AQ
Rubex
teniposide
TheraCys
thiotepa
TICE BCG
Toposar injection
VePesid injection

VePesid Oral
Vumon injection

Carcinoma (Colorectal)
Adrucil injection
Efudex Topical
Ergamisol
Fluoroplex Topical
fluorouracil
Folex PFS
Hydrea
hydroxyurea
levamisole hydrochloride
methotrexate
Rheumatrex
streptozocin
Zanosar

Carcinoma (Esophagus)
Adriamycin PFS
Adriamycin RDF
Adrucil injection
carboplatin
doxorubicin hydrochloride
Efudex Topical
Fluoroplex Topical
fluorouracil
Paraplatin
Rubex

Carcinoma (Gallbladder)
floxuridine
FUDR

Carcinoma (Gastrointestinal Tract)
Adrucil injection
Efudex Topical
floxuridine
Fluoroplex Topical
fluorouracil
FUDR
mitomycin
Mutamycin
pentagastrin
Peptavlon

Carcinoma (Liver)
Adriamycin PFS
Adriamycin RDF
Adrucil injection
doxorubicin hydrochloride
floxuridine
fluorouracil
FUDR
Rubex
streptozocin
Zanosar

Carcinoma (Pancreatic)
Adriamycin PFS
Adriamycin RDF
Adrucil injection
doxorubicin hydrochloride
fluorouracil
streptozocin
mitomycin
Mutamycin
Rubex
Zanosar

Carcinoma (Renal)
aldesleukin
Alkaban-AQ
Amen Oral
CeeNu Oral
Curretab Oral
Cycrin Oral
Depo-Provera injection
lomustine
medroxyprogesterone acetate
Megace
megestrol acetate
Proleukin
Provera Oral
Velban
vinblastine sulfate

Carcinoma (Stomach)
Adriamycin PFS
Adriamycin RDF
Adrucil injection

cisplatin
doxorubicin hydrochloride
fluorouracil
Folex PFS
methotrexate
mitomycin
Mutamycin
Platinol
Platinol-AQ
Rubex

Carcinoma (Testis)
Adriamycin PFS
Adriamycin RDF
Alkaban-AQ
Blenoxane
bleomycin sulfate
carboplatin
chlorambucil
cisplatin
Cosmegen
cyclophosphamide
Cytoxan injection
Cytoxan Oral
dactinomycin
doxorubicin hydrochloride
etoposide
Folex PFS
Ifex injection
ifosfamide
Leukeran
methotrexate
Mithracin
Neosar injection
Oncovin injection
Paraplatin
Platinol
Platinol-AQ
plicamycin
Rubex
Toposar injection
Velban
VePesid injection
VePesid Oral

vinblastine sulfate
Vincasar PFS injection
vincristine sulfate

Cholelithiasis
Actigall
chenodiol
Moctanin
monoctanoin
ursodiol

Cholestasis
AquaMEPHYTON injection
Konakion injection
MCT oil
medium chain triglycerides
Mephyton Oral
phytonadione

Cirrhosis
Alka-Mints
Amitone
Aquasol A
azathioprine
Cal Carb-HD
Calci-Chew
Calciday-667
Calciferol injection
Calciferol Oral
Calci-Mix
calcium carbonate
calcium citrate
calcium glubionate
calcium lactate
Cal-Plus
Caltrate 600
Caltrate, Jr.
cholestyramine resin
Chooz
Citracal
Dicarbosil
Drisdol Oral
Equilet
ergocalciferol
Florical

Gencalc 600
Imuran
Mallamint
Neo-Calglucon
Nephro-Calci
Os-Cal 500
Oyst-Cal 500
Oystercal 500
Palmitate-A 5000
Questran
Questran Light
Rolaids Calcium Rich
Tums
Tums E-X Extra Strength Tablet
Tums Extra Strength Liquid
vitamin A

Cirrhosis (Primary Biliary)
Cuprimine
Depen
penicillamine

Citrobacter Infection
amikacin sulfate
Amikin injection
cefixime
Cefizox
Cefobid
cefoperazone sodium
cefotaxime sodium
ceftazidime
ceftizoxime sodium
ceftriaxone sodium
Ceptaz
Claforan
Fortaz
Garamycin injection
gentamicin sulfate
imipenem/cilastatin
Jenamicin injection
Mezlin
mezlocillin sodium
moxalactam
Moxam
Nebcin injection

netilmicin sulfate
Netromycin injection
Pentacef
piperacillin sodium
piperacillin sodium and tazobactam
  sodium
Pipracil
Primaxin
Rocephin
Suprax
Tazicef
Tazidime
Ticar
ticarcillin and clavulanic acid
ticarcillin disodium
Timentin
tobramycin
Zosyn

Clostridium Difficile Infection
Baci-IM injection
bacitracin
Flagyl Oral
Lyphocin injection
Metro I.V. injection
metronidazole
Protostat Oral
Vancocin injection
Vancocin Oral
Vancoled injection
vancomycin hydrochloride

Clostridium Perfringens Infection
Achromycin V Oral
Beepen-VK Oral
Betapen-VK Oral
Bio-Tab Oral
chloramphenicol
Chloromycetin
Cleocin HCl
Cleocin Pediatric
Cleocin Phosphate

clindamycin
Doryx Oral
Doxy Oral
Doxychel injection
Doxychel Oral
doxycycline
Flagyl Oral
imipenem/cilastatin
Ledercillin VK Oral
Metro I.V. injection
metronidazole
Monodox Oral
Nor-tet Oral
Panmycin Oral
PenVee K Oral
penicillin g, parenteral, aqueous
penicillin v potassium
Pfizerpen injection
Primaxin
Protostat Oral
Robicillin VK Oral
Robitet Oral
Sumycin Oral
Teline Oral
Tetracap Oral
tetracycline
Tetralan Oral
Tetram Oral
V-Cillin K Oral
Veetids Oral
Vibramycin injection
Vibramycin Oral
Vibra-Tabs

Clostridium Tetani Infection
Flagyl Oral
Hyper-Tet
Metro I.V. injection
metronidazole
penicillin g, parenteral, aqueous
Pfizerpen injection
Protostat Oral
tetanus immune globulin, human

Colitis (Ulcerative)
Acthar
Aristocort tablet
Aristospan
Articulose-50 injection
Asacol Oral
Azulfidine
Azulfidine EN-tabs
betamethasone
Celestone
Cortef
corticotropin
cortisone acetate
Cortone Acetate injection
Cortone Acetate Oral
Decadron
Delta-Cortef Oral
Deltasone Oral
Depo-Medrol injection
dexamethasone
Dipentum
H.P. Acthar Gel
Haldrone
Hydeltrasol injection
Hydeltra-T.B.A. injection
hydrocortisone
Kenacort syrup
Kenacort tablet
Kenalog injection
Key-Pred injection
Key-Pred-SP injection
Liquid Pred Oral
Medrol Oral
mesalamine
methylprednisolone
Meticorten Oral
olsalazine sodium
Orasone Oral
paramethasone acetate
Pediapred Oral
Pentasa Oral
Predaject injection
Predalone injection

Predcor injection
Predicort-50 injection
Prednicen-M Oral
Prednisol TBA injection
prednisolone
prednisone
Prelone Oral
Rowasa Rectal
Solu-Medrol injection
Stemex
Sterapred Oral
sulfasalazine
triamcinolone

Constipation

Alophen pills
Alphamul
Alramucil
bisacodyl
Bisacodyl Uniserts
Bisco-Lax
Black Draught
calcium polycarbophil
Carter's Little Pills
cascara sagrada
castor oil
Cephulac
Cholac
Cholan-HMB
Chronulac
Citrucel
Clysodrast
Colace
Colax
Constilac
Constulose
Correctol
Correctol Extra Gentle
DC 240 Softgel
Decholin
dehydrocholic acid
Dialose Plus capsule
Dialose Plus tablet
Diocto

Diocto C
Diocto-K
Diocto-K Plus
Dioctolose Plus
Dioeze
Disanthrol
Disolan
Disonate
Docucal-P
docusate
docusate and casanthranol
docusate and phenolphthalein
DOK
DOS Softgel
Doxidan
DSMC Plus
D-S-S
D-S-S Plus
Dulcagen
Dulcolax
Duphalac
Effer-Syllium
Emulsoil
Enulose
Equalactin tablet
Espotabs
Evac-U-Gen
Evac-U-Lax
Evalose
Ex-Lax
Ex-Lax, Extra Gentle Pills
Feen-a-Mint
Feen-a-Mint Pills
Femilax
Fiberall Chewable tablet
Fiberall powder
Fiberall wafer
FiberCon tablet
Fiber-Lax tablet
FiberNorm
Fleet Babylax Rectal
Fleet Enema
Fleet Flavored Castor Oil

Fleet Laxative
Fleet Phospho-Soda
Genasoft Plus
glycerin
Haley's M-O
Heptalac
Hydrocil
Kasof
Konsyl
Konsyl-D
Konsyl Fiber
lactulose
Lactulose PSE
Lax-Pills
Maalox Daily Fiber Therapy
magnesium hydroxide
magnesium hydroxide and mineral oil
  emulsion
magnesium oxide
magnesium sulfate
malt soup extract
Maltsupex
Maox
Medilax
Metamucil
Metamucil Instant Mix
methylcellulose
Mitrolan Chewable tablet
Modane
Modane Bulk
Modane Plus
Modane Soft
Mylanta Natural Fiber Supplement
Neoloid
Ophthalgan Ophthalmic
Osmoglyn Ophthalmic
Perdiem Plain
Peri-Colace
Phenolax
phenolphthalein
Phillips' LaxCaps
Phillips' Milk of Magnesia
Pro-Cal-Sof

Pro-Sof Plus
Prulet
psyllium
Purge
Regulace
Regulax SS
Reguloid
Regutol
Restore
Sani-Supp Suppository
senna
Senna-Gen
Senokot
Senolax
Serutan
Siblin
Silace
Silace-C
sodium phosphate
sorbitol
Sulfalax
Surfak
Syllact
Unilax
V-Lax
X-Prep Liquid

Cornybacterium Infection Other Than C. Jeikeium

E.E.S. Oral
E-Mycin Oral
Eryc Oral
EryPed Oral
Ery-Tab Oral
Erythrocin Oral
erythromycin
Ilosone Oral
PCE Oral
penicillin g, parenteral, aqueous
Pfizerpen injection

Crohn Disease

Acthar
Asacol Oral

Azulfidine
Azulfidine EN-tabs
Cortef
corticotropin
Deltasone Oral
Dipentum
H.P. Acthar gel
hydrocortisone
Hydrocortone Acetate
Hydrocortone Phosphate
Liquid Pred Oral
mesalamine
Meticorten Oral
olsalazine sodium
Orasone Oral
Pentasa Oral
Prednicen-M Oral
prednisone
Rowasa Rectal
Solu-Cortef
Sterapred Oral
sulfasalazine

Cryptorchidism
A.P.L.
Chorex
chorionic gonadotropin
Choron
Follutein
Glukor
Gonic
Pregnyl
Profasi HP

Diarrhea
attapulgite
Bacid
Bismatrol
bismuth subgallate
bismuth subsalicylate
calcium polycarbophil
Children's Kaopectate
colistin sulfate
Coly-Mycin S Oral

Devrom
Diar-aid
Diasorb
difenoxin and atropine
diphenoxylate and atropine
Donnagel
Donnapectolin-PG
Equalactin tablet
Fiberall Chewable tablet
FiberCon tablet
Fiber-Lax tablet
FiberNorm
hyoscyamine, atropine, scopolamine,
   kaolin, and pectin
hyoscyamine, atropine, scopolamine,
   kaolin, pectin, and opium
Imodium
Imodium A-D
Kaodene
kaolin and pectin
kaolin and pectin with opium
Kaopectate Advanced Formula
Kaopectate II
Kaopectate Maximum Strength
   caplets
Kao-Spen
Kapectolin
Kapectolin PG
Konsyl Fiber
Lactinex
lactobacillus
Lofene
Logen
Lomanate
Lomodix
Lomotil
Lonox
loperamide hydrochloride
Low-Quel
Mitrolan Chewable tablet
More-Dophilus
Motofen
octreotide acetate

opium tincture
paregoric
Parepectolin
Pepto Diarrhea Control
Pepto-Bismol
Rheaban
Sandostatin

Diarrhea (Bacterial)
Mycifradin Sulfate Oral
Neo-fradin Oral
neomycin sulfate
Neo-Tabs Oral

Diarrhea (Bile Acids)
cholestyramine resin
Questran
Questran Light

Diarrhea (Travelers)
Bactrim
Bactrim DS
Bismatrol
bismuth subgallate
bismuth subsalicylate
Cipro injection
Cipro Oral
ciprofloxacin hydrochloride
Cotrim
Cotrim DS
co-trimoxazole
Devrom
Pepto-Bismol
Septra
Septra DS
Sulfamethoprim
Sulfatrim
Sulfatrim DS
Uroplus DS
Uroplus SS

Diverticulitis
amikacin sulfate
Amikin injection
ampicillin

ampicillin and sulbactam
bacampicillin hydrochloride
cefmetazole sodium
cefoxitin sodium
Cleocin HCl
Cleocin Pediatric
Cleocin Phosphate
clindamycin
Flagyl Oral
Garamycin injection
gentamicin sulfate
Jenamicin injection
Marcillin
Mefoxin
Metro I.V. injection
metronidazole
Nebcin injection
netilmicin sulfate
Netromycin injection
Omnipen
Omnipen-N
piperacillin sodium and tazobactam
    sodium
Polycillin
Polycillin-N
Principen
Protostat Oral
Spectrobid
ticarcillin and clavulanic acid
Timentin
tobramycin
Totacillin
Totacillin-N
Unasyn
Zefazone
Zosyn

Duodenal Ulcer
Axid
calcium carbonate and simethicone
Carafate
cimetidine
famotidine
magaldrate

magaldrate and simethicone
magnesium hydroxide
magnesium oxide
Maox
nizatidine
pentagastrin
Pepcid AC Acid Controller
Pepcid I.V.
Pepcid Oral
Peptavlon
Phillips' Milk of Magnesia
ranitidine hydrochloride
Riopan
Riopan Plus
sucralfate
Tagamet
Tagamet HB
Titralac Plus Liquid
Zantac injection
Zantac Oral

Dysentery
Achromycin V Oral
furazolidone
Furoxone
Nor-tet Oral
Panmycin Oral
Robitet Oral
Sumycin Oral
Teline Oral
Tetracap Oral
tetracycline
Tetralan Oral
Tetram Oral

Dysuria
Azo-Standard
flavoxate hydrochloride
Geridium
phenazopyridine hydrochloride
Prodium
Pyridiate
Pyridium
sulfamethoxazole and
    phenazopyridine

sulfisoxazole and phenazopyridine
Urispas

Entamoeba Histolytica Infection
Flagyl Oral
Humatin
Metro I.V. injection
metronidazole
paromomycin sulfate
Protostat Oral

Enterobacter Infection
amikacin sulfate
Amikin injection
Azactam
aztreonam
Bactrim
Bactrim DS
carbenicillin
Cefizox
cefotaxime sodium
ceftazidime
ceftizoxime sodium
ceftriaxone sodium
Ceptaz
chloramphenicol
Chloromycetin
Cipro injection
Cipro Oral
ciprofloxacin hydrochloride
Claforan
colistimethate sodium
Coly-Mycin M Parenteral
Cotrim
Cotrim DS
co-trimoxazole
cycloserine
Floxin injection
Floxin Oral
Fortaz
Furadantin
Furalan
Furan
Furanite

Garamycin injection
gentamicin sulfate
Geocillin
imipenem/cilastatin
imipenem/cilastatin
Jenamicin injection
lomefloxacin hydrochloride
Macrobid
Macrodantin
Maxaquin Oral
Mezlin
mezlocillin sodium
nalidixic acid
Nebcin injection
NegGram
netilmicin sulfate
Netromycin injection
nitrofurantoin
norfloxacin
Noroxin Oral
ofloxacin
Pentacef
piperacillin sodium
piperacillin sodium and tazobactam
    sodium
Pipracil
Primaxin
Rocephin
Septra
Septra DS
Seromycin Pulvules
Sulfamethoprim
Sulfatrim
Sulfatrim DS
Tazicef
Tazidime
Ticar
ticarcillin and clavulanic acid
ticarcillin disodium
Timentin
tobramycin
Uroplus DS
Uroplus SS
Zosyn

Enterococcus Infection
ampicillin
Beepen-VK Oral
Betapen-VK Oral
Garamycin injection
gentamicin sulfate
Jenamicin injection
Ledercillin VK Oral
Lyphocin injection
Marcillin
Omnipen
Omnipen-N
Pen.Vee K Oral
penicillin g, parenteral, aqueous
penicillin v potassium
Pfizerpen injection
Polycillin
Polycillin-N
Principen
Robicillin VK Oral
streptomycin sulfate
Totacillin
Totacillin-N
Vancocin injection
Vancocin Oral
Vancoled injection
vancomycin hydrochloride
V-Cillin K Oral
Veetids Oral

Enuresis
belladonna
Concentraid Nasal
DDAVP injection
DDAVP Nasal
desmopressin acetate
Ditropan
imipramine
Janimine Oral
oxybutynin chloride
Tofranil injection
Tofranil Oral
Tofranil-PM Oral

Epididymitis

amikacin sulfate
Amikin injection
amoxicillin
Amoxil
ampicillin
Bactrim
Bactrim DS
Biomox
Bio-Tab Oral
cefixime
Cefizox
Cefobid
cefoperazone sodium
cefotaxime sodium
ceftazidime
ceftizoxime sodium
ceftriaxone sodium
Ceptaz
Cipro injection
Cipro Oral
ciprofloxacin hydrochloride
Claforan
Cotrim
Cotrim DS
co-trimoxazole
Doryx Oral
Doxy Oral
Doxychel injection
Doxychel Oral
doxycycline
enoxacin
Floxin injection
Floxin Oral
Fortaz
Garamycin injection
gentamicin sulfate
Jenamicin injection
lomefloxacin hydrochloride
Marcillin
Maxaquin Oral
Monodox Oral
moxalactam

Moxam
nalidixic acid
Nebcin injection
NegGram
netilmicin sulfate
Netromycin injection
norfloxacin
Noroxin Oral
ofloxacin
Omnipen
Omnipen-N
Penetrex Oral
Pentacef
Polycillin
Polycillin-N
Polymox
Principen
Rocephin
Septra
Septra DS
Sulfamethoprim
Sulfatrim
Sulfatrim DS
Suprax
Tazicef
Tazidime
tobramycin
Totacillin
Totacillin-N
Trimox
Uroplus DS
Uroplus SS
Vibramycin injection
Vibramycin Oral
Vibra-Tabs
Wymox

Epiglottitis

ampicillin
Cefizox
cefotaxime sodium
Ceftin Oral
ceftizoxime sodium
ceftriaxone sodium

cefuroxime
chloramphenicol
Chloromycetin
Claforan
Kefurox injection
Marcillin
Mezlin
mezlocillin sodium
Omnipen
Omnipen-N
piperacillin sodium
piperacillin sodium and tazobactam
  sodium
Pipracil
Polycillin
Polycillin-N
Principen
Rocephin
ticarcillin and clavulanic acid
Timentin
Totacillin
Totacillin-N
Zinacef injection
Zosyn

Escherichia Coli Infection

Achromycin V Oral
amikacin sulfate
Amikin injection
amoxicillin
amoxicillin and clavulanic acid
Amoxil
ampicillin
Ancef
Augmentin
Azactam
aztreonam
Bactrim
Bactrim DS
Biocef
Biomox
Bio-Tab Oral
carbenicillin
Ceclor

cefaclor
cefadroxil monohydrate
Cefadyl
cefamandole nafate
Cefanex
cefazolin sodium
cefixime
Cefizox
Cefobid
cefonicid sodium
cefoperazone sodium
cefotaxime sodium
cefoxitin sodium
cefpodoxime proxetil
cefprozil
ceftazidime
Ceftin Oral
ceftizoxime sodium
ceftriaxone sodium
cefuroxime
Cefzil
cephalexin monohydrate
cephalothin sodium
cephapirin sodium
cephradine
Ceptaz
chloramphenicol
Chloromycetin
Cinobac Pulvules
cinoxacin
Cipro injection
Cipro Oral
ciprofloxacin hydrochloride
Claforan
colistimethate sodium
colistin sulfate
Coly-Mycin M Parenteral
Coly-Mycin S Oral
Cotrim
Cotrim DS
co-trimoxazole
cycloserine
Declomycin
demeclocycline hydrochloride

Doryx Oral
Doxy Oral
Doxychel injection
Doxychel Oral
doxycycline
Duricef
enoxacin
Fortaz
Furadantin
Furalan
Furan
Furanite
Garamycin injection
gentamicin sulfate
Geocillin
imipenem/cilastatin
Jenamicin injection
Keflex
Keflin injection
Keftab
Kefurox injection
Kefzol
Lorabid
loracarbef
Macrobid
Macrodantin
Mandol
Marcillin
Mefoxin
Mezlin
mezlocillin sodium
Monocid
Monodox Oral
moxalactam
Moxam
Mycifradin Sulfate Oral
nalidixic acid
Nebcin injection
NegGram
Neo-fradin Oral
neomycin sulfate
Neo-Tabs Oral
netilmicin sulfate
Netromycin injection

nitrofurantoin
norfloxacin
Noroxin Oral
Nor-tet Oral
Omnipen
Omnipen-N
oxytetracycline hydrochloride
Panmycin Oral
Penetrex Oral
Pentacef
piperacillin sodium
piperacillin sodium and tazobactam
 sodium
Pipracil
Polycillin
Polycillin-N
Polymox
Primaxin
Principen
Robitet Oral
Rocephin
Septra
Septra DS
Seromycin Pulvules
Sulfamethoprim
Sulfatrim
Sulfatrim DS
Sumycin Oral
Suprax
Tazicef
Tazidime
Teline Oral
Terramycin I.M. injection
Terramycin Oral
Tetracap Oral
tetracycline
Tetralan Oral
Tetram Oral
Ticar
ticarcillin and clavulanic acid
ticarcillin disodium
Timentin
tobramycin
Totacillin

Totacillin-N
Trimox
Ultracef
Uri-Tet Oral
Uroplus DS
Uroplus SS
Vantin
Velosef
Vibramycin injection
Vibramycin Oral
Vibra-Tabs
Wymox
Zartan
Zinacef injection
Zolicef
Zosyn

Esophageal Reflux

aluminum hydroxide and magnesium
  trisilicate
bethanechol chloride
cimetidine
cisapride
Clopra
Duvoid
famotidine
Gaviscon tablet
Gaviscon-2 tablet
lansoprazole
Maxolon
metoclopramide
Myotonachol
Octamide
omeprazole
Pepcid AC Acid Controller
Pepcid I.V.
Pepcid Oral
Prevacid
Prilosec
Propulsid
ranitidine hydrochloride
Reglan
Tagamet
Tagamet HB

Urecholine
Zantac injection
Zantac Oral

Esophageal Varices

Ethamolin injection
ethanolamine oleate
Pitressin injection
sodium tetradecyl sulfate
Sotradecol injection
vasopressin

Fusobacterium Infection

ampicillin
ampicillin and sulbactam
bacampicillin hydrochloride
Beepen-VK Oral
Betapen-VK Oral
chloramphenicol
Chloromycetin
Cleocin HCl
Cleocin Pediatric
Cleocin Phosphate
clindamycin
Flagyl Oral
Ledercillin VK Oral
Marcillin
Metro I.V. injection
metronidazole
Mezlin
mezlocillin sodium
Omnipen
Omnipen-N
Pen.Vee K Oral
penicillin g, parenteral, aqueous
penicillin v potassium
Pfizerpen injection
piperacillin sodium
piperacillin sodium and tazobactam
  sodium
Pipracil
Polycillin
Polycillin-N
Principen

Protostat Oral
Robicillin VK Oral
Spectrobid
Ticar
ticarcillin and clavulanic acid
ticarcillin disodium
Timentin
Totacillin
Totacillin-N
Unasyn
V-Cillin K Oral
Veetids Oral
Zosyn

Gag Reflex Suppression

Americaine
benzocaine
Dyclone
dyclonine hydrochloride
Hurricaine
lidocaine hydrochloride
Pontocaine Topical
tetracaine hydrochloride
Xylocaine

Gas Pains

aluminum hydroxide, magnesium
    hydroxide, and simethicone
calcium carbonate and simethicone
Di-Gel
Flatulex
Gas-Ban DS
Gas-X
Gelusil
Maalox Anti-Gas
Maalox Plus
magaldrate and simethicone
Magalox Plus
Mylanta
Mylanta Gas
Mylanta-II
Mylicon
Phazyme
Riopan Plus

Silain
simethicone
Titralac Plus Liquid

Gastric Ulcer

Axid
calcium carbonate and simethicone
cimetidine
Cytotec
famotidine
magaldrate
magaldrate and simethicone
magnesium hydroxide
magnesium oxide
Maox
misoprostol
nizatidine
Pepcid AC Acid Controller
Pepcid I.V.
Pepcid Oral
Phillips' Milk of Magnesia
ranitidine hydrochloride
Riopan
Riopan Plus
Tagamet
Tagamet HB
Titralac Plus Liquid
Zantac injection
Zantac Oral

Gastritis

Aludrox
aluminum hydroxide and magnesium
    hydroxide
cimetidine
hyoscyamine, atropine, scopolamine,
    kaolin, and pectin
Maalox
Maalox Therapeutic Concentrate
ranitidine hydrochloride
Tagamet
Tagamet HB
Zantac injection
Zantac Oral

Gastrointestinal Reflux Disease

Axid
cimetidine
cisapride
famotidine
lansoprazole
nizatidine
omeprazole
Pepcid AC Acid Controller
Pepcid I.V.
Pepcid Oral
Prevacid
Prilosec
Propulsid
ranitidine hydrochloride
Tagamet
Tagamet HB
Zantac injection
Zantac Oral

Haemophilus Ducreyi Infection

amoxicillin and clavulanic acid
Augmentin
Bactrim
Bactrim DS
ceftriaxone sodium
Cipro injection
Cipro Oral
ciprofloxacin hydrochloride
Cotrim
Cotrim DS
co-trimoxazole
E.E.S. Oral
E-Mycin Oral
Eryc Oral
EryPed Oral
Ery-Tab Oral
Erythrocin Oral
erythromycin
Ilosone Oral
PCE Oral
Rocephin

Septra
Septra DS
Sulfamethoprim
Sulfatrim
Sulfatrim DS
Uroplus DS
Uroplus SS

Haemophilus Influenzae Infection

amoxicillin
amoxicillin and clavulanic acid
Amoxil
ampicillin
ampicillin and sulbactam
Augmentin
bacampicillin hydrochloride
Bactrim
Bactrim DS
Biomox
Ceclor
cefaclor
cefamandole nafate
cefixime
Cefizox
cefmetazole sodium
Cefobid
cefonicid sodium
cefoperazone sodium
cefotaxime sodium
cefpodoxime proxetil
cefprozil
ceftazidime
Ceftin Oral
ceftizoxime sodium
ceftriaxone sodium
cefuroxime
Cefzil
Ceptaz
chloramphenicol
Chloromycetin
Cipro injection
Cipro Oral
ciprofloxacin hydrochloride

Claforan
Cotrim
Cotrim DS
co-trimoxazole
erythromycin and sulfisoxazole
Eryzole Oral
Floxin injection
Floxin Oral
Fortaz
haemophilus b conjugate vaccine
HibTITER
Kefurox injection
lomefloxacin hydrochloride
Mandol
Marcillin
Maxaquin Oral
Monocid
moxalactam
Moxam
ofloxacin
OmniHIB
Omnipen
Omnipen-N
Pediazole Oral
Pediazole Oral
PedvaxHIB
Pentacef
piperacillin sodium and tazobactam
    sodium
Polycillin
Polycillin-N
Polymox
Principen
Prohibit
Rocephin
Septra
Septra DS
Spectrobid
Sulfamethoprim
Sulfatrim
Sulfatrim DS
Suprax
Tazicef
Tazidime

ticarcillin and clavulanic acid
Timentin
Totacillin
Totacillin-N
Trimox
Unasyn
Uroplus DS
Uroplus SS
Vantin
Wymox
Zefazone
Zinacef injection
Zosyn

Helicobacter Pylori Infection
Achromycin V Oral
amoxicillin
Amoxil
Biomox
Bismatrol
bismuth subgallate
bismuth subsalicylate
Devrom
Flagyl Oral
Metro I.V. injection
metronidazole
Nor-tet Oral
Panmycin Oral
Pepto-Bismol
Polymox
Protostat Oral
Robitet Oral
Sumycin Oral
Teline Oral
Tetracap Oral
tetracycline
Tetralan Oral
Tetram Oral
Trimox
Wymox

Hemorrhoids
Anucort-HC suppository
Anuprep HC suppository

Anusol-HC 1
Anusol-HC 2.5%
Anusol-HC suppository
benzocaine
Cortaid with aloe
Corticaine Topical
Cortifoam
Dermtex HC with aloe
dibucaine
dibucaine and hydrocortisone
Enzone
Hemril-HC Uniserts
hydrocortisone
Itch-X
Lanacane
Nupercainal Topical
Phicon
Pontocaine Topical
PrameGel
Pramosone
pramoxine and hydrocortisone
pramoxine hydrochloride
Prax
Proctofoam
Proctofoam-HC
tetracaine hydrochloride
Tronolane
Tronothane
Tucks
Witch Hazel
Zone-A Forte

Hepatic Coma
Cephulac
Cholac
Chronulac
Constilac
Constulose
Duphalac
Enulose
Evalose
Heptalac
Humatin
kanamycin sulfate

Kantrex injection
Kantrex Oral
lactulose
Lactulose PSE
Mycifradin Sulfate Oral
Neo-fradin Oral
neomycin sulfate
Neo-Tabs Oral
paromomycin sulfate

Hepatitis a
Gamastan
Gammar
Havrix
hepatitis A vaccine
immune globulin, intramuscular

Hepatitis b
Engerix-B
H-BIG
hepatitis B immune globulin
hepatitis B vaccine
Hep-B-Gammagee
HyperHep
interferon alfa-2b
Intron A
Recombivax HB

Hepatitis c
interferon alfa-2b
Intron A

Hiccups
chlorpromazine hydrochloride
Ormazine
Thorazine
triflupromazine hydrochloride
Vesprin

Hyperacidity
Alka-Mints
Alternagel
Alu-Cap
Aludrox
aluminum carbonate
aluminum hydroxide

aluminum hydroxide and magnesium
   hydroxide
aluminum hydroxide and magnesium
   trisilicate
aluminum hydroxide, magnesium
   hydroxide, and simethicone
Alu-Tab
Amitone
Amphojel
Basaljel
Cal Carb-HD
Calci-Chew
Calciday-667
Calci-Mix
calcium carbonate
calcium carbonate and simethicone
calcium lactate
Cal-Plus
Caltrate 600
Caltrate, Jr.
Chooz
Dialume
Dicarbosil
Di-Gel
dihydroxyaluminum sodium
   carbonate
Equilet
Florical
Gas-Ban DS
Gaviscon tablet
Gaviscon-2 tablet
Gelusil
Gencalc 600
Maalox
Maalox Plus
Maalox Therapeutic Concentrate
magaldrate
magaldrate and simethicone
Magalox Plus
magnesium hydroxide
magnesium oxide
Mallamint
Maox

Mylanta
Mylanta-II
Nephro-Calci
Nephrox suspension
Neut injection
Os-Cal 500
Oyst-Cal 500
Oystercal 500
Phillips' Milk of Magnesia
Riopan
Riopan Plus
Rolaids
Rolaids Calcium Rich
sodium bicarbonate
Titralac Plus Liquid
Tums
Tums E-X Extra Strength tablet
Tums Extra Strength Liquid

Inflammatory Bowel Disease

Acthar
Adlone injection
A-methaPred injection
Asacol Oral
Azulfidine
Azulfidine EN-tabs
betamethasone
Celestone
Cortef
Cortenema
corticotropin
depMedalone injection
Depoject injection
Depo-Medrol injection
Depopred injection
Dipentum
D-Med injection
Duralone injection
H.P. Acthar gel
hydrocortisone
Medralone injection
Medrol Oral
mesalamine
methylprednisolone

M-Prednisol injection
olsalazine sodium
Pentasa Oral
Rowasa Rectal
Solu-Medrol injection
sulfasalazine

Irritable Bowel Syndrome

Alramucil
atropine sulfate
Banthine
Barbidonna
Barophen
belladonna
Bentyl Hydrochloride Oral
clidinium and chlordiazepoxide
Clindex
Clinoxide
Clipoxide
dicyclomine hydrochloride
Di-Spaz Oral
Donnapine
Donna-Sed
Donnatal
Effer-Syllium
Fiberall powder
Fiberall wafer
Hydrocil
hyoscyamine, atropine, scopolamine,
    and phenobarbital
Hyosophen
Kinesed
Konsyl
Konsyl-D
Librax
Lidox
Maalox Daily Fiber Therapy
Malatal
Metamucil
Metamucil Instant Mix
methantheline bromide
Modane Bulk
Mylanta Natural Fiber Supplement
Perdiem Plain
Pro-Banthine

propantheline bromide
psyllium
Reguloid
Relaxadon
Restore
Serutan
Siblin
Spasmolin
Spasmophen
Spasquid
Susano
Syllact
V-Lax

Kidney Stone

allopurinol
Bicitra
Calcibind
cellulose sodium phosphate
citric acid bladder mixture
Cuprimine
Depen
K-Phos Neutral
Lopurin
Neutra-Phos
Oracit
penicillamine
Polycitra
potassium citrate
potassium phosphate
potassium phosphate and sodium
    phosphate
Renacidin
sodium citrate and citric acid
sodium citrate and potassium citrate
    mixture
Thiola
tiopronin
Urocit-K
Uro-KP-Neutral
Zyloprim

Klebsiella Infection

Achromycin V Oral
amikacin sulfate

Amikin injection
Ancef
Azactam
aztreonam
Bactrim
Bactrim DS
Biocef
Bio-Tab Oral
carbenicillin
Ceclor
cefaclor
cefadroxil monohydrate
Cefadyl
cefamandole nafate
Cefanex
cefazolin sodium
cefixime
Cefizox
cefmetazole sodium
Cefobid
cefonicid sodium
cefoperazone sodium
cefotaxime sodium
cefoxitin sodium
cefprozil
ceftazidime
Ceftin Oral
ceftizoxime sodium
ceftriaxone sodium
cefuroxime
Cefzil
cephalexin monohydrate
cephalothin sodium
cephapirin sodium
cephradine
Ceptaz
chloramphenicol
Chloromycetin
Cinobac Pulvules
cinoxacin
Cipro injection
Cipro Oral
ciprofloxacin hydrochloride
Claforan

colistimethate sodium
Coly-Mycin M Parenteral
Cotrim
Cotrim DS
co-trimoxazole
Declomycin
demeclocycline hydrochloride
Doryx Oral
Doxy Oral
Doxychel injection
Doxychel Oral
doxycycline
Duricef
Dynacin Oral
enoxacin
Floxin injection
Floxin Oral
Fortaz
Furadantin
Furalan
Furan
Furanite
Garamycin injection
gentamicin sulfate
Geocillin
imipenem/cilastatin
Jenamicin injection
Keflex
Keflin injection
Keftab
Kefurox injection
Kefzol
lomefloxacin hydrochloride
Lorabid
loracarbef
Macrobid
Macrodantin
Mandol
Maxaquin Oral
Mefoxin
Mezlin
mezlocillin sodium
Minocin IV injection
Minocin Oral

minocycline hydrochloride
Monocid
Monodox Oral
moxalactam
Moxam
nalidixic acid
Nebcin injection
NegGram
netilmicin sulfate
Netromycin injection
nitrofurantoin
norfloxacin
Noroxin Oral
Nor-tet Oral
ofloxacin
Panmycin Oral
Penetrex Oral
Pentacef
piperacillin sodium
piperacillin sodium and tazobactam
  sodium
Pipracil
Primaxin
Primaxin
Robitet Oral
Rocephin
Septra
Septra DS
Sulfamethoprim
Sulfatrim
Sulfatrim DS
Sumycin Oral
Suprax
Tazicef
Tazidime
Teline Oral
Tetracap Oral
tetracycline
Tetralan Oral
Tetram Oral
ticarcillin and clavulanic acid
Timentin
tobramycin
Ultracef

Uroplus DS
Uroplus SS
Velosef
Vibramycin injection
Vibramycin Oral
Vibra-Tabs
Zartan
Zefazone
Zinacef injection
Zolicef
Zosyn

Malabsorption

Aquasol A
Chroma-Pak
Iodopen
M.T.E.-4
M.T.E.-5
M.T.E.-6
Molypen
Multe-Pak-4
Neotrace-4
P.T.E.-4
P.T.E.-5
Palmitate-A 5000
Pedte-Pak-5
Pedtrace-4
Sele-Pak
Selepen
trace metals
Trace-4
vitamin A
Zinca-Pak

Malnutrition

Adeflor
Amino-Opti-E Oral
Apatate
Aquasol E Oral
Chromagen OB
Chroma-Pak
cysteine hydrochloride
Filibon
Florvite
Gevrabon

glucose polymers
Iodopen
Lederplex
Lipovite
LKV-Drops
M.T.E.-4
M.T.E.-5
M.T.E.-6
M.V.C. 9 + 3
M.V.I. Concentrate
M.V.I. Pediatric
M.V.I.-12
MCT Oil
medium chain triglycerides
Mega-B
Megaton
Moducal
Molypen
Mucoplex
Multe-Pak-4
Multi Vit Drops
Natabec
Natabec FA
Natabec Rx
Natalins
Natalins Rx
Neotrace-4
NeoVadrin
NeoVadrin B Complex
Nestrex
Niferex-PN
Orazinc Oral
Orexin
P.T.E.-4
P.T.E.-5
Pedtê-Pak-5
Pedtrace-4
Polycose
Poly-Vi-Flor
Poly-Vi-Sol
Pramet FA
Pramilet FA
Prenavite
pyridoxine hydrochloride

Secran
Sele-Pak
Selepen
Stuart Prenatal
Stuartnatal 1+1
Sumacal
Surbex
thiamine hydrochloride
trace metals
Trace-4
Tri-Vi-Flor
Verazinc Oral
Vi-Daylin
Vi-Daylin/F
vitamin A
vitamin B complex
vitamin E
vitamin, multiple (injectable)
vitamin, multiple (pediatric)
vitamin, multiple (prenatal)
zinc sulfate
Zinca-Pak
Zincate Oral

Motion Sickness

Antivert
Benadryl Oral
Bonine
Bucladin-S Softab
buclizine hydrochloride
cyclizine hydrochloride
dimenhydrinate
diphenhydramine hydrochloride
Dramamine II
Dramamine Oral
Marezine
meclizine hydrochloride
Phenameth Oral
Phenazine injection
Phenergan injection
Phenergan Oral
Prometh injection
promethazine hydrochloride
Prorex injection

Prothazine injection
Prothazine Oral
scopolamine
Transderm Scop Patch
TripTone Caplets
V-Gan injection

Nausea

Arrestin
Calm-X Oral
Cesamet
chlorpromazine hydrochloride
Clopra
Compazine injection
Compazine Oral
Compazine Rectal
cyclizine hydrochloride
dimenhydrinate
Dimetabs Oral
diphenidol hydrochloride
Dramamine Oral
dronabinol
droperidol
Emecheck
Emetrol
Inapsine
Marezine
Marinol
Marmine Oral
Maxolon
metoclopramide
nabilone
Naus-A-Way
Nausetrol
Norzine
Octamide
ondansetron hydrochloride
Ormazine
Pediatric Triban
perphenazine
Phenameth Oral
Phenazine injection
Phenergan injection
Phenergan Oral

Phenergan Rectal
phosphorated carbohydrate solution
prochlorperazine
Prometh injection
promethazine hydrochloride
Prorex injection
Prothazine injection
Prothazine Oral
Reglan
Tebamide
Tega-Vert Oral
T-Gen
thiethylperazine maleate
Thorazine
Ticon
Tigan
Torecan
Triban
triflupromazine hydrochloride
Trilafon
Trimazide
trimethobenzamide hydrochloride
TripTone caplets
Vesprin
V-Gan injection
Vontrol
Zofran injection
Zofran Oral

Nephrotic Syndrome

Alazide
Aldactazide
Aquatag
Aquatensen
Aquazide-H
azathioprine
bendroflumethiazide
benzthiazide
bumetanide
Bumex
chlorambucil
chlorothiazide
chlorthalidone
cyclophosphamide

Cytoxan injection
Cytoxan Oral
Delta-Cortef Oral
Deltasone Oral
Demadex injection
Demadex Oral
Diaqua
Diucardin
Diurigen
Diuril
Dyazide
Enduron
Esidrix
Exna
Ezide
furosemide
Hydeltrasol injection
Hydeltra-T.B.A. injection
Hydrex
hydrochlorothiazide
hydrochlorothiazide and reserpine
hydrochlorothiazide and
   spironolactone
hydrochlorothiazide and triamterene
HydroDIURIL
hydroflumethiazide
Hydro-Par
Hydropres
Hydro-Serp
Hydroserpine
Hydro-T
Hygroton
Imuran
indapamide
Key-Pred injection
Key-Pred-SP injection
Lasix injection
Lasix Oral
Leukeran
Liquid Pred Oral
Lozol
Marazide
Maxzide

Metahydrin
methyclothiazide
Meticorten Oral
metolazone
Mictrin
Mykrox
Naqua
Naturetin
Neosar injection
Orasone Oral
Oretic
Pediapred Oral
Predicort-50 injection
Prednicen-M Oral
Prednisol TBA injection
prednisolone
prednisone
Prelone Oral
Proaqua
Saluron
Spironazide
Spirozide
Sterapred Oral
Thalitone
torsemide
trichlormethiazide
Zaroxolyn

Neurogenic Bladder

Anaspaz
Banthine
Cystospaz
Cystospaz-M
Ditropan
Donnamar
ED-SPAZ
Gastrosed
hyoscyamine sulfate
Levbid
Levsin
Levsin/SL
Levsinex
methantheline bromide
oxybutynin chloride

Obesity

Acutrim Precision Release
Adipex-P
amphetamine sulfate
benzphetamine hydrochloride
Control
Desoxyn
Dexatrim
Dexedrine
dextroamphetamine sulfate
Dextrostat
Didrex
diethylpropion hydrochloride
Fastin
fenfluramine hydrochloride
Ionamin
Mazanor
mazindol
methamphetamine hydrochloride
phentermine hydrochloride
phenylpropanolamine hydrochloride
Pondimin
Sanorex
Stay Trim Diet Gum
Tenuate
Tepanil
Westrim LA
Zantryl

Pancreatitis

Banthine
methantheline bromide
Pro-Banthine
propantheline bromide

Paralytic Ileus

dexpanthenol
Ilopan injection
Ilopan-Choline Oral
Panthoderm cream

Peptic Ulcer

Anaspaz
anisotropine methylbromide
atropine sulfate
Banthine
Barbidonna
Barophen
belladonna
Cantil
Carafate
cimetidine
clidinium and chlordiazepoxide
Clindex
Clinoxide
Clipoxide
Cystospaz
Cystospaz-M
Daricon
Donnamar
Donnapine
Donna-Sed
Donnatal
ED-SPAZ
famotidine
Gastrosed
glycopyrrolate
hyoscyamine sulfate
hyoscyamine, atropine, scopolamine,
  and phenobarbital
Hyosophen
Kinesed
lansoprazole
Levbid
Levsin
Levsin/SL
Levsinex
Librax
Lidox
Malatal
mepenzolate bromide
methantheline bromide
methscopolamine bromide
omeprazole
oxyphencyclimine hydrochloride
Pamine
Pathilon
Pepcid AC Acid Controller
Pepcid I.V.

Pepcid Oral
Prevacid
Prilosec
Pro-Banthine
propantheline bromide
ranitidine hydrochloride
Relaxadon
Robinul
Robinul Forte
Spasmolin
Spasmophen
Spasquid
sucralfate
Susano
Tagamet
Tagamet HB
tridihexethyl chloride
Valpin 50
Zantac injection
Zantac Oral

Peritonitis

ampicillin and sulbactam
bacampicillin hydrochloride
cefoxitin sodium
Cleocin HCl
Cleocin Pediatric
Cleocin Phosphate
clindamycin
Flagyl Oral
Garamycin injection
gentamicin sulfate
Jenamicin injection
Mefoxin
Metro I.V. injection
metronidazole
piperacillin sodium and tazobactam
    sodium
Protostat Oral
Spectrobid
ticarcillin and clavulanic acid
Timentin
Unasyn
Zosyn

Pharyngitis

Achromycin V Oral
amoxicillin
Amoxil
ampicillin
Beepen-VK Oral
Betapen-VK Oral
Bicillin C-R 900/300 injection
Bicillin C-R injection
Bicillin L-A injection
Biocef
Biomox
Bio-Tab Oral
Ceclor
cefaclor
cefadroxil monohydrate
Cefanex
cefpodoxime proxetil
cefprozil
Ceftin Oral
cefuroxime
Cefzil
cephalexin monohydrate
cephradine
Crysticillin A.S. injection
Declomycin
demeclocycline hydrochloride
Doryx Oral
Doxy Oral
Doxychel injection
Doxychel Oral
doxycycline
Duricef
Dynacin Oral
E.E.S. Oral
E-Mycin Oral
Eryc Oral
EryPed Oral
Ery-Tab Oral
Erythrocin Oral
erythromycin
Ilosone Oral
Keflex
Keftab

Kefurox injection
Ledercillin VK Oral
Lorabid
loracarbef
Marcillin
Minocin IV injection
Minocin Oral
minocycline hydrochloride
Monodox Oral
Nor-tet Oral
Omnipen
Omnipen-N
oxytetracycline hydrochloride
Panmycin Oral
PCE Oral
Pen.Vee K Oral
penicillin g benzathine
penicillin g benzathine and procaine
  combined
penicillin g procaine
penicillin v potassium
Permapen injection
Pfizerpen-AS injection
Polycillin
Polycillin-N
Polymox
Principen
Robicillin VK Oral
Robitet Oral
Sumycin Oral
Teline Oral
Terramycin I.M. injection
Terramycin Oral
Tetracap Oral
tetracycline
Tetralan Oral
Tetram Oral
Totacillin
Totacillin-N
Trimox
Ultracef
Uri-Tet Oral
Vantin

V-Cillin K Oral
Veetids Oral
Velosef
Vibramycin injection
Vibramycin Oral
Vibra-Tabs
Wycillin injection
Wymox
Zartan
Zinacef injection

Proctitis
Asacol Oral
mesalamine
Pentasa Oral
Rowasa Rectal

Prostatitis
Bactrim
Bactrim DS
carbenicillin
Cipro injection
Cipro Oral
ciprofloxacin hydrochloride
Cotrim
Cotrim DS
co-trimoxazole
enoxacin
Floxin injection
Floxin Oral
Furadantin
Furalan
Furan
Furanite
Geocillin
lomefloxacin hydrochloride
Macrobid
Macrodantin
Maxaquin Oral
nitrofurantoin
ofloxacin
Penetrex Oral
Septra
Septra DS

Sulfamethoprim
Sulfatrim
Sulfatrim DS
Uroplus DS
Uroplus SS

Proteus Mirabilis Infection

amikacin sulfate
Amikin injection
amoxicillin
Amoxil
ampicillin
ampicillin and sulbactam
Ancef
Azactam
aztreonam
bacampicillin hydrochloride
Bactrim
Bactrim DS
Biocef
Biomox
Ceclor
cefaclor
cefadroxil monohydrate
Cefadyl
cefamandole nafate
Cefanex
cefazolin sodium
cefixime
Cefizox
cefmetazole sodium
Cefobid
cefonicid sodium
cefoperazone sodium
cefoxitin sodium
cefpodoxime proxetil
cefprozil
ceftazidime
Ceftin Oral
ceftizoxime sodium
ceftriaxone sodium
cefuroxime
Cefzil
cephalexin monohydrate

cephalothin sodium
cephapirin sodium
cephradine
Ceptaz
chloramphenicol
Chloromycetin
Cipro injection
Cipro Oral
ciprofloxacin hydrochloride
Cotrim
Cotrim DS
co-trimoxazole
Duricef
enoxacin
Floxin injection
Floxin Oral
Fortaz
Garamycin injection
gentamicin sulfate
imipenem/cilastatin
Jenamicin injection
Keflex
Keflin injection
Keftab
Kefurox injection
Kefzol
lomefloxacin hydrochloride
Lorabid
loracarbef
Mandol
Marcillin
Maxaquin Oral
Mefoxin
Mezlin
mezlocillin sodium
Monocid
moxalactam
Moxam
nalidixic acid
Nebcin injection
NegGram
netilmicin sulfate
Netromycin injection

norfloxacin
Noroxin Oral
ofloxacin
Omnipen
Omnipen-N
Penetrex Oral
Pentacef
piperacillin sodium
piperacillin sodium and tazobactam
    sodium
Pipracil
Polycillin
Polycillin-N
Polymox
Primaxin
Principen
Rocephin
Septra
Septra DS
Spectrobid
Sulfamethoprim
Sulfatrim
Sulfatrim DS
Suprax
Tazicef
Tazidime
Ticar
ticarcillin and clavulanic acid
ticarcillin disodium
Timentin
tobramycin
Totacillin
Totacillin-N
Trimox
Ultracef
Unasyn
Uroplus DS
Uroplus SS
Vantin
Velosef
Wymox
Zartan
Zefazone

Zinacef injection
Zolicef
Zosyn

Pseudomonas Aeruginosa Infection

amikacin sulfate
Amikin injection
Azactam
aztreonam
carbenicillin
Cefobid
cefoperazone sodium
ceftazidime
Ceptaz
Cipro injection
Cipro Oral
ciprofloxacin hydrochloride
enoxacin
Floxin injection
Floxin Oral
Fortaz
Furadantin
Furalan
Furan
Furanite
Garamycin injection
gentamicin sulfate
Geocillin
imipenem/cilastatin
Jenamicin injection
lomefloxacin hydrochloride
Macrobid
Macrodantin
Maxaquin Oral
Mezlin
mezlocillin sodium
Nebcin injection
netilmicin sulfate
Netromycin injection
nitrofurantoin
norfloxacin
Noroxin Oral
ofloxacin

Penetrex Oral
Pentacef
piperacillin sodium
piperacillin sodium and tazobactam
    sodium
Pipracil
Primaxin
Tazicef
Tazidime
Ticar
ticarcillin and clavulanic acid
ticarcillin disodium
Timentin
tobramycin
Zosyn

Relapsing Fever (Borrelia Recurrentis)

Achromycin V Oral
Bio-Tab Oral
chloramphenicol
Chloromycetin
Declomycin
demeclocycline hydrochloride
Doryx Oral
Doxy Oral
Doxychel injection
Doxychel Oral
doxycycline
Dynacin Oral
E.E.S. Oral
E-Mycin Oral
Eryc Oral
EryPed Oral
Ery-Tab Oral
Erythrocin Oral
erythromycin
Ilosone Oral
Minocin IV injection
Minocin Oral
minocycline hydrochloride
Monodox Oral
Nor-tet Oral

oxytetracycline hydrochloride
Panmycin Oral
PCE Oral
penicillin g, parenteral, aqueous
Pfizerpen injection
Robitet Oral
Sumycin Oral
Teline Oral
Terramycin I.M. injection
Terramycin Oral
Tetracap Oral
tetracycline
Tetralan Oral
Tetram Oral
Uri-Tet Oral
Vibramycin injection
Vibramycin Oral
Vibra-Tabs

Salivation (Excessive)

Anaspaz
atropine sulfate
Cystospaz
Cystospaz-M
Donnamar
ED-SPAZ
Gastrosed
glycopyrrolate
hyoscyamine sulfate
Levbid
Levsin
Levsin/SL
Levsinex
Robinul
Robinul Forte
scopolamine

Salmonella Infection

amoxicillin
Amoxil
ampicillin
Bactrim
Bactrim DS
Biomox

Cefizox
Cefobid
cefoperazone sodium
ceftazidime
ceftizoxime sodium
ceftriaxone sodium
Ceptaz
chloramphenicol
Chloromycetin
Cipro injection
Cipro Oral
ciprofloxacin hydrochloride
Cotrim
Cotrim DS
co-trimoxazole
Floxin injection
Floxin Oral
Fortaz
lomefloxacin hydrochloride
Marcillin
Maxaquin Oral
moxalactam
Moxam
ofloxacin
Omnipen
Omnipen-N
Pentacef
Polycillin
Polycillin-N
Polymox
Principen
Rocephin
Septra
Septra DS
Sulfamethoprim
Sulfatrim
Sulfatrim DS
Tazicef
Tazidime
Totacillin
Totacillin-N
Trimox

Uroplus DS
Uroplus SS
Wymox

Shigella Infection
ampicillin
Bactrim
Bactrim DS
Cefizox
Cefobid
cefoperazone sodium
ceftazidime
ceftizoxime sodium
ceftriaxone sodium
Ceptaz
Cipro injection
Cipro Oral
ciprofloxacin hydrochloride
co-trimoxazole
Cotrim
Cotrim DS
Floxin injection
Floxin Oral
Fortaz
lomefloxacin hydrochloride
Marcillin
Maxaquin Oral
moxalactam
Moxam
ofloxacin
Omnipen
Omnipen-N
Pentacef
Polycillin
Polycillin-N
Principen
Rocephin
Septra
Septra DS
Sulfamethoprim
Sulfatrim
Sulfatrim DS
Tazicef

Tazidime
Totacillin
Totacillin-N
Uroplus DS
Uroplus SS

Sjögren Syndrome
Moi-Stir
Orex
saliva substitute
Salivart
Xero-Lube

Staphylococcal Saprophyticus Infection
ampicillin
Bactrim
Bactrim DS
Cotrim
Cotrim DS
co-trimoxazole
Furadantin
Furalan
Furan
Furanite
Macrobid
Macrodantin
Marcillin
nitrofurantoin
Omnipen
Omnipen-N
Polycillin
Polycillin-N
Principen
Septra
Septra DS
Sulfamethoprim
Sulfatrim
Sulfatrim DS
Totacillin
Totacillin-N
Uroplus DS
Uroplus SS

Trichinosis
mebendazole
Mintezol
thiabendazole
Vermox

Ureaplasma Urealyticum Infection
Achromycin V Oral
azithromycin
Biaxin Filmtabs
clarithromycin
dirithromycin
Dynabac
E.E.S. Oral
E-Mycin Oral
Eryc Oral
EryPed Oral
Ery-Tab Oral
Erythrocin Oral
erythromycin
Ilosone Oral
Nor-tet Oral
Panmycin Oral
PCE Oral
Robitet Oral
Sumycin Oral
Teline Oral
Tetracap Oral
tetracycline
Tetralan Oral
Tetram Oral
Zithromax

Urethritis (Gonococcal)
ceftriaxone sodium
Rocephin

Urethritis (Nongonococcal)
Achromycin V Oral
E.E.S. Oral
E-Mycin Oral
Eryc Oral
EryPed Oral

Ery-Tab Oral
Erythrocin Oral
erythromycin
Ilosone Oral
Nor-tet Oral
Panmycin Oral
PCE Oral
Robitet Oral
Sumycin Oral
Teline Oral
Tetracap Oral
tetracycline
Tetralan Oral
Tetram Oral

Urinary Bladder Spasm
Banthine
methantheline bromide
Pro-Banthine
propantheline bromide

Urinary Retention
bethanechol chloride
Ditropan
Duvoid
Myotonachol
neostigmine
oxybutynin chloride
Prostigmin injection
Prostigmin Oral
Urecholine

Urinary Tract Infection, Catheter-associated
ampicillin
Lyphocin injection
Marcillin
Omnipen
Omnipen-N
Polycillin
Polycillin-N
Principen
Totacillin
Totacillin-N

Vancocin injection
Vancocin Oral
Vancoled injection
vancomycin hydrochloride

Urinary Tract Infection, Chronic Urea-splitting
acetohydroxamic acid
Lithostat

Urinary Tract Infection, Perinephric Abscess
Ancef
Bactrim
Bactrim DS
cefazolin sodium
Cotrim
Cotrim DS
co-trimoxazole
Kefzol
Septra
Septra DS
Sulfamethoprim
Sulfatrim
Sulfatrim DS
Uroplus DS
Uroplus SS
Zolicef

Urinary Tract Infection, Pyelonephritis
ampicillin
Bactrim
Bactrim DS
Cotrim
Cotrim DS
co-trimoxazole
Garamycin injection
gentamicin sulfate
Jenamicin injection
Marcillin
Omnipen
Omnipen-N
Polycillin

Polycillin-N
Principen
Septra
Septra DS
Sulfamethoprim
Sulfatrim
Sulfatrim DS
Totacillin
Totacillin-N
Uroplus DS
Uroplus SS

Urinary Tract Infection, Uncomplicated

amoxicillin
Amoxil
Bactrim
Bactrim DS
Biomox
Cotrim
Cotrim DS
co-trimoxazole
Polymox
Septra
Septra DS
Sulfamethoprim
Sulfatrim
Sulfatrim DS
Trimox
Uroplus DS
Uroplus SS
Wymox

Urinary Tract Infection (Unspecific)

citric acid bladder mixture
Gantrisin Oral
Hiprex
methenamine
Proloprim
Renacidin
Renoquid
sulfacytine

sulfamethoxazole and phenazopyridine
sulfisoxazole
sulfisoxazole and phenazopyridine
trimethoprim
Trimpex
Urex

Vomiting

Anxanil
Arrestin
Atarax
Atozine
Cesamet
chlorpromazine hydrochloride
Compazine injection
Compazine Oral
Compazine Rectal
dimenhydrinate
diphenidol hydrochloride
Dramamine Oral
dronabinol
droperidol
Durrax
E-Vista
hydroxyzine
Hy-Pam
Hyzine-50
Inapsine
Marinol
nabilone
Neucalm
Norzine
ondansetron hydrochloride
Ormazine
Pediatric Triban
perphenazine
Phenameth Oral
Phenazine injection
Phenergan injection
Phenergan Oral
Phenergan Rectal
prochlorperazine
Prometh injection

promethazine hydrochloride
Prorex injection
Prothazine injection
Prothazine Oral
Quiess
Rezine
Tebamide
T-Gen
thiethylperazine maleate
Thorazine
Ticon
Tigan
Torecan
Triban
triflupromazine hydrochloride
Trilafon
Trimazide
trimethobenzamide hydrochloride
TripTone Caplets
Vamate
Vesprin
V-Gan injection
Vistacon-50
Vistaject-25
Vistaject-50
Vistaquel
Vistaril
Vistazine
Vontrol
Zofran injection
Zofran Oral

Zollinger-Ellison Syndrome

calcium carbonate and simethicone
cimetidine
Cytotec
famotidine
lansoprazole
magaldrate
magaldrate and simethicone
magnesium hydroxide
magnesium oxide
Maox
misoprostol
omeprazole
pentagastrin
Pepcid AC Acid Controller
Pepcid I.V.
Pepcid Oral
Peptavlon
Phillips' Milk of Magnesia
Prevacid
Prilosec
ranitidine hydrochloride
Riopan
Riopan Plus
streptozocin
Tagamet
Tagamet HB
Titralac Plus Liquid
Zanosar
Zantac injection
Zantac Oral

Common Terms by Procedure

Upper Endoscopic, Esophageal, and Cholangiopancreatography Procedure Terms

achalasia dilator
alligator jaws forceps
Amsterdam biliary stent
angularis
antrum of stomach
Bernstein test
BICAP cautery
biliary ampulla
biliary tree
biliary balloon dilator
biliary dilator catheter
biliary endoprosthesis
biopsy forceps
bipolar hemostasis probe
Blakemore-Sengstaken tube
blind technique
body of stomach
bougie á boule
bougie dilator
bullet-tip catheter
C-loop
cannulation
Cantor tube
cardia
cholangiogram
CLOtest
common bile duct
cone-tip catheter
Cotton cannulatome
cutting wire
cystic duct
duodenal bulb
duodenoscope
Eder-Puestow dilator
endoprosthesis
endoscopic retrograde
    cholangiopancreatography (ERCP)

endoscopic ultrasound
esophageal introitus
esophageal prosthesis
esophageal motility perfused catheter
esophageal varices
esophagogastroduodenoscope
fluoroscopy
flush injection
French esophageal dilator
French external diameter instrument
French heavy dilator
fundus
Geenan cytology brush
Glidewire
grasp tripod forceps
guidewire
heater probe
Helicobacter pylori
24-hour esophageal pH probe
incisor
incisura
J-turn of the scope
Linton-Nachlas tube
Maloney dilator
manual lithotriptor
metal ball-tip catheter
Microvasive Altertome
Minnesota tube
modified Sacks-Vine push-pull
    technique
nasobiliary drainage
Nd:YAG laser
needle-tip catheter
needle papillotome
Olympus GIF-100 video
    esophagogastroduodenoscope
overtube

papillotome
papillotomy
pelican biopsy forceps
Pentax video duodenoscope
Pentax video gastroscope
percutaneous endoscopic jejunostomy
  (PEJ)
percutaneous endoscopic gastrostomy
  (PEG)
perfused catheter pull-through
pigtail biliary stent
pneumostatic dilatation
postbulbar descending duodenum
pyloric intubation
pylorus
rat-tooth forceps

retroflexion
Savary dilator
Savary-Gilliard dilator
sclerotherapy needle
shark-tooth forceps
side-viewing endoscope
sphincter of Oddi manometry
sphincterotome
sphincterotomy
squamocolumnar junction
stent
taper-tip catheter
through-the-scope (TTS)
W-shaped forceps
Z-line pristine

Esophageal Manometric Study Terms

acid reflux event
antireflux measure
aperistalsis
average peak pressure (mm Hg)
average esophageal sphincter pressure
  average
classification, i.e., III B23a
distal body
double-peaked waves
duration (HH:MM)
esophageal motility study
esophageal body
fraction time pH
gastroesophageal reflux
hydrochloric acid perfusion
lower esophageal sphincter (LES)
lower esophageal sphincter pressure
  (LESP)
mean wave amplitude (normal value
  < 135 > 35 mm Hg/30 waves)
mean wave duration (normal value
  < 5.6 sec/30 waves)
motor responses (normal value
  < 3/30 swallows)

Narco esophageal motility machine
peak maximum pressure (mm Hg)
peristaltic performance
pharyngeal contraction
postprandial acid reflux
pressure
provocative testing
proximal body
rapid pull-through (normal value
  10–37 mm Hg)
reflux episode
regurgitation
simultaneous sequences—85.7%
  peristalsis
supine acid reflux
total acid reflux
total time pH
triple-peaked contraction waves
upper esophageal sphincter
  relaxation
upright acid reflux
water probe

Cholecystectomy and Cholangiogram Terms

anterior rectus sheath
Avitene
Balfour retractor
Balfour retractor with fenestrated
  blade
bayonet forceps
Cholangiocath
cholangiocatheter
cholecystoduodenal ligament
common bile duct
common hepatic duct
Crile forceps
Cushing dressing forceps
cystic artery
cystic duct
cystic duct Cholangiocath
Doyen intestinal forceps
Foley catheter
foramen of Winslow
Frazier suction tip
free flow
French-eye Vital needle holder
fundus-to-duct dissection
gallbladder bed
gallbladder fossa
gallbladder infundibulum
gallbladder ring clamp
gut
Hartmann pouch
hemostatic clamp
hepatoduodenal peritoneal reflection
Jackson-Pratt drain
Jarit mosquito forceps

Kelly forceps
Lahey thoracic clamp
laparotomy pad
Ligaclip
liver margin
Mayo scissors
Mayo scoop
Metzenbaum scissors
midclavicular line
Mixter ligature-carrying clamp
mosquito forceps
Ochsner forceps
Péan forceps
rectus sheath
red rubber catheter
Renografin solution
Rochester-Ochsner forceps
Rochester-Péan forceps
round ligament
sludge
Stille Super Cut scissors
subcostal incision
subcostal trocar
subhepatic region
T tube
T-tube drain
Thrombostat
towel clip
transhepatic cholangiography
trocar
umbilical area
Weck clip
xiphoid

Lower Endoscopy, Colonoscopy, and Sigmoidoscopy Terms

anoscope
bipolar electrocautery
colon motility catheter
colonoscope
colonoscopist
crescent snare
Crohn disease
decompression catheter
digital rectal examination
diverticula (plural)
diverticulum (singular)
endoscopist
external hemorrhoid
flexible sigmoidoscope
GoLytely bowel prep
hematochezia
heme-negative stool
heme-positive stool
Hemoccult test
hexagon snare
hot biopsy forceps
ileocecal valve

ileoscopy
internal hemorrhoid
lubricated gloved finger
monopolar electrocautery
oval snare
overtube
Pentax video colonoscope
polypectomy snare
polypectomy
random biopsy
rectosphincter manometric study,
    rectosphincteromanometric study
retroflex view
rigid sigmoidoscope
snare
still photography
stool aspirate
terminal ileum
tripod
video photography
videoscope
wire snare

Colonic Manometric Study Terms

colonic dysmotility
colonic motility
fasting recording
high-amplitude propagated
   contractions (HAPC)

phasic contraction
tonic contraction
water-perfused manometry catheter

Vasectomy Terms

dissecting instrument
grasping instrument
no-scalpel vasectomy instrument
RB1 needle

scrotum
vas deferens
vas-dissecting instrument

Transurethral Resection of Prostate (TURP) and Cystoscopy Terms

Adson clamp
Adson forceps
Alexander elevator
Allis clamp
anterior urethral approach
Army-Navy retractor
Babcock clamp
bilobar hyperplasia
bilobar hypertrophy
bladder light reflex
bladder outlet obstruction
Bovie electrocautery
Bovie holder
Brown Buerger cystoscope
bulbomembranous area of urethra
bulldog clamp
calculus
cellules (plural)
continuous bladder irrigation (CBI)
Crile angle retractor
curved hemostat
Cushing forceps
Deaver retractor
diverticula (plural)
diverticulum (singular)
dorsal lithotomy position
Ellik evacuator
Foley catheter
Foroblique resectoscope
Frazier suction tube
French caliber
French cystoscope
Gerald forceps
Gil-Vernet retractor
hemostat
Herrick kidney clamp
Iglesias fiberoptic resectoscope
Iglesias resectoscope sheath
indigo carmine dye
kidney pedicle clamp

Kocher clamp
lithotomy position
long scalpel
long tissue forceps
malleable retractor
Maxaquin
Mayo-Hegar needle holder
Mayo scissors
McBurney retractor
McCarthy panendoscope
median bar formation
Metzenbaum scissors
microscopic hematuria
Millin bladder retractor
Millin forceps
Moynihan clamp
nocturia
Pfister-Schwartz basket
Poole suction tube
Potts forceps
prostate-specific antigen (PSA)
prostatic capsule
prostatic chips
prostatic fossa
prostatic hyperplasia
prostatic hypertrophy
prostatic urethra
Randall stone forceps
resectoscope
resectoscope loop
resectoscope sheath
retrograde pyelogram
ribbon retractor
Richardson retractor
right-angle clamp
sponge forceps
staghorn calculus
stent
stone retrieval balloon
stone extraction

stone retrieval basket
Storz cystoscope
straight hemostat
subcostal space
suture scissors
Timberlake obturator
towel clip
trabeculation
trigonitis
trilobar hyperplasia
trilobar hypertrophy
tubing clamp
ureteral catheter
ureteroscope sheath

urethrotome
urinary spurt
urine reflux
Van Buren sound
verumontanum
vesical mucosa
vesical neck
Vim-Silverman needle
Walther sound
wire scissors
working bridge
Xylocaine jelly
Young needle holder
Young prostatic retractor

Renal Transplant and Dialysis Access Terms

antecubital fossa
arteriotomy
axilla plexus
Bentson guidewire
bilateral carotid duplex ultrasound
bilateral renal ultrasound
cadaveric kidney
celiac axis
common iliac artery
digital subtraction angiography
external iliac artery
external iliac vein
external oblique aponeurosis
French pigtail catheter
inferior epigastric artery
inferior epigastric vein
internal iliac artery
internal iliac vein
internal oblique aponeurosis
intravenous urogram
kidney biopsy
living-related donor

median cubital vein
oblique planes with magnification
overhead spot films
perfusion
psoas muscle
rectus muscle
rectus sheath
renal arteriogram
renal ultrasound
reperfusion
retroperitoneum
round ligament
Satinsky clamp
Seldinger technique
spatulated
transversalis fascia
transversus abdominis
ureteric vessel
vascular access
vascular clamp
vascular loop
venotomy

Appendix 4
Sample Reports of Common Procedures
Sample Upper Endoscopy with Biopsy

TITLE OF OPERATION Upper endoscopy with biopsy.

PROCEDURE IN DETAIL Upper endoscopy indicated in patient with dyspepsia refractory to H2 blockers. Following administration of Demerol 75 mg, Versed 5 mg, and droperidol 1.2 mg, the esophagus was examined with Olympus GIF-100 with findings of normal mucosa. There was a small hiatal hernia located 42 cm from the incisors. The stomach revealed a 1-cm ulcer on the incisura. The ulcer was biopsied 4 times and a CLOtest was performed. The duodenum was normal without ulcerations.

IMPRESSION Gastric ulcer with biopsies pending to rule out gastric malignancy. A CLOtest is pending to exclude Helicobacter pylori infection.

RECOMMENDATIONS Continue full-dose H2 blockers for 8 weeks with follow-up endoscopy at that time to assess ulcer healing. If H. pylori is positive, would treat with triple antibiotics.

Sample Esophagogastroduodenoscopy

TITLE OF OPERATION Esophagogastroduodenoscopy to duodenal bulb.

PROCEDURE IN DETAIL Medications: Demerol 100 mg IV and Versed 5 mg IV. The patient was brought to the endoscopy suite, placed in the left lateral decubitus position, and the Pentax video gastroscope was introduced into the oropharynx under direct visualization. The vocal cords appeared normal. The posterior pharynx revealed no abnormalities. The esophagus was intubated without difficulty revealing normal pinkish-gray mucosa throughout the entire length of the esophagus. The squamocolumnar junction was at 41 cm from the incisors, was slightly irregular but sharp and intact. The stomach was entered without difficulty revealing normal rugal folds that flattened with air insufflation. The body of the stomach appeared normal. The antrum revealed some erythematous streaks emanating from the pylorus. No erosions and no ulcers were seen. The duodenal bulb was examined and a large, ulcerated mass likely representing extension of pancreatic carcinoma was found. A biopsy was taken and forwarded to pathology. The second and third portion of the duodenum appeared normal. The endoscope was withdrawn into the stomach. The endoscope was retroflexed revealing normal cardia and fundus. The endoscope was then straightened and withdrawn. The patient tolerated the procedure well.

Sample Endoscopic Retrograde Cholangiopancreatography (ERCP)

TITLE OF OPERATION Endoscopic retrograde cholangiopancreatography (ERCP).

PROCEDURE IN DETAIL The patient was examined and thought to be medically fit for endoscopy. Informed consent was obtained from the patient. The risks and benefits and possible complications including sepsis, pancreatitis, perforation, and bleeding were discussed and the patient agreed to proceed. Medications administered: Demerol 75 mg, Versed 8 mg, Glucagon 1.5 mg IV, and Unasyn 1.5 g IV. With the patient in the prone position, the Pentax video duodenoscope was passed into the esophagus under direct visualization without difficulty. The scope was advanced into the stomach and through the pylorus into the second portion of the duodenum. In the second portion of the duodenum, a large diverticulum was noted. The biliary ampulla was not readily identified; however, bile was seen coming from the diverticulum and, after careful examination, the ampulla was seen in the diverticulum. It was very difficult to maintain position to manage adequate visualization of the ampulla. A microinvasive altertome was initially used to cannulate the ampulla. Initially, the pancreatic duct was cannulated and had a normal appearance in the head and into the body. Since this was not the duct of interest, further injection was not performed. Several attempts were made to reposition or obtain a better angle on the ampulla and finally cannulation of the bile duct was obtained. Fluoroscopic and radiologic images were difficult to visualize. The common bile duct, common hepatic duct, and intrahepatic system were dilated. The common bile duct measured approximately 1.5 cm. Because of the severe difficulty of maintaining cannulation and the patient being uncomfortable from the air needed to keep the diverticulum opened, the procedure was terminated. The scope was then withdrawn and removed. The patient tolerated the procedure well and there were no immediate complications.

Sample Esophageal Manometric Study

TITLE OF OPERATION Esophageal manometry studies.

HISTORY/INDICATIONS This esophageal motility was performed for evaluation of dysphagia to solids, chest pain, and regurgitation of 5 years' duration.

Medications: None
Biopsies: No
Brushings: No
Photographs: No

FINDINGS
The esophageal manometry was measured, each of the 10 wet swallows had
    normal peristaltic activity.
There were no simultaneous waves or multi-peaked waves.
The mean average was 84 mmHg.
The mean duration was 4.7.
Both of these were normal.
The lower esophageal sphincter pressure was measured and was elevated at a
    pressure of 95 mmHg.
No relaxation of the sphincter; it appeared normal on rapid pull-throughs but a
    slow pull through was not analyzed.
Testing with acid profusion caused burning in the throat after 1 minute.
The normal range for lower esophageal sphincter pressure is 10–35 mmHg.

IMPRESSION Hypertensive lower sphincter pressure.
    Normal esophageal motility.
    Rapid response to acid profusion.

ESOPHAGEAL BODY
Normal	Abnormal
_____	_____ aperistalsis
_____	_____ proximal body
_____	_____ distal body

_____ mean wave amplitude (mmHg/#waves) _____
    (Normal value > 35 or < 135/30 waves)
_____ mean wave duration (sec/#waves) _____
    (Normal value < 5.6/30 waves)
_____ abnormal motor responses (#/# swallows) _____
    (Normal value < 3/30 swallows)
_____ triple-peaked contraction waves (#) _____
    (Normal value none)

LOWER ESOPHAGEAL SPHINCTER (LES)

Normal   Abnormal

_____   _____ pressure
_____   _____ relaxation
rapid pull through (mmHg) _____
(Normal values 10–37 mmHg)
estimated from stations _____

PROVOCATIVE TESTING

hydrochloric acid perfusion   positive _____   negative _____
Others: balloon   positive _____   negative _____

Sample Laparoscopic Cholecystectomy

TITLE OF OPERATION Laparoscopic cholecystectomy.

PROCEDURE IN DETAIL Under general endotracheal anesthesia, the abdomen and genitalia were prepped and draped. A Foley catheter was inserted. Using a blunt trocar, a small incision was made in the infraumbilical area and the fascia was opened. The blunt trocar was inserted. The camera was inserted through this trocar. Another 10-mm trocar was placed in the subcostal space about 2 inches lateral to the midline. On the right side, two 5-mm trocars were placed, one in the posterior axillary line and one in the midclavicular line on the right side. A grasper was used to grab the fundus of the gallbladder and also the Hartmann pouch pulling the cystic artery and duct into tension and visibility. Using a dissector, the cystic duct and artery were dissected and mobilized. Two surgical clips were placed on the cystic ducts and the cystic duct was transected with scissors. Three surgical clips were also placed on the cystic artery, and this was transected also. Using coagulating current with a coagulator, the gallbladder was removed from its gallbladder bed. Some bleeding points from the liver surface were coagulated. The gallbladder was then removed through the superior 10-mm trocar. In the process the gallbladder ruptured, and the stone, which was mostly a cholesterol stone, broke down leaving some stones in the intra-abdominal area. Broken stones were removed using graspers and dissectors until 95% of all stones were removed. Only those of small sandy-like material were not able to be removed, and these were evacuated using suction after copious irrigation. The gallbladder bed was checked for bleeding. The trocars were removed. The abdominal cavity was deflated. The fascia was closed using 0 Vicryl in the infraumbilical area and subcostal area following removal of the trocar. The skin was closed using subcuticular and 4–0 Vicryl. Sterile dry dressings were applied. The patient was then awakened, extubated, and taken to the recovery room in satisfactory condition.

Sample Cholecystectomy with Operative Cholangiogram

TITLE OF OPERATION Cholecystectomy with operative cholangiogram.

PROCEDURE IN DETAIL The patient was placed under general anesthesia in the supine position and was prepped and draped in the usual manner. A right subcostal incision was made through all layers, with exploration revealing the above-noted observations. Using very meticulous blunt and sharp dissection, the cystic duct, cystic artery, and common bile duct were visualized, identified, and isolated. The cystic duct was ligated adjacent to the common duct. An operative cholangiogram was then performed using standard technique, with no evidence of filling defect in the retained common duct. The cystic artery was likewise divided between ligatures. A fundus-to-duct dissection was then performed, with the gallbladder being excised intact. Hemostasis in the gallbladder fossa was achieved with cautery, followed by Thrombostat, as well as Avitene, to provide hemostasis. A separate stab wound was made and a drain was inserted. Closure was achieved utilizing a #0 continuous chromic suture for approximation of the peritoneum and multiple interrupted figure-of-eight sutures of #0 Prolene for approximation of the fascia. The skin was closed with skin clips. Sterile dry dressings were applied and the patient was taken to the recovery room in apparent satisfactory condition.

Sample Colonoscopy

TITLE OF OPERATION Colonoscopy.

PROCEDURE IN DETAIL The patient was examined and thought to be medically fit for endoscopy. Consent was obtained from the patient. Following administration of Fentanyl 0.1 mg and Versed 1.5 mg and with the patient in the left lateral decubitus position, digital rectal examination was performed and showed blood. The Pentax video colonoscope was passed into the rectum. The rectal mucosa was covered with blood. No obvious bleeding source was detected in the rectum. The scope was advanced into the sigmoid colon which showed diverticulosis. There was no evidence of an active diverticular bleed. In the sigmoid colon there was also a 2– to 2.5–cm polyp that was biopsied. This also did not appear to be a bleeding source. The scope was advanced through the remainder of the sigmoid colon, descending transverse, and ascending colon to the tip of the cecum. There was blood throughout the entire colon. No arteriovenous malformations were noted. There was no obvious bleeding source seen. Areas were flushed and the underlying mucosa revealed good vascular pattern. There was no evidence of any ischemic changes or ulcerations present. We were unable to intubate the terminal ileum because of the angle of the ileocecal valve. The scope was slowly withdrawn, a careful examination was performed, and no other abnormalities were seen. Retroflexion was performed and showed no evidence of carcinoma or other abnormality. The scope was then removed. The patient tolerated the procedure well. There were no immediate complications.

Sample Sigmoidoscopy

TITLE OF OPERATION Sigmoidoscopy to 60 cm from anus.

PREOPERATIVE HISTORY A 74-year-old male.

INDICATIONS FOR PROCEDURE
1. Rectal bleeding
2. Cardiogenic shock
3. Radiation proctitis. Status post laser 10/95 with continued blood per rectum

MEDICATIONS USED Demerol 100 mg IV, Versed 4 mg IV

DESCRIPTION OF ENDOSCOPIC PROCEDURE Rectum examined with findings of multiple telangiectasias. Still photography and laser ablation were performed. Large internal hemorrhoids were found. The sigmoid colon was examined, with findings of superficially located hemorrhage(s) and vascular deformity. Pale denuded mucosa from 5–50 cm loss of vascular pattern, superficial hemorrhage.

COMPLICATIONS Procedure was well tolerated with no complications.

MATERIAL TO LAB FOR EXAMINATION No biopsy or cytology performed.

FINAL DISPOSITION Remain in CT ICU.

ENDOSCOPIC DIAGNOSES
1. Rule out ischemic colitis.
2. Radiation prostatitis.
3. Radiation colitis.
4. Internal hemorrhoids noted.

Sample Colonic Manometric Study

TITLE OF OPERATION Colonic manometric studies.

MAXIMUM RESTING PRESSURE	L 33 mmHg R 40 mmHg A 11 mmHg P 23 mmHg
MAXIMUM SQUEEZE PRESSURE	L 101 mmHg R 132 mmHg A 46 mmHg P 85 mmHg
SPHINCTER LENGTH	L 2.5 cm R 2.9 cm A 1.8 cm P 2.2 cm

Balloon expulsion $\pm$ BR (+)
Rectosphincteric reflex $\pm$ (+)
Min. sensory rectal vol.   20 cc

ELECTROPHYSIOLOGY

SINGLE FIBER EMG

EAS PR
Fiber Density _____ _____ (1.5 +/- 0.16)
Mapping Deficiency (external sphincter)
L _____
R _____
A _____
P _____
Nerve Conduction: Pudendal Nerve Latency L 1.9 ms R 2.1 ms (2.0 +/- 0.2)

IMPRESSIONS 1. Low rest pressures in the anterior, posterior and left lateral
quadrants.
2. Low squeeze pressures in the anterior quadrant.
3. Short sphincter length in the anterior and posterior quadrant.

No evidence of neurogenic incontinence.
Probable anterior sphincter injury.
Able to expel a rectal balloon, which is not consistent with nonrelaxing puborectalis.

RECOMMENDATIONS 1. Continue workup for incontinence.
2. Consider transrectal ultrasound for sphincter
mapping if surgical repair is a consideration.

Sample Cystoscopy, Right Retrograde Pyelogram, Stone Basketing

TITLE OF OPERATION

1. Cystoscopy.
2. Right retrograde pyelogram.
3. Stone basketing.

FINDINGS FROM SURGERY The anterior urethral approach was normal and inspection of the bladder was normal. The right retrograde pyelogram demonstrated a 3-mm calculus in the distal right ureter with high-grade obstruction.

PROCEDURE IN DETAIL The patient was placed in the lithotomy position after routine prep and drape in sterile fashion. A #21 French cystoscope was advanced under direct vision through the urethra into the bladder with the findings as above. The bladder was entirely normal with the findings above. Through the working bridge of the cystoscope, a cone-tipped catheter was inserted in the right ureteral orifice and 10 cc of contrast was injected and retrograde studies were obtained. Through the working bridge of the cystoscope, a Pfister-Schwartz basket was passed under fluoroscopic control into the right ureter and the stone was engaged and removed with one pass of the basket. This completed the procedure. No stent was retained. The patient tolerated the procedure with no complications.

Sample Transurethral Resection of Prostate

TITLE OF OPERATION   Transurethral resection of prostate.

PROCEDURE IN DETAIL   The patient was taken to the operating room where he received spinal anesthesia without incident. He was placed in the lithotomy position and was prepped and draped in the usual sterile fashion. The meatus was dilated with Van Buren sounds to #30. Then the resectoscope sheath was introduced into the bladder without difficulty. The bladder was then inspected and the ureteric orifices were easily visualized. The bladder demonstrated grade 3/4 trabeculation. There was no evidence of stone or tumor noted. The tissue in the prostatic fossa was quite irregular and predominant around the verumontanum towards the apex. Resection was begun on the left side. Resection progressed from the 5 o'clock position back to the 1 o'clock position. The right side was resected in a similar fashion from the 7 o'clock to 11 o'clock positions. The tissue anteriorly was resected carefully down to the capsule. Next, the floor of the prostatic fossa was carefully resected without any undermining or perforation. Very careful resection of the tissue around the verumontanum was carried out with particular care being taken so as not to go beyond the level of the veru, thus avoiding sphincteric damage. The prostatic fossa was noted to be wide open and there was no tissue remaining on the side of the veru. All the tissue chips were irrigated out of the bladder. The ureteric orifices were rechecked and were intact. A 24 French Foley catheter was introduced into the bladder and irrigation was started. The irrigant output cleared up immediately on slight traction. A Foley catheter was taped to the patient's right leg. Continuous irrigation was carried on while the patient was being transferred to the recovery room. Estimated blood loss was less than 100 cc. There were no complications. The surgical specimen consisted of less than 10 g of prostatic tissue, which was sent to pathology for final examination.

Sample Vasectomy

TITLE OF OPERATION   Vasectomy.

PROCEDURE IN DETAIL   The patient was placed in the supine position after his scrotum had been shaved and prepped. He was draped in the usual sterile fashion. Then, 1 cc of 1% plain Xylocaine was infiltrated into the scrotal skin and vas deferens for local anesthesia. Next, utilizing the no-scalpel vasectomy instruments, the right vas deferens was mobilized and secured with the vas-grasping instrument. A small puncture was made with the vas-dissecting instrument and the vas deferens was brought up out of the scrotum through the small puncture wound. The vas deferens was ligated on both ends and divided. A small segment of the vas deferens was cauterized. The proximal end of the vas deferens was closed into the sheath of the vas deferens utilizing a 4–0 chromic stitch with RB1 needle. This effectively separated the two ends of the vas deferens with a layer of healthy tissue. Hemostasis is excellent at this time and the right vas deferens is returned to the scrotum.

Next, 1 cc of plain Xylocaine was infiltrated into the left scrotal skin and vas deferens for local anesthesia. The left vas deferens was then likewise mobilized and secured with the vas-grasping instrument. The dissecting instrument was used to dissect away the sheath of the vas deferens. It was then again mobilized and brought up out of the scrotal wound and the grasping instrument was reapplied. The vas deferens was ligated and a small segment was removed and sent for pathologic examination. The cut ends are then cauterized and the proximal end was closed within the sheath of the vas utilizing a 4–0 chromic stitch separating the two ends of the cut vas deferens with normal healthy tissue. Hemostasis is excellent at this point and the left vas deferens is returned to the scrotum. Pressure was applied to the small puncture wound for several minutes. Hemostasis was excellent and required no sutures. Neosporin was applied to the wound as well as a gauze dressing and scrotal support. The patient was again instructed to restrict his activities and apply ice for 48 hours, to keep the wound dry for 72 hours, and return to the office in 1 week for wound check.

Sample Renal Transplant

TITLE OF OPERATION   Living-related renal transplantation.

PROCEDURE IN DETAIL   The patient was taken to the operating room and positioned on the operating room table in the supine position with arms abducted at 90°. General endotracheal anesthesia was induced. Vascular access was obtained. A Foley catheter was inserted into the urinary bladder. The bladder was washed with an antibiotic that contained normal saline and then filled with approximately 30 cc of neomycin solution. The abdomen was then prepared with Betadine and draped in the usual sterile fashion. A curvilinear incision was made in the right lower quadrant, extending from midline to a point along the lateral edge of the rectus sheath, approximately at the level of the bottom of the rib cage. This incision was carried down through the subcutaneous fat using electrocautery. The anterior rectus sheath was divided using electrocautery. The external oblique aponeurosis, the internal oblique aponeurosis, and the transversalis fascia were all divided using electrocautery. The rectus muscle was retracted medially. The peritoneum was dissected away from the anterior abdominal wall and also retracted medially. In the course of this dissection, the inferior epigastric artery and veins were ligated and divided, as was the round ligament. With retraction of the peritoneum and the abdominal wall superiorly and medially, the psoas muscles and the internal and external iliac artery and vein were seen. The external iliac vein was dissected from surrounding tissues. Two small branches were ligated and divided. The common iliac artery was also dissected from surrounding tissue in preparation for anastomosis. The fascia overlying the urinary bladder was also dissected away on the anterolateral surface of the bladder.

The kidney was recovered in the adjoining operating room and it has two renal arteries, a single renal vein, and a single ureter. The kidney appeared to be of good quality. It was brought to the operating room. On the back table, the two renal arteries were spatulated and a single orifice was made by rejoining the spatulated portion of the arteries using running sutures of 8–0 Prolene. The kidney was then brought to the operating field and implanted in the following fashion. The patient was heparinized with 4000 units of IV heparin. A Satinsky clamp was placed on the external iliac vein. A longitudinal venotomy was performed and an end-to-side anastomosis between the renal vein and iliac vein was constructed using a running stitch of 6–0 Prolene. Next, a second Satinsky clamp was placed on the common iliac artery. The arteriotomy was made and end-to-side anastomosis was constructed between the ends of the conjoined renal arteries and the common iliac artery using a running stitch of 7–0 Prolene. Both anastomoses were checked for water tightness and found to be satisfactory. The kidney was reperfused with arterial blood. The clamps were removed and the kidney immediately took on a good color. Within approximately 10 minutes, it began making urine. The ureter was then inspected and found to be satisfactory. There were two good blood vessels on either side of the ureter. The point of transection was selected and the ureteric vessels were individually ligated and divided using 4–0 silk ties. The ureter was then transected and spatulated. The muscle overlying the mucosa of the urinary bladder was divided using electrocautery. The mucosa of the bladder was opened and an end-to-side anastomosis was constructed between the ureter and the urinary bladder using a running stitch of 6–0 Maxon. The muscle of the bladder wall was then closed over the ureteric anastomosis using interrupted stitches of 5–0 Maxon. The retroperitoneum was then irrigated. Several bleeders were controlled using electrocautery. When adequate hemostasis was achieved, closure was undertaken.

Closure consisted of two layers laterally. The deep layer consists of the transversus abdominis and internal oblique fascia. The superficial layer laterally consists of the external oblique aponeurosis. A single layer closure over the rectus muscle was constructed with a single layer of running 0 Prolene in the rectus sheath. Subcutaneous tissue was irrigated and the skin was approximated with skin staples. The patient tolerated the procedure well and was making large amounts of urine by the conclusion of the operation. The patient was extubated in the operating room and taken to the recovery room in satisfactory condition.

Sample Insertion PTFE Graft Fistula

TITLE OF OPERATION Insertion arteriovenous PTFE graft fistula for permanent dialysis access.

PROCEDURE IN DETAIL With the patient in the supine position and anesthesia standby, the left arm and axilla were prepped with Betadine and draped with sterile towels. With a total of 30 cc of 1.5% Xylocaine with epinephrine percutaneously, the left axilla plexus was infiltrated achieving anesthesia to the entire left arm. At the antecubital fossa, a modified transverse skin incision was placed in the subcutaneous tissue. The fascia was incised and it was found that the median cubital vein was rather small and did not qualify as site for anastomosis. The search was continued for the deeper venous system and the aponeurosis of the biceps was divided. A good-sized branch of the deep venous system was mobilized and controlled with a vascular loop proximally and distally. A second incision was placed at the wrist level along the course of the radial artery extending through the subcutaneous tissue. The fascia was excised. The radial artery was identified. Bleeding was controlled with vascular loop proximally and distally as well. Between the two incisions, a subcutaneous tunnel was created to about 6 mm and the graft was inserted. The proximal end of the graft was trimmed and tapered and, with 5–0 Prolene, an extension anastomosis was established between the graft and the vein. Having the first anastomosis completed, attention was now given to the radial artery which was occluded proximally and distally. Arteriotomy was performed. The distal end of the graft was trimmed and tapered and, with 5–0 Prolene, an extension anastomosis was established between the graft and the radial artery. Having the two anastomoses completed, all the occluding vascular clamps and loops were removed. Perfusion of the graft was completed with good palpable pulses present in both ends of the graft. The wound was irrigated and suctioned, assuring no active bleeding and no leak. Now the closure of the incision was started, subcutaneous tissues were reapproximated, and the skin was closed with 4–0 nylon sutures. Sterile dressing was applied and the patient was transferred to the recovery room in satisfactory condition. All instrument, sponge, and needle counts were correct. Estimated blood loss was about 10 cc.